The Companion to Specialist Surgical Practice eLibrary

Series edited by

O. James Garden and Simon Paterson-Brown

The content of all eight volumes of the Fifth Edition of the **Companion to Specialist Surgical Practice** is now available both in print and as part of an electronic library. Your purchase of this book allows you to download the fully searchable contents to your desktop, laptop, tablet or smartphone.

Your **Companion to Specialist Surgical Practice eLibrary** is portable: the titles in the series download to your device or you can access online so they are with you whenever you need them.

Your eBook is much more than just 'pictures of pages':

- customize your page views
- search in single books that you have purchased or across any volumes in the series in your collection
- highlight and take searchable notes, and even print and copy-and-paste with bibliographic support
- utilize reference lists linked where available to Medline citations (including authors, title, source, and often an abstract) to journal articles and an indication of free electronic full-text availability.

To purchase other eBooks in the **Companion to Specialist Surgical Practice eLibrary** please visit www.elsevierhealth.com/companionseries

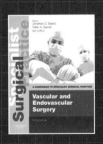
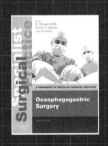
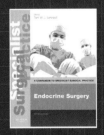
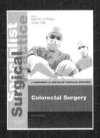
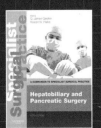
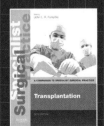
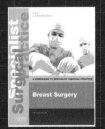
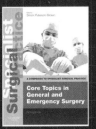

LATER EDITION AVAILABLE OCTOBER 2018

Hepatobiliary and Pancreatic Surgery

OF01032

A COMPANION TO SPECIALIST SURGICAL PRACTICE

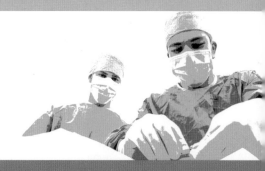

Series Editors
O. James Garden
Simon Paterson-Brown

Hepatobiliary and Pancreatic Surgery

FIFTH EDITION

Edited by

O. James Garden
BSc MBChB MD FRCS(Glas) FRCS(Ed) FRCP(Ed) FRACS(Hon) FRCSC(Hon) FRSE
Regius Professor of Clinical Surgery, Clinical Surgery School of Clinical Sciences,
The University of Edinburgh; Honorary Consultant Surgeon,
Royal Infirmary of Edinburgh, Edinburgh, UK

Rowan W. Parks
MBBCh BAO MD FRCSI FRCS(Ed)
Professor of Surgical Sciences, Clinical Surgery School of Clinical Sciences,
The University of Edinburgh; Honorary Consultant Surgeon,
Royal Infirmary of Edinburgh, Edinburgh, UK

SAUNDERS

ELSEVIER

Edinburgh   London   New York   Oxford   Philadelphia   St Louis   Sydney   Toronto   2014

SAUNDERS

ELSEVIER

Fifth edition © 2014 Elsevier Limited. All rights reserved.

First edition 1997
Second edition 2001
Third edition 2005
Fourth edition 2009
Fifth edition 2014
    Reprinted 2014, 2016

ISBN 978-0-7020-4961-3
e-ISBN 978-0-7020-4969-9

British Library Cataloguing in Publication Data
A catalogue record for this book is available from the British Library

Library of Congress Cataloging in Publication Data
A catalog record for this book is available from the Library of Congress

Notice

your source for books,
journals and multimedia
in the health sciences

www.elsevierhealth.com

Working together
to grow libraries in
developing countries

www.elsevier.com • www.bookaid.org

The
Publisher's
policy is to use
**paper manufactured
from sustainable forests**

Printed in China

Commissioning Editor: Laurence Hunter
Development Editor: Lynn Watt
Project Manager: Vinod Kumar Iyyappan
Designer/Design Direction: Miles Hitchen
Illustration Manager: Jennifer Rose
Illustrator: Antbits Ltd

Contents

Contents

Contributors

René Adam, MD, PhD
Professor of Surgery, Universite Paris-Sud;
Centre Hepato-Biliaire, Hôpital Paul Brousse,
University Paris-Sud, Paris, France

Kai Bachmann, MD
Department of General, Visceral and
Thoracic Surgery, University Medical Center,
Hamburg-Eppendorf, Germany

John A.C. Buckels, CBE, MD, FRCS
Professor of Hepatobiliary and Transplant Surgery
Liver Unit, University Hospital Birmingham NHS Trust
Queen Elizabeth Hospital, Birmingham, UK

Olivier R.C. Busch, MD, PhD
Gastrointestinal Surgeon, Department of Surgery,
Academic Medical Center, Amsterdam, The
Netherlands

C. Ross Carter, MBChB, FRCS, MD, FRCS(Gen)
Consultant Pancreaticobiliary Surgeon, West of
Scotland Pancreatic Unit, Glasgow Royal Infirmary,
Glasgow, UK

Steve M.M. de Castro, MD, PhD
Chief Surgery Resident, Department of Surgery,
Academic Medical Center, Amsterdam, The
Netherlands

**Kevin C. Conlon, MA, MCh, MBA, FRCSI, FACS,
FRCS, FTCD**
Chair of Surgery, Professorial Surgical Unit, University
of Dublin, Trinity College; St Vincent's University
Hospital, Dublin, Ireland

Saxon Connor, MBChB, FRACS
HPB Surgeon, General Surgery, Christchurch
Hospital, Christchurch, New Zealand

Otto M. van Delden, MD, PhD
Interventional Radiologist, Department of Radiology,
Academic Medical Center, Amsterdam, The
Netherlands

Euan J. Dickson, MBChB, MD, FRCS
Consultant Surgeon, West of Scotland Pancreatic
Unit, Glasgow Royal Infirmary, Glasgow, UK

Declan F.J. Dunne, MBChB(Hons), MRCS
Surgical Research Fellow, University of Liverpool;
Department of Hepatobiliary Surgery, Aintree
University Hospital, Liverpool, UK

Olivier Farges, MD, PhD
Professor of Surgery, Department of Hepato-biliary
and Pancreatic Surgery and Liver Transplantation,
Hôpital Beaujon, Université Paris 7, Paris, France

Stuart J. Forbes, FRCP(Ed), PhD
Professor of Transplantation and Regenerative Medicine,
MRC Centre for Regenerative Medicine, Edinburgh, UK,

Steven Gallinger, MD, MSc, FRCSC
Professor of Surgery, Division of General Surgery
Toronto General Hospital, University Health Network,
University of Toronto, Toronto, Canada

**O. James Garden, BSc, MBChB, MD,
FRCS(Glas), FRCS(Ed), FRCP(Ed) FRACS(Hon),
FRCSC(Hon), FRSE**
Regius Professor of Clinical Surgery, Clinical Surgery,
School of Clinical Sciences and Community Health,
The University of Edinburgh; Honorary Consultant
Surgeon, Royal Infirmary of Edinburgh, Edinburgh, UK

Jean-François Gigot, MD, PhD, FRCS
Professor of Surgery, Division of HBP Surgery,
Department of Abdominal Surgery and Transplantation,
Cliniques Universitaires Saint-Luc, Université
Catholique de Louvain (UCL), Brussels, Belgium

Dirk J. Gouma, MD, PhD
Professor of Surgery, Chair of the Department of
Surgery, Academic Medical Center, Amsterdam,
The Netherlands

Geoffrey H. Haydon, MBChB, MSc, MD, FRCP
Consultant Hepatologist, Liver Unit, Queen Elizabeth
Hospital, University Hospital Birmingham NHS Trust,
Birmingham, UK

**John R. Isaac, MBBS, MMed(Surgery),
FRCS(Edin), FRCS(Glasg), FAMS**
Hepato-Pancreatico-Biliary and Liver Transplant
Surgeon, Liver Unit, Queen Elizabeth Hospital, University
Hospital Birmingham NHS Trust, Birmingham, UK

Contributors

Jakob R. Izbicki, MD, FACS
Department of General, Visceral and
Thoracic Surgery, University Medical Center,
Hamburg-Eppendorf, Germany

William R. Jarnagin, MD, FACS
Enid A. Haupt Chair in Surgery, Professor of Surgery;
Chief, HPB Service, Department of Surgery, Memorial
Sloan-Kettering Cancer Center, New York, NY, USA

Robert P. Jones, BSc (Hons), MBChB
Surgical Research Fellow, University of Liverpool;
Northwestern Hepatobiliary Unit, Aintree University
Hospital, Liverpool, UK

Zaheer S. Kanji, MD, BSc, BMedSci
Research Fellow, Samuel Lunenfeld Research
Institute of Mount Sinai Hospital, University of
Toronto, Toronto, Canada; Resident Physician,
Division of General Surgery, University of British
Columbia, Vancouver, Canada

Michael E. Kelly, BA, MBBCh, BAO, MRCS
Adelaide & Meath Hospital, Tallaght, Dublin,
Ireland

Alexandra M. Koenig, MD
Department of General, Visceral and Thoracic
Surgery, University Medical Center, Hamburg-
Eppendorf, Germany

Chetana Lim, MD
Department of Hepato-biliary and Pancreatic
Surgery and Liver Transplantation, Hôpital Beaujon,
Université Paris 7, Paris, France

Lynn Mikula, MD, MSc
Consulting General Surgeon, Peterborough, Ontario,
Canada

Carol-Anne Moulton, MBBS, MEd, PhD, FRACS
Associate Professor of Surgery, Division of General
Surgery, Toronto General Hospital, University Health
Network, University of Toronto, Toronto, Canada

Colin J. McKay, MBChB, MD, FRCS
Consultant Surgeon, West of Scotland Pancreatic
Unit, Glasgow Royal Infirmary Glasgow, UK

Shishir K. Maithel, MD, FACS
Assistant Professor of Surgery, Division of Surgical
Oncology, Department of Surgery, Emory University
School of Medicine, Atlanta, GA, USA

Leslie K. Nathanson, MBChB, FRACS
Consultant Surgeon, Royal Brisbane and Women's
Hospital, Herston, Australia

Simon P. Olliff, MRCP, FRCR
Consultant Radiologist, Department of Radiology,
Queen Elizabeth Hospital, Birmingham, UK

**Rowan W. Parks, MBBCh, BAO, MD, FRCSI,
FRCS(Ed)**
Professor of Surgical Sciences, Clinical Surgery,
School of Clinical Sciences and Community Health,
The University of Edinburgh; Honorary Consultant
Surgeon, Royal Infirmary of Edinburgh,
Edinburgh, UK

Graeme J. Poston, MBBS, MS, FRCS
Professor of Surgery, University of Liverpool;
Northwestern Hepatobiliary Unit, Aintree University
Hospital, Liverpool, UK

Richard T. Schlinkert, MD, FACS
Professor of Surgery, Mayo Clinic College of
Medicine; Consultant Surgeon, Department of
Surgery, Mayo Clinic Arizona, Phoenix, AZ, USA

**Steven M. Strasberg, MD, FRCS(C), FACS,
FRCS(Ed)**
Pruett Professor of Surgery, Section of Hepato-
Pancreato-Biliary Surgery, Washington University in
Saint Louis, St Louis, MO, USA

Chee-Chee H. Stucky, MD
Surgical Resident, General Surgery, Mayo Clinic
Arizona, Phoenix, AZ, USA

**Benjamin M. Stutchfield, BSc, MBChB, MSc,
MRCS(Ed)**
Clinical Research Fellow, MRC Centre for
Regenerative Medicine, The University of Edinburgh,
Edinburgh, UK

Benjamin N.J. Thomson, MBBS, DMedSc, FRACS
Head of Specialist General Surgery, Royal Melbourne
Hospital, Parkville, Victoria, Australia

**Stephen J. Wigmore, BSc(Hons), MBBS, MD,
FRCSEd, FRCS(Gen Surg)**
Professor of Transplantation Surgery, Clinical Surgery,
School of Clinical Sciences and Community Health,
The University of Edinburgh; Clinical Director General
Surgery and Transplantation, Royal Infirmary of
Edinburgh, Edinburgh, UK

Series Editors' preface

It is now some 17 years since the first edition of the *Companion to Specialist Surgical Practice* series was published. We set ourselves the task of meeting the educational needs of surgeons in the later years of specialist surgical training, as well as consultant surgeons in independent practice who wished for contemporary, evidence-based information on the subspecialist areas relevant to their general surgical practice. The series was never intended to replace the large reference surgical textbooks which, although valuable in their own way, struggle to keep pace with changing surgical practice. This Fifth Edition has also had to take due account of the increasing specialisation in 'general' surgery. The rise of minimal access surgery and therapy, and the desire of some subspecialties such as breast and vascular surgery to separate away from 'general surgery', may have proved challenging in some countries, but has also served to emphasise the importance of all surgeons being aware of current developments in their surgical field. As in previous editions, there has been increasing emphasis on evidence-based practice and contributors have endeavoured to provide key recommendations within each chapter. The e-Book versions of the textbook have also allowed the technophile improved access to key data and content within each chapter.

We remain indebted to the volume editors and all the contributors of this Fifth Edition. We have endeavoured where possible to bring in new blood to freshen content. We are impressed by the enthusiasm, commitment and hard work that our contributors and editorial team have shown and this has ensured a short turnover between editions while maintaining as accurate and up-to-date content as is possible. We remain grateful for the support and encouragement of Laurence Hunter and Lynn Watt at Elsevier Ltd. We trust that our original vision of delivering an up-to-date affordable text has been met and that readers, whether in training or independent practice, will find this Fifth Edition an invaluable resource.

O. James Garden BSc, MBChB, MD, FRCS(Glas), FRCS(Ed), FRCP(Ed), FRACS(Hon), FRCSC(Hon), FRSE
Regius Professor of Clinical Surgery, Clinical Surgery School of Clinical Sciences, The University of Edinburgh and Honorary Consultant Surgeon, Royal Infirmary of Edinburgh

Simon Paterson-Brown MBBS, MPhil, MS, FRCS(Ed), FRCS(Engl), FCS(HK)
Honorary Senior Lecturer, Clinical Surgery School of Clinical Sciences, The University of Edinburgh and Consultant General and Upper Gastrointestinal Surgeon, Royal Infirmary of Edinburgh

Editors' preface

This Fifth Edition of *Hepatobiliary and Pancreatic Surgery* continues to build on the strong foundations of previous contributors since the First Edition appeared in 1997. My colleague, Professor Rowan Parks has joined me as Editor of this volume in an effort to bring fresh thought regarding content and format. Each edition delivers refinement and updates to existing chapters, which have been updated extensively. We have endeavoured to secure leading international contributors who will keep the reader at the forefront of those rapidly developing areas of HPB surgery.

The content is as comprehensive as any previous edition although we have not attempted to duplicate some areas of the speciality which are addressed in the *Endocrine* or *Transplantation* Volumes. All chapters have been brought up to date with new evidence base and references. We have endeavoured to maintain a uniform style and we are grateful to our contributors for allowing us to make various amendments of content to achieve this.

Acknowledgements

We are grateful to colleagues at Elsevier for trying to keep us on schedule and for addressing issues of style, formatting and layout. We would wish to acknowledge the tremendous support and tolerance shown by our families in allowing us to deliver this volume and take us to 20 years of the Companion Series.

O. James Garden
Rowan W. Parks
Edinburgh

Evidence-based practice in surgery

Critical appraisal for developing evidence-based practice can be obtained from a number of sources, the most reliable being randomised controlled clinical trials, systematic literature reviews, meta-analyses and observational studies. For practical purposes three grades of evidence can be used, analogous to the levels of 'proof' required in a court of law:

1. **Beyond all reasonable doubt.** Such evidence is likely to have arisen from high-quality randomised controlled trials, systematic reviews or high-quality synthesised evidence such as decision analysis, cost-effectiveness analysis or large observational datasets. The studies need to be directly applicable to the population of concern and have clear results. The grade is analogous to burden of proof within a criminal court and may be thought of as corresponding to the usual standard of 'proof' within the medical literature (i.e. $P<0.05$).

2. **On the balance of probabilities.** In many cases a high-quality review of literature may fail to reach firm conclusions due to conflicting or inconclusive results, trials of poor methodological quality or the lack of evidence in the population to which the guidelines apply. In such cases it may still be possible to make a statement as to the best treatment on the 'balance of probabilities'. This is analogous to the decision in a civil court where all the available evidence will be weighed up and the verdict will depend upon the balance of probabilities.

3. **Not proven.** Insufficient evidence upon which to base a decision, or contradictory evidence.

Depending on the information available, three grades of recommendation can be used:

a. Strong recommendation, which should be followed unless there are compelling reasons to act otherwise.

b. A recommendation based on evidence of effectiveness, but where there may be other factors to take into account in decision-making, for example the user of the guidelines may be expected to take into account patient preferences, local facilities, local audit results or available resources.

c. A recommendation made where there is no adequate evidence as to the most effective practice, although there may be reasons for making a recommendation in order to minimise cost or reduce the chance of error through a locally agreed protocol.

✔✔ Evidence where a conclusion can be reached **'beyond all reasonable doubt'** and therefore where a **strong recommendation** can be given.
  This will normally be based on evidence levels:
- Ia. Meta-analysis of randomised controlled trials
- Ib. Evidence from at least one randomised controlled trial
- IIa. Evidence from at least one controlled study without randomisation
- IIb. Evidence from at least one other type of quasi-experimental study.

✔ Evidence where a conclusion might be reached **'on the balance of probabilities'** and where there may be other factors involved which influence the recommendation given. This will normally be based on less conclusive evidence than that represented by the double tick icons:
- III. Evidence from non-experimental descriptive studies, such as comparative studies and case–control studies
- IV. Evidence from expert committee reports or opinions or clinical experience of respected authorities, or both.

Evidence which is associated with either a **strong recommendation** or **expert opinion** is highlighted in the text in panels such as those shown above, and is distinguished by either a double or single tick icon, respectively. The references associated with double-tick evidence are highlighted in the reference lists at the end of each chapter along with a short summary of the paper's conclusions where applicable.

The reader is referred to Chapter 1, 'Evidence-based practice in surgery' in the volume, *Core Topics in General and Emergency Surgery* of this series, for a more detailed description of this topic.

1

Liver function and failure

Stephen J. Wigmore
Benjamin M. Stutchfield
Stuart J. Forbes

Overview of liver functions and evolution

The liver is the largest solid organ in the human body. It has a unique structure with a dual blood supply, being approximately one-third from the hepatic artery and two-thirds from portal venous blood. Within the liver substance blood flows through sinusoids between plates of hepatocytes to drain into central veins, which in turn join the hepatic veins draining into the vena cava. The liver is a major site of protein synthesis exporting plasma proteins to maintain oncotic pressure and coagulation factors. Acute phase proteins that act as antiproteases, opsonins and metal ion carriers are synthesised by the liver in response to injury or infection. Numerous immune cells populate the liver and the resident tissue macrophages, the Kupffer cells, form an important component of the innate immune system. Nutrients are extracted from portal blood by the liver and processed, and the liver acts as an important reservoir for glycogen. Waste products are either modified in the liver for excretion by the kidneys or are excreted into bile. Many drugs are taken up by the liver and metabolised, giving either active metabolites or inactive metabolites for excretion. In man, as in many vertebrates, the liver's capacity for metabolism and clearance far exceeds what is required for day-to-day life. It is possible that in evolutionary terms this ability offers a survival advantage in terms of survival of poisoning, starvation or trauma.

Symptoms of liver failure: acute and chronic

In the acute setting, liver failure can present with a number of symptoms, but it is important to note that not all of these may be present at the same time. Typically, a patient with acute liver failure after surgery, transplantation or in acute poisoning will be confused or mentally slow as a result of encephalopathy, which may progress to loss of consciousness and a need to protect the airway by intubation and mechanical ventilation. Patients are often not immediately jaundiced, but jaundice may develop over the course of several days. Patients may be hypoglycaemic and the requirement for intravenous infusion of dextrose is a sinister development and an indicator of severe acute liver failure. Coagulopathy may develop, with evidence of bruising or bleeding from line sites or surgical scars. Severe acute liver failure can be assessed using the King's College Hospital criteria, which were designed to predict mortality in paracetomol- and non-paracetomol-dependent acute liver failure.[1] Later, this scoring system was adopted in the UK to determine criteria indicating likely benefit from liver transplantation. In the surgical patient, the development of acute liver failure is usually more gradual and less dramatic; a useful scoring system for liver dysfunction in the acute setting has been reported by Schindl et al.[2] (see Box 1.1).

Box 1.1 • Definition of postoperative hepatic dysfunction based on results from blood tests and clinical observation

Total serum bilirubin (μmol/L)
≤20
21–60
>60

Prothrombin time (seconds above normal)
<4
4–6
>6

Serum lactate (mmol/L)
≤1.5
1.6–3.5
>3.5

Encephalopathy grade
No
1 and 2
3 and 4
0
1
2

Severity of hepatic dysfunction
None (0), mild (1–2), moderate (3–4), severe (>4)

Adapted from Schindl MJ, Redhead DN, Fearon KC et al. The value of residual liver volume as a predictor of hepatic dysfunction and infection after major liver resection. Gut 2005; 54:289–96. With permission from the BMJ Publishing Group Ltd.

Common causes of acute liver failure: hepatic insufficiency following liver resections

Liver resection is the only treatment with the potential to cure patients with cancers that have originated in the liver itself (primary liver cancer) or that have originated elsewhere and have subsequently spread to the liver (metastatic liver cancer). Equally, it is a preferred therapy in patients with tumours in the liver that are benign, but with the potential of malignant transformation (uncertain benign primary liver tumours). Liver resection of even major parts of the liver (up to 70%) is feasible, because the liver has a remarkable capacity to regenerate. Within 6–8 weeks following 60–70% hepatectomy, the liver has regained nearly its original size and weight.

The most common cause of metastatic liver cancers is primary colorectal cancer, and it is estimated that in the West there is a yearly incidence of 300 new cases of liver metastases from colorectal origin per million population. The current estimate is that this should lead to approximately 100–150 patients per million eligible for liver resection for this indication. To this should be added the patients with primary benign and malignant liver tumours, and hence about 150–200 liver resections should probably be performed per million population each year.

Ever since the first liver resection by Langenbuch in 1887, this procedure has remained a major undertaking and even in the recent past, liver resection was still a dangerous surgical procedure with a high mortality of 20–30% in the 1970s. This was mainly due to excessive intraoperative bleeding but, over the subsequent decades, the procedure has become increasingly safe due to improvements in surgical and anaesthetic techniques. At present, mortality rates are reported to be well below 5%. Currently, the single most important cause of lethal outcome following surgical removal of major parts of the liver is liver failure. For this reason, many researchers and clinicians have attempted to design methods to identify patients at risk of liver failure (and hence mortality) following liver resection. The development of such a method has been hampered by several factors, as outlined below.

The critical point determining lethal outcome following liver resection has been a failure of the residual liver to function properly. Therefore, focus in this research area has always been in identifying a single liver function test that identifies those patients that have a liver with limited function. This has proven exceedingly difficult, and hence such a test is not available for a number of reasons.

First, as outlined above, the liver has a remarkable capacity to regenerate very rapidly, which underlines that there is tremendous overcapacity of several liver functions. In this context, it is known that it is entirely safe in most instances to resect 50% of the liver, because the residual half liver will simply take over all vital liver functions such as clearing bacteria, urea synthesis and synthesis of crucial proteins. From this, it has been estimated that a crucial liver function such as urea synthesis has an overcapacity of 300%, which implies that a static preoperative liver function test will be unable to assess this particular function. An alternative and innovative strategy would be to give a challenge to the liver and measure the ability of the liver to respond or cope – a dynamic test.

✓✓ The critical minimum residual liver volume has been estimated to be approximately 25% after resection.[2]

The second crucial problem has been that there is only a poor correlation between volume and function. However, it is still unclear why some patients with smaller hepatic remnants do not develop liver failure whilst some with greater residual volumes do. These observations suggest, however, that peri- and intraoperative events superimposed on the innate hepatic capacity to withstand injury play a role. Hepatic insufficiency in this situation may arise either if not enough liver volume is left after partial hepatectomy or if the residual volume does not function properly. A functional limitation may arise, for example, in patients that have received aggressive chemotherapy in order to reduce the number and size of metastases prior to surgical treatment by liver resection. One of the factors contributing to defective defence may be preoperative fasting,[3] but equally prior chemotherapy and pre-existent steatosis may play a role.

A third important aspect is that during liver surgery deliberate hypotension and temporary hepatic blood inflow occlusion (the so-called Pringle manoeuvre) are used by many surgeons to reduce blood loss during liver surgery (15 minutes ischaemia, 5 minutes reperfusion (15/5 Pringle)). Other surgeons do not use this manoeuvre, assuming that it causes oxidative stress and ischaemia/reperfusion (I/R) injury.[4,5] There is little doubt that this procedure does cause oxidative stress and I/R injury; however, the consequence of this is variable. In a situation where defence mechanisms against oxidative stress are deficient it may adversely affect liver function. In this situation hepatic steatosis may constitute an additional predisposing factor to damage by ischaemia/reperfusion.

✓✓ Ischaemia/reperfusion is, on the other hand, the basis of ischaemic preconditioning, a process in which temporary clamping and release of the liver blood flow has been shown to be beneficial in terms of increasing resistance to subsequent injury.[6]

In this situation it is assumed that defence mechanisms against oxidative stress are adequate and are indeed enhanced by short-term I/R injury.[7]

The above three factors explain why it has been exceedingly difficult hitherto to design a proper liver function test that reliably singles out those patients at risk of liver failure following liver resection. The term 'liver function' is a rather crude denominator for a range of functions that includes ammonia detoxification, urea synthesis, protein synthesis and breakdown, bile synthesis and secretion, gluconeogenesis and detoxification of drugs, bacteria and bacterial toxins.

Chronic liver failure

The clinical signs of chronic liver failure are often insidious and can also be related to the type of disease.

Cirrhosis is associated with a failure of hepatic function and the consequences of increased hepatic vascular resistance. Metabolic impairment is manifest by jaundice, coagulopathy, impaired ammonia clearance and encephalopathy, hypoalbuminaemia and oedema. The presence of increased vascular resistance is associated with the development of splenomegaly, ascites and gastro-oesophageal or abdominal wall varices. The slow progression of many chronic liver diseases, over years, implies a gradual, almost incremental, loss of liver cell mass or function. There are many causes of liver failure, including hepatitis B and C virus, autoimmune diseases such as primary biliary cirrhosis, primary sclerosing cholangitis and autoimmune hepatitis, alcoholic liver disease, Wilson's disease, α_1-antitrypsin deficiency and others. All are associated with chronic or repeated cell injury and attempts at repair. The fibrosis and scarring associated with this regeneration and repair lead to the clinical condition termed cirrhosis, with a typically small shrunken irregular liver and an increased risk of cancer.

The Child–Pugh score for chronic liver disease[8] has served as a useful means of categorising patients based on the severity of their liver disease. It employs five clinical measures of liver disease and each measure is scored 1–3, with 3 indicating the most severe derangement (Table 1.1).

Metabolic liver function

The liver plays a central role in fat, carbohydrate and protein metabolism, as well as in acid–base homeostasis. In the context of liver failure, disturbances of fat metabolism are probably not crucially important. With respect to carbohydrate metabolism, it is well known that the liver plays a central role in the conversion of lactate to glucose. Part of this lactate is formed due to anaerobic metabolism of, amongst others, glucose in skeletal muscle. This metabolic route of glucose to lactate (muscle) and then back to glucose (liver) is very important for glycaemic homeostasis and is called the Cori cycle. Failure of the liver will be witnessed by lactic acidosis and hypoglycaemia.

Next to its role in carbohydrate metabolism, the liver plays a central function in nitrogen homeostasis. Hepatic synthesis and breakdown of proteins

Table 1.1 • Child-Pugh score for chronic liver disease

Measure	1 point	2 points	3 points	Units
Bilirubin (total)	<34 (<2)	34–50 (2–3)	>50 (>3)	μmol/L (mg/dL)
Serum albumin	>35	28–35	<28	g/L
INR	<1.7	1.71–2.20	>2.20	No unit
Ascites	None	Suppressed with medication	Refractory	No unit
Hepatic encephalopathy	None	Grade I–II (or suppressed with medication)	Grade III–IV (or refractory)	No unit

and amino acids, and detoxification and clearance of nitrogenous waste products of amino acid and protein metabolism in other organs are of central importance. For example, the gut uses the amino acid glutamine as a fuel for enterocytes, which give rise to the production of waste end-products of intestinal metabolism, like ammonia. This ammonia is then transported by the portal vein to the liver, where it is detoxified by the formation of urea.

Liver failure gives rise to multiple abnormalities in nitrogen metabolism, some of which are thought to play a crucial role in the characteristic syndrome of hepatic encephalopathy that accompanies liver failure. Hepatic encephalopathy is a reversible neuropsychiatric syndrome, with a probably multifactorial cause.[9] The current belief is that ammonia is one of the key components in the aetiology of hepatic encephalopathy[10] because liver failure is usually associated with moderate to severe hyperammonaemia. Hyperammonaemia leads to increased brain uptake of ammonia, followed by detoxification of ammonia in the brain by coupling to glutamate to form glutamine. This process consumes glutamate (an important excitatory neurotransmitter) and leads to the formation of glutamine, which acts as an osmolite causing brain oedema.

One other well-known metabolic abnormality during liver failure is an imbalance in plasma amino acids, notably the ratio between the branched chain amino acids (BCAAs) and the aromatic amino acids (AAAs).

✔✔ Some 30 years ago, Fischer and colleagues published their 'unified hypothesis on the pathogenesis of hepatic encephalopathy',[11] based on the observation that, during hepatic failure, plasma levels of BCAAs were decreased and the AAAs were increased.[11–13]

These changes in plasma levels were thought to be caused by increased BCAA catabolism in muscle and decreased AAA breakdown in the failing liver.[14] A reduction in the insulin–glucagon ratio in this situation may play a key role in disturbing the balance between anabolism and catabolism. Accumulation of AAAs in the circulation in combination with the increased breakdown of BCAAs, particularly in skeletal muscle, would, according to this hypothesis, give rise to a decrease in the BCAA to AAA ratio, the so-called Fischer ratio. The increase in plasma AAAs in combination with increased blood–brain barrier permeability for neutral amino acids has been suggested to contribute to an increased influx of AAAs in the brain, since they compete for the same amino acid transporter. This, in turn, would lead to imbalances in neurotransmitter synthesis and accumulation of false neurotransmitters such as octopamine in the brain, which may contribute to hepatic encephalopathy.[15]

Measuring liver volume

Advances in imaging have permitted the development of in vivo imaging of the liver. Three-dimensional models of the liver can be constructed from computed tomography (CT) or other cross-sectional imaging modalities, such as magnetic resonance imaging (MRI). The volume of the liver can then be calculated based on known separation of image slices combined with planar mapping of cross-sectional areas. In addition, such three-dimensional computer models can be simulated to map the effects of surgery by performing virtual hepatic resection, and studies have demonstrated that there is a good correlation between computer modelling and actual resection weight of surgical liver specimens (**Fig. 1.1**).[2,16]

This technology is useful as a research tool because it allows liver function to be put into the direct context of

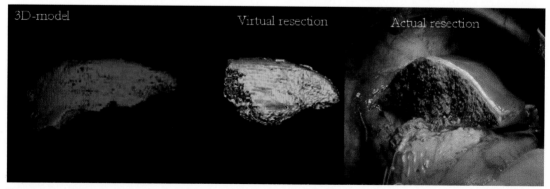

Figure 1.1 • Three-dimensional reconstruction of the liver preoperatively (red) showing tumours (green). Computer prediction of residual liver volume based on virtual hepatectomy of 3-D model (yellow) and actual photograph of resection showing residual liver segments. Reproduced from Schindl MJ, Redhead DN, Fearon KC et al. The value of residual liver volume as a predictor of hepatic dysfunction and infection after major liver resection. Gut 2005; 54:289–96. With permission from the BMJ Publishing Group Ltd.

the volume of functioning liver tissue. In addition, this technology is useful for predicting the need for reconstruction of venous territories of the liver in split liver transplantation. Usually, liver volumetry is performed on software directly linked to the hardware MRI or CT. In recent years, however, stand-alone software has become available, which makes it possible to perform hepatic volumetry remote from the radiological hardware. Examples of such software are the freely downloadable program ImageJ (for Windows-based PCs) and OsiriX (for Apple Macintosh). Our group has recently shown that the ImageJ software is very useful in measuring liver volumes in patients referred with a CT undertaken in the referring centre[17] (**Figs 1.2** and **1.3**).

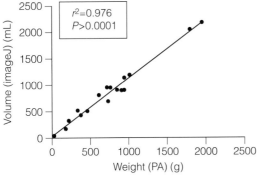

$r^2 = 0.976$
$P > 0.0001$

Figure 1.2 • Correlation between volume of resection calculated with ImageJ and actual measured weights of the resection specimens ($n = 15$, Pearson's test).[14] Reproduced with permission from World J Surg.

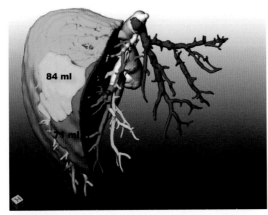

84 ml

Figure 1.3 • Mapping the territory of the right hepatic lobe drained by the middle hepatic vein. The numbers represent the volumes of the territories at risk if segment 5 and 8 tributaries of the middle hepatic vein were not reconstructed in a potential right lobe living-donor liver transplant. Image reproduced with permission of MeVis imaging technologies, Bremen, Germany Kindly provided by H. Lang and A. Radtke, Plainz, Germany.

Blood tests of liver function

As part of many blood chemistry analyses, it is possible to request liver function tests. These tests refer to the transaminases, alkaline phosphatase, γ-glutamyl transferase and bilirubin. These tests are not truly measures of function but do give an indication of processes going on within the liver. Aspartate aminotransferase and alanine aminotransferase are hepatocyte enzymes that are released in conditions in which hepatocytes are damaged or killed, such as ischaemic injury, hepatitis, severe sepsis and in response to cancer. Liver-specific alkaline phosphatase is expressed predominantly in the biliary epithelium and is elevated in conditions such as cholangitis or biliary obstruction. γ-Glutamyl transferase is expressed by both hepatocytes and biliary epithelium, and can also be induced by high alcohol consumption.

Biochemical markers of true liver function vary depending on whether acute or chronic liver failure or injury is being considered (Table 1.2).

Tests of liver function measuring substance clearance

The ability to accurately predict postoperative outcome based on preoperative liver function would be a valuable addition to preoperative assessment. However, while various tests have been developed to assess liver function there is little evidence that these tests have sufficient sensitivity or specificity to predict postoperative outcome at an individual patient level. The tests currently in common use include the indocyanine green (ICG) clearance test, hepatobiliary scintigraphy with radioisotope clearance, lidocaine clearance test, the aminopyrine breath test and the galactose elimination test. These tests aim to provide an indicator of dynamic liver function, in that they can provide real-time assessment of liver

Table 1.2 • Blood tests useful to assess function in acute and chronic liver injury

	Acute	**Chronic**
Albumin	–	+++
Prothrombin time	+++	+++
Bilirubin	+	+++
Lactate	++	–
Glucose requirement	++	–
Ammonia	+	+

function in response to a challenge. However, none of these tests challenge the liver to demonstrate its full functional capacity. Serum bilirubin and clotting factors provide a static indirect estimation of liver metabolism and synthetic function, but are influenced by a range of other factors that limit their relevance and suitability to predict postoperative outcome. The most commonly used test for liver function prior to liver resections is the ICG clearance test.

Indocyanine green (ICG)

ICG is a compound that is used widely to measure liver function. It is rapidly cleared from blood by hepatocytes and is excreted into bile without enterohepatic circulation. Hepatocytes are so effective at clearing ICG from the circulation that the major limiting factor to its clearance is liver blood flow. This is thought to be reduced in cirrhosis. ICG clearance can be measured as 'disappearance' from the blood or can also be measured as accumulation in bile. Liver dysfunction is suggested by a slower rate of clearance from the blood and is usually expressed as percentage retention at 5 or 15 minutes after injection. Continuous measurement of ICG clearance can also be performed, which offers the potential improvement in accuracy by measurement of area under the clearance curve (**Fig. 1.4**). In some centres ICG clearance is routinely performed during preoperative work-up with cut-off values set for which patients are 'safe' to proceed to resection. However, there is no evidence to suggest that outcomes are improved in centres that use this test compared to centres that do not. In chronic liver disease, discriminative ability of ICG clearance is greatest in those with intermediate to severe liver failure. Addition of this test to the MELD score (Model for End-stage Liver Disease) can improve prognostic accuracy for patients with intermediate to severe liver dysfunction.[18] However, given the relationship with hepatic blood flow, caution should be exercised when interpreting ICG clearance in the context of abnormally high cardiac output.

Hepatobiliary scintigraphy

Using a radiolabelled tracer that is eliminated exclusively by the liver, such as [^{99m}Tc]mebrofenin, blood clearance and hepatic uptake can be measured using a gamma camera to provide an indication of hepatic function. Hepatobiliary scintigraphy may improve predictive value compared to future liver remnant volume, especially in patients with uncertain quality of liver parenchyma.[19] However, HBS has not been widely used preoperatively, there is no evidence that it outperforms ICG clearance and the requirement for a nuclear medicine facility on-site may limit its application.

Lidocaine (MEG-X)

Lidocaine, also known as monoethylglycinexylidide (MEG-X), is a local anaesthetic that is taken up by the liver and undergoes biotransformation by a cytochrome P450 enzyme, CYP1A2. The rate of disappearance of lidocaine from plasma correlates with liver function; however, measurement of lidocaine is more complex than that of ICG.

Aminopyrine breath test

The aminopyrine breath test was the first breath test that has been proposed for the assessment of liver function in patients with liver disease. The test uses $^{13}C_2$-aminopyrine, which is a stable, non-radioactive, isotopically labelled compound eliminated almost exclusively by the liver. Following oral intake, the compound is taken up by the gut and then transported to the liver, where it is metabolised by microsomal cytochrome P450 function. This metabolism will liberate $^{13}CO_2$, which can be measured non-invasively in exhaled air. This test is not readily available at the bedside and requires fairly sophisticated apparatus to measure stable isotopic enrichment in the exhaled air. Induction of microsomal metabolism by various drugs may constitute a problem.

Urea synthesis

In the recent past, we have explored the feasibility of measuring urea synthesis using stable isotopes and relating this to liver volume in patients undergoing liver resection.[20] This study was conducted against the background of the notion that liver failure is almost always accompanied by hyperammonaemia, related to a presumed failure of hepatic

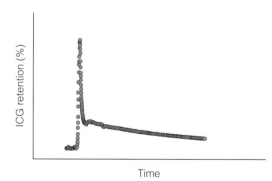

Figure 1.4 • Typical ICG clearance curve for a subject with healthy liver function.

urea synthesis. Using stable isotopically ^{13}C-labelled urea, urea synthesis was measured before and after major hepatic resection, and liver volumes before and after resection with CT scans.

✓✓ Major hepatic resection did not affect total body ureagenesis, because the synthesis of urea per gram of residual liver went up and increased 2.6-fold.[20] Therefore, it is unlikely that urea synthesis is a limiting factor in the initial aetiology of liver failure and this test is not likely to contribute to predicting liver failure following liver resection.

Glutathione synthesis

Unfortunately, most of the above tests focus on very specific functions or pathways. None of them assesses the main hepatic protection system against many diverse forms of stress and intoxications: the intracellular content and synthesis of glutathione (GSH). It is generally accepted that GSH plays a key role in the protection of the liver against many forms of stress, ischaemia and toxic compounds such as paracetamol. Unfortunately, there is currently no adequate test to assess hepatic GSH synthesis and metabolism in vivo in humans, even though such a test would be of great clinical importance. We have previously explored the feasibility of measuring GSH synthesis in vivo during liver surgery in humans using stable isotopically labelled ^{2}H$_2$-glycine, a component of GSH (γ-glutamyl-cysteinyl-glycine), but this approach was not suitable, because part of the deuterium label of glycine was lost (unpublished data). Future research will have to focus on designing a test that is both dynamic and which focuses on the GSH system, making it possible to determine liver function correlated to liver volume, and assess an individual's risk of developing liver failure following liver resection.

Measuring liver blood flow

Blood flow in the splanchnic area, particularly the gut and liver, can be measured in a number of ways. These can basically be either invasive (i.e. intraoperative) or non-invasive. During surgery, when the abdomen is opened, blood flow can be measured in the portal vein and in the main hepatic artery. Portal vein blood flow measurements provide predominantly information on the flow across the intestines. By summing up the blood flow in the hepatic artery and the portal vein, total hepatic blood flow can be calculated. Theoretically, this could also be achieved by measuring hepatic venous outflow, but this is impractical in humans because of the short common outflow tract of the three hepatic veins.

Non-invasive MRI-based techniques are being developed that may offer improved accuracy of measurement of liver blood flow and the potential for repeat measurements.[21] The ratio of portal vein to hepatic artery blood flow changes with increasing resistance of the liver and may indicate the development of fibrosis or cirrhosis. Methodology for assessing the importance of blood flow as a predictor of liver parenchymal condition has not been fully evaluated but may provide a means of assessing safety of surgery and regenerative capacity in some patients.

Such measurements of hepatic and portal arterial blood flow can be obtained using 6–8 mm and 12–14 mm handle ultrasonic flow probes, respectively (Transonic Systems, Kimal PLC, Uxbridge, UK). Essentially, the vessels have to be dissected free for this flow measurement and the three-quarters circular probe is applied to the vessel. These probes are believed to provide the most accurate technique for assessing flow in relatively small vessels. However, there is considerable variability in measurement related to Doppler ultrasound signal strength and coupling with the vessel wall. Also, there are likely to be changes in diameter of the artery, in particular related to its handling during surgery. The advantage is that repeated measurements can be obtained and that the surgeon can operate this application without help from a radiologist. Likewise, post-resection blood flow measurements can be taken before closure of the abdomen, typically 1–2 hours after the first measurement. This gives an impression of blood flow across the residual liver following major resections.

During liver surgery, organ blood flow can also be measured by means of colour Doppler ultrasound scanning (e.g. Aloka Prosound SSD 5000; Aloka Co. Ltd, Tokyo, Japan). A 5-MHz probe is used to trace the vessels and calculate the cross-sectional area. Then, time-averaged mean velocities of the bloodstream are measured at the point where the cross-sectional area of the portal vein and hepatic artery is taken. For accurate velocity measurements, care must be taken to keep the angle between the ultrasonic beam direction and blood flow direction below 60°. The cross-sectional area of the vessel is calculated by drawing an area ellipse at the same point as where the velocity was measured. Portal venous and hepatic arterial blood flows can then be measured proximal to their hilar bifurcations. In the case of an accessory hepatic artery, both arteries should obviously be measured.[22,23] In our experience, this method gives roughly the same values as the ultrasonic flow measurement described above. Theoretically, it is possible to perform such flow measurements preoperatively or postoperatively using a percutaneous approach, although the measurement in the hepatic artery requires a skilled ultrasonographer.

In recent years, technical improvements in hardware and software applications for MRI have made it possible to measure blood flow in the portal vein and hepatic artery in a non-invasive manner. By linking this method of flow measurement to hepatic volumetry using MRI, blood flow per volume unit of liver can be calculated.[24,25] It has been suggested that MRI may provide a more accurate and reliable assessment of portal vein and hepatic artery blood flow than ultrasonography, particularly given the wide interobserver variability seen with the latter technique.[21] Although limited to the preoperative period, MRI flow studies may provide complementary information to intraoperative ultrasonography as required.

A further technique that is emerging is the use of near-infrared spectroscopy. This technique measures absorption of near-infrared wavelength light and from this can be calculated tissue oxygenation, since haemoglobin oxygenation status alters absorption of this wavelength light. This technique is more useful for estimating tissue oxygenation and perfusion at a sinusoidal level, but could potentially be combined with other measures to estimate liver blood flow.[26]

Effect of major liver resection on hepatic blood flow

Direct measurement of hepatic artery and portal vein blood flow before and after liver resection reveals interesting results. When expressed as absolute values portal blood flow does not change whereas hepatic artery blood flow falls. Typically, portal vein flow is approximately 840 mL/min and post-resection 805 mL/min. Using this method, hepatic artery flow pre-resection is about 450 mL/min and post-resection 270 mL/min. When these flows are expressed in relation to the preoperative liver volume and residual postoperative liver volume, it can be seen that the blood flow per gram of liver tissue increases in portal flow from a mean 0.55 mL/min per g liver to 1.09 mL/min per g liver and the hepatic artery flow remains relatively constant (**Fig. 1.5**). In experimental research, pressure measurements can also be obtained using radial artery invasive monitoring to estimate hepatic artery pressure and direct portal vein pressure measurement using a small needle coupled to a pressure transducer similar to that used for measuring central venous pressure. The combination of flow and pressure measurement then allows calculation of hepatic sinusoidal resistance (Fig. 1.5).

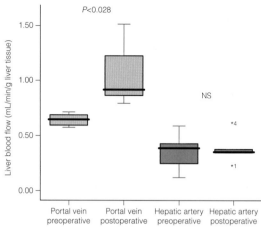

Figure 1.5 • Directly measured blood flow intraoperatively in six patients during major hepatic resection. Measurements were taken from the main portal vein and the main hepatic artery simultaneously using multichannel Transonics ultrasound flow probes. During the liver resection one branch of each of the portal vein and hepatic artery is ligated. The post-resection blood flow measurement has been taken just before closure of the abdomen, typically 1–2 hours after the first measurement. Results are expressed per gram of liver tissue.

Effect of major liver resection on innate immunity

The liver forms an important part of the innate immune system by producing acute-phase proteins and other opsonins, proteins that bind to bacteria facilitating their phagocytosis. In addition, 85% of the reticuloendothelial system is located in the liver (Kupffer cells) and clearly surgical resection will involve a reduction of this cell mass.

It is not unreasonable to expect that major liver resection might result in some impairment of innate immunity. Our group has previously demonstrated that major liver resection is associated with increased frequency of infection as well as increased likelihood of objective evidence of liver function impairment.[2]

In a separate study, our group has also shown that major liver resection is associated with a temporary defect in the ability of the reticuloendothelial system to clear albumin microspheres that were used as a surrogate for bacteria.

✔ Loss of approximately 50% of liver volume, such as might occur during a right hepatectomy, is associated with impairment of reticuloendothelial cell clearance equivalent to that of non-surgical patients with Child C chronic liver disease.[27]

The liver also synthesises and exports many acute-phase proteins involved in innate immunity or homeostasis. C-reactive protein, for example, binds to phosphoryl choline moieties of encapsulated bacteria and acts as an opsonin, promoting phagocytosis. Mannan-binding lectin, complement fragments and α_1-acid glycoprotein (orosomucoid) can also act as opsonins. Transferrin and caeruloplasmin are important in the binding and carriage of free metal ions and α_1-antitrypsin and α_1-antichymotrypsin act as antiproteases. Liver failure or liver surgery may be associated with a reduction in synthesis of some of these acute-phase proteins (mannan-binding lectin, haptoglobin, α-fetuin and fibronectin), whereas the concentrations of others may be increased despite a reduction in functional liver tissue (C-reactive protein, liver fatty acid-binding protein; unpublished data). The exact significance of these changes is unclear but may contribute to a global impairment in innate immunity in the injured liver.

Liver regeneration

The liver is unique in that it is the only organ in the adult that is capable of regenerating or renewing itself to restore the ratio between pre-injury liver volume and body weight. Knowledge of the capacity for the liver to regenerate is presumed to be ancient and is the basis for the punishment meted out by Zeus to Prometheus, who according to Greek mythology was chained to a rock and had his liver eaten daily by a vulture (only for it to regenerate overnight). This continued for several years until the vulture was finally killed by Heracles, who also released Prometheus. While the speed of liver regeneration is exaggerated in this myth, it is true that it is an extremely rapid process. In the context of surgery, liver regeneration happens very rapidly, with most of the cell division required for regeneration occurring within 72 hours of injury. Full liver function and volume are usually restored within 6–12 weeks. In chronic injury or in the presence of fibrosis, liver regeneration can be chaotic with repeated insults causing scarring, and nodular regeneration with disordered architecture leading to cirrhosis.

Molecular signals for hepatic regeneration

At a cellular level, liver regeneration depends on the co-existence of three key factors: changes in the microenvironment of the liver cell supporting growth, the ability of differentiated hepatocytes to proliferate and inhibition of processes, linking injury to programmed cell death.

Stimuli for liver regeneration stimulate transcription factors that turn on a variety of genes expressing growth factors. Although not direct growth factors, the hormones insulin and adrenaline potentiate the effects of growth factors on hepatocyte regeneration. All elements of the liver are required to regenerate; however, the coordination of these processes is complex. Removal of the stimulus for regeneration by growth to pre-injury capacity and transforming growth factor-β act as brakes that slow regeneration of liver elements (**Fig. 1.6**).

> ✅ Macrophage-derived Wnt signalling directs hepatic progenitor cells to become hepatocytes in chronic liver injury by maintaining progenitor cell expression of Numb (a cell fate determinant).[28] Targeting progenitor cells may offer the potential to enhance regeneration of the chronically injured liver.

Barriers to hepatic regeneration include cirrhosis and fibrosis and ongoing liver injury such as might occur with biliary obstruction or sepsis.

Cell populations involved in liver regeneration

Histology of normal liver regeneration following resection or acute injury shows the presence of high mitotic rates in mature hepatocytes. Normally, these cells are mitotically quiescent but can move into S phase extremely rapidly. For example, following 70% hepatectomy in rat approximately 30–40% of hepatocytes are seen to be undergoing mitosis within 48 hours of surgery and indeed the liver will regain its normal size within 10 days. The situation is more complex in chronically injured liver (e.g. cirrhotic liver); here, the hepatocytes are less able to undergo mitosis and are frequently in cell cycle arrest. Furthermore, the accumulation of excess scar tissue deposited in cirrhosis contributes to the inability of the liver to respond to injury and regenerate effectively. In this setting a second population of cells becomes activated and can contribute to parenchymal regeneration. These intrahepatic cells are located in the canal of Hering (the most distal branch of the biliary tree); termed hepatic progenitor cells (HPCs), they are bipotential and are capable of giving rise to both biliary and hepatocyte populations under the influence of macrophage-derived factors (see above). This response is seen in chronic or severe injury and sometimes appears as a ductular reaction. Although it is now recognised that the HPCs can regenerate the liver in chronic liver disease, whether these progenitor cells are capable of responding to the acute demands of major hepatic resection is as yet unknown. It is also worth noting that there is an increasing recognition that intrahepatic stem cells are a likely source of a significant proportion of liver cancers. The role

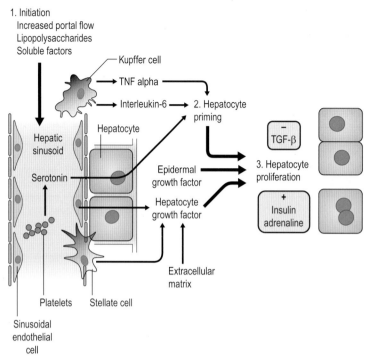

Figure 1.6 • Schematic of some of the factors known to regulate liver regeneration.

of circulating extrahepatic cells in liver regeneration has received interest recently and the potential bone marrow origin of hepatocytes has been suggested. However, if this phenomenon occurs at all, it is extremely rare. The bone marrow does, however, supply macrophages and myofibroblasts that are involved in the liver's scarring response to injury. The relationship between bone marrow-derived cells and the response to injury is complex, with different macrophage subtypes shown to either promote fibrosis or repair. However, administration of bone marrow-derived macrophages to the fibrotic liver via the portal vein has been shown to reduce fibrosis and improve markers of regeneration in preclinical models.[29] The use of bone marrow populations to stimulate liver regeneration in both animal models and clinical studies is likely to be an area of future development (see later).

Consequences of surgery

Unfortunately, at present it is unclear what the key mechanisms of liver failure are, and why the liver usually regenerates but sometimes progresses into liver failure. It is believed that ischaemia/reperfusion (I/R) injury plays an important role in the sequence of events leading to liver failure. Hepatic resections are major surgical procedures, often leading to significant blood loss. In order to reduce blood loss, central venous pressure is reduced during liver surgery and hepatobiliary surgeons frequently occlude hepatic blood inflow

temporarily (Pringle manoeuvre). Obviously, all these factors may contribute to I/R injury in the liver. A key component of I/R injury is the generation of oxygen free radicals. The latter can induce ischaemic necrosis and caspase-dependent apoptosis, and may contribute to failure of vital metabolic synthetic pathways. However, it remains to be investigated which one of these plays a key role during liver failure. In this context, it has been proposed that the balance between hepatocyte regeneration and apoptosis can be tipped towards either side by hepatic defence mechanisms against oxygen free radical damage. Also, oxygen free radicals play a role in determining whether apoptosis or ischaemic necrosis occurs in the liver. Apparently, the equilibrium between oxygen free radicals and their scavengers plays a pivotal role in determining whether regeneration or decay occurs. Glutathione (GSH) is the principal oxygen free radical scavenger in the liver and the principal defence mechanism against I/R damage. Hepatic GSH levels decrease following I/R damage, inflammation and nutritional deprivation. It seems conceivable that a reduction in liver volume following surgery contributes to insufficient hepatic free radical scavenging capacity as a consequence of reduced GSH synthesis. I/R injury may aggravate this situation.

Small-for-size syndrome

The original descriptions of small-for-size syndrome described a condition arising in split liver transplantation characterised by the development of ascites, portal hypertension and liver dysfunction in an otherwise healthy transplanted portion of liver. The underlying cause for this syndrome is believed to relate to blood flow and the failure of a small liver volume to cope with often very high blood flows of patients with previous chronic liver disease undergoing transplantation. The validity of this hypothesis was supported by the observation that partial diversion of portal blood flow into the graft using a portocaval shunt could limit or prevent the development of small-for-size syndrome. Subsequently, other manoeuvres have also been effected, such as ligation or embolisation of the splenic artery, which works in the same way by reducing portal vein flow.

In patients undergoing even very major liver resection it is rare to develop small-for-size syndrome. Some patients do, however, develop ascites, jaundice and chronic liver dysfunction, and it is more likely that this syndrome is more dependent on a failure to regenerate than on excessive blood flow.

Hepatic steatosis

Fat infiltration of the liver is an increasing problem with increased prevalence of obesity and the metabolic syndrome (obesity and type 2 diabetes). Macroscopically the liver may appear enlarged, pale or yellow coloured with rounded edges. Microscopically the liver can have microsteatosis (small fat droplets within every hepatocyte) or macrosteatosis (regional infiltration of hepatocytes with large fat droplets) (see **Fig. 1.7**).

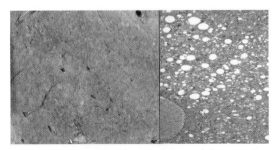

Figure 1.7 • Macroscopic and microscopic images of steatotic liver.

Assessment of steatosis

Assessment of hepatic steatosis is notoriously difficult. Experienced surgeons can estimate liver fat by judging the size, rounded or sharp edges of the liver and its appearance. Even using colour as an estimate is prone to error, as can be seen in **Fig. 1.8**.

The gold standard for hepatic fat assessment is histology. Trucut or wedge biopsies can be assessed by a pathologist and a reliable estimate of the percentage fat content produced. In addition, useful information including the distribution – macrosteatosis or microsteatosis – and the presence of fibrosis or inflammation can be provided. New MRI techniques are, however, challenging the accuracy of pathological assessment of steatosis and offer the potential advantage of being non-invasive.[30]

Chemotherapy-induced liver changes

Increased usage of chemotherapy in the neoadjuvant context has revealed changes in the liver associated with chemotherapy, particularly oxaliplatin and irinotecan. These range from a soft, fragile pale liver to steatosis, steatohepatitis and sinusoidal dilatation. Surgery should be deferred until 6 weeks after chemotherapy and studies, although conflicting, suggest that tolerance of major liver resection may be reduced and complications more frequent in individuals who have received chemotherapy. A study by Mehta et al. showed that oxaliplatin-based chemotherapy was associated with increased blood loss and prolonged hospital stay.[31]

Portal vein embolisation

Morbidity and mortality after hepatectomy have constituted a limitation on the number of patients eligible for resection, and currently only 8% of patients with colorectal hepatic metastases are candidates for curative liver resection. Liver function is correlated with liver volume, and consequently hepatic insufficiency in this situation may arise because not enough functional liver volume is left after surgical removal of part of the liver. Interestingly, following removal of part of the liver, the residual liver usually regenerates to the point where the preoperative liver weight–body weight ratio is regained. This notion has led to the belief that if it were possible to increase preoperatively the volume of

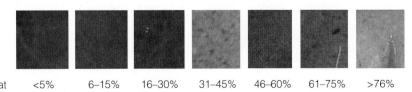

| % fat | <5% | 6–15% | 16–30% | 31–45% | 46–60% | 61–75% | >76% |

Figure 1.8 • Physical appearance of livers with varying fat content confirmed by histology to demonstrate the poor correlation between colour and objective measurement of fat content.

the future residual liver, it would be possible to perform more extensive liver resections and hence cure more patients. It has long been recognised that interruption of one part of the liver portal blood flow usually leads to hypertrophy of normally vascularised liver. This has been observed in patients with Klatskin tumours, which have a tendency to invade the portal vein, causing ipsilateral atrophy and contralateral hypertrophy. This concept has subsequently been harnessed by manoeuvres such as embolising the right portal vein prior to surgical resection. This leads to hypertrophy of the left liver lobe prior to surgery and facilitates the subsequent safe extensive resection of the right liver (extended right hepatectomy) 6 weeks later (**Fig. 1.9**). This phenomenon has been harnessed to maximise the residual functional liver volume of patients who are predicted to have a small remnant liver volume. This approach is fully based on the concept that, in the normal liver, volume is correlated to function and hence liver failure occurs when residual liver volume is too small. A completely different and novel approach would be to improve liver function per volume unit of liver. Recent evidence from studies using mebrofenin suggests that functional improvement of the future liver remnant following portal vein embolisation (PVE) may precede changes in liver volume.[32] This important observation suggests that surgery earlier after PVE may be possible. Limitations to PVE-induced hypertrophy include pre-existing hepatic fibrosis or cirrhosis and technical or anatomical inability to completely obstruct a major portal vein branch.

Technique

The most common technique of PVE is to puncture a branch of the vein using a percutaneous approach. A venogram is obtained to demonstrate all of the relevant branches and then the branch to be embolised is cannulated and coils and embolic material delivered to obstruct portal flow. A check angiogram can be performed to demonstrate success of the technique. Usually either a left or right main branch is occluded. To obtain hypertrophy of segments 2 and 3 in large right-sided tumours, it is not sufficient to embolise just the right portal vein and it is recommended that the branches supplying segment 4 should also be embolised. Patients usually tolerate PVE remarkably well, presumably because of the dual blood supply of the liver, and complications are uncommon. Significant hypertrophy can be achieved, as can be seen in **Fig. 1.10**.

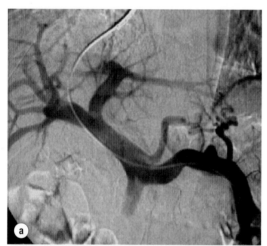

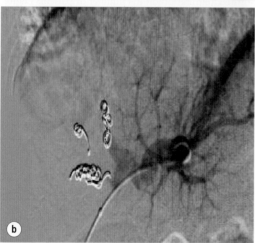

Figure 1.9 • Portal venograms showing the main left and right branches prior to embolisation **(a)**, and after embolisation of the right portal vein **(b)**.

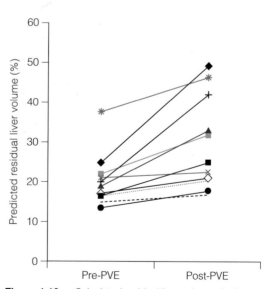

Figure 1.10 • Calculated residual liver volumes before and after portal vein embolisation (PVE) in patients scheduled to undergo major liver resection.

Therapy for liver failure

N-Acetyl cysteine

Glutathione depletion is a major problem in patients with paracetamol (acetaminophen) toxicity. N-Acetyl cysteine has been used for many years as a treatment for early paracetamol poisoning. It is thought to act by replenishing glutathione stores and by providing alternative thiol groups to which damaging reactive oxygen species can bind. The realisation that reactive oxygen species can be generated by conditions other than paracetamol poisoning such as sepsis and ischaemia/reperfusion has led to N-acetyl cysteine being used in a more general way to support patients with early evidence of liver dysfunction or failure.

Nutritional support in liver failure

The role of nutritional support in acute liver failure is uncertain, largely because of a lack of evidence in the world literature. Enteral nutrition is known to preserve gut barrier function and thus might be considered to be beneficial in the context of liver failure. In addition, the provision of energy might be considered beneficial in the context of glycogen storage failure, and to fuel the regeneration of liver tissue and recover function. The limited ability of the failing liver to handle nitrogen and synthesise urea (potentially exacerbating encephalopathy) would argue against excessive provision of proteins unless these were in a form where they did not contribute to the circulating ammonia load.

Artificial extracorporeal liver support

For the vast majority of patients who take toxic doses of paracetamol, suffer alcohol-induced liver injury or develop liver dysfunction following liver resection, the regenerative capacity of the liver is sufficient to prevent irretrievable liver failure and death. However, when this regenerative capacity is overwhelmed treatment strategies to temporarily or permanently replace the failing liver are required. The ability to provide short-term extracorporeal liver support, either during the wait for transplantation or to facilitate liver regeneration and avoid transplantation, is an attractive option. A range of devices have been developed, either focusing on the detoxification functions of liver (artificial liver support) or also incorporating bioreactors intended to also perform synthetic liver functions (bioartificial liver support). Assessment of efficacy has been hampered by the limited number of randomised controlled trials and small sample size, but a recent meta-analysis does suggest overall survival benefit in acute liver failure.[33]

Artificial liver support

Artificial systems include the MARS (Molecular Adsorbent Recirculating System) device, Prometheus and the BioLogic-DT (now called the Liver Dialysis Device, currently being redesigned). The greatest experience has been with the MARS device, which deploys an albumin dialysis circuit to remove both water-soluble and protein-bound toxins.[34] Thus, a low Fischer ratio can be corrected by recirculating albumin dialysis.[35] Because the system preferentially removes AAAs, compared with BCAAs, the Fischer ratio significantly increases, predominantly by the removal of AAAs in a small series of patients.[35–38] MARS has been shown to be useful in fulminant hepatic failure, by attenuating the increase in intracranial pressure, which plays a major role in this situation.[32] There may also be an effect on survival and improvement of degree of hepatic encephalopathy in patients with acute or chronic liver failure.[37,39] Equally, the system has been tested on artificial neuronal networks showing a normalisation of abnormal signals if the medium (plasma derived from rats with liver failure) was pretreated with MARS. The role of MARS in a more chronic situation of mild hepatic encephalopathy, when correction of an abnormal Fischer ratio would likely be more important if this were a major pathogenetic factor, is still largely unknown and deserves further study.[40] It has been suggested that the role of MARS and bioartificial liver support systems should be limited to carefully designed clinical trials.[41] It is currently uncertain how hepatic excretory assistance devices, such as MARS, compare with bioartificial liver assistance devices, which in addition to their excretory functions aim to provide biosynthetic capacity.[37]

Bioartificial liver systems

Bioartificial systems incorporate a bioreactor containing either human hepatoblastoma cell lines (e.g. the HepatAssist device) or porcine hepatocytes (e.g. the ELAD – Extracorporeal Liver Assist Device), through which the patient's blood is perfused. An additional filter component may be included to aid detoxification and improve bioreactor survival.

One of the major problems with these systems is what type of cells to use, and a variety of different approaches have been taken. Animal hepatocytes perform many of the same functions as human hepatocytes, although some of the proteins produced are obviously different. Human immortalised cell lines are an attractive proposition and some of the more differentiated cell lines can replicate many of the normal hepatocyte functions. Regardless, the true functionality of these cells in the clinical setting is uncertain. The design of bioartificial liver systems is challenging and the large surface area of hepatocytes needed to be effective is difficult. Engineering scaffolds of membranes or tubules has been the most popular approach. In normal liver, hepatocytes are polarised and have an epithelial surface. However, it is still to be determined how to recreate this polarity and its absolute importance has yet to be defined. Hepatocytes proliferate and function better in association with non-parenchymal cells; however, the creation of co-cultures in reactors produces its own problems. Cells must maintain viability or be able to be replenished to provide liver support over a prolonged period of time. In addition, very sick patients require a short time period to set up the support system, and the reactor must be easy to use by critical care nurses, safe from contamination and not overly expensive. For all of these reasons, bioartificial liver systems remain a tantalising prospect that has yet to break through into routine clinical practice.

Liver transplantation

Irreversible acute or chronic liver failure is amenable to treatment by liver transplantation. It is extremely uncommon for patients who have undergone liver resection to subsequently require or proceed to liver transplantation. The most obvious reason for this is that many patients who undergo liver resection do so for metastatic or primary liver cancer and transplantation would be contraindicated because of the risk of immunosuppression and aggressive recrudescence of the tumour. A number of patients with bile duct injury have progressed to transplantation, usually in a chronic setting following the development of biliary stricture, cholangitis and secondary biliary cirrhosis. Similarly, a number of patients who have undergone a 'cancer resection' for what turned out to be a benign biliary stricture, perhaps as part of primary sclerosing cholangitis, fail to regenerate their livers and may progress to transplantation.

Cell therapy for liver failure: general principles

A number of key principles have operated as key drivers for the development of cell therapies for clinical treatment of liver failure. Firstly, it is recognised that the injured liver usually provides a rich environment stimulating tissue regeneration and the liver can normally 'heal' itself. Secondly, in animal models there is evidence that stem cells or non-parenchymal cells can support regeneration of hepatocytes. Thirdly, it is recognised that the difference between liver failure and compensated liver function in terms

of cellular functional equivalents is probably very small. Finally, it would be preferable to support the liver by techniques that were within the body rather than using extracorporeal devices. This desire has stimulated research into therapeutic application of cell or stem cell transplantation.

The dual goals of stem cell therapy in the context of acute liver failure or injury are to promote rapid recovery of hepatocyte function and to allow regeneration of liver tissue without excessive scarring. Direct administration of hepatocytes or stem cell-derived hepatocytes to the injured liver has been met with little success in preclinical studies. However, using bone marrow-derived cells to support endogenous processes may support the regenerating liver, enabling effective regeneration.[42]

Haemopoetic stem cell therapy for liver disease in humans

There are several reports in the scientific literature of bone marrow (BM) stem cell therapy in patients with advanced liver disease. It was first reported that BM stem cells could increase the liver's ability to regenerate in patients who were undergoing hepatic resection for various liver cancers sited in the right lobe. Here the patients underwent embolisation of the right branch of the portal vein prior to surgery to stimulate compensatory hypertrophy of the left lobe. Autologous CD133-positive BM stem cells were injected into the blood vessels that supply the left liver lobe shortly after the surgery and accelerated regeneration of the non-embolised section of the liver was seen compared with control patients.[43] However, it must be stated that this was a small non-randomised study. The second report used BM stem cells in patients with liver cirrhosis.[44] CD34-positive stem cells were isolated from the patients' own blood following granulocyte colony-stimulating factor (GCSF)-induced haematopoietic stem cell mobilisation and were re-injected into the blood supply to the liver – preliminary evidence appeared to show that improvement in liver function in three out of five of the patients occurred during this therapy. In the third study, patients with liver cirrhosis had mononuclear cells isolated from their own BM during general anaesthesia.[45] These cells were re-injected into the patient's bloodstream and again the patient's liver function appeared to improve. Although these studies are very encouraging, they are preliminary, of small numbers and non-randomised. Furthermore, in none of these studies were the cells marked to enable identification either by radiological tracking or in biopsies of the liver tissue. Therefore, a number of important questions are unanswered. It is not certain that these cells definitely settled in the liver over a period of time, whether some of the cells engrafted other organs in the body and by what mechanisms the cells were having their positive effects within the recipients' livers.

Future developments

The ability to exert greater control in modulating liver volume and function in the surgical patient would be a major advantage. Preoperative functional enhancement might expand the group of patients who would be amenable to surgery, while postoperative intervention might be useful in liver resection, transplantation and acute liver failure as a means of rescuing a failing liver. The potential to use autologous stem cells derived from bone marrow to stimulate liver regeneration is enormous if its positive effects are seen in larger randomised studies.

Key points

- Conventional measures of liver function are poor and take no account of liver volume.
- Liver resection leaving a residual liver volume of <25% is associated with a high risk of liver dysfunction and infection.
- In patients with chronic liver disease smaller resections can be dangerous.
- The combination of liver dysfunction and sepsis can be fatal.
- Preoperative portal vein embolisation and newer regenerative strategies may improve the safety of liver surgery.

References

1. O'Grady JG, Alexander GJ, Hayllar KM, et al. Early indicators of prognosis in fulminant hepatic failure. Gastroenterology 1989;97:439–45.

2. Schindl MJ, Redhead DN, Fearon KC, et al. The value of residual liver volume as a predictor of hepatic dysfunction and infection after major liver resection. Gut 2005;54:289–96.
   The first paper providing strong evidence of an association between residual liver volume and clinical infection.

3. van Hoorn EC, van Middelaar-Voskuilen MC, van Limpt CJ, et al. Preoperative supplementation with a carbohydrate mixture decreases organ dysfunction-associated risk factors. Clin Nutr 2005;24:114–23.

4. Kretzschmar M, Kruger A, Schirrmeister W. Hepatic ischemia–reperfusion syndrome after partial liver resection (LR): hepatic venous oxygen saturation, enzyme pattern, reduced and oxidized glutathione, procalcitonin and interleukin-6. Exp Toxicol Pathol 2003;54:423–31.

5. Garcea G, Gescher A, Steward W, et al. Oxidative stress in humans following the Pringle manoeuvre. Hepatobil Pancreat Dis Int 2006;5:210–4.

6. Clavien PA, Yadav S, Sindram D, et al. Protective effects of ischemic preconditioning for liver resection performed under inflow occlusion in humans. Ann Surg 2000;232:155–62.
   The first randomised clinical trial demonstrating benefit in clinical markers from ischaemic preconditioning of the liver in patients undergoing liver resection.

7. Patel A, van de Poll MC, Greve JW, et al. Early stress protein gene expression in a human model of ischemic preconditioning. Transplantation 2004;78(27):1479–87.

8. Pugh RN, Murray-Lyon IM, Dawson JL, et al. Transection of the oesophagus for bleeding oesophageal varices. Br J Surg 1973;60:646–9.

9. Albrecht J, Jones EA. Hepatic encephalopathy: molecular mechanisms underlying the clinical syndrome. J Neurol Sci 1999;170:138–46.

10. Shawcross D, Jalan R. The pathophysiologic basis of hepatic encephalopathy: central role for ammonia and inflammation. Cell Mol Life Sci 2005;62:2295–304.

11. James JH, Ziparo V, Jeppsson B, Fischer JE. Hyperammonaemia, plasma amino acid imbalance, and blood–brain amino acid transport: a unified theory of portal–systemic encephalopathy. Lancet 1979;2:772–5.
    Explanation of the relationship between the urea cycle and hepatic encephalopathy.

12. Fischer JE, Yoshimura N, Aguirre A, et al. Plasma amino acids in patients with hepatic encephalopathy. Effects of amino acid infusions. Am J Surg 1974;127:40–7.

13. Soeters PB, Fischer JE. Insulin, glucagon, amino-acid imbalance, and hepatic encephalopathy. Lancet 1976;2:880–2.

14. Fischer JE, Rosen HM, Ebeid AM, et al. The effect of normalization of plasma amino acids on hepatic encephalopathy in man. Surgery 1976;80:77–91.

15. Fischer JE, Baldessarini RJ. False neurotransmitters and hepatic failure. Lancet 1971;2:75–80.

16. Wigmore SJ, Redhead DN, Yan XJ, et al. Virtual hepatic resection using three-dimensional reconstruction

of helical computed tomography angioportograms. Ann Surg 2001;233:221–6.

17. Dello SA, van Dam RM, Slangen JJ, et al. Liver volumetry plug and play: do it yourself with ImageJ. World J Surg 2007;31:2215–21.

18. Zipprich A, Kuss O, Rogowski S, et al. Incorporating indocyanin green clearance into the Model for End Stage Liver Disease (MELD-ICG) improves prognostic accuracy in intermediate to advanced cirrhosis. Gut 2010;59(7):963–8.

19. Bennink RJ, Dinant S, Erdogan D, et al. Preoperative assessment of postoperative remnant liver function using hepatobiliary scintigraphy. J Nucl Med 2004;45:965–71.

20. van de Poll MC, Wigmore SJ, Redhead DN, et al. Effect of major liver resection on hepatic ureagenesis in humans. Am J Physiol Gastrointest Liver Physiol 2007;293:G956–62.
   Clinical experimental study demonstrating the relationship between liver volume and urea synthesis in patients undergoing varying degrees of liver resection.

21. Vermeulen MA, Ligthart-Melis GC, Buijsman R, et al. Accurate perioperative flow measurement of the portal vein and hepatic and renal artery: a role for preoperative MRI? Eur J Radiol 2012;81(9):2042–8.

22. van de Poll MC, Ligthart-Melis GC, Boelens PG, et al. Intestinal and hepatic metabolism of glutamine and citrulline in humans. J Physiol 2007;581:819–27.

23. van de Poll MC, Siroen MP, van Leeuwen PA, et al. Interorgan amino acid exchange in humans: consequences for arginine and citrulline metabolism. Am J Clin Nutr 2007;85:167–72.

24. Barbaro B, Manfredi R, Bombardieri G, et al. Correlation of MRI liver volume and Doppler sonographic portal hemodynamics with histologic findings in patients with chronic hepatitis C. J Clin Ultrasound 2000;28:461–8.

25. Nanashima A, Shibasaki S, Sakamoto I, et al. Clinical evaluation of magnetic resonance imaging flowmetry of portal and hepatic veins in patients following hepatectomy. Liver Int 2006;26:587–94.

26. El-Desoky AE, Seifalian A, Cope M, et al. Changes in tissue oxygenation of the porcine liver measured by near-infrared spectroscopy. Liver Transpl Surg 1999;5:219–26.

27. Schindl MJ, Millar AM, Redhead DN, et al. The adaptive response of the reticuloendothelial system to major liver resection in humans. Ann Surg 2006;243:507–14.

28. Boulter L, Govaere O, Bird TG, et al. Macrophage-derived Wnt opposes Notch signaling to specify hepatic progenitor cell fate in chronic liver disease. Nat Med 2012;18(4):572–9.

29. Thomas JA, Pope C, Wojtacha D, et al. Macrophage therapy for murine liver fibrosis recruits host effector cells improving fibrosis, regeneration, and function. Hepatology 2011;53(6):2003–15.

30. Raptis DA, Fischer MA, Nanz D, et al. MRI as the new reference standard in quantifying liver steatosis: the need for international guidelines. Gut 2012;61(9):1370–1.

31. Mehta NN, Ravikumar R, Coldham CA, et al. Effect of preoperative chemotherapy on liver resection for colorectal liver metastases. Eur J Surg Oncol 2008;34:782–6.

32. de Graaf W, van Lienden KP, van den Esschert JW, et al. Increase in future remnant liver function after preoperative portal vein embolization. Br J Surg 2011;98(6):825–34.

33. Stutchfield BM, Simpson K, Wigmore SJ. Systematic review and meta-analysis of survival following extracorporeal liver support. Br J Surg 2011;98(5):623–31.

34. Tan HK. Molecular adsorbent recirculating system (MARS). Ann Acad Med Singapore 2004;33:329–35.

35. Loock J, Mitzner SR, Peters E, et al. Amino acid dysbalance in liver failure is favourably influenced by recirculating albumin dialysis (MARS). Liver 2002;22(Suppl. 2):35–9.

36. Awad SS, Swaniker F, Magee J, et al. Results of a phase I trial evaluating a liver support device utilizing albumin dialysis. Surgery 2001;130:354–62.

37. Mitzner S, Loock J, Peszynski P, et al. Improvement in central nervous system functions during treatment of liver failure with albumin dialysis MARS – a review of clinical, biochemical, and electrophysiological data. Metab Brain Dis 2002;17:463–75.

38. Steczko J, Bax KC, Ash SR. Effect of hemodiabsorption and sorbent-based pheresis on amino acid levels in hepatic failure. Int J Artif Organs 2000;23:375–88.

39. Boyle M, Kurtovic J, Bihari D, et al. Equipment review: the molecular adsorbents recirculating system (MARS). Crit Care 2004;8:280–6.

40. Hassanein TI, Tofteng F, Brown Jr RS, et al. Randomized controlled study of extracorporeal albumin dialysis for hepatic encephalopathy in advanced cirrhosis. Hepatology 2007;46:1853–62.

41. Ferenci P, Kramer L. MARS and the failing liver – Any help from the outer space? Hepatology 2007;46:1682–4.

42. Stutchfield BM, Forbes SJ, Wigmore SJ. Prospects for stem cell transplantation in the treatment of hepatic disease. Liver Transpl 2010;16(7):827–36.

43. am Esch 2nd. JS, Knoefel WT, Klein M, et al. Portal application of autologous CD133+ BM cells to the liver: a novel concept to support hepatic regeneration. Stem Cells 2005;23:463–70.

44. Gordon MY, Levicar N, Pai M, et al. Characterisation and clinical application of human CD34+ stem/progenitor cell populations mobilised into the blood by G-CSF. Stem Cells 2006;24:1822–30.

45. Terai S, Ishikawa T, Omori K, et al. Improved liver function in liver cirrhosis patients after autologous bone marrow cell infusion therapy. Stem Cells 2006;24:2292–8.

2

Hepatic, biliary and pancreatic anatomy

Steven M. Strasberg

The aim of this chapter is to provide the basic anatomical foundation for performing liver, biliary and pancreatic surgery. Surgically unimportant anatomical features are omitted, but anatomical distortions due to pathological processes are included. A key point of hepato-pancreato-biliary (HPB) surgical anatomy is that whilst there is a **prevailing pattern** of anatomy, i.e. a pattern that is most commonly found, variations from the prevailing pattern termed **anomalies** are frequent. Every surgical operation in this area should be conducted with this fact in mind.

Liver

Overview of hepatic anatomy and terminology

Modern hepatic anatomy is concerned mainly with internal vascular and biliary structures rather than surface markings. Ramifications of the hepatic artery and bile ducts are regular and virtually identical. The portal vein on the left side of the liver is a vessel with unusual morphology, consequent to its need to perform different functions in the foetus and in the postnatal period. Consequently, the Brisbane 2000 Terminology of Hepatic Anatomy and Resections of the International Hepato-Pancreato-Biliary Association used in this chapter is primarily based on hepatic artery and bile duct ramifications.[1]

Divisions of the liver based on the hepatic artery

The primary (first-order) division of the proper hepatic artery is into the right and left hepatic arteries (**Fig. 2.1**). These branches supply arterial inflow to the right and left hemilivers or livers (**Fig. 2.2**). The plane between the two distinct zones of vascular supply is called a watershed. The border or watershed of the first-order division is called the **midplane of the liver**. It intersects the gallbladder fossa and the fossa for the inferior vena cava (IVC) (Fig. 2.2). The right liver usually has a larger volume than the left liver (60:40), although this is variable.

The second-order divisions (Figs 2.1 and **2.3**) of the hepatic artery supply four distinct zones of the liver. Each is referred to as a **section**. The right liver is divided into two sections, the **right anterior section** and the **right posterior section**. These sections are supplied by the right anterior sectional hepatic artery and the right posterior sectional hepatic artery (Fig. 2.1). The plane between these sections is the **right intersectional plane**. The right intersectional plane does not have any surface markings to indicate its position. The left liver is also divided into two sections, the **left medial section** and the **left lateral section** (Fig. 2.3), which are supplied by the left medial sectional hepatic artery and the left lateral sectional hepatic artery (Fig. 2.1). The plane between these sections is referred to as the left intersectional plane. It does have surface markings indicating its position – the umbilical fissure and

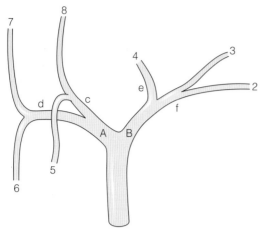

Figure 2.1 • Ramification of the hepatic artery in the liver. The prevailing pattern is shown. The first-order division of the proper hepatic artery is into the right **(a)** and left **(b)** hepatic arteries, which supply right and left hemilivers (Fig. 2.2), respectively. The second-order division of the hepatic arteries, supplies the four sections (Fig. 2.3). The third-order division, shown in orange, supplies the segments (Fig. 2.4). Since the left medial section and segment 4 are the same, the artery is shown as being both sectional and segmental (red/orange). The caudate lobe is supplied by branches from **(a)** and **(b)**. Bile duct anatomy and nomenclature is similar to that of the hepatic artery. © Washington University in St Louis.

the line of attachment of the falciform ligament to the anterior surface of the liver.

The third-order divisions of the hepatic artery divide the right and left hemilivers into **segments** (Sg) 2–8 (Figs 2.1 and **2.4**). Each of the segments has its own feeding segmental artery. The left lateral section is divided into Sg2 and Sg3. The pattern or ramification of vessels within the left medial section does not permit subdivision of this section into segments, each with its own arterial blood supply. Therefore the left medial section and Sg4 are synonymous. However, Sg4 is arbitrarily divided into superior (4a) and inferior (4b) parts without an exact anatomical plane of separation based on internal ramification of vessels. The right anterior section is divided into two segments, Sg5 and Sg8. The right posterior section is divided into Sg6 and Sg7. The planes between segments are referred to as intersegmental planes. The ramifications of the bile ducts are identical to that described for the arteries, as are the zones of the liver drained by the respective ducts.

Segment 1 (caudate lobe) is a distinct portion of the liver, separate from the right and left hemilivers (**Fig. 2.5**). It is appropriately referred to as a lobe since it is demarcated by visible fissures. It consists of three parts: the bulbous left part (Spiegelian lobe), which grips the left side of the vena cava and is readily visible through the lesser omentum; the paracaval portion, which lies anterior to the vena

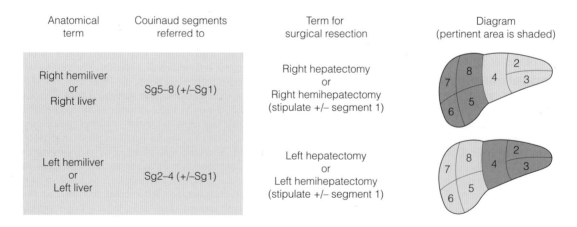

Anatomical term	Couinaud segments referred to	Term for surgical resection	Diagram (pertinent area is shaded)
Right hemiliver or Right liver	Sg5–8 (+/–Sg1)	Right hepatectomy or Right hemihepatectomy (stipulate +/– segment 1)	
Left hemiliver or Left liver	Sg2–4 (+/–Sg1)	Left hepatectomy or Left hemihepatectomy (stipulate +/– segment 1)	

Border or watershed: The border or watershed of the first-order division which separates the two hemilivers is a plane which intersects the gallbladder fossa and the fossa for the IVC and is called the midplane of the liver.

Figure 2.2 • Nomenclature for first-order division anatomy (hemilivers or livers) and resections. © Washington University in St Louis.

Second-order division
(second-order division based on bile ducts and hepatic artery)

Anatomical term	Couinaud segments referred to	Term for surgical resection	Diagram (pertinent area is shaded)
Right anterior section	Sg 5,8	Add (-ectomy) to any of the anatomical terms as in Right anterior sectionectomy	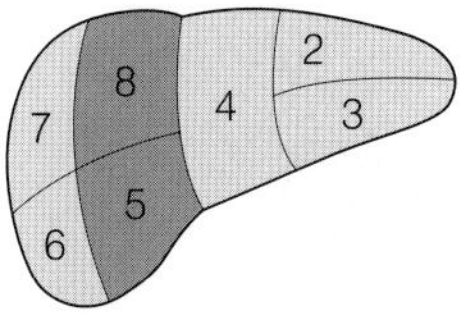
Right posterior section	Sg 6,7	Right posterior sectionectomy	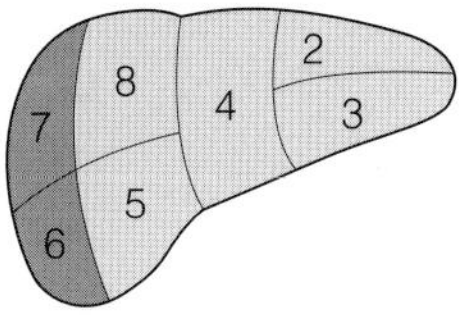
Left medial section	Sg 4	Left medial sectionectomy or Resection segment 4 (also see third order) or Segmentectomy 4 (also see third order)	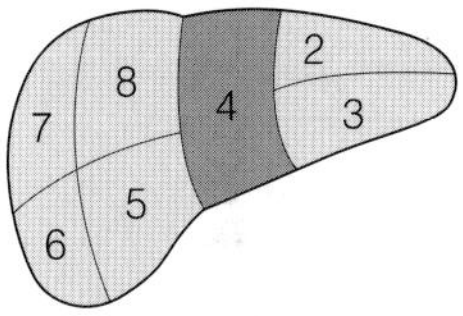
Left lateral section	Sg 2,3	Left lateral sectionectomy or Bisegmentectomy 2,3 (also see third order)	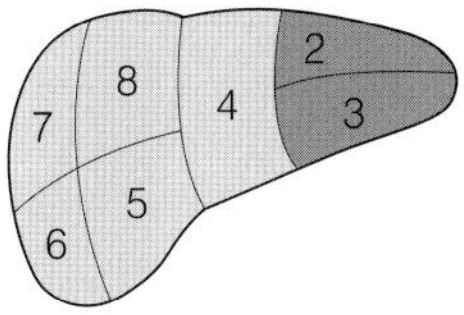

Other sectional liver resections

	Sg 4–8 (+/–Sg1)	Right trisectionectomy (preferred term) or Extended right hepatectomy or Extended right hemihepatectomy (stipulate +/– segment 1)	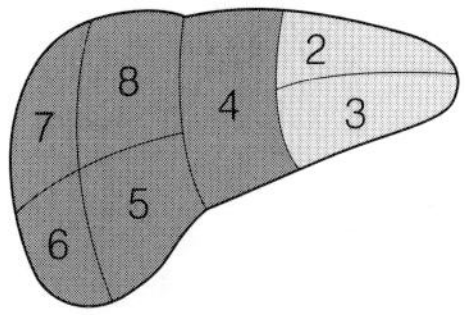
	Sg 2,3,4,5,8 (+/–Sg1)	Left trisectionectomy (preferred term) or Extended left hepatectomy or Extended left hemihepatectomy (stipulate +/– segment 1)	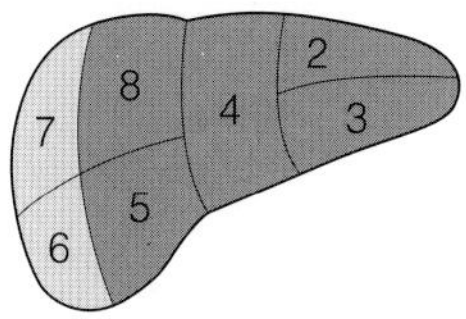

Border or watershed: The borders or watersheds of the sections are planes referred to as the right and left intersectional planes. The left intersectional plane passes through the umbilical fissure and the attachment of the falciform ligament. There is no surface marking of the right intersectional plane.

Figure 2.3 • Nomenclature for second-order division anatomy (sections) and resections including extended resections. © Washington University in St Louis.

Third-order division

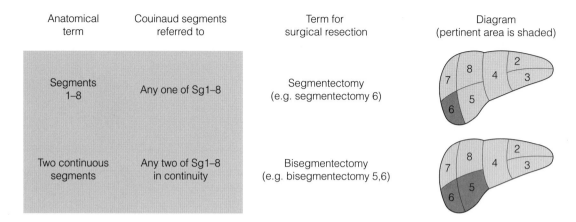

Anatomical term	Couinaud segments referred to	Term for surgical resection	Diagram (pertinent area is shaded)
Segments 1–8	Any one of Sg1–8	Segmentectomy (e.g. segmentectomy 6)	
Two continuous segments	Any two of Sg1–8 in continuity	Bisegmentectomy (e.g. bisegmentectomy 5,6)	

Border or watershed: The borders or watersheds of the segments are planes referred to as intersegmental planes.

Figure 2.4 • Nomenclature for third-order division anatomy (segments) and resections. © Washington University in St Louis.

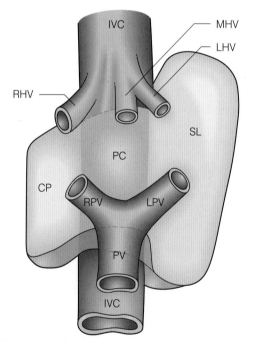

Figure 2.5 • Schematic representation of the anatomy of the caudate lobe. The caudate lobe consists of three parts: the caudate process (CP), on the right, the paracaval portion anterior to the vena cava (PC) and the bulbous left part (Spiegelian lobe, SL). IVC, inferior vena cava; PV, portal vein; RHV, MHV, LHV, right hepatic, middle hepatic and left hepatic veins, respectively. © Washington University in St Louis.

cava; and the caudate process, on the right. The caudate process merges indistinctly with the right hemiliver. The caudate lobe is situated posterior to the hilum and the portal veins. Lying anterior and superior to the paracaval portion are the hepatic veins, which limit the upper extent of the caudate lobe[2,3] (Fig. 2.5). The caudate receives vascular supply from both right and left hepatic arteries (and portal veins). Caudate bile ducts drain into both right and left hepatic ducts.[3] The caudate lobe is drained by several short caudate veins that enter the IVC directly from the caudate lobe. Their number and size are variable. Occasionally caudate veins are quite short and wide, and therefore must be isolated and divided cautiously. Commonly, these veins enter the IVC on either side of the midplane of the vessel, an anatomical feature that normally allows the creation of a tunnel behind the liver on the surface of the IVC without encountering the caudate veins. The 'hanging manoeuvre' is performed by lifting up on a tape placed through this tunnel (see below).

Resectional terminology

The terminology of hepatic resections is based upon the terminology of hepatic anatomy. Resection of one side of the liver is called a hepatectomy or hemihepatectomy (Fig. 2.2). Resection of the right side of the liver is a right hepatectomy or hemihepatectomy and resection of the left side of the liver is a left hemihepatectomy or hepatectomy. Resection of a liver section is referred to as a sectionectomy

(Fig. 2.3). Resection of the liver to the left side of the umbilical fissure is a left lateral sectionectomy. The other sectionectomies are named accordingly, e.g. right anterior sectionectomy. Resection of the right hemiliver plus Sg4 is referred to as a right trisectionectomy (Fig. 2.3). Similarly, resection of the left hemiliver plus the right anterior section is referred to as a left trisectionectomy.

Resection of one of the numbered segments is referred to as a segmentectomy (Fig. 2.4). Resection of the caudate lobe can be referred to as a caudate lobectomy or resection of Sg1. It is always appropriate to refer to a resection by the numbered segments. For instance, it would be appropriate to call a left lateral sectionectomy a resection of Sg2 and Sg3.

Surgical anatomy for liver resections

Hepatic arteries and liver resections

In the prevailing anatomical pattern, the coeliac artery terminates to divide into splenic and common hepatic arteries. Rarely, the hepatic artery arises directly from the aorta. The common hepatic artery runs for 2–3 cm anteriorly and to the right to ramify into gastroduodenal and proper hepatic arteries. The proper hepatic artery enters the hepatoduodenal ligament and normally runs for 2–3 cm along the left side of the common bile duct and terminates by dividing into the right and left hepatic arteries, the right immediately passing behind the common hepatic duct. The terms "common" and "proper" in respect to hepatic arteries while correct are not intuitive and the arteries are sometimes confused in the literature. The four sectional arteries arise from the right and left arteries 1–2 cm from the liver. While this is the commonest pattern, variations from this pattern are also very common (**Fig. 2.6**). The surgeon is wise not to make assumptions regarding hepatic arteries based on size or position, but rely instead on complete dissection, trial occlusions and radiological support. When an artery appears unusually large it is especially important to dissect until identification is unquestionable.

'Replaced' arteries are surgically important anomalies. 'Replaced' means that the artery supplying a particular volume of liver is in an unusual location and also that it is the sole supply to that volume of liver. 'Aberrant' means the structure is in an unusual location. While the definition of 'aberrant' does not state whether the structure provides sole supply, it is usually considered to be synonymous with 'replaced' in respect to these arteries. 'Accessory' refers to an artery that is additional, i.e. is present in addition to the normal structure and as a result is *not* the sole supply to a volume.

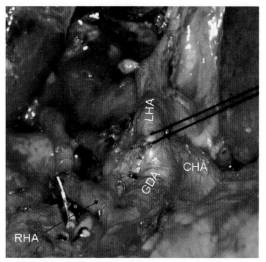

Figure 2.6 • A most dangerous arterial anatomy. The right hepatic artery (RHA) arises from the gastroduodenal artery (GDA). There is no proper hepatic artery. The left hepatic artery (LHA) could easily be mistaken for the proper hepatic artery. Ligation of the GDA would lead to arterial devascularisation of the right liver. © Washington University in St Louis.

Consequently, ligation of an accessory artery does not result in ischaemia.

In about 25% of patients, part or all of the liver is supplied by a replaced (or aberrant) artery. The **replaced right hepatic artery** arises from the superior mesenteric artery. It runs from left to right behind the lower end of the common bile duct to emerge and course on its right posterior border. It may supply a segment, section or the entire right hemiliver. Rarely, this artery supplies the entire liver and then it is called a **replaced hepatic artery**. The **replaced left hepatic artery** arises from the left gastric artery and courses in the lesser omentum in conjunction with vagal branches to the liver (hepatic nerve). As with the right artery it may supply a segment, section (usually the left lateral section), hemiliver or very rarely the whole liver. Sometimes left hepatic arteries arising from the left gastric artery are actually accessory rather than replaced and exist in conjunction with normally situated left hepatic arteries. Knowledge of these particular arterial variations is of importance not only in hepatobiliary surgery, including transplantation, but also in gastric surgery and pancreatic surgery. Transection of the left gastric artery at its origin during gastrectomy may cause ischaemic necrosis of the left hemiliver if a replaced left artery is present. The same may occur on the right side as a result of injury to a replaced right artery. Also, these vessels need to be preserved and perfused during donor hepatectomy. Sometimes there is no proper hepatic artery because the entire liver is supplied by right or left replaced arteries or both. This anomaly may be suspected when, on opening the peritoneum at the base of the right side of the hepatoduodenal ligament, the portal vein is immediately apparent instead of the hepatic artery.

Replaced arteries may confer an advantage during surgery. For instance, when a replaced left artery supplies the left lateral section it is possible to resect the entire proper hepatic artery when performing a right trisectionectomy for hilar cholangicarcinoma. The replaced right artery is sometimes invaded by pancreatic head tumours and is in danger of injury during pancreato-duodenectomy. This is only a brief description of replaced arteries. There are many variations of replaced arteries, especially on the right, depending on the relationships of the artery to the pancreatic head and neck, the bile duct and the portal vein.[4]

In performing hepatectomies by the standard technique of isolating individual structures instead of pedicles it is critical to correctly identify the particular artery(ies) supplying the volume of liver to be resected. One important anatomical point is that an artery located to the right side of the bile duct always supplies the right side of the liver, but arteries found on the left side of the bile duct may supply either side of the liver. Therefore, when using the individual vessel ligation method it is important to be aware of the position of the common hepatic duct. A trial occlusion of an artery with an atraumatic clamp should always be performed in order to be sure that there is a good pulse to the side of the liver to be retained.

Bile ducts and liver resections

Prevailing pattern and important variations of bile ducts draining the right hemiliver

Normally only a short portion of the right hepatic duct, about 1 cm, is in an extrahepatic position. The prevailing pattern of bile duct drainage from the right liver is shown in **Fig. 2.7a**. The segmental ducts from Sg6 and Sg7 (called **B6, B7**) unite to form the **right posterior sectional bile duct** and the segmental ducts from Sg5 and Sg8 (**B5, B8**) unite to form the **right anterior sectional bile duct** (Fig. 2.7a). The sectional ducts unite to form the **right hepatic duct**, which unites with the left hepatic duct at the **confluence** to form the common hepatic duct.

There are two important sets of biliary anomalies on the right side of the liver. The first involves insertion of a right sectional duct into the left bile duct. This is a common anomaly. The right posterior sectional duct inserts into the left hepatic duct in 20% of individuals (**Fig. 2.7b**) and the right anterior bile duct does so in 6% (**Fig. 2.7c**). In these situations there is no right hepatic duct. A right sectional bile duct inserting into the left hepatic duct is in danger of injury during left hepatectomy if the left duct is divided at its termination. Therefore, when performing left hepatectomy, the left hepatic duct should be divided close to the umbilical fissure to avoid injury to a right sectional duct.

The second important anomaly is insertion of a right bile duct into the biliary tree at a lower level than the prevailing site of confluence. Low union may affect the right hepatic duct, a sectional right duct (usually the anterior one), a segmental duct or a subsegmental duct. A right bile duct unites with the common hepatic duct below the prevailing site of confluence in about 2% of individuals. Sometimes the duct unites with the cystic duct and then with the common hepatic duct. The latter anomaly places the aberrant duct at great risk of injury during laparoscopic cholecystectomy.

Very rarely the right hepatic duct terminates in the gallbladder. This may be congenital or acquired. In the latter case a gallstone has effaced a cystic duct which united with the right hepatic duct, giving the appearance that it joins the gallbladder. An extremely rare anomaly is the absent common hepatic duct. In these cases the right and left hepatic duct

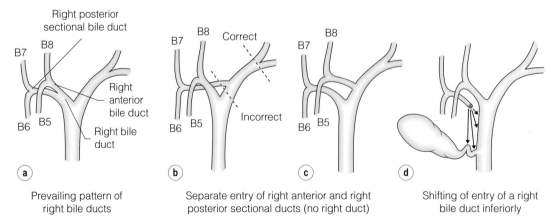

(a) Prevailing pattern of right bile ducts

(b) Separate entry of right anterior and right posterior sectional ducts (no right duct)

(c)

(d) Shifting of entry of a right bile duct inferiorly

Figure 2.7 • Prevailing pattern **(a)** and important variations **(b–d)** of bile ducts draining the right hemiliver (see text). © Washington University in St Louis.

enters the gallbladder and the duct emerging from the gallbladder runs downward to join with the duodenum.[5] In the presence of these anomalies, which would be extremely difficult to detect, a complete cholecystectomy will result in ductal injury. These ducts should not be confused with ducts of Luschka (see below).

The right **posterior** sectional duct normally hooks over the origin of the right *anterior* sectional portal vein ('Hjortsjo's crook'),[6] where it is in danger of being injured if the right anterior sectional pedicle is clamped too close to its origin (**Fig. 2.8**).

Prevailing pattern and important variations of bile ducts draining the left hemiliver

The prevailing pattern of bile duct drainage from the left liver is shown in **Fig. 2.9a**. It is present in only 30% of individuals, i.e. variations (anomalies) are present in the majority of individuals. In the prevailing pattern, the segmental ducts from Sg2 and Sg3 (**B2, B3**) unite to form the **left lateral sectional bile duct**. This duct passes behind the umbilical portion of the portal vein and unites with the duct from segment 4 (**B4**; also called the left medial sectional duct since section and segment are synonymous for this volume of liver). The site of union of these ducts to form the left hepatic duct lies about one-third of

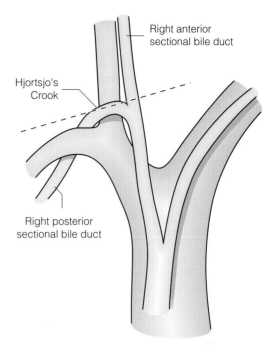

Figure 2.8 • Hjortsjo's crook. Note that the right posterior sectional bile duct (RPSBD) crosses the origin of the right anterior sectional portal vein. © Washington University in St Louis.

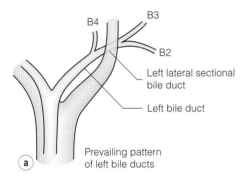

(a) Prevailing pattern of left bile ducts

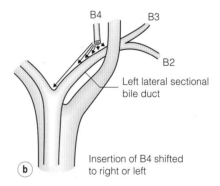

(b) Insertion of B4 shifted to right or left

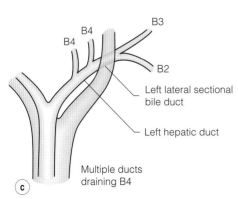

(c) Multiple ducts draining B4

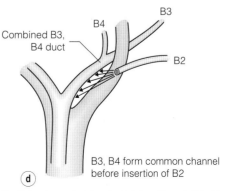

(d) B3, B4 form common channel before insertion of B2

Figure 2.9 • Prevailing pattern **(a)** and important variations **(b–d)** of bile ducts draining the left hemiliver. © Washington University in St Louis.

the distance between the umbilical fissure and the midplane of the liver. The left hepatic duct continues from this point for 2–3 cm along the base of segment 4 to its confluence with the right hepatic duct. Note that it is in an extrahepatic position and that it has a much longer extrahepatic course than the right bile duct. The extrahepatic position of the left hepatic duct is a key anatomical feature, which makes this section of duct the prime site for high biliary–enteric anastomoses.

The main anomalies of the left ductal system involve variations in site of insertion of B4 (**Fig. 2.9b**), multiple ducts coming from B4 (**Fig. 2.9c**) and primary union of B3 and B4 with subsequent union of B2 (**Fig. 2.9d**). B4 may join the left lateral sectional duct to the left or right of its point of union in the prevailing pattern (Fig. 2.9b); in the former case the insertion of B4 is at the umbilical fissure and in the latter the insertion may occur at any place to the right of the prevailing location up to the point where the left hepatic duct normally unites with the right hepatic duct. In the latter instance, which according to Couinaud is present in 8% of individuals, there is no left hepatic duct. Instead there is a confluence of three ducts, the left lateral sectional duct, B4 and the right hepatic duct to form the common hepatic duct. These variations are important in split liver transplantation and in diagnosis and repair of biliary injuries.

The bile duct to Sg3 has been used to perform biliary bypass and can be isolated by following the superior surface of the ligamentum teres down to isolate the portal pedicle to Sg3. The technique is less commonly used now that internal endoscopic bypass has been developed.

Prevailing pattern of bile ducts draining the caudate lobe (Sg1)

Normally, two to three caudate ducts enter the biliary tree. Their orifices are usually located posteriorly on the left duct, right duct or right posterior sectional duct.

Portal veins and liver resections

On the right side of the liver the portal vein divisions correspond to those of the hepatic artery and bile duct, and they supply the same hepatic volumes. Therefore, there is a right portal vein that supplies the entire right hemiliver (**Fig. 2.10**). It divides into two sectional and four segmental veins, as do the arteries and bile ducts. On the left side of the liver, however, the left portal vein is quite unusual because of the fact that its structure was adapted to function in utero as a conduit between the umbilical vein and the ductus venosus, whilst postnatally the direction of flow is reversed. The left portal vein consists of a **horizontal or transverse portion**, which is located under Sg4, and a **vertical part or umbilical portion**,

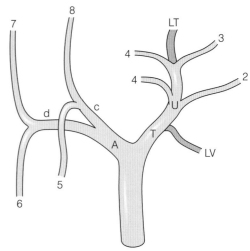

Figure 2.10 • Ramification of the portal vein in the liver. The portal vein divides into right (A) and left (T) branches. The branches in the right liver correspond to those of the hepatic artery and bile duct (Fig. 2.1). The branching pattern on the left is unique. The left portal vein has transverse (T) and umbilical portions (U). The transition point between the two parts is marked by the attachment of the ligamentum venosum (LV). All major branches come off the umbilical portion (see text). The vein ends blindly in the ligamentum teres (LT). © Washington University in St Louis.

which is situated in the umbilical fissure (Fig. 2.10). Unlike the right portal vein, neither portion of the left portal vein actually enters the liver, but rather they lie directly on its surface. Often the umbilical portion is hidden by a bridge of tissue passing between left medial and lateral sections. This bridge of liver tissue may be as thick as 2 cm or only be a fibrous band. The junction of the transverse and umbilical portions of the left portal vein is marked by the attachment of a stout cord – the ligamentum venosum. This structure, the remnant of the foetal ductus venosus, runs in the groove between the left lateral section and the caudate lobe and attaches to the left hepatic vein/IVC junction.

Ramification of the left portal vein (Figs 2.10 and **2.11**)

The transverse portion of the left portal vein sends only a few small branches to Sg4. Large branches from the portal vein to the left liver arise exclusively beyond the attachment of the ligamentum venosum, i.e. from the umbilical part of the vein.[7] These branches come off both sides of the vein – those arising from the right side pass into Sg4 and those from the left supply Sg2 and Sg3. There is usually only one branch to Sg2 and Sg3, but often there is more than one branch to Sg4. The left portal vein terminates in the ligamentum teres at the free edge of the left liver. Note that the umbilical portion of

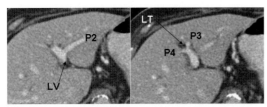

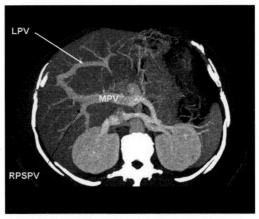

Figure 2.11 • Ramification of the left portal vein as seen on CT. Note the branches to segments 2–4 and the ligamentum teres (LT). The arrow points to the ligamentum venosum (LT) and the groove between the left lateral section and the caudate lobe. This is also the site of origin of the ligamentum venosum, where the transverse portion of the left portal vein becomes the umbilical portion of the vein, proving conclusively that the branch to Sg2 is not part of a terminal division of the transverse portion of the vein as might be concluded from case studies (also see Ref. 7). © Washington University in St Louis.

Figure 2.12 • Absent extrahepatic left portal vein, a rare and very dangerous anomaly. Three-dimensional reconstruction of CT scan. Note that the main portal vein (MPV) enters the right liver, gives off the right posterior sectional portal vein (RPSPV) and some branches to the right anterior section, then proceeds to the left as an internal left portal vein (LPV). © Washington University in St Louis.

the portal vein has a unique pattern of ramification. The pattern is similar to an air-conditioning duct that sends branches at right angles from both of its sides to supply rooms (segments), tapering as it does so, finally to end blindly (in the ligamentum teres). Other vascular and biliary structures normally ramify by dividing into two other structures at their termination and not by sending out branches along their length.

Although the divisions of the portal vein are unusual, for the embryonic reasons described above, it is uncommon to have variations from this pattern. Probably the most common variation is absence of the right portal vein. In these cases the right posterior and right anterior sectional portal veins originate independently from the main portal vein. Under these circumstances the anterior sectional vein is usually quite high in the porta hepatis and may not be obvious. An unsuspecting surgeon may divide the posterior sectional vein thinking that it is the right portal vein and become confused when the anterior sectional vein is subsequently revealed during hepatic transection.

A rare but potentially devastating anomaly is the absent extrahepatic left portal vein (**Fig. 2.12**). The apparent right vein is really the main portal vein, a structure that enters the liver, gives off branches to the right liver and then loops back within the liver substance to supply the left side. The vein looks like a right vein in terms of position but is larger. Transection results in total portal vein disconnection from the liver. This anomaly should always be searched for on computed tomography (CT) as right hepatectomy is not usually possible when it is present. The presence of the transverse portion of the left vein at the base of Sg4, which then enters the umbilical fissure, precludes the presence of this anomaly.

The portal vein branches to Sg4 may be isolated in the umbilical fissure on the right side of the umbilical portion of the left portal vein. The veins here are associated with the bile ducts and the arteries passing to Sg4, i.e. they enter sheaths as they go into the liver substance. Isolation in this location may provide extra margin when resecting a tumour in Sg4 that impinges upon the umbilical fissure. Normally the branches to Sg4 are isolated after dividing the parenchyma of the liver of Sg4 close to the umbilical fissure, an approach that is used to avoid injury to the umbilical portion of the left portal vein. Injury to this vein could, of course, deprive Sg2 and Sg3 of portal vein supply as well as Sg4. For instance, if this occurs when performing a right trisectionectomy, the only portion of the liver to be retained would be devascularised of portal vein flow. However, isolation of these structures within the umbilical fissure does provide an extra margin of clearance on tumours and can be done safely if care is taken to ascertain the position of the portal vein. Likewise, it is possible to isolate the portal vein branches going into Sg2 and Sg3 in the umbilical fissure and to extend a margin when resecting a tumour in the left lateral section. For the same reasons given above, caution must be taken when doing this in order not to injure the umbilical portion of the portal vein. In order to access the portal vein in this location it is usually necessary to divide the bridge of liver tissue, between the left medial and lateral sections. This is done by passing a blunt instrument behind the bridge before dividing it, usually with cautery. Note that arteries and bile ducts passing to the left lateral section are in danger of being injured as one isolates the most posterior–superior portion of the bridge. To facilitate passage of an instrument behind the bridge, the peritoneum at the base of the bridge may be opened in a preliminary step. The instrument being passed behind the bridge should never be forced.

Hepatic veins and liver resection (Fig. 2.13)

There are normally three large hepatic veins. These run in the midplane of the liver (middle hepatic vein), the right intersectional plane (right hepatic vein) and the left intersectional plane (left hepatic vein). The left hepatic vein actually begins in the plane between Sg2 and Sg3 and travels in that plane for most of its length. It becomes quite a large vein even in that location. It leaves the plane between Sg2 and Sg3 and enters the left intersectional plane about 1 cm from where it terminates by uniting with the middle hepatic vein to form a common channel that enters the IVC. It receives the umbilical vein from Sg4 in its short course in the left intersectional plane (Figs 2.13 and **2.14**). Note that this is the same plane in which the umbilical portion of the left portal vein lies. It is important not to confuse the 'umbilical portion of the left portal vein' with the 'umbilical vein'. The latter is a tributary of

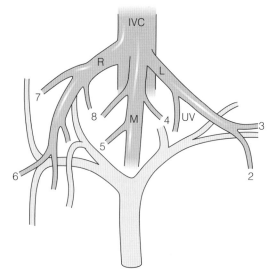

Figure 2.13 • Hepatic veins. There are normally three hepatic veins: right (R), middle (M) and left (L). Note the segments drained. UV is the umbilical vein, which normally drains part of Sg4 into the left hepatic vein. The latter is proof that the terminal portion of the left vein lies in the intersectional plane of the left liver. © Washington University in St Louis.

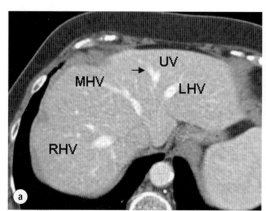

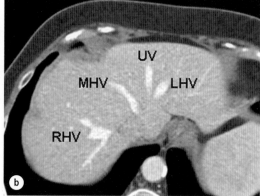

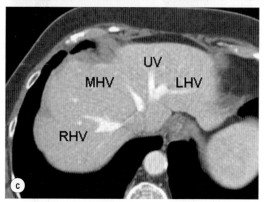

Figure 2.14 • Prevailing pattern of the umbilical vein (UV). **(a)** Umbilical vein forming from tributaries draining both the left lateral section and the left medial section. **(b)** Umbilical vein coursing in the plane of the umbilical fissure dividing the left lateral and left medial sections. **(c)** Umbilical vein uniting with the left hepatic vein (LHV), which then runs a short 1-cm course in the plane of the umbilical fissure before joining the IVC. The umbilical vein is normally smaller than in this example. MHV, middle hepatic vein; RHV, right hepatic vein. © Washington University in St Louis.

the left hepatic vein that normally drains the most leftward part of Sg4.[8,9] The left and middle hepatic veins usually fuse at a distance of about 1–2 cm from the IVC, so that when viewed from within the IVC there are only two hepatic vein openings. Rarely, hepatic veins join the IVC above the diaphragm.

In about 10% of individuals there is more than one large right hepatic vein. In these people, in addition to the right superior hepatic vein (normally called the right hepatic vein), which enters the IVC just below the level of the diaphragm, there is a right inferior hepatic vein that enters the IVC 5–6 cm below this level. In the presence of this vein, resections of Sg7 and Sg8 may be performed, including resection of the right superior vein, without compromising the venous drainage of Sg5 and Sg6.

The caudate lobe is drained by its own veins – several short veins that enter the IVC directly from the caudate lobe. When performing a classical right hepatectomy, caudate veins are divided in the preliminary stage of the dissection. As dissection moves up the anterior surface of the vena cava to isolate the right hepatic vein, one encounters a bridge of tissue lateral to the IVC referred to as the 'inferior vena caval ligament'.[10] It connects the posterior portion of the right liver to the caudate lobe behind the IVC. This bridge of tissue usually consists of fibrous tissue, but occasionally is a bridge of liver parenchyma. It limits exposure of the right side of the IVC at a point just below the right hepatic vein and must be divided in order to isolate the right vein extrahepatically. This must be done with care as the ligament may contain a large vein and forceful dissection of the ligament may also result in injury to the right lateral side of the IVC. Isolation of the right hepatic vein is also aided by clearing the areolar tissue between the right and middle hepatic veins down to the level of the IVC when exposing these veins from above.

Another approach to right hepatectomy is to leave division of the caudate and right hepatic veins until after the liver is transected. In this case a clamp may be passed up along the anterior surface of the vena from below to emerge between the right and middle hepatic veins. Once an umbilical tape is passed, the liver may be hung to facilitate transection ('hanging manoeuvre').[11] This is possible since caudate veins usually lie lateral to the midplane of the vena cava, as noted above.

The left and middle veins can also be isolated prior to division of the liver. There are several ways to achieve this anatomically. One method is to divide all the caudate veins as well as the right hepatic vein. This exposes the entire anterior surface of the retrohepatic vena cava and leaves the liver attached to the vena cava only by the middle and left hepatic veins, which are then easily isolated. This is suitable when performing a right hepatectomy or extended right hepatectomy, especially when the caudate lobe is also to be resected. The advantage of having control of these veins during operations on the right liver is that total vascular occlusion is possible without occlusion of the IVC and haemodynamically the effect is not much different from occlusion of the main portal pedicle alone (Pringle manoeuvre).

In performing a left hepatectomy the right hepatic vein is conserved and a different anatomical approach to isolation of the left and middle hepatic veins is required. They may be isolated from the left side by dividing the ligamentum venosum, where it attaches to the left hepatic vein, then dividing the peritoneum at the superior tip of the caudate lobe and gently passing an instrument on the anterior surface of the vena cava to emerge between the middle and right veins and/or between the left and middle veins. Again, care needs to be applied when performing this manoeuvre in order to avoid injury to the structures.

Isolation of the vena cava above and below the hepatic veins is also a technique that should be in the armamentarium of every surgeon performing major hepatic resection. It is not usually necessary when performing standard liver resections but surgeons should be familiar with the anatomical technique of doing so. Isolation of the vena cava superior to the hepatic veins is done by dividing the left triangular ligament and the lesser omentum, being careful to first look for a replaced left hepatic artery. Next the peritoneum on the superior border of the caudate lobe is divided and a finger is passed behind the vena cava to come out just inferior to the crus of the diaphragm. The crus of the diaphragm makes an easily identified column on the right side. This column passes across the right side of the vena cava and dissection of the space inferior to this column and behind the vena cava facilitates passage of the finger from the left side to the right side in the space behind the vena cava. Isolation of the vena cava below the liver is more straightforward but one should be aware of the position of the adrenal vein and in some cases it is necessary to isolate the adrenal vein if bleeding is persisting after occlusion of the vena cava above and below the liver.

Finally, the surgeon should be aware that during transection of the liver large veins will be encountered in certain planes of transection. For instance, in its passage along the midplane the middle hepatic vein usually receives two large tributaries, one from Sg5 inferiorly and the other from Sg8 superiorly (Fig. 2.12). Both are routinely encountered in performing right hepatectomy. The venous drainage of the right side of the liver is highly variable and additional large veins, including one from Sg6, may also enter the middle hepatic vein.

The plate/sheath system of the liver

The system of fibrous plates and sheaths that lies on the ventral surface of the liver and extends into it is of great importance in liver surgery. The plate/sheath system can be understood by first imagining a shirt with the front cut away to leave only the back and the sleeves (**Fig. 2.15**, inset).[12] If the shirt were made of fibrous tissue the back of the shirt would be a plate and the sleeves would be sheaths. The true plate/sheath system is more complex, as there are four plates (hilar, cystic, umbilical and arantian) and several sheaths[3] (Fig. 2.15). The hilar plate is the most important plate in liver surgery. It is a mostly flat structure, which lies principally in the coronal plane, posterior to the main bilovascular structures in the porta hepatis. However, its upper border is curved, so that it has the shape of a toboggan when viewed in the sagittal plane. This upper curved edge lies superior to the right and left bile ducts, the most superior structures in the porta hepatis. It is this taut, firm, upper curved edge of the hilar plate that is dissected free from the underside of the liver when 'lowering the hilar plate'.

The sheath of the right portal pedicle extends off the hilar plate like a sleeve into the liver surrounding the portal structures, i.e. portal vein, hepatic artery and bile duct. The combined structure is referred to as a 'portal pedicle'. As the right portal pedicle enters the liver it divides into a right anterior and right posterior portal pedicle supplying the respective sections, and then segmental pedicles supplying the four segments. On the left side, only the segmental structures are sheathed. There is no sheathed main portal pedicle because the main portal vein, proper hepatic artery and common hepatic duct are not close enough to the liver to be enclosed in a sheath.

The cystic plate is the ovoid fibrous sheet on which the gallbladder lies (Fig. 2.15). When performing a cholecystectomy this plate is normally left behind. In its posterior extent the cystic plate narrows to become a stout cord that attaches to the anterior surface of the sheath of the right portal pedicle. The latter is a point of anatomical importance for the surgeon wishing to expose the anterior surface of the right portal pedicle, since this cord must be divided to do so, as we have described.[13] With severe chronic inflammation the cystic plate may become shortened and thickened so that the distance between the top of the cystic plate and the right portal

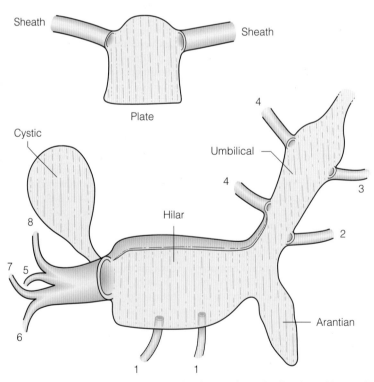

Figure 2.15 • Plate/sheath system of the liver with inset showing a schematic of a plate with two sheaths (see text). Reproduced from Strasberg SM, Linehan DC, Hawkins WG. Isolation of right main and right sectional portal pedicles for liver resection without hepatotomy or inflow occlusion. J Am Coll Surg 2008; 206:390–6. With permission of the Journal of the American College of Surgeons.

pedicle is likewise much shorter than usual. This places the structures in the right pedicle in danger during cholecystectomy when dissection is performed 'top down' as a primary strategy. The other plates are the umbilical and arantian, which underlie the umbilical portion of the left portal vein and the ligamentum venosum, respectively (Fig. 2.15). The other sheaths carry segmental bilovascular pedicles of the left liver and caudate lobe.

In performing a right hepatectomy there are two methods of managing the right-sided portal vessels and bile ducts. The first is to isolate the hepatic artery, portal vein and bile duct individually and either control them or ligate them extrahepatically, and the second is to isolate the entire portal pedicle and staple the pedicle. Isolation of the right portal pedicle can be performed by making hepatotomies above the right portal pedicle in Sg4 and in the gallbladder fossa after removing the gallbladder. A finger is passed through the hepatotomy to isolate the right portal pedicle. This technique usually requires inflow occlusion. It can also be done without inflow occlusion by lowering the hilar plate and coming around the right portal pedicle directly on its surface, as we have described (**Fig. 2.16**).[12] It is advisable to divide caudate veins in the area below the vena caval ligament before performing pedicle isolation, since haemorrhage from these veins can be considerable if they are injured during isolation of the right portal pedicle. The advantage of pedicle isolation over isolation of individual vessels and the bile duct is that sectional resections require isolation of

pedicles (Fig. 2.16).[12] Furthermore, pedicle isolation is much easier to do laparoscopically than individual structure isolation.

Liver capsule and attachments

The liver is encased in a thin fibrous capsule that covers the entire organ except for a large bare area posteriorly where the organ is in contact with the IVC and with the diaphragm to the right of the IVC. The bare area stretches superiorly to include the termination of the three hepatic veins and ends in a point, which is also where the attachment of the falciform ligament ends. The limit of the bare area, where the peritoneum passes between the body wall and the liver, is called the coronary ligament. It is one of three structures that connect the liver to the abdominal wall 'dorsally', the other two being the right and left triangular ligaments. The liver also has another bare area, best thought of as a bare crease, where the hepatoduodenal ligament and the lesser omentum attach on the 'ventral' surface. It is through this crease that the portal structures enter the liver at the hilum (hilum = 'a crease on a seed'). The other ligamentous structures of interest to surgeons are the ligamentum teres, falciform ligament and the ligamentum venosum. The ligamentum teres (teres = 'round') is the obliterated left umbilical vein and runs in the free edge of the falciform ligament from the umbilicus to the termination of the umbilical portion of the left portal vein. The falciform (falciform = 'scythe shaped') is the filmy fold that runs between the anterior abdominal wall

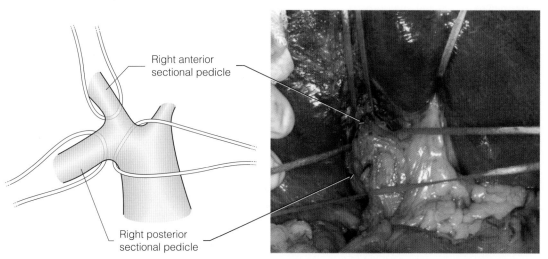

Right anterior sectional pedicle

Right posterior sectional pedicle

Figure 2.16 • Isolation of right portal pedicle and sectional pedicles by technique of dissection on surface of pedicles. No inflow occlusion or separate hepatotomies are used (see Ref. 12). The umbilical tape in the upper right of the photograph is around the bridge of liver tissue over the umbilical fissure. Reproduced from Strasberg SM, Linehan DC, Hawkins WG. Isolation of right main and right sectional portal pedicles for liver resection without hepatotomy or inflow occlusion. J Am Coll Surg 2008; 206:390–6. With permission of the Journal of the American College of Surgeons.

above the umbilicus and attaches to the anterior surface of the liver between the left medial and left lateral sections.

Surface anatomy

Numerous terms for surface anatomy exist. They are of minimal surgical importance. Since the term 'lobe' has been used in different ways by various anatomists and surgeons it is best avoided except in reference to the caudate lobe. Fissure and scissure or scissura are similarly confusing terms since they apply only to clefts in casts of the liver. The ligaments of the liver are of surgical importance and are described under capsule and attachments.

Pathological conditions may distort or alter the position of normal hepatic structures. Tumours may push vessels so that they are stretched and curved over the surface of the tumour, narrowing or occluding them by direct pressure. Tumours may partially or completely occlude vessels by mural invasion, by inducing bland thrombi or by entering the lumen and producing tumour thrombi. They may cause bile ducts to dilate to a size many times normal. Atrophy of liver volume will be induced by processes that occlude either the portal vein or bile duct. Since the liver will undergo hyperplasia to maintain a constant volume of liver cells, atrophy of one part of the liver is usually accompanied by growth of another. If the right portal vein is occluded by a tumour, the right liver will atrophy and the left liver will grow. When seen from below, this process will exert a counter-clockwise rotational effect on the porta hepatis, rotating the bile duct posteriorly, the hepatic artery to the right, and the portal vein to the left and anteriorly.

Gallbladder and extrahepatic bile ducts

Gallbladder

The gallbladder lies on the cystic plate. The edge of the gallbladder forms one side of the hepatocystic triangle. The other two sides are the right side of the common hepatic duct and the liver. Eponyms covering this anatomy (Calot, Moosman, etc.) are confusing and should be abandoned. The hepatocystic triangle contains the cystic artery and cystic node and a portion of the right hepatic artery, as well as fat and fibrous tissue. Clearance of this triangle along with isolation of the cystic duct and elevation of the base of the gallbladder off the lower portion of the cystic plate gives the 'critical view of safety' that we have described for identification of the cystic structures during laparoscopic cholecystectomy.[14]

A large number of curiosities of the gallbladder, e.g. the phrygian cap, have been described. The following are anomalies of importance to the biliary surgeon.

Agenesis of the gallbladder

Agenesis occurs in about 1 in 8000 patients. It can be difficult to recognise. An ultrasonographer may describe a 'shrunken' gallbladder. When agenesis is suspected it may be confirmed by axial imaging. If doubt remains, laparoscopy is definitive.

Double gallbladder

This is also a very rare anomaly but can be the cause of persistent symptoms after resection of one gallbladder. A gallbladder may also be bifid, which usually does not cause symptoms, or have an hourglass constriction, which may cause symptoms due to obstruction of the upper segment.

Cystic duct

This structure is normally 1–2 cm in length and 2–3 mm in diameter. It joins the common hepatic duct at an acute angle to form the common bile duct. The cystic duct normally joins the common hepatic duct approximately 4 cm above the duodenum. However, the cystic duct may enter at any level up to the right hepatic duct and down to the ampulla. The cystic duct may also join the right hepatic duct either when the right duct is in its normal position or in an aberrant location.

There are three patterns of confluence of the cystic duct and common hepatic duct (**Fig. 2.17**). In the

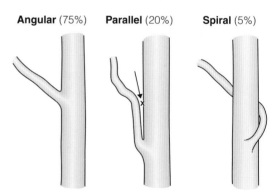

Figure 2.17 • The three types of cystic duct/common hepatic duct confluence. The parallel union confluence is shown in the middle. Dissection of this type of cystic duct (arrow) may lead to injury to the side of the common hepatic duct. During laparoscopic cholecystectomy this is often a cautery injury. Adapted from Warrren KW, McDonald WM, Kune GA. Bile duct strictures: New concepts in the management of an old problem. In: Irvine WT (ed.) Modern trends in surgery. London: Butterworth, 1966. With permission from Elsevier.

20% of patients in whom there is a parallel union, the surgeon approaching the common hepatic duct by dissecting the cystic duct is prone to injure the side of the former structure (Fig. 2.17). Also, when making a choledochotomy at this level the incision should be started slightly to the left side of the mid-plane of the bile duct in order to avoid entering a septum between the two fused cystic/common hepatic ducts. When performing cholecystectomy the cystic duct should be occluded in such a way that there is a visible section of cystic duct below the clip closest to the common bile duct.

Although a gallbladder with two cystic ducts has been described, the author has not seen convincing proof that this anomaly actually exists. If it does, it must be an anomaly of extreme rarity. When two 'cystic ducts' are identified, it is likely that the cystic duct is congenitally short or has been effaced by a stone and that the two structures thought to be dual cystic ducts are, in fact, the common bile duct and the common hepatic duct.

Cystic artery

The cystic artery is about 1 mm in diameter and normally arises from the right hepatic artery in the hepatocystic triangle. The cystic artery may arise from a right hepatic artery that runs anterior to the common hepatic duct. The cystic artery may also arise from the right hepatic artery on the left side of the common hepatic duct and run anterior to this duct, while the right hepatic artery runs behind it. Such cystic arteries tend to tether the gallbladder and make dissection of the hepatocystic triangle more difficult. The cystic artery may arise from an aberrant right hepatic artery coming off the superior mesenteric artery (SMA). In this case the cystic artery and not the cystic duct tends to be in the free edge of the fold leading from the hepatoduodenal ligament to the gallbladder. This should be suspected whenever the 'cystic duct' looks smaller than the 'cystic artery'.

Normally the cystic artery runs for 1–2 cm to meet the gallbladder superior to the insertion of the cystic duct. The artery ramifies into an anterior and posterior branch at the point of contact with the gallbladder and these branches continue to divide on their respective surfaces. Sometimes the cystic artery divides into branches before the gallbladder edge is reached. In that case the anterior branch may be mistaken to be the cystic artery proper and the posterior branch will not be discovered until later in the dissection, when it may be divided inadvertently. The artery may ramify into several branches before arriving at the gallbladder, giving the impression that there is no cystic artery. The anterior and posterior branches may arise independently from the right hepatic artery, giving rise to two distinct cystic arteries.

Multiple small cystic veins drain into intrahepatic portal vein branches by passing into the liver around or through the cystic plate. Sometimes there are cystic veins in the hepatocystic triangle that run parallel to the cystic artery to enter the main portal vein.

The **cystic plate** has been described above. Small bile ducts may penetrate the cystic plate to enter the gallbladder. These 'ducts of Luschka' are very small, usually submillimetre accessory ducts. However, when divided during a cholecystectomy postoperative bilomas may occur. Bilomas and haemorrhage may also be caused by penetration of the cystic plate during dissection. In about 10% of patients there is a large peripheral bile duct immediately deep to the plate, disruption of which will cause copious bile drainage. The origin of the middle hepatic vein is also in this location, and if it is injured massive haemorrhage may ensue. There is areolar tissue between the muscularis of the gallbladder and the cystic plate. At the top of the gallbladder the layer is very thin. As one progresses downwards the areolar layer thickens. If dissection from the top of the gallbladder downward is carried out leaving the areolar tissue on the cystic plate one will arrive to the posterior surface of the cystic artery and cystic duct. Conversely, if it is carried out downward on the cystic plate leaving the areolar tissue on the gallbladder one will arrive at the surface of the right portal pedicle. If this is not anticipated, structures in the right portal pedicle may be injured. Therefore, the proper plane of dissection is between the gallbladder and the areolar tissue.

Extrahepatic bile ducts

The common hepatic duct (CHD) is a structure formed by the union of the right and left hepatic ducts. The union normally occurs at the right extremity of the base of Sg4 anterior and superior to the bifurcation of the portal vein. The CHD travels in the right edge of the hepatoduodenal ligament for 2–3 cm, where it joins with the cystic duct to form the common bile duct (CBD). The latter has a supraduodenal course of 3–4 cm and then passes behind the duodenum to run in or occasionally behind the pancreas to enter the second portion of the duodenum. Details of its lower section and relation to the pancreatic duct are described in the final section of this chapter. The external diameter of the common bile duct varies from 5 to 13 mm when distended to physiological pressures. However, the duct diameter at surgery, i.e. in fasting patients with low duct pressures, may be as small as 3 mm. Radiologically, the internal duct diameter is measured on fasting patients. Under these conditions the upper limit is normally about 8 mm. Size should never be used as a sole criterion for identifying a bile duct. Caution is required in situations in which a structure seems larger than expected. Although the cystic duct may be enlarged due to passage of stones, the surgeon should take extra precautions before dividing a 'cystic duct' that is greater than 2 mm in diameter because the common bile duct can be 3 mm in diameter and aberrant ducts may be smaller.

Anomalies of extrahepatic bile ducts

As already noted, there are biliary anomalies of the right and left ductal systems that can affect the outcome of hepatic surgery. The same is true for biliary surgery. The most important clinical anomaly is low insertion of right hepatic ducts referred to above. Because of its low location, it may be mistaken to be the cystic duct and be injured. This is even more likely to occur when the cystic duct unites with an aberrant duct as opposed to joining the common hepatic duct. Left hepatic ducts can also join the common hepatic duct at a low level. They are less prone to be injured since the dissection during cholecystectomy is on the right side of the biliary tree.

Extrahepatic arteries

The course of these arteries has been described above. Anomalies of the hepatic artery may be important in gallbladder surgery. Normally the right hepatic artery passes posterior to the bile duct (80%) and gives off the cystic artery in the hepatocystic triangle. However, in 20% of cases the right hepatic artery runs anterior to the bile duct. The right hepatic artery may lie very close to the gallbladder and chronic inflammation can draw the right hepatic artery directly on to the gallbladder, where it lies in an inverse U-loop and is prone to injury. In the 'classical injury' in laparoscopic cholecystectomy, in which the common bile duct is mistaken for the cystic duct, an associated right hepatic artery injury is very common.

Blood supply of bile ducts

Many studies, dating back to the 19th century, have examined the blood supply of the extrahepatic bile ducts in cadaveric specimens. A key observation made by Rappaport is that the bile ducts are supplied by the hepatic artery only,[15] unlike the liver, which has a dual blood supply from the artery and the portal vein. The arterial blood supply can be thought of as having three anatomical elements. The first consists of afferent vessels from the hepatic artery and its branches (**Fig. 2.18a**). The second element is longitudinal arteries that run parallel to the long axis of the bile ducts and that receive blood from the afferent vessels (**Fig. 2.18b**). The third element, an arterial plexus encasing the bile ducts, receives blood from the marginal arteries (**Fig. 2.18c**). Tiny branches of the plexus pierce the bile duct wall to supply the capillaries of the bile duct.

The afferent vessels are branches of the hepatic arteries and less commonly of the superior mesenteric artery or other upper abdominal arteries. The most constant and important artery supplying the bile duct is the posterior superior pancreatico-duodenal artery, usually the first branch of the gastroduodenal artery. Arterial twigs pass to the duct as the artery winds around the lower end of the duct. These branches supply much of the retroduodenal and intrapancreatic bile duct, but also ascend the bile duct to supply the supraduodenal bile duct. The lowest portion of the duct near the ampulla is also supplied by the anterior superior pancreatic artery from the inferior pancreatico-duodenal artery. Other vessels that commonly send afferents to the supraduodenal duct are the proper hepatic artery, cystic artery and artery to Sg4. Furthermore, body wall collaterals such as phrenic arteries can at times supply the bile ducts (as well as the liver) since bile duct infarction is much more common when there is occlusion of the common hepatic artery after a transplant than it is in an in situ liver. The notion that the extrahepatic bile duct is supplied by arteries that join it only at the bottom and top of its course is incorrect. Supplying arteries from the cystic artery, right and left hepatic arteries and proper hepatic artery may join it in its mid course.

The afferent vessels usually empty into longitudinal or 'marginal' arteries that run parallel to the long axis of the bile ducts (also called 'marginal anastomotic loop').[16] These vessels are disposed at 3 and 9 or, less commonly, at 12 o'clock on the common bile duct/common hepatic duct, or run across the top of the confluence and the right and left bile ducts. This 'hilar marginal artery' has been called the 'caudate arcade' or 'communicating arcade'. This artery is of great importance in maintaining blood supply to the liver when one hepatic artery (right or left) is occluded.[17]

The third element of this system is the 'epicholedochal plexus', a fine arterial plexus that lies on and surrounds the entire common bile duct and the left and right bile ducts. The latter is the hilar component of the epicholedochal plexus. The vessels of the plexus tend to run along the long axis of the ducts so that on the common duct many of the vessels are vertical while those around the confluence and the right and left ducts are disposed horizontally. In the portion of the biliary tree that lies adjacent to the hilar plate or which has entered the fibrous sheaths, the epicholedochal plexus lies between the sheath and the wall of the bile duct. Dissection in this plane has the potential to devascularise bile ducts.[18]

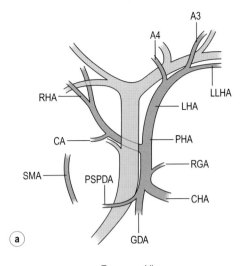

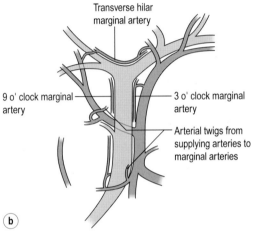

(a)

Figure 2.18 • (a) The supplying arteries. All arteries shown can all give twigs to the marginal arteries or in some cases directly supply the epicholedochal plexus. A2, A3, A4, arteries to segments 2, 3 and 4; CA, cystic artery; CHA, common hepatic artery; GDA, gastroduodenal artery; LHA, left hepatic artery; LLSA, left lateral sectional artery; PHA, proper hepatic artery; PSPDA, posterior superior pancreaticoduodenal artery, the most important and constant artery; RHA, right hepatic artery. Replaced arteries arising from the superior mesenteric artery may also supply the bile ducts. **(b)** Marginal arteries. Marginal arteries are disposed at 3 and 9 o'clock (and occasionally at 12 o'clock) on the common bile duct/common hepatic duct. The hilar marginal artery runs across the top of the confluence of the right and left hepatic ducts. **(c)** Epicholedochal plexus. The epicholedochal plexus is supplied by the marginal arteries. Adapted from Strasberg SM, Helton WS An analytical review of vasculobiliary injury in laparoscopic and open cholecystectomy. HPB 2011; 13(1):1–14. With permission from John Wiley & Sons.

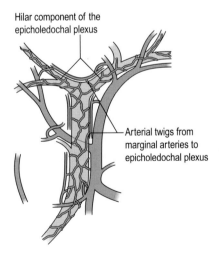

(b)

(c)

Transection of the bile duct may result in ischaemia of the duct. For instance, if the duct is transected at the level of the duodenum, ischaemia of a portion of the bile duct above this level may occur since blood flow originating from the superior pancreato-duodenal artery and passing up along the marginal artery is cut off. Similarly, in a high transection at the level of the confluence, the lower cut end of the duct may become ischaemic. This problem is thought to be an important contributory cause to the frequent failure of choledocho-choledochotomy as a form of biliary reconstruction. To avoid this problem hepatico-jejunostomy is used and the bile duct is trimmed back to within 1 cm of the confluence.

Pancreas

The pancreas is a retroperitoneal organ lying obliquely across the upper abdomen so that the tail is superior to the head. It is formed by the fusion of ventral and dorsal buds in utero, the ventral pancreas rotating to come behind and fuse with the dorsal pancreas. On average it is 22 cm in length. The head of the pancreas is discoid in shape and terminates inferiorly and medially in the hook-like uncinate process. The neck, body and tail are shaped like a flattened cylinder, sometimes somewhat triangular in cross-section with a flat anterior and pointed posterior surface. These divisions of the organ are somewhat arbitrary; the neck of the pancreas sits anterior to the superior mesenteric and portal veins. Normally the consistency of the gland is soft.

Pancreatic ducts

The prevailing anatomical pattern of the pancreatic duct is the result of union of the ventral duct (Wirsung) with the dorsal duct (Santorini), along with partial regression of the dorsal duct in the head. The 'genu' of the duct (genu = knee) is the bend in the duct concave inferiorly where the ventral duct joins the dorsal. In the prevailing pattern both ducts communicate with the duodenum, the dorsal duct entering at the minor papilla about 2 cm above and 5 mm anterior to the major papilla. Other ductal patterns are possible that involve various degrees of dominance or regression of the portions of the ducts in the head of the pancreas. For instance, the ducts may not unite, resulting in separate drainage from the ventral and dorsal pancreas (pancreas divisum), the dorsal duct may lose its connection to the duodenum, or the dorsal duct in the head may lose its connection to the rest of the ductal system and drain only a small section of the head into the duodenum. Alternatively, the ventral duct may regress and the dorsal duct drain more or all of the pancreas through the minor ampulla. The uncinate process is served by its own duct, which joins the main pancreatic duct 1–2 cm from its entry into the duodenum.

The pancreatic duct (and pancreas) are often referred to as proximal (head) and distal (tail). These are confusing terms – as are the terms proximal and distal bile duct. Adding to the confusion is that the 'distal' bile duct is near the ampulla, but that site is 'proximal' regarding the pancreatic duct. Instead, that part of the bile duct should be referred to as the pancreatic portion or lower bile duct, while that near the confluence should be called the upper extrahepatic or hilar bile duct. In the case of the pancreas, the duct should be referred to as the 'pancreatic head duct', 'pancreatic body duct', etc.

The ventral duct usually joins the common bile duct to form a common channel several millimetres from the ampulla of Vater, usually within the wall of the duodenum. The bile duct traverses the duodenal wall obliquely and the pancreatic duct at a right angle. Each duct and the common channel have their own sphincters. The sphincters can be palpated from within the duodenum and form part of the raised 'major papilla' at whose apex the opening of the common channel can be seen. The common channel may be longer or absent, with both ducts entering the duodenum separately, the pancreatic duct more inferiorly. In performing a sphincteroplasty, it is advisable to open the common opening superiorly (10–12 o'clock position in the mobilised duodenum) to avoid the orifice of the pancreatic duct (4 o'clock). The ampulla is normally at the midpoint of the second part of the duodenum. It is rarely higher but can be as low as the midpoint of the third part of the duodenum. When the dorsal duct has its own communication with the duodenum, it is found at the 'minor papilla', about 2 cm proximal and 1 cm anterior to the major papilla.

Blood supply of the pancreas

The arterial supply of the pancreas consists of two vascular systems, one supplying the head and uncinate, and the other the body and tail. The neck is a watershed between these two areas of supply.[4] The head and uncinate process are supplied by the pancreatico-duodenal arcade, which consists of two to several loops of vessels that arise from the superior pancreatico-duodenal (branch of gastroduodenal) and inferior pancreatico-duodenal (branch of the SMA). The arcades run on the anterior and posterior surface of the pancreas next to the duodenum, the anterior arcade lying somewhat closer to the duodenum. The second system arises from the splenic artery, which gives rise to three arteries into the dorsal surface of the gland (**Fig. 2.19**). The dorsal pancreatic artery is

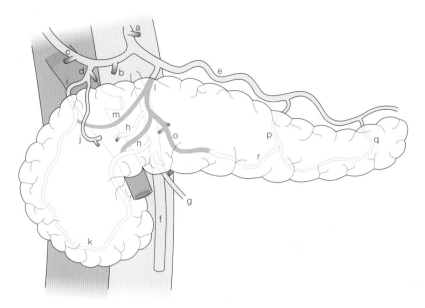

Figure 2.19 • Arterial blood supply to the pancreas. The dorsal pancreatic artery is shown shaded. Alternative origins of the artery are shown as black stumps. Key: a, coeliac artery; b, common hepatic artery; c, right hepatic artery; d, gastroduodenal artery; e, splenic artery; f, superior mesenteric artery; g, middle colic artery; h, right hepatic artery (aberrant); i, superior pancreatico-duodenal artery; j, right gastroepiploic artery; k, inferior pancreatico-duodenal artery; l, dorsal pancreatic artery (DPA); m, right anastomotic branch of DPA to superior part of pancreatico-duodenal arcade; o, left anastomotic branch of DPA becomes transverse pancreatic artery; p, pancreatica magna artery; q, caudal pancreatic artery; r, transverse pancreatic artery. © Washington University in St Louis.

the most medial of the three and the most important. It anastomoses with the pancreatico-duodenal arcade in the neck of the pancreas. It is the most aberrant artery in the upper abdomen and may arise from vessels that are routinely occluded during pancreatico-duodenectomy, which may account in part for fistula formation after this procedure.

Venous drainage generally follows arterial supply. The veins of the body and tail of the pancreas drain into the splenic vein, where it lies partly embedded in the posterior surface of the gland. These veins are short and fragile. The head and uncinate process veins drain into the superior mesenteric vein (SMV) and portal vein on the right lateral side of these structures. Uncinate veins often drain into a large first jejunal tributary vein, which then empties into the SMV. This vein usually passes behind the SMA. A nearly constant posterior superior pancreatico-duodenal vein enters the right lateral side of the portal vein at the level of the duodenum.

Lymphatics of the pancreas

For surgical purposes the lymphatic drainage of the pancreas is best considered in relation to the two main surgical procedures, resection of the pancreatic head and resection on the pancreatic body and tail. The aim of lymphatic resection during these procedures is to resect the primary lymph nodes, i.e. those nodes that receive lymph directly from pancreatic tissue (N1 nodes) as opposed to nodes that receive drainage from N1 nodes (N2 nodes). There is a ring of nodes around the pancreas that drain the adjacent sections of the gland (N1 nodes).[19] These in turn drain into nodes along the SMA, coeliac artery and aorta (axial nodes). The axial nodes, which are N2 for most areas of the pancreas, are also N1 for portions of the pancreatic head, body and uncinate process that lie close to the aorta. The lymphatics of the body and tail are shown in **Fig. 2.20**. The lymphatics of the head and uncinate process drain into a nodal ring for this part of the gland, consisting of lymph nodes in the pancreatico-duodenal groove anteriorly and posteriorly, into subpyloric nodes inferiorly, into nodes adjacent to the common bile duct and hepatic artery superiorly, and into nodes along the SMA medially. These are N1, but as noted above so are some of the axial nodes. The standard node dissection for a Whipple procedure removes all of these nodal groups. This removes the N1 nodes unless there is direct lymphatic drainage to the left side of the SMA or to nodes around the coeliac artery, which does occur in a small proportion of patients.

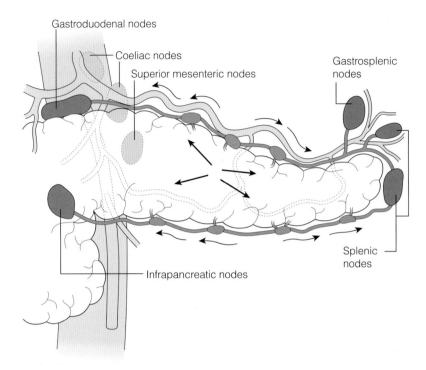

Figure 2.20 • Lymphatic drainage of the body and tail of the pancreas. The intraparenchymal lymphatics from the four quadrants empty into lymphatic vessels on the superior and inferior borders of the pancreas (arrows). Small nodes are found along these vessels. The lymph flows to the nodes of the 'ring'. These are N1 nodes, although some of the lymph may have passed through the smaller nodes as described. The nodes of the ring empty into nodes along the SMA, coeliac artery and aorta. The latter are therefore N2 nodes, but they are also N1 nodes for the more central part of the pancreas. © Washington University in St Louis.

Anatomical relations and ligaments of the pancreas

The pancreas is a deeply seated organ that, unlike the liver and most of the biliary tree, is not obvious when opening the abdomen. The anatomical relations of the pancreas are very important in pancreatic surgery. The structures emphasised in the following section are those that are commonly invaded by tumours.

The pancreas lies in the anterior pararenal space anterior to the anterior renal fascia and behind the peritoneum. Posteriorly, the pancreas is related from right to left to the right kidney and perinephric fat, IVC and right gonadal vein, aorta, left renal vein (slightly inferior), **retropancreatic fat**, the **left adrenal gland** and the superior pole of the left kidney. All of the former structures lie in the perirenal space and behind the anterior renal fascia. In the case of oncological resections the plane of dissection should be behind the anterior renal fascia in order to maximise the chance of obtaining negative margins as described for the radical antegrade modular pancreato-splenectomy (RAMPS) procedure.[20]

The **SMV** and **portal vein** are posterior relations of the neck of the pancreas, and **splenic vein** of the body and tail. The **SMA** is a posterior relation of the junction of the neck and body of the gland lying posterior and to the right of the SMV. The SMA and SMV are both related to the uncinate process and give branches into (SMA) and receive tributaries from (SMV) the uncinate process. Often the uncinate veins enter a large tributary of the SMV, the first jejunal vein, which also abuts the uncinate process. These short arteries and veins are of importance surgically as they are divided when the head of the pancreas is resected. The **coeliac artery** rises vertically superior to the SMA close to the superior edge of the pancreas, where it gives off the common hepatic artery and the **splenic artery**. The former runs anteriorly and to the left in approximation to the superior border of the pancreas. At the point where the artery passes in front of the portal vein, it divides into the **gastroduodenal artery**, which passes anterior to the neck of the pancreas, sometimes buried within it. It terminates in the right gastroepiploic artery that rises in a fold of tissue toward the pylorus, a fold that also contains the right gastroepiploic vein and subpyloric nodes. The splenic artery snakes along the superior border of the pancreas to leave it 2–3 cm from the termination of the pancreas. The head of the pancreas is wrapped in the first three parts of the duodenum and the tail ends in relation to the splenic hilum. There is variability in the proximity of the tail of the pancreas to the spleen. In some cases the pancreas terminates 2 cm from the splenic substance and in others it abuts it. The anterior surface of the body and tail of the pancreas is covered by peritoneum, which is the posterior wall of the lesser sac, and then by the posterior wall of the stomach anterior to this. The transverse mesocolon is related to the inferior border of the pancreas, and the right and left extremities of the transverse colon are related to the head and tail of the gland. The inferior mesenteric vein is related to the inferior border of the neck of the pancreas and may pass behind it to enter the splenic vein or turn medially to enter the SMV.

The pancreas is normally accessed surgically by entering the lesser sac either by division of the greater omentum below the gastroepiploic arcade or by releasing the greater omentum from its attachment to the transverse colon. When the lesser sac is entered the anterior surface of the neck, body and tail are often visible, but may be obscured by congenital filmy adhesions to the posterior wall of the stomach. To expose the head of the pancreas it is necessary to mobilise the right side of the transverse

colon and hepatic flexure inferiorly and to divide the right gastroepiploic vein. The latter crosses the inferior border of the pancreas to join with the middle colic vein to form the gastrocolic trunk, which then enters the SMV. For complete exposure, e.g. for a Frey procedure, the right gastroepiploic artery is also divided and it and the subpyloric nodes are swept upwards off the pancreas. To access the SMV at the inferior border of the pancreas the peritoneum at the inferior border of the neck is divided and the dissection is carried inferiorly and laterally to open a groove between the uncinate process and the mesentery. Division of the right gastroepiploic vein at the inferior border of the pancreas greatly facilitates this manoeuvre. Normally no veins enter the SMV or portal vein from the posterior surface of the neck of the pancreas. Consequently the neck of the pancreas can be separated from the anterior surface of the SMV/portal vein in this avascular plane. The peritoneum at the inferior border of the neck, body and tail of the pancreas is avascular, and there are few vascular connections between the back of the body and tail of the pancreas and retroperitoneal tissues. As a result the pancreas may be readily dissected free from retroperitoneum. The splenic vein is partly embedded in the back of the pancreas from the point that it reaches the gland on the left to about 1 cm from its termination at its confluence with the SMV.

Key points

- A prevailing pattern of hepatic, biliary and pancreatic anatomy exists but variations (anomalies) are frequent.
- All HBP operations should be conducted with the strong suspicion that an anatomical anomaly may be present.

References

1. Terminology Committee of the IHPBA. The Brisbane 2000 Terminology of Liver Anatomy and Resections. HPB 2000;2:333–9.

2. Healey JEJ, Schroy PC. Anatomy of the biliary ducts within the human liver; analysis of the prevailing pattern of branchings and the major variations of the biliary ducts. Arch Surg 1953;66:599–616.

3. Couinaud C. Le Foie. Etudes anatomiques et chirugicales. Paris: Masson & Cie; 1957.

4. Michels NA. Blood supply and anatomy of the upper abdominal organs. Philadelphia: JB Lippincott; 1955.

5. Moosman DA. The surgical significance of six anomalies of the biliary duct system. Surg Obst Gynec 1970;131:655–60.

6. Hjortsjo C-H. The topography of the intrahepatic duct systems. Acta Anat (Basel) 1951;11: 599–615.

7. Botero AC, Strasberg SM. Division of the left hemiliver in man – segments, sectors, or sections. Liver Transpl Surg 1998;4:226–31.

8. Masselot R, Leborgne J. Anatomical study of hepatic veins. Anat Clin 1978;1:109–25.

9. Kawasaki S, Makuuchi M, Miyagawa S, et al. Extended lateral segmentectomy using intraoperative ultrasound to obtain a partial liver graft. Am J Surg 1996;171:286–8.

10. Makuuchi M, Yamamoto J, Takayama T, et al. Extrahepatic division of the right hepatic vein in hepatectomy. Hepatogastroenterology 1991;38:176–9.

11. Belghiti J, Guevara OA, Noun R, et al. Liver hanging maneuver: a safe approach to right hepatectomy

without liver mobilization. J Am Coll Surg 2001;193:109–11.

12. Strasberg SM, Linehan DC, Hawkins WG. Isolation of right main and right sectional portal pedicles for liver resection without hepatotomy or inflow occlusion. J Am Coll Surg 2008;206: 390–6.

13. Strasberg SM, Picus DD, Drebin JA. Results of a new strategy for reconstruction of biliary injuries having an isolated right-sided component. J Gastrointest Surg 2001;5:266–74.

14. Strasberg SM, Brunt LM. Rationale and use of the critical view of safety in laparoscopic cholecystectomy. J Am Coll Surg 2010;211:132–8.

15. Rappaport AM, Kawamura T, Knoblauch M, et al. Effects of arterial or portal ischemia on survival and metabolism of partially and totally depancreatized dogs. Z Exp Chir 1975;8:326–42.

16. Northover JMA, Terblanche J. A new look at the arterial supply of the bile duct in man and its surgical implications. Br J Surg 1979;66:379–84.

17. Gunji H, Cho A, Tohma T, et al. The blood supply of the hilar bile duct and its relationship to the communicating arcade located between the right and left hepatic arteries. Am J Surg 2006;192: 276–80.

18. Nery JR, Frasson E, Rilo HL, et al. Surgical anatomy and blood supply of the left biliary tree pertaining to partial liver grafts from living donors. Transplant Proc 1990;22:1492–6.

19. O'Morchoe CC. Lymphatic system of the pancreas. Microsc Res Tech 1997;37:456–77.

20. Mitchem JB, Hamilton N, Gao F, et al. Long-term results of resection of adenocarcinoma of the body and tail of the pancreas using radical antegrade modular pancreatosplenectomy procedure. J Am Coll Surg 2012;214:46–52.

3

Staging and assessment of hepatobiliary malignancies

Steve M.M. de Castro
Otto M. van Delden
Dirk J. Gouma
Olivier R.C. Busch

Introduction

Selection in patients with hepato-pancreato-biliary (HPB) malignancy is of the utmost importance. Patient selection should ideally identify those who might benefit from surgery and those who will not. Palliation for the majority of patients with unresectable or incurable disease utilises minimally invasive techniques (i.e. endoscopic or percutaneous biliary stenting, radiochemotherapy). Technological advances have changed the approach to evaluate patients with suspected HPB disease. Modern state-of-the-art imaging now allows physicians to focus on two key questions in patients with suspected HPB tumours. Is there really a malignant tumour present? If so, can it be removed with an R0 resection?

This chapter focuses on the diagnostic work-up of patients with the most common HPB malignancies and discusses the staging and assessment of resectability.

Colorectal liver metastases

Imaging of colorectal liver metastases (CRLMs) is important in patient assessment in several aspects. Firstly, to detect as many liver metastases as possible with their exact location within the liver, in order to maximise the chance of achieving complete clearance of disease at surgery. Secondly, to characterise any benign liver lesions that may be present, so as to avoid unnecessary surgical procedures.

Transabdominal ultrasound

Ultrasound has a diagnostic sensitivity of 36–61% for detecting lesions measuring 1–2 cm, even when performed by experienced radiologists.[1] It is very useful in guiding fine-needle aspiration (FNA) to confirm unresectability by cytopathology. However, FNA has a risk of seeding metastases in up to10% of patients and a risk of a false-negative result, which does not justify its use in candidates for potentially curative therapy.[2]

A meta-analysis of the performance of ultrasound for CRLMs found a pooled sensitivity of 63% (95% confidence interval (CI) 56–70%; five studies) with a specificity of 97.6% (95% CI 95.6–99.5%; four studies).[3]

Ultrasound can be very useful as a problem-solving tool when computed tomography (CT) or magnetic resonance imaging (MRI) is uncertain. A targeted ultrasound of a suspicious lesion can often discriminate between a benign and malignant lesion.

> ✓✓ MRI, though not as widely available as CT, is the preferred first-line modality for evaluating CRLM; it provides anatomical detail and has a high detection rate, even for lesions less than 10mm in diameter. FDG-PET is valuable in the evaluation of extrahepatic disease.

Computed tomography and magnetic resonance imaging

Nowadays, CT is the most commonly used imaging modality for staging and follow-up of these patients. Current multidetector scanners allow for multiplanar reformatting with the same resolution as the original axial images. This may improve detection and characterisation of small lesions.[3] Multiplanar reformatting also enables the demonstration of hepatic arterial, venous and portal anatomy, which can be useful in preoperative planning.[4] CT allows for accurate volumetric assessment of tumour size, liver volume to be resected and future liver remnant volume.[5]

A multiphase contrast-enhanced CT should be performed to stage liver metastases. The study should include an unenhanced, arterial, portovenous and delayed phase. CRLMs may show an enhancing rim on arterial phase imaging and are hypodense on portovenous phase imaging (**Fig. 3.1**). A slice thickness of 2–4 mm is recommended for axial viewing.

A meta-analysis on the performance of CT found a pooled sensitivity of 74.8% (95% CI 71.2–78.3%; 12 studies) and specificity of 95.6% (95% CI 93.4–97.8%; seven studies).[3]

The standard MRI protocol includes T2-weighted, unenhanced T1-weighted and dynamic contrast-enhanced T1-weighted sequences. T2-weighted images are used for the detection and characterisation of lesions (haemangioma, cyst).[6,7]

A meta-analysis on the performance of MRI found a pooled sensitivity of 81.1% (95% CI 76.0–86.1%; five studies) and specificity of 97.2% (95% CI 94.5–99.9%; two studies).[3] On per lesion analysis, MRI appeared to be the modality showing higher sensitivities across individual studies compared to CT. Pooled data showed comparable results, with MRI having a combined sensitivity of 88% and accuracy of 87% compared to CT with sensitivity of 74% and accuracy of 78%. Therefore, most centres choose the imaging technique of their preference.

Subgroup analyses of these studies showed that MRI has better sensitivity at picking up the smaller lesions <1 cm compared to CT and also positron emission tomography (PET)-CT.[8] The majority of lesions missed by CT and PET-CT were micrometastases of <1 cm. This meta-analysis concludes that MRI is preferred as a first-line modality for evaluating the liver. It has high overall sensitivity and specificity estimates and can accurately depict lesions smaller than 10 mm. Secondly, it provides excellent anatomical details.

Positron emission tomography

Fluorine-18-2-fluoro-2-deoxy-D-glucose (FDG)-PET is a well-established non-invasive functional scanning method, where a labelled glucose molecule is injected intravenously. The principle of FDG-PET is that malignant cells have a higher glucose uptake than regular cells. The scanner performs a rapid non-invasive interrogation of glycolytic activity throughout the whole body in a single imaging session. Besides being used for the detection of primary malignant tumours, it also can be used to detect regional and distant metastases, to differentiate benign from malignant disease or recurrent cancer from treatment-related scarring, and to evaluate response to therapy.

With the PET-CT combination it is possible to produce fusion images with high-resolution anatomical localisation of CT together with the functional data of FDG-PET. This combination of scanning characteristics is becoming more widely available (**Fig. 3.2**).

Kinkel et al.[9] performed a meta-analysis and concluded that, at equivalent specificity, PET-CT is more sensitive than ultrasound (US), CT and MRI for the detection of hepatic metastases from gastrointestinal cancers.

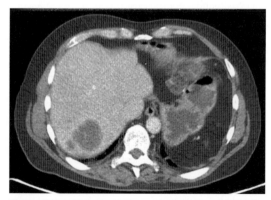

Figure 3.1 • Patient with liver metastases in segment 7 and small adjacent satellite lesion on CT.

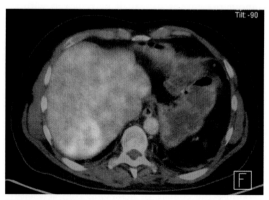

Figure 3.2 • PET-CT of same patient with CRLMs showing two distinct lesions.

✔✔ Bipat et al.[10] performed a meta-analysis and concluded that PET-CT is the most sensitive diagnostic tool for the detection of hepatic metastases from colorectal cancer on a per-patient basis, but not on a per-lesion basis. The authors suggest that in patients requiring further work-up, FDG-PET can be used as a second-line modality because both sensitivity and specificity were high and FDG-PET plays a role in detecting extrahepatic disease.

Mainenti et al.[11] found that PET-CT showed a trend to perform better than the other modalities. The pooled estimates of a meta-analysis for PET-CT was 93.8% (95% CI 90.0–97.7; six studies) and specificity per patient was 98.7% (95% CI 97.2–100%; six studies).[3]

Diagnostic laparoscopy and laparoscopic ultrasound

Diagnostic laparoscopy is used to detect small peritoneal metastases or subcapsular liver metastases, which can be missed on non-invasive imaging. The addition of laparoscopic ultrasound (LUS) may increase the detection of small intrahepatic metastases. There are not many prospective studies on these specific patients and most retrospective series also include patients with other liver tumours.

✔✔ Recent prospective studies have reported a limited benefit and found that an unnecessary laparotomy can be prevented in 10–13% of patients with CRLMs,[12,13] which is considerably lower than in earlier reports, where the figure varies from 12% to 33%.[14–16]

One reason for the lower yield might be that the indications for resection for metastases have changed towards a more aggressive approach for multiple lesions and bilobar disease. Furthermore, the use of local ablative techniques such as radiofrequency ablation (RFA) in combination with resection and downsizing with chemotherapy has extended the possibilities for surgical treatment. Currently the only absolute restrictions for curative resection include unresectable extrahepatic dissemination and limited function of the (future) liver remnant. The varying definition of unresectablility has a linear correlation with the yield of laparoscopy. In addition, improved cross-sectional imaging techniques in recent years have also decreased the yield of diagnostic laparoscopy.

Several centres favour the selective use of laparoscopy. Jarnagin et al.[13] have described a clinical risk score (CRS) that predicted survival after hepatic resection and was also suitable in identifying high-risk patients most likely to benefit from laparoscopy. In a study of 103 patients, occult unresectable disease was found in 12% of patients with a low score versus 42% of patients with a high score.[13,17] Similarly, in a series of 200 patients, a detection rate of only 6% was reported in patients with the lowest CRS, whereas this was 75% for the highest CRS scores.[14] Another study demonstrated a yield of 50% in a selected group of patients, while in the group of 49 patients selected for direct surgical exploration, 46 patients (94%) were eventually resected.[15]

Staging and assesment of resectability

✔✔ Factors that have favourable impact on survival are tumour-free resection margin, low level of carcinoembryonic antigen (CEA), single metastatic deposit and node-negative disease.[18]

The significance of resection margins of less than 10 mm is not clear.[19] The results of this meta-analysis demonstrate that a negative margin of 1 cm or more confers a survival advantage when compared with subcentimeter negative margins. The management of synchronous liver metastases and extrahepatic abnormalities (particularly the hilar lymph nodes) is also unclear. There is a huge variation in techniques for resection (anatomical vs. non-anatomical, vena cava reconstruction, etc.). Although promising, clear results on the effectiveness of combination treatments with (neo)adjuvant chemotherapy are still lacking.

The optimal selection of patients for hepatic resection is evolving, and the criteria for resectability differ among individual liver surgeons.

✔✔ A consensus statement in 2005 defined resectability as absence of non-treatable extrahepatic disease, fitness for surgery, ability to leave 30% of residual liver parenchyma in healthy livers or disease in no more than six segments.[20]

Modern multidisciplinary consensus defines resectable CRLM simply as tumours that can be resected completely, leaving an adequate liver remnant.[21] Before surgical exploration, most surgeons would require that there was no radiographic evidence of involvement of the hepatic artery, major bile ducts, main portal vein, or coeliac/para-aortic lymph nodes, and an adequate predicted functional hepatic remnant.[22]

✔✔ Some centres with extensive expertise do perform resections directly adjacent to major vascular structures with margins less than 10 mm; however, a margin of 10 mm is still recommended.[19]

In the presence of a limited number of lesions in the lung, liver resection is generally performed first. After radical resection of liver metastases, resection of the lung can follow. There is no reason to refrain from liver resection in a patient with advanced age who has good general (cardiopulmonary) fitness. Risk scoring systems (such as the clinical risk score[23] and others[24–26]) to predict which patients with CRLMs are most likely to benefit from resection are of uncertain clinical utility, particularly since most patients undergo different neoadjuvant chemotherapy regimens. Some studies have shown that the risk scoring system needs refinement[27,28] and that the outcome in patients treated by neoadjuvant chemotherapy was not predicted by the traditional clinical scoring system, but rather by response to chemotherapy as evaluated by CT and PET-CT.[29]

Resection of synchronous metastases should be considered in selected patients. Other strategies such as RFA, portal vein embolisation and isolated liver perfusion fall beyond the scope of this chapter.

Hepatocellular carcinoma

The diagnosis of hepatocellular carcinoma (HCC) is challenging as it has a variable imaging appearance and because lesion detection is difficult against the inhomogeneous background of liver cirrhosis with dysplastic and regenerating nodules mimicking HCC.

Transabdominal ultrasound

Transabdominal ultrasound is recommended by the European Associasion for the Study of the Liver (EASL), the American Association for the Study of Liver Disease (AASLC) and the Asian Pacific Association for the Study of Liver Disease (APASL) as a surveillance tool for patients at high risk of developing HCC. Meta-regression analysis has demonstrated a significantly higher sensitivity for early HCC with US every 6 months than with annual surveillance.[30]

Computed tomography and magnetic resonance imaging

Multiphase contrast-enhanced CT or MRI should be performed when evaluating HCC. The hallmark of HCC on CT and MRI is strong arterial enhancement (**Fig. 3.3**) and washout of contrast agent in the delayed phase (**Fig. 3.4**).[31] This feature in particular enables differentiation from intrahepatic cholangiocarcinoma, which shows delayed enhancement.[32]

HCC arising in a non-cirrhotic liver is often large, due to its long asymptomatic course and late presentation.[33] This contrasts with the multifocal tumours more commonly found in patients with chronic liver disease, who are often in surveillance programmes. Large HCCs may demonstrate a

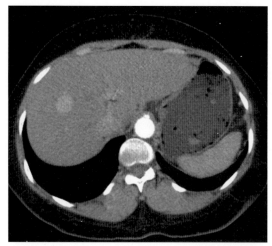

Figure 3.3 • CT image of patient with HCC in the liver showing arterial enhancement of the lesion.

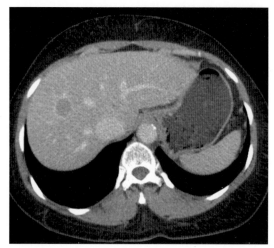

Figure 3.4 • CT image of same patient with HCC in the liver showing venous washout of the lesion with enhancing rim.

number of characteristic appearances on CT, which make differentiation from other causes of focal liver masses relatively straightforward. These features include mosaic appearance, with fibrous septa separating areas of variable attenuation which represent internal regions of haemorrhage, necrosis, fatty degeneration and fibrosis. The fibrous capsule has a low attenuation on unenhanced images and enhances on the portal venous phase.

A number of benign lesions, including haemangiomas, focal confluent fibrosis, peliosis, benign regenerative nodules and transient hepatic attenuation difference, can mimic small HCC lesions on CT.[34]

On MRI, HCCs can have a variable appearance on unenhanced T1-weighted images and typically show an increased signal on T2-weighted images.[35] Following gadolinium administration, HCC demonstrates characteristic early enhancement on arterial phase imaging[36] and washout on delayed images, resulting in a hypo-intense lesion compared to the surrounding parenchyma.[37]

Diagnostic laparoscopy and laparoscopic ultrasound

Laparoscopic evaluation can avoid exploratory laparotomy in 45–63% of patients with unresectable disease.[38,39] The procedure has been shown to be accurate in assessing the presence of advanced intrahepatic disease and the quality of the liver remnant, but it was less sensitive in determining the extent of local invasion, especially in large (>10 cm) tumours. Another study clearly reported the value of LUS in detecting small HCCs; 134 new nodules were visualised with this technique in 64 of 186 (34%) patients in

whom 28 nodules (in 23 patients) were histologically diagnosed as HCC.[40] Of these 23 patients, 18 were diagnosed as having a solitary HCC before laparoscopy. Similarly, new lesions of histologically proven HCC were found in 22% of patients.[41] Even when preoperative staging includes a CT, LUS was superior in detecting additional tumours.[42] Ultrasound confirmed all 201 tumours seen on CT and detected 21 additional tumours (9.5%) in 11 patients (20%).

Staging and assesment of resectability

Tumour staging to select a treatment regimen is complicated by the fact that many of the staging systems (including the TNM staging system of the American Joint Committee on Cancer (AJCC) – see Table 3.1) are based on surgical

Table 3.1 • TNM staging for hepatocellular cancer

Primary tumour (T)

TX	Primary tumour cannot be assessed
T0	No evidence of primary tumour
T1	Solitary tumour without vascular invasion
T2	Solitary tumour with vascular invasion or multiple tumours none more than 5 cm
T3a	Multiple tumours more than 5 cm
T3b	Single tumour or multiple tumours of any size involving a major branch of the portal vein or hepatic vein
T4	Tumour(s) with direct invasion of adjacent organs other than the gallbladder or with perforation of visceral peritoneum

Regional lymph nodes (N)

NX	Regional lymph nodes cannot be assessed
N0	No regional lymph node metastasis
N1	Regional lymph node metastasis

Distant metastasis (M)

M0	No distant metastasis
M1	Distant metastasis

Fibrosis score (F)*

F0	Fibrosis score 0–4 (none to moderate fibrosis)
F1	Fibrosis score 5–6 (severe fibrosis or cirrhosis)

Anatomical stage/prognostic groups				5-year survival after resection,[†] $n=13772$[91]
Stage I	T1	N0	M0	70
Stage II	T2	N0	M0	58
Stage IIIA	T3a	N0	M0	41
Stage IIIB	T3b	N0	M0	
Stage IIIC	T4	N0	M0	
Stage IVA	Any T	N1	M0	25
Stage IVB	Any T	Any N	M1	15

Note: cTNM is the clinical classification, pTNM is the pathological classification.

*The fibrosis score as defined by Ishak is recommended because of its prognostic value in overall survival. This scoring system uses a 0–6 scale.

[†] Data from AJCC sixth edition.

Modified from the AJCC Cancer Staging Manual, seventh edition (2010), published by Springer, New York.

findings, while surgery is applicable to only about 5% of these patients. Others recommend the Barcelona Clinic Liver Cancer (BCLC) staging system.[43] The Barcelona algorithm does not address the value of resection for some subgroups of patients with HCC who may potentially benefit from this approach, including some patients defined as being 'early stage' (with a single tumour size >2 cm or multiple nodules) and 'intermediate stage' (patients who have multinodular tumours but a good performance status). The Milano/Mazzaferro criteria for liver transplantation for HCC (i.e. solitary tumour ≤5 cm or up to three tumours all ≤3 cm) are widely accepted.[44] However, according to the Barcelona algorithm, only selected patients with three nodules ≤3 cm (those without 'associated diseases') should also undergo liver transplantation.[43] The American Hepato-Pancreato-Biliary Association (AHPBA)/ American Joint Commission on Cancer (AJCC) Consensus Conference on HCC in 2002 concluded that no single staging system could be used to accurately stage patients across the spectrum of HCCs.[44,45]

The ideal patient for resection has a solitary HCC confined to the liver that shows no radiographic evidence of invasion of the hepatic vasculature, no evidence of portal hypertension and well-preserved hepatic function. According to the current TNM/UICC staging system for HCC (Table 3.1), most consider stage IIIB, IIIC, IVA or IVB disease to be incurable by resection. However, hepatic resection for stage IIIB, IIIC and IVA disease may be considered in some centres of excellence as clinical benefits, and long-term survival can be achieved in a selected minority of patients.

Assessment of hepatic reserve is paramount to selection for resection. Postoperative mortality is twice as high in cirrhotic as in non-cirrhotic patients unless proper patient selection is applied. For patients with cirrhosis, surgical resection can safely be performed in those with Child–Pugh class A disease. These patients should undergo assessment of liver volumetry and remaining function. Other indications for therapies such as liver transplantation, RFA, ablation and arterial chemoembolisation are discussed elsewhere.

> ✔✔ Interval US at 6 months is recommended as a screening tool, while CT and MRI are most useful to confirm the diagnosis. Laparoscopic staging is useful in these patients since these tumours tend to be at high risk of being unresectable. The value of laparoscopy is further increased due to its capacity to aid guided biopsies of the future liver remnant in patients with cirrhosis.

Pancreatic and periampullary carcinoma

Most pancreatic tumours are located in the head of the pancreas (60–65%), while 20% are present in the body and 10% in the tail region. Unfortunately only a minority (5–20%) of pancreatic tumours are resectable. Tumours in the pancreatic head often present earlier due to compression of the adjacent common bile duct causing obstructive jaundice. Therefore these tumours are often smaller at time of presentation and more often resectable. These smaller tumours (<2 cm) without liver metastases have better 5-year survival.[46] Hence, by accurately detecting and staging smaller tumours, imaging has the potential to influence survival.

The goal of imaging for pancreatic tumours is twofold. The first is to accurately identify tumours with local invasion or distant metastasis to tailor the treatment strategy, and the second is to accurately image the anatomical variations prior to resection.

Transabdominal ultrasound

This is usually the first screening examination of the abdomen in patients with obstructive jaundice. It is a useful diagnostic modality with a reasonable sensitivity (>90%) for detecting bile duct obstruction, determining the level of the obstruction (e.g. intrahepatic, proximal or distal) and identifying the presence of gallstone disease.[47] Transabdominal ultrasound is cost-effective, widely available but highly operator dependent and often limited by the inability to adequately visualise the pancreas due to bowel gas interference. The goal of ultrasound is therefore to primarily establish a differential diagnosis among the various causes of obstructive jaundice and in identifying liver metastases. Ultrasound is highly sensitive in detecting gallbladder stones (>90%),[48] but this sensitivity drops to 50–75% for the detection of bile duct stones.[49] On ultrasound, a pancreatic tumour appears as a hypoechoic (poorly reflective) mass. A tell-tale sign suggestive of malignant obstruction is the combined presence of a dilated common bile duct and pancreatic duct (double duct sign).

> ✔✔ Ultrasound is able to detect most pancreatic masses of at least 3 cm, as was shown in a meta-analysis of 14 studies.[50] Pancreatic tumours (irrespective of size) yielded a sensitivity of 76% and a specificity of 75%.

However, these results are from studies performed in centres with significant experience in the diagnostic work-up of patients with pancreatic cancer.

Doppler ultrasound can show vascular involvement of portal and mesenteric veins.

Additionally, transabdominal ultrasound has a high sensitivity for detecting liver metastases and ascites, and an FNA can be performed. Sensitivity for liver lesions depends on the size of the lesion and is >90% for lesions larger than 2 cm, 60% for lesions of 1–2 cm and 20% for lesions <1 cm in diameter.[1]

Computed tomography and magnetic resonance imaging

CT is the most widely used imaging modality for pancreatic disease and staging pancreatic tumours. Modern multidetector CT enables evaluation of the vascular and ductal structures, and mapping of the anatomy and anatomical variations. The most important goal of CT imaging, besides the detection of tumours, is the assessment of resectability.

Tumour conspicuity depends heavily on CT scanning phases. Currently, a combination of pancreatic and portal phase CT is the optimal technique for pancreatic lesions. The best oral contrast is water. The optimal CT section thickness is 2 mm.

The arterial phase optimally demonstrates the arterial vessels (superior mesenteric artery, coeliac artery and hepatic artery) and their relation to the pancreatic tumour (**Fig. 3.5**). The portal venous phase demonstrates the portal and superior mesenteric veins and the junction (the confluence) at the pancreatic neck (**Fig. 3.6**). The parenchymal phase is between these two phases and demonstrates pancreatic adenocarinoma as a hypovascular tumour compared to the rest of the parenchyma.

Tumours in the head of the pancreas usually cause dilatation of the common bile duct (CBD). The double duct sign appears when both the CBD and the pancreatic duct are dilated. Smooth dilatation is more suggestive of malignancy, whereas irregular

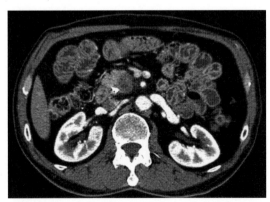

Figure 3.5 • CT image of patient with pancreatic head mass with no vascular involvement.

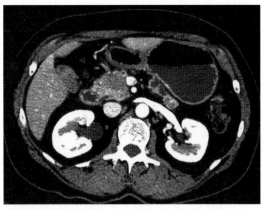

Figure 3.6 • CT image of patient with pancreatic head mass with portal vein contact of approximately 90 degrees.

or beaded dilatation is more suggestive of pancreatitis. Tumours that extend beyond the contours of the pancreas with infiltration of the peripancreatic fat are seen as blurring of the normal dark peripancreatic fat. The sensitivity and specificity of CT for detection of a pancreatic head mass were 91% and 85%, respectively, versus 84% and 82% for MRI in a pooled meta-analysis.[50] The meta-analysis found that CT was significantly better than MRI and US.

CT has been reported to have a positive predictive value of 100%, negative predictive value of 56% and overall accuracy of 70% for unresectable pancreatic carcinoma.[51] This ability to predict unresectability preoperatively is superior to the ability to predict resectability, particularly because the detection of small (<5 mm) liver and peritoneal metastases is limited.

Endoscopic retrograde cholangiopancreatography (ERCP)

ERCP has been performed as an initial investigation in patients with obstructive jaundice for many years. However, the advent of improved non-invasive diagnostic modalities such as CT, MRI and endoscopic ultrasound (EUS) has led to less frequent use of invasive ERCP. Endoscopic retrograde cholangiopancreatography is associated with a morbidity of 5–10% and a mortality of 0.1–1%. The most common complications include pancreatitis (5–10%), bleeding (1–2%) and perforation (<0.3%).[52]

✓✓ A recent randomised controlled trial showed that early surgery without preoperative biliary drainage did not increase the risk of complications after surgery, as compared with preoperative biliary drainage.[53]

Magnetic resonance cholangiopancreaticography (MRCP) closely mimics the imaging capacity of ERCP but is non-invasive. One advantage of MRCP is that information regarding the tumour and its relation to surrounding structures is also obtained during the same examination. In addition, distant metastases can be detected with MRI. The results of MRCP in visualisation of the biliary system are similar to ERCP in clinical studies, with a sensitivity of 71–93% versus 81–86% and specificity of 92–94% versus 82–100%. When comparing ERCP with EUS, the sensitivity was 75–89% versus 85–89% and specificity was 65–92% versus 80–96%.[54] There are no known direct comparisons between ERCP and CT. If an ERCP is performed, it is possible to perform brush cytology, bile aspiration cytology and even intraductal biopsies. These examinations are highly sensitive but lack specificity.

The detection rate of malignancy was not significantly different for brush cytology compared to bile cytology (sensitivity of 33–100% versus specificity of 6–50%, respectively) and also not significantly different for FNA cytology compared to brush cytology (25–91% versus 8–56%, respectively). Forceps biopsy versus brush cytology was also not significantly different (43–81% versus 18–53%, respectively).[54] Other new modalities such as intraductal cholangiopancreaticoscopy and intraductal endosonography have yet to be proven in larger series.

Endoscopic ultrasound

EUS allows a sonographic transducer to be placed in close proximity to the pancreas. In doing so, interference from overlying bowel gas is eliminated and higher frequencies can be used, resulting in markedly improved resolution. EUS was considered superior to the other imaging modalities prior to the recent refinements made in CT,[55] because most current CT studies date from the period 1994–2000. EUS was considered more sensitive in one systematic review describing nine studies of EUS compared to CT for diagnostic effectiveness.[56] The most valuable role of EUS in these studies was in detecting small tumours (<2 cm). The pooled sensitivity was 85% with a specificity of 94%, but heterogeneity was an issue in this pooled analysis. FNA can be performed when in doubt with a lower risk of causing peritoneal carcinomatosis than with transabdominal aspiration. A study in 62 patients with pancreatic cancer that compared EUS, CT and MRI with the gold standard of surgery found that a sequential approach consisting of helical CT as an initial test and EUS as a confirmatory technique when in doubt seemed to be the most reliable and cost-effective strategy.[57] Thus, EUS is not mandatory in the work-up of patients with pancreatic cancer. In those cases with potentially resectable tumours,

an EUS-guided (FNA) biopsy has a pooled sensitivity for malignant cytology of 85% (95% CI 84–86%) and a pooled specificity of 98% (95% CI 97–99%).[58] The major limitations of this technology are operator dependence and a limited field of visualisation for the detection of distant metastases. This modality should be used on a selective basis (e.g. to obtain preoperative tissue biopsy for patients scheduled for neoadjuvant therapy) and in centres with experience.

Positron emission tomography

Preliminary reports indicate that FDG-PET may provide additional information regarding the M status of a patient and can change the therapeutic option in up to 16% of patients.[59] A meta-analysis of PET scanning in patients with a positive, negative and inconclusive CT found sensitivity and specificity of 92% and 68%, respectively, after a positive CT, 73% and 86%, respectively, after a negative CT, and 100% and 68%, respectively, after an inconclusive CT.[60] Its usefulness will vary depending upon the pretest probability of the patient and the results of CT. FDG-PET is most often used for response evaluation in neoadjuvant chemoradiotherapy trials.

Diagnostic laparoscopy and laparoscopic ultrasound

Despite best efforts, there are still unexpected occasions when the intraoperative findings are contrary to those reported by the preoperative investigations, especially with regard to resectability. These patients consequently undergo an unnecessary laparotomy, along with its accompanying risks, albeit small, of postoperative morbidity and mortality. The quality of life becomes further diminished in a patient population whose survival is already limited. The detection of small liver and peritoneal metastases (**Fig. 3.7**) is an important motivation for performing diagnostic laparoscopy, since this might avoid open exploration. CT has excellent accuracy in predicting unresectability; however, sensitivity for assessment of resectability remains much lower. This is due to its inability to detect very small liver lesions (<1 cm) or peritoneal deposits.

Despite the logical rationale behind its use, laparoscopy continues to provoke considerable debate. Advocates have reported that laparoscopy can identify occult metastases, which were not detected by a preceding CT, in 30% of patients.[61] Consequently, the resection rates after laparoscopy have been reported to be 75–92%.[62] Because of these results, some centres strongly recommend the use of diagnostic laparoscopy as a routine procedure.

Critics argue that routine laparoscopy is not cost-effective. With the newer generations of CT

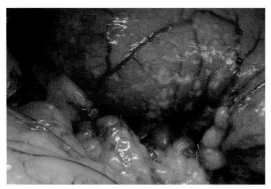

Figure 3.7 • Peritoneal metastases on the first part of the duodenum found during laparotomy in a patient with a periampullary carcinoma.

scanners, the incidence of missed hepatic or peritoneal metastases is less than 20%. The implication is that performing routine laparoscopy adds unnecessary surgical time and expense to the remaining 80% of patients with resectable disease or, if locally unresectable, precludes them from surgical palliation, which is considered superior.[63,64]

The yield of additional laparoscopic staging is influenced greatly by the quality of the prelaparoscopic staging process. Incorrect staging with poor quality CT, for example, results in an overestimation in the yield of diagnostic laparoscopy and LUS. While the most important objective in laparoscopy is to prevent an unnecessary laparotomy, a number of patients do need a subsequent laparotomy for further palliation (e.g. bypass procedure for gastrointestinal obstruction). The limited detection rate

for unresectable metastatic disease and the likely absence of a large gain after switching from surgical to endoscopic palliation prompted many centres not to routinely perform laparoscopy in patients with peripancreatic carcinoma.[64] In a study assessing 233 patients with upper gastrointestinal malignancy, of whom 114 patients had a periampullary tumour, laparotomy was avoided initially in 17 patients (15%), but five of these patients subsequently required laparotomy for duodenal obstruction.[61] This reduced the overall efficacy of laparoscopy in preventing unnecessary laparotomies from 15% to 11%. In a more recent study of 297 patients, the laparoscopic yield decreased to 13% (39 patients), probably due to improved radiological staging techniques.[64] This, combined with an increasingly critical view of resectability and palliation, has resulted in a decreased benefit of laparoscopic staging.

> ✔ Diagnostic laparoscopy is advised to identify true locally advanced disease when chemoradiation is considered to 'downstage' the tumour. This is important to exclude patients with metastases not seen on preoperative imaging.

Staging and assesment of resectability

Staging is according to the TNM atlas, seventh edition, 2009 (Tables 3.2–3.4). Most clinicians agree that a tumour is considered incurable if there are distant metastases (liver, lung, lymph nodes outside the (radical) lymph node dissection area as defined

Table 3.2 • TNM staging system for exocrine and endocrine tumours of the pancreas

Primary tumour (T)	
TX	Primary tumour cannot be assessed
T0	No evidence of primary tumour
Tis	Carcinoma in situ*
T1	Tumour limited to the pancreas, 2 cm or less in greatest dimension
T2	Tumour limited to the pancreas, more than 2 cm in greatest dimension
T3	Tumour extends beyond the pancreas but without involvement of the coeliac axis or the superior mesenteric artery
T4	Tumour involves the coeliac axis or the superior mesenteric artery (unresectable primary tumour)
Regional lymph nodes (N)	
NX	Regional lymph nodes cannot be assessed
N0	No regional lymph node metastasis
N1	Regional lymph node metastasis
Distant metastasis (M)	
M0	No distant metastasis
M1	Distant metastasis

(Continued)

Table 3.2 • (*cont.*) TNM staging system for exocrine and endocrine tumours of the pancreas

Anatomical stage/prognostic groups				5-year survival after resection,[†] n=21 512[92]
Stage 0	Tis	N0	M0	
Stage IA	T1	N0	M0	31
Stage IB	T2	N0	M0	27
Stage IIA	T3	N0	M0	16
Stage IIB	T1	N1	M0	8
	T2	N1	M0	
	T3	N1	M0	
Stage III	T4	Any N	M0	7
Stage IV	Any T	Any N	M1	3

Note: cTNM is the clinical classification, pTNM is the pathological classification.
*This includes lesions classified as PanIn III classification.
[†] Data from AJCC sixth edition.
Modified from the AJCC Cancer Staging Manual, seventh edition (2010), published by Springer, New York.

Table 3.3 • TNM staging for ampullary carcinoma

Primary tumour (T)	
TX	Primary tumour cannot be assessed
T0	No evidence of primary tumour
Tis	Carcinoma in situ
T1	Tumour limited to the ampulla of Vater or sphincter of Oddi
T2	Tumour invades duodenal wall
T3	Tumour invades pancreas
T4	Tumour invades peripancreatic soft tissues or other adjacent organs or structures other than pancreas
Regional lymph nodes (N)	
NX	Regional lymph nodes cannot be assessed
N0	No regional lymph node metastasis
N1	Regional lymph node metastasis
Distant metastasis (M)	
M0	No distant metastasis
M1	Distant metastasis

Anatomical stage/prognostic groups				5-year survival after resection,* n=1301[93]
Stage 0	Tis	N0	M0	
Stage IA	T1	N0	M0	60
Stage IB	T2	N0	M0	57
Stage IIA	T3	N0	M0	30
Stage IIB	T1	N1	M0	22
	T2	N1	M0	
	T3	N1	M0	
Stage III	T4	Any N	M0	27
Stage IV	Any T	Any N	M1	0

Note: cTNM is the clinical classification, pTNM is the pathological classification.
*Data from AJCC sixth edition.
Modified from the AJCC Cancer Staging Manual, seventh edition (2010), published by Springer, New York.

Table 3.4 • TNM staging system for distal cholangiocarcinoma

Primary tumour (T)	
TX	Primary tumour cannot be assessed
T0	No evidence of primary tumour
Tis	Carcinoma in situ
T1	Tumour confined to the bile duct histologically
T2	Tumour invades beyond the wall of the bile duct
T3	Tumour invades the gallbladder, pancreas, duodenum, or other adjacent organs without involvement of the coeliac axis, or the superior mesenteric artery
T4	Tumour involves the coeliac axis, or the superior mesenteric artery
Regional lymph nodes (N)	
NX	Regional lymph nodes cannot be assessed
N0	No regional lymph node metastasis
N1	Regional lymph node metastasis
Distant metastasis (M)	
M0	No distant metastasis
M1	Distant metastasis

Anatomical stage/prognostic groups				**5-year survival after resection,* n = 779[94]**
Stage 0	Tis	N0	M0	
Stage IA	T1	N0	M0	60
Stage IB	T2	N0	M0	
Stage IIA	T3	N0	M0	39
Stage IIB	T1	N1	M0	
	T2	N1	M0	
	T3	N1	M0	
Stage III	T4	Any N	M0	34
Stage IV	Any T	Any N	M1	10

Note: cTNM is the clinical classification, pTNM is the pathological classification.
*Data from AJCC sixth edition.
Modified from the AJCC Cancer Staging Manual, seventh edition (2010), published by Springer, New York.

by Pedrazzoli et al.[65]) or if there is local invasion into arterial structures such as superior mesenteric artery, coeliac trunk or common hepatic artery (Table 3.5).

✅ Arterial resections with reconstruction have been described in small retrospective studies, with almost no survival benefit, but increased mortality and morbidity, 21–40% and 2–35%, respectively.[66]

Criteria to assess vascular ingrowth on CT include tumour involvement of any of the major pancreatic vessels (coeliac artery, hepatic artery, superior mesenteric artery, superior mesenteric vein or portal vein) that exceeds one-half of the circumference of the vessels (**Fig. 3.8**). This is especially specific for the involved arteries. Contour deformity, obliteration and thrombosis of the veins is also highly suspicious of vascular involvement.[67] Additional radiological

Table 3.5 • Resectability of pancreatic tumours

Resectable	Borderline	Unresectable
No tumour abutment with vessel	>90° tumour abutment with PV of SMV	>180° tumour abutment with PV or SMV
	>5 mm length of PV or SMV contact	PV/SMV constriction or thrombus or teardrop deformation of SMV
		Any ingrowth in SMA
No distant metastasis		Distant metastasis

PV, portal vein; SMA, superior mesenteric artery; SMV, superior mesenteric vein.

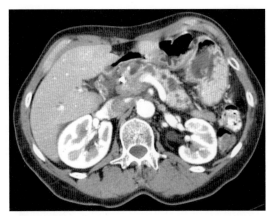

Figure 3.8 • CT image of patient with pancreatic head mass with portal contact of more than 180 degrees.

features that suggest vascular invasion include perivascular cuffing, described as increased attenuation of the normal perivascular fat, and the presence of dilated collateral veins. The 'teardrop' sign, which describes the deformity of the otherwise round shape of the superior mesenteric vein, suggests venous invasion. Nevertheless, there is much debate over the exact definition of vascular involvement.

Successful resection of (a part of) the superior mesenteric vein or portal vein has been described and could be an advantage, provided that an R0/R1 resection can be achieved. In a review by Ramacciato et al.,[68] 12 series are described with a total of 399 patients; the morbidity rate was 16.7–54% and mortality rate 0–7.7%, with a median survival of 13–22 months and a 5-year survival of 9–18%. Muller et al.[69] also described 110 patients following resection of venous invasion with a morbidity rate of 41.8% and mortality rate of 3.6%. The survival was not increased by the addition of a venous resection with bypass, because earlier local recurrence and/or distant metastases arose in this group of patients compared to patients who had no invasion of the vein.

✔✔ Glanemann et al.[70] reported morbidity rates of 21–42% and mortality rates of 0–5.9% when pooling a series of 1967 patients with simultaneous venous vessel resection described throughout the literature. The 5-year survival in this study ranged from 7% to 20%. The systematic review of Siriwardana and Siriwardena[66] found no benefit from resection of venous structures with invasion.

Size is the only characteristic of a pancreatic tumour that can be determined preoperatively. A review by Garcea et al.[71] analysed studies and used the size measured at histopathology. In these studies the cut-off value varied, but most studies suggested 2 cm. In all these studies, the median survival of patients with tumours <2 cm is 35.5 months versus 14 months for larger tumours. Although the studies varied in quality, this meta-analysis concluded that size (<2 cm or >2 cm) is an (independent) prognostic factor for median survival (odds ratio (OR) = 2.52, 95% CI 1.95–3, P <0.001). One relatively small study used size of the tumour on preoperative imaging and found that prognosis correlated with the size determined on CT.[72]

✔✔ Staging and assessment of patients with pancreatic or periampullary tumours is important because distant metastasis and frank vascular ingrowth precludes a curative resection. A pancreas protocol CT is the most important factor in the staging and assessment of pancreatic cancer.

✔ There is still some controversy over the degree of vascular ingrowth and tumour resectability. It is clear that obvious vascular involvement precludes a curative resection. Patients with borderline tumours could benefit from limited vascular resection and should undergo explorative laparotomy.

Proximal bile duct tumours

Patients with proximal bile duct tumours generally present with jaundice. Patients with jaundice and a hilar stricture will either have a benign biliary stricture or a malignancy that has obstructed the hepatic confluence.[73,74] The differential diagnosis includes benign biliary strictures (postoperative bile duct injury, primary sclerosing cholangitis, HIV cholangiopathy, Mirizzi syndrome) or another malignancy such as gallbladder cancer or lymphoma. Diagnosis of a hilar cholangiocarcinoma can be challenging, particularly in patients with primary sclerosing cholangitis, with multiple stenosis and mass lesions often identified on imaging without significant intrahepatic biliary dilation.

Transabdominal ultrasound

Abdominal ultrasound is often the first diagnostic study to confirm biliary duct dilatation, identify the level of obstruction and exclude gallstones.[75] Duplex ultrasound has also been useful to assess vascular involvement.[76]

Computed tomography and magnetic resonance imaging

CT is used to establish the presence of a tumour, its location as well as local spread, vascular ingrowth and metastases. Magnetic resonance cholangiography is comparable to ERCP in the detection of biliary malignancy. An advantage offered by magnetic resonance cholangiography is that it can identify the luminal involvement and thus give a better staging of the tumour without cannulation of the bile ducts and risk of infection. It allows visualisation of both the obstructed and non-obstructed ducts, and gives important information such as the extent of tumour within the biliary tree and in periductal tissue, vascular and nodal involvement, lobar atrophy, invasion of adjacent liver parenchyma and distant metastases, without the risk of biliary intubation.[77] If imaging studies demonstrate a focal stenotic lesion of the bile duct in the absence of previous biliary tract surgery, an assumptive diagnosis of hilar cholangiocarcinoma is made until proven otherwise.[74]

Endoscopic retrograde cholangiopancreatography

ERCP and percutaneous transhepatic cholangiography (PTC) both allow for the collection of tissue samples for pathology and bile for cytology. The value of cytology has recently been stressed.[78] Non-invasive imaging does not allow tissue diagnosis, but histological confirmation is not mandatory before surgical exploration. It is notable that, in patients that require biliary drainage preoperatively, PTC is preferable to ERCP, as it allows selective evaluation of the intrahepatic biliary tree much more clearly.

Positron emission tomography

PET has been shown to have a high sensitivity for diagnosing biliary malignancy. The limitation of the method is that patients with an inflammatory process of the biliary tree (as in primary sclerosing cholangitis) can have false-positive findings. In a prospective study by Kim et al.,[79] PET proved significantly more accurate in identifying distant metastases compared with CT (58% vs. 0%). Other studies have confirmed the usefulness of PET for detecting metastases not found by other imaging,[80] ultimately influencing clinical management in up to 25% of patients.[81] The sensitivity of FDG-PET for detecting primary intrahepatic cholangiocarcinoma has been estimated at 78%.[81] However, Petrowsky et al.[82] found PET-CT to be more sensitive (93% vs. 55%) and specific (80% vs. 33%) in detecting intrahepatic compared to extrahepatic cholangiocarcinoma.[78] Another limitation reported by Kluge et al.[83] was a sensitivity

of 92% in detecting hilarcholangiocarcinoma, but the rate of detection of extrahepatic tumours was dependent on the shape of the tumour.

Diagnostic laparoscopy and laparoscopic ultrasound

Information on the additional value of diagnostic laparoscopy for malignant proximal bile duct obstruction is limited.

✅ In a pilot study, advanced disease was diagnosed in 19 of 47 patients (40%) by laparoscopy.[84]

These results were explained by a change in diagnosis after laparoscopy from a primary bile duct tumour to locally invasive gallbladder cancer. Another study of 110 consecutive patients confirmed these data.[85] Laparoscopy revealed histologically proven incurable disease in 44 patients (41%). Of the 65 patients who underwent laparotomy, 35 patients (54%) were unresectable. Although laparotomy was avoided in 41% of cases, laparoscopy was unable to assess resectability correctly in 44% of patients. These findings are in agreement with the study from the Memorial Sloan Kettering Cancer Center involving 100 patients with carcinoma of the extrahepatic biliary tree.[86] Thirty-five patients (35%) were identified as having unresectable disease at laparoscopy. Of the 65 patients who underwent laparotomy, a further 34 tumours (52%) were unresectable, resulting in an overall accuracy of 51%. Finally, in a series of 401 patients with hepatobiliary cancer, the highest yield for laparoscopy was found in patients with biliary cancer, but the study emphasised that the surgeon's preoperative impression of resectability was as important as the laparoscopic staging procedure itself.[12] Recently, a study found that the yield has decreased to 12% in recent years due to better preoperative imaging.[87]

LUS has not been very useful in staging the local tumour spread of proximal bile duct cancer. A previous study confirmed that patients with unresectable disease most often had locally advanced tumours, but LUS did not contribute to the assessment of resectability in these patients.[86] Furthermore, extensive biliary and vascular involvement can be determined with high accuracy (91%) using external colour Doppler ultrasound, as well as thin-slice contrast-enhanced multislice CT.[88] The additional value of LUS is therefore too low for it to be performed routinely.

Staging and assesment of resectability

The American Joint Committee on Cancer (AJCC) TNM staging system is most commonly used to stage hilar cholangiocarcinoma (Table 3.6). However, this system is based on pathology criteria and does not provide information on the potential for resectability. Therefore, other staging systems have been used to predict resectability and to assess the extent of resection. The Bismuth–Corlette classification (**Fig. 3.9**) stratifies patients based on extent of biliary involvement by tumour. In brief: type I tumours are below the confluence of the left and right hepatic duct; type II tumours reach the confluence; type IIIa and IIIb tumours occlude the common hepatic duct and either the right or left hepatic duct, respectively; and type IV tumours involve the confluence and both the right and left hepatic ducts.

The preoperative clinical T staging system (Table 3.7) as proposed by Jarnagin and colleagues[89,90] defines both the radial and longitudinal extension of hilar cholangiocarcinoma, which are critical factors in the determination of resectability. This Memorial Sloan-Kettering Cancer Center (MSKCC) staging system incorporates three factors based on preoperative imaging studies: (1) location and extent of ductal involvement; (2) presence or absence of portal vein invasion; and (3) presence or absence of hepatic lobar atrophy. Criteria for unresectable disease include locally advanced tumour extending to secondary biliary radicles (i.e. sectional bile ducts (right anterior, right posterior, left lateral and left medial) bilaterally), to unilateral sectional bile ducts with contralateral portal vein branch involvement, encasement or occlusion

Table 3.6 • TNM staging system for perihilar cholangiocarcinoma

Primary tumour (T)			
TX	Primary tumour cannot be assessed		
T0	No evidence of primary tumour		
Tis	Carcinoma in situ		
T1	Tumour confined to the bile duct, with extension up to the muscle layer or fibrous tissue		
T2a	Tumour invades beyond the wall of the bile duct to surrounding adipose tissue		
T2b	Tumour invades adjacent hepatic parenchyma		
T3	Tumour invades unilateral branches of the portal vein or hepatic artery		
T4	Tumour invades main portal vein or its branches bilaterally; or the common hepatic artery; or the second-order biliary radicals bilaterally; or unilateral second-order biliary radicals with contralateral portal vein or hepatic artery involvement		
Regional lymph nodes (N)			
NX	Regional lymph nodes cannot be assessed		
N0	No regional lymph node metastasis		
N1	Regional lymph node metastasis (including nodes along the cystic duct, common bile duct, hepatic artery and portal vein)		
N2	Metastasis to periaortic, pericaval, superior mesenteric artery and/or coeliac artery lymph nodes		
Distant metastasis (M)			
M0	No distant metastasis		
M1	Distant metastasis		
Anatomical stage/prognostic groups			
Stage 0	Tis	N0	M0
Stage I	T1	N0	M0
Stage II	T2a–b	N0	M0
Stage IIIA	T3	N0	M0
Stage IIIB	T1–3	N1	M0
Stage IVA	T4	N0–1	M0
Stage IVB	Any T	N2	M0
	Any T	Any N	M1

Note: cTNM is the clinical classification, pTNM is the pathological classification.
Modified from the AJCC Cancer Staging Manual, seventh edition (2010), published by Springer, New York.

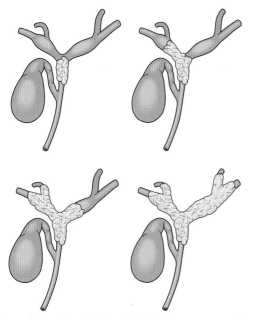

of the main portal vein proximal to its bifurcation, atrophy of one hepatic lobe with contralateral portal vein involvement, or atrophy of one hepatic lobe with contralateral tumour extension to sectional bile ducts. A recently designed new system of staging incorporates the size of the tumour, the extent of the disease in the biliary system, the involvement of the hepatic artery and portal vein, the involvement of lymph nodes, distant metastases, and the volume of the putative remnant liver after resection (Table 3.8). These staging systems are relatively new and have to be proven in future studies.

☑☑ Staging and assessment of proximal bile duct tumours is difficult and usually consists of a combination of tests including US, CT and MRI. More invasive tests should be performed only if necessary, in order to avoid procedure-related complications and delay of surgery. Preoperative biopsies and brushings are not always reliable and should not delay surgery.

☑☑ The older staging and classification systems were of limited use in guiding preoperative decision-making. This led to the development of new modified clinical staging systems that have overcome these limitations and can aid with preoperative decision-making.

Figure 3.9 • Classification of Klatskin tumours according to Bismuth–Corlette, types I, II, IIIa and IV. Type I and II tumours are limited to the confluence of the right and left hepatic duct. In type III tumours, the segmental branches of the right or left hepatic duct are involved (type IIIa or IIIb respectively). In type IV tumours, the tumour extends into the segmental branches of both right and left hepatic duct.

Table 3.7 • Jarnagin–Blumgart Clinical T staging system[89]

	Biliary involvement	**PV involvement**	**Lobar atrophy**
T1	Hilus ± unilateral sectional bile ducts	No	No
T2	Hilus ± unilateral sectional bile ducts	+ Ipsilateral	± Ipsilateral
T3	Hilus + bilateral sectional bile ducts	Yes/no	Yes/no
	Hilus + unilateral sectional bile ducts	+ Contralateral	Yes/no
	Hilus + unilateral bile ducts	Yes/no	+ Contralateral
	Hilus ± unilateral sectional bile ducts	Bilateral	Yes/no

Sectional bile ducts = right anterior, right posterior, left medial, left lateral. PV, portal vein.

Table 3.8 • Classification system proposed by DeOliveira et al.*, [95]

Bile duct (B)†		
B1		Common bile duct
B2		Hepatic duct confluence
B3	R	Right hepatic duct
B3	L	Left hepatic duct
B4		Right and left hepatic duct
Tumour size (T)		
T1		<1 cm
T2		1–3 cm
T3		≥3 cm

(*Continued*)

Table 3.8 • (cont.) Classification system proposed by DeOliveira et al.[*,95]

Tumour form (F)		
Sclerosing		Sclerosing (or periductal)
Mass		Mass forming (or nodular)
Mixed		Sclerosing and mass forming
Polypoid		Polypoid (or intraductal)
Involvement (>180°) of the portal vein (PV)		
PV0		No portal involvement
PV1		Main portal vein
PV2		Portal vein bifurcation
PV3	R	Right portal vein
PV3	L	Left portal vein
PV4		Right and left portal veins
Involvement (>180°) of the hepatic artery (HA)		
HA0		No arterial involvement
HA1		Proper hepatic artery
HA2		Hepatic artery bifurcation
HA3	R	Right hepatic artery
HA3	L	Left hepatic artery
HA4		Right and left hepatic artery
Liver remnant volume (V)		
V0		No information on the volume needed (liver resection not foreseen)
V%	Indicate segments	Percentage of the total volume of a putative remnant liver after resection
Underlying liver disease (D)		
		Fibrosis
		Non-alcoholic steatohepatitis
		Primary sclerosing cholangitis
Lymph nodes (N)[‡]		
N0		No lymph node involvement
N1		Hilar and/or hepatic artery lymph node involvement
N2		Periaortic lymph node involvement
Metastases (M)[§]		
M0		No distant metastases
M1		Distant metastases (including liver and peritoneal metastases)

[*] 'R' indicates right and 'L' indicates left.
[†] Based on the Bismuth classification.
[‡] Based on the Japanese Society of Biliary Surgery classification.
[§] Based on the TNM classification.

Key points

- CT or MRI should be performed for staging patients with HCC or CRLMs depending on local expertise.
- A PET scan provides useful information in the work-up of patients with CRLMs that can serve to reduce the number of unnecessary laparotomies.
- Abdominal ultrasound has a high accuracy in identifying biliary obstruction and stone disease but is of limited use in the detection and staging of pancreatic tumours.

- CT is the test of choice for the diagnostic work-up and staging of pancreatic tumours.
- The accuracy of non-invasive imaging with CT, MRI/MRCP and EUS is superior to more invasive ERCP for the diagnosis of malignant bile duct obstruction.
- FDG-PET plays no routine role in patients with a pancreatic mass because it is associated with high false-negative results.
- EUS is most accurate in detecting smaller tumours and to differentiate between focal pancreatitis and malignancy.
- Diagnostic laparoscopy and LUS has limited yield for patients with colorectal liver malignancy and pancreatic cancer but is useful in patients with hepatocellucar carcinoma. The role of diagnostic laparoscopy for proximal bile duct tumours is uncertain.
- The presence of vascular invasion and hepatocellular function determine the treatment of patients with cancer of the proximal biliary tract.
- Surgery for HPB tumours demands careful multidisciplinary preoperative assessment of risk factors and subsequent selection of patients. This should be done in a multidisciplinary meeting that includes HPB specialists in the field of medical oncology, radiotherapy, gastroenterology, (interventional) radiology and surgery.

References

1. Hagspiel KD, Neidl KF, Eichenberger AC, et al. Detection of liver metastases: comparison of superparamagnetic iron oxide-enhanced and unenhanced MR imaging at 1.5 T with dynamic CT, intraoperative US, and percutaneous US. Radiology 1995;196(2):471–8.

2. Ohlsson B, Nilsson J, Stenram U, et al. Percutaneous fine-needle aspiration cytology in the diagnosis and management of liver tumours. Br J Surg 2002;89(6):757–62.

3. Floriani I, Torri V, Rulli E, et al. Performance of imaging modalities in diagnosis of liver metastases from colorectal cancer: a systematic review and meta-analysis. J Magn Reson Imaging 2010;31(1):19–31.

4. Sahani D, Mehta A, Blake M, et al. Preoperative hepatic vascular evaluation with CT and MR angiography: implications for surgery. Radiographics 2004;24(5):1367–80.

5. Yim PJ, Vora AV, Raghavan D, et al. Volumetric analysis of liver metastases in computed tomography with the fuzzy C-means algorithm. J Comput Assist Tomogr 2006;30(2):212–20.

6. Bennett GL, Petersein A, Mayo-Smith WW, et al. Addition of gadolinium chelates to heavily T2-weighted MR imaging: limited role in differentiating hepatic hemangiomas from metastases. Am J Roentgenol 2000;174(2):477–85.

7. Schima W, Saini S, Echeverri JA, et al. Focal liver lesions: characterization with conventional spin-echo versus fast spin-echo T2-weighted MR imaging. Radiology 1997;202(2):389–93.

8. Wiering B, Krabbe PF, Jager GJ, et al. The impact of fluoro-18-deoxyglucose-positron emission tomography in the management of colorectal liver metastases. Cancer 2005;104(12):2658–70.

9. Kinkel K, Lu Y, Both M, et al. Detection of hepatic metastases from cancers of the gastrointestinal tract by using noninvasive imaging methods (US, CT, MR imaging, PET): a meta-analysis. Radiology 2002;224(3):748–56.

10. Bipat S, van Leeuwen MS, Comans EF, et al. Colorectal liver metastases: CT, MR imaging, and PET for diagnosis – meta-analysis. Radiology 2005;237(1):123–31.

11. Mainenti PP, Mancini M, Mainolfi C, et al. Detection of colo-rectal liver metastases: prospective comparison of contrast enhanced US, multidetector CT, PET/CT, and 1.5 Tesla MR with extracellular and reticulo-endothelial cell specific contrast agents. Abdom Imaging 2010;35(5):511–21.

12. D'Angelica M, Fong Y, Weber S, et al. The role of staging laparoscopy in hepatobiliary malignancy: prospective analysis of 401 cases. Ann Surg Oncol 2003;10(2):183–9.

13. Jarnagin WR, Conlon K, Bodniewicz J, et al. A clinical scoring system predicts the yield of diagnostic laparoscopy in patients with potentially resectable hepatic colorectal metastases. Cancer 2001;91(6):1121–8.

14. Mann CD, Neal CP, Metcalfe MS, et al. Clinical Risk Score predicts yield of staging laparoscopy in patients with colorectal liver metastases. Br J Surg 2007;94(7):855–9.

15. Metcalfe MS, Close JS, Iswariah H, et al. The value of laparoscopic staging for patients with colorectal metastases. Arch Surg 2003;138(7):770–2.

16. Jarnagin WR, Bodniewicz J, Dougherty E, et al. A prospective analysis of staging laparoscopy in

patients with primary and secondary hepatobiliary malignancies. J Gastrointest Surg 2000;4(1):34–43.

17. Grobmyer SR, Fong Y, D'Angelica M, et al. Diagnostic laparoscopy prior to planned hepatic resection for colorectal metastases. Arch Surg 2004;139(12):1326–30.

18. Abbas S, Lam V, Hollands M. Ten-year survival after liver resection for colorectal metastases: systematic review and meta-analysis. ISRN Oncol 2011;2011:763245.

19. Dhir M, Lyden ER, Wang A, et al. Influence of margins on overall survival after hepatic resection for colorectal metastasis: a meta-analysis. Ann Surg 2011;254(2):234–42.

20. Poston GJ, Adam R, Alberts S, et al. OncoSurge: a strategy for improving resectability with curative intent in metastatic colorectal cancer. J Clin Oncol 2005;23(28):7125–34.

21. Berri RN, Abdalla EK. Curable metastatic colorectal cancer: recommended paradigms. Curr Oncol Rep 2009;11(3):200–8.

22. Adam R, de Haas RJ, Wicherts DA, et al. Is hepatic resection justified after chemotherapy in patients with colorectal liver metastases and lymph node involvement? J Clin Oncol 2008;26(22):3672–80.

23. Fong Y, Fortner J, Sun RL, et al. Clinical score for predicting recurrence after hepatic resection for metastatic colorectal cancer: analysis of 1001 consecutive cases. Ann Surg 1999;230(3):309–18.

24. Konopke R, Kersting S, Distler M, et al. Prognostic factors and evaluation of a clinical score for predicting survival after resection of colorectal liver metastases. Liver Int 2009;29(1):89–102.

25. Nagashima I, Takada T, Matsuda K, et al. A new scoring system to classify patients with colorectal liver metastases: proposal of criteria to select candidates for hepatic resection. J Hepatobiliary Pancreat Surg 2004;11(2):79–83.

26. Nordlinger B, Guiguet M, Vaillant JC, et al. Surgical resection of colorectal carcinoma metastases to the liver. A prognostic scoring system to improve case selection, based on 1568 patients. Association Francaise de Chirurgie. Cancer 1996;77(7):1254–62.

27. Reissfelder C, Rahbari NN, Koch M, et al. Validation of prognostic scoring systems for patients undergoing resection of colorectal cancer liver metastases. Ann Surg Oncol 2009;16(12):3279–88.

28. Zakaria S, Donohue JH, Que FG, et al. Hepatic resection for colorectal metastases: value for risk scoring systems? Ann Surg 2007;246(2):183–91.

29. Small RM, Lubezky N, Shmueli E, et al. Response to chemotherapy predicts survival following resection of hepatic colo-rectal metastases in patients treated with neoadjuvant therapy. J Surg Oncol 2009;99(2):93–8.

30. Santi V, Trevisani F, Gramenzi A, et al. Semiannual surveillance is superior to annual surveillance for the detection of early hepatocellular carcinoma and patient survival. J Hepatol 2010;53(2):291–7.

31. Baron RL, Oliver III JH, Dodd III GD, et al. Hepatocellular carcinoma: evaluation with biphasic, contrast-enhanced, helical CT. Radiology 1996;199(2):505–11.

32. Rimola J, Forner A, Reig M, et al. Cholangiocarcinoma in cirrhosis: absence of contrast washout in delayed phases by magnetic resonance imaging avoids misdiagnosis of hepatocellular carcinoma. Hepatology 2009;50(3):791–8.

33. Iannaccone R, Piacentini F, Murakami T, et al. Hepatocellular carcinoma in patients with nonalcoholic fatty liver disease: helical CT and MR imaging findings with clinical–pathologic comparison. Radiology 2007;243(2):422–30.

34. Ariff B, Lloyd CR, Khan S, et al. Imaging of liver cancer. World J Gastroenterol 2009;15(11):1289–300.

35. Beavers KL, Semelka RC. MRI evaluation of the liver. Semin Liver Dis 2001;21(2):161–77.

36. Hussain SM, Zondervan PE, Ijzermans JN, et al. Benign versus malignant hepatic nodules: MR imaging findings with pathologic correlation. Radiographics 2002;22(5):1023–36.

37. Semelka RC, Helmberger TK. Contrast agents for MR imaging of the liver. Radiology 2001;218(1):27–38.

38. Lo CM, Lai EC, Liu CL, et al. Laparoscopy and laparoscopic ultrasonography avoid exploratory laparotomy in patients with hepatocellular carcinoma. Ann Surg 1998;227(4):527–32.

39. De Castro SM, Tilleman EH, Busch OR, et al. Diagnostic laparoscopy for primary and secondary liver malignancies: impact of improved imaging and changed criteria for resection. Ann Surg Oncol 2004;11(5):522–9.

40. Ido K, Nakazawa Y, Isoda N, et al. The role of laparoscopic US and laparoscopic US-guided aspiration biopsy in the diagnosis of multicentric hepatocellular carcinoma. Gastrointest Endosc 1999;50(4):523–6.

41. Montorsi M, Santambrogio R, Bianchi P, et al. Laparoscopy with laparoscopic ultrasound for pretreatment staging of hepatocellular carcinoma: a prospective study. J Gastrointest Surg 2001;5(3):312–5.

42. Foroutani A, Garland AM, Berber E, et al. Laparoscopic ultrasound vs triphasic computed tomography for detecting liver tumors. Arch Surg 2000;135(8):933–8.

43. Llovet JM, Di Bisceglie AM, Bruix J, et al. Design and endpoints of clinical trials in hepatocellular carcinoma. J Natl Cancer Inst 2008;100(10):698–711.

44. Liu CL, Fan ST, Lo CM, et al. Management of spontaneous rupture of hepatocellular carcinoma: single-center experience. J Clin Oncol 2001;19(17):3725–32.

45. Henderson JM, Sherman M, Tavill A, et al. AHPBA/AJCC consensus conference on staging

of hepatocellular carcinoma: consensus statement. HPB (Oxford) 2003;5(4):243–50.

46. Nix GA, Dubbelman C, Wilson JH, et al. Prognostic implications of tumor diameter in carcinoma of the head of the pancreas. Cancer 1991;67(2):529–35.

47. Laing FC, Jeffrey Jr. RB, Wing VW, et al. Biliary dilatation: defining the level and cause by real-time US. Radiology 1986;160(1):39–42.

48. Shea JA, Berlin JA, Escarce JJ, et al. Revised estimates of diagnostic test sensitivity and specificity in suspected biliary tract disease. Arch Intern Med 1994;154(22):2573–81.

49. Cronan JJ. US diagnosis of choledocholithiasis: a reappraisal. Radiology 1986;161(1):133–4.

50. Bipat S, Phoa SS, van Delden OM, et al. Ultrasonography, computed tomography and magnetic resonance imaging for diagnosis and determining resectability of pancreatic adenocarcinoma: a meta-analysis. J Comput Assist Tomogr 2005;29(4):438–45.

51. Kalra MK, Maher MM, Mueller PR, et al. State-of-the-art imaging of pancreatic neoplasms. Br J Radiol 2003;76(912):857–65.

52. Loperfido S, Angelini G, Benedetti G, et al. Major early complications from diagnostic and therapeutic ERCP: a prospective multicenter study. Gastrointest Endosc 1998;48(1):1–10.

53. van der Gaag NA, Rauws EA, van Eijck CH, et al. Preoperative biliary drainage for cancer of the head of the pancreas. N Engl J Med 2010;362(2):129–37.

54. Agency for Healthcare Research and Quality. Evidence report/technology assessment: Number 50 Endoscopic retrograde cholangiopancreatography. Summary. Agency for Healthcare Research and Quality; 2002.

55. Long EE, Van DJ, Weinstein S, et al. Computed tomography, endoscopic, laparoscopic, and intraoperative sonography for assessing resectability of pancreatic cancer. Surg Oncol 2005;14(2):105–13.

56. Dewitt J, Devereaux BM, Lehman GA, et al. Comparison of endoscopic ultrasound and computed tomography for the preoperative evaluation of pancreatic cancer: a systematic review. Clin Gastroenterol Hepatol 2006;4(6):717–25.

57. Soriano A, Castells A, Ayuso C, et al. Preoperative staging and tumor resectability assessment of pancreatic cancer: prospective study comparing endoscopic ultrasonography, helical computed tomography, magnetic resonance imaging, and angiography. Am J Gastroenterol 2004;99(3):492–501.

58. Hewitt MJ, McPhail MJ, Possamai L, et al. EUS-guided FNA for diagnosis of solid pancreatic neoplasms: a meta-analysis. Gastrointest Endosc 2012;75(2):319–31.

59. Heinrich S, Goerres GW, Schafer M, et al. Positron emission tomography/computed tomography influences on the management of resectable pancreatic cancer and its cost-effectiveness. Ann Surg 2005;242(2):235–43.

60. Orlando LA, Kulasingam SL, Matchar DB. Meta-analysis: the detection of pancreatic malignancy with positron emission tomography. Aliment Pharmacol Ther 2004;20(10):1063–70.

61. Jimenez RE, Warshaw AL, Rattner DW, et al. Impact of laparoscopic staging in the treatment of pancreatic cancer. Arch Surg 2000;135(4):409–14.

62. Jimenez RE, Warshaw AL. Fernandez-Del Castillo C. Laparoscopy and peritoneal cytology in the staging of pancreatic cancer. J Hepatobiliary Pancreat Surg 2000;7(1):15–20.

63. Van Heek NT, De Castro SM, van Eijck CH, et al. The need for a prophylactic gastrojejunostomy for unresectable periampullary cancer: a prospective randomized multicenter trial with special focus on assessment of quality of life. Ann Surg 2003;238(6):894–902.

64. Nieveen van Dijkum EJ, Romijn MG, Terwee CB, et al. Laparoscopic staging and subsequent palliation in patients with peripancreatic carcinoma. Ann Surg 2003;237(1):66–73.

65. Pedrazzoli S, Pasquali C, Sperti C. General aspects of surgical treatment of pancreatic cancer. Dig Surg 1999;16(4):265–75.

66. Siriwardana HP, Siriwardena AK. Systematic review of outcome of synchronous portal-superior mesenteric vein resection during pancreatectomy for cancer. Br J Surg 2006;93(6):662–73.

67. Lu DS, Vedantham S, Krasny RM, et al. Two-phase helical CT for pancreatic tumors: pancreatic versus hepatic phase enhancement of tumor, pancreas, and vascular structures. Radiology 1996;199(3):697–701.

68. Ramacciato G, Mercantini P, Petrucciani N, et al. Does portal–superior mesenteric vein invasion still indicate irresectability for pancreatic carcinoma? Ann Surg Oncol 2009;16(4):817–25.

69. Muller MW, Friess H, Koninger J, et al. Factors influencing survival after bypass procedures in patients with advanced pancreatic adenocarcinomas. Am J Surg 2008;195(2):221–8.

70. Glanemann M, Shi B, Liang F, et al. Surgical strategies for treatment of malignant pancreatic tumors: extended, standard or local surgery? World J Surg Oncol 2008;6:123.

71. Garcea G, Dennison AR, Pattenden CJ, et al. Survival following curative resection for pancreatic ductal adenocarcinoma. A systematic review of the literature. JOP 2008;9(2):99–132.

72. Phoa SS, Tilleman EH, van Delden OM, et al. Value of CT criteria in predicting survival in patients with potentially resectable pancreatic head carcinoma. J Surg Oncol 2005;91(1):33–40.

73. Allema JH, Reinders ME, van Gulik TM, et al. Results of pancreaticoduodenectomy for ampullary

carcinoma and analysis of prognostic factors for survival. Surgery 1995;117(3):247–53.

74. Wetter LA, Ring EJ, Pellegrini CA, et al. Differential diagnosis of sclerosing cholangiocarcinomas of the common hepatic duct (Klatskin tumors). Am J Surg 1991;161(1):57–62.

75. Saini S. Imaging of the hepatobiliary tract. N Engl J Med 1997;336(26):1889–94.

76. Hann LE, Greatrex KV, Bach AM, et al. Cholangiocarcinoma at the hepatic hilus: sonographic findings. Am J Roentgenol 1997;168(4):985–9.

77. Manfredi R, Barbaro B, Masselli G, et al. Magnetic resonance imaging of cholangiocarcinoma. Semin Liver Dis 2004;24(2):155–64.

78. Boberg KM, Jebsen P, Clausen OP, et al. Diagnostic benefit of biliary brush cytology in cholangiocarcinoma in primary sclerosing cholangitis. J Hepatol 2006;45(4):568–74.

79. Kim JY, Kim MH, Lee TY, et al. Clinical role of ^{18}F-FDG PET-CT in suspected and potentially operable cholangiocarcinoma: a prospective study compared with conventional imaging. Am J Gastroenterol 2008;103(5):1145–51.

80. Moon CM, Bang S, Chung JB, et al. Usefulness of ^{18}F-fluorodeoxyglucose positron emission tomography in differential diagnosis and staging of cholangiocarcinomas. J Gastroenterol Hepatol 2008;23(5):759–65.

81. Corvera CU, Blumgart LH, Akhurst T, et al. ^{18}F-fluorodeoxyglucose positron emission tomography influences management decisions in patients with biliary cancer. J Am Coll Surg 2008;206(1):57–65.

82. Petrowsky H, Wildbrett P, Husarik DB, et al. Impact of integrated positron emission tomography and computed tomography on staging and management of gallbladder cancer and cholangiocarcinoma. J Hepatol 2006;45(1):43–50.

83. Kluge R, Schmidt F, Caca K, et al. Positron emission tomography with [^{18}F]fluoro-2-deoxy-D-glucose for diagnosis and staging of bile duct cancer. Hepatology 2001;33(5):1029–35.

84. Nieveen van Dijkum EJ, de Wit LT, van Delden OM, et al. Staging laparoscopy and laparoscopic ultrasonography in more than 400 patients with upper gastrointestinal carcinoma. J Am Coll Surg 1999;189(5):459–65.

85. Tilleman EH, De Castro SM, Busch OR, et al. Diagnostic laparoscopy and laparoscopic ultrasound for staging of patients with malignant proximal bile duct obstruction. J Gastrointest Surg 2002;6(3):426–30.

86. Weber SM, DeMatteo RP, Fong Y, et al. Staging laparoscopy in patients with extrahepatic biliary carcinoma. Analysis of 100 patients. Ann Surg 2002;235(3):392–9.

87. Ruys AT, Busch OR, Gouma DJ, et al. Staging laparoscopy for hilar cholangiocarcinoma: is it still worthwhile? Ann Surg Oncol 2011;18(9):2647–53.

88. Smits NJ, Reeders JW. Imaging and staging of biliopancreatic malignancy: role of ultrasound. Ann Oncol 1999;10(Suppl. 4):20–4.

89. Jarnagin WR, Fong Y, DeMatteo RP, et al. Staging, resectability, and outcome in 225 patients with hilar cholangiocarcinoma. Ann Surg 2001;234(4):507–17.

90. Burke EC, Jarnagin WR, Hochwald SN, et al. Hilar cholangiocarcinoma: patterns of spread, the importance of hepatic resection for curative operation, and a presurgical clinical staging system. Ann Surg 1998;228(3):385–94.

91. Minagawa M, Ikai I, Matsuyama Y, et al. Staging of hepatocellular carcinoma: assessment of the Japanese TNM and AJCC/UICC TNM systems in a cohort of 13,772 patients in Japan. Ann Surg 2007;245(6):909–22.

92. Bilimoria KY, Bentrem DJ, Ko CY, et al. Validation of the 6th edition AJCC Pancreatic Cancer Staging System: report from the National Cancer Database. Cancer 2007;110(4):738–44.

93. O'Connell JB, Maggard MA, Manunga Jr. J, et al. Survival after resection of ampullary carcinoma: a national population-based study. Ann Surg Oncol 2008;15(7):1820–7.

94. Miyakawa S, Ishihara S, Horiguchi A, et al. Biliary tract cancer treatment: 5,584 results from the Biliary Tract Cancer Statistics Registry from 1998 to 2004 in Japan. J Hepatobiliary Pancreat Surg 2009;16(1):1–7.

95. DeOliveira ML, Schulick RD, Nimura Y, et al. New staging system and a registry for perihilar cholangiocarcinoma. Hepatology 2011;53(4):1363–71.

4

Benign liver lesions

Rowan W. Parks
O. James Garden
Jean-Francois Gigot

Introduction

Benign liver lesions are common and may be difficult to differentiate from primary and secondary hepatic tumours. Such may be identified as an incidental finding when radiological investigation is undertaken for unrelated intra-abdominal disease or when coexistent hepatic pathology is present, giving rise to problems of diagnosis and management. Although these lesions may be of congenital origin, most are of unknown aetiology. They generally are asymptomatic but, since they are often slow growing, they may produce symptoms caused by mass effect or compression of adjacent organs. Rarely, such lesions may give rise to acute symptoms resulting from necrosis, thrombosis, haemorrhage or rupture.

Routine liver function tests are invariably normal unless the lesion compresses the biliary confluence or common bile duct, and are therefore of value in guiding the clinician towards a diagnosis of benign disease. Nonetheless, complications such as haemorrhage and necrosis may be associated with increases in serum transaminase levels. Elevation in tumour markers and the development of paraneoplastic syndromes such as erythrocytosis, hyperglycaemia and hypercalcaemia are observed rarely.

Characterisation of hepatic lesions is provided by imaging tests of the liver. Ultrasonography (US), computed tomography (CT) and magnetic resonance imaging (MRI) are the cornerstones of diagnosis and often complement one another. More recently, positron emission tomography (PET) has shown promise. Abdominal US will differentiate cystic forms from solid lesions, whereas CT and MRI using intravenous contrast and delayed imaging will not only detect the number and size of the lesions, but also allow further characterisation. Haemangioma and focal nodular hyperplasia are relatively easily confirmed by modern imaging techniques, whereas differentiation of liver cell adenoma from well-differentiated hepatocellular carcinoma remains challenging.

Biopsy should only be performed in those patients who are being considered candidates for surgical intervention and only where the results of biopsy might influence further management. Biopsy is contraindicated for patients with suspected haemangioma, haemangioendothelioma and cysts suspected of being echinococcal in origin. Needle biopsy or fine-needle aspiration cytology of suspected hypervascular solid tumours may result in haemorrhage, sampling error, misdiagnosis and needle-tract tumour seeding. Tissue from a haemangioma may resemble fibrosis, and focal nodular hyperplasia may resemble cirrhosis. Needle samples of hepatic adenoma may be interpreted as normal tissue and may be difficult to differentiate from well-differentiated hepatocellular carcinoma. In selected patients with tumours of unclear nature, biopsy may be useful by a percutaneous approach for deep-sited lesions or by a laparoscopic approach for superficial and accessible lesions.

The general surgeon should be thoroughly familiar with the gross appearance, clinical significance and natural history of these benign lesions as the treatment strategy may vary from simple observation (of focal nodular hyperplasia) to complex radical hepatic resection (of hepatocellular adenoma). Most symptomatic benign liver lesions are excised; however, hepatic resection, if performed without the proper indications, can prove hazardous.

Classification

Although a variety of benign liver tumours have been described, many are rare and a detailed description of these various lesions is beyond the scope of the current text (Box 4.1). The majority of benign hepatic lesions encountered in clinical practice include haemangioma, liver cell adenoma, focal nodular hyperplasia, bile duct hamartoma and hepatic cysts. For completeness, a brief résumé is provided of less common and miscellaneous lesions that may give rise to diagnostic and management dilemmas.

Box 4.1 • Classification of benign tumours of the liver

Epithelial tumours
Hepatocellular
- Nodular transformation
- Focal nodular hyperplasia
- Hepatocellular adenoma

Cholangiocellular
- Bile duct adenoma
- Biliary cystadenoma

Mesenchymal tumours
Tumours of adipose tissue
- Lipoma
- Myelolipoma
- Angiomyolipoma

Tumours of muscle tissue
- Leiomyoma

Tumours of blood vessels
- Infantile haemangioendothelioma

Haemangioma
- Hereditary haemorrhagic telangiectasia
- Peliosis hepatic

Tumours of mesothelial tissue
- Benign mesothelioma

Mixed mesenchymal and epithelial tumours
- Mesenchymal hamartoma
- Benign teratoma

Miscellaneous
- Adrenal rest tumour
- Pancreatic heterotopia
- Inflammatory pseudotumour

Reproduced from Ishak KG, Goodman ZD. Benign tumours of the liver. In: Berk JE (ed.) Bockus gastroenterology, 4th edn. Philadelphia: WB Saunders, 1985. With permission from Elsevier.

Haemangiomas

Haemangiomas are the most common benign hepatic tumours of mesenchymal origin. Small capillary haemangiomas are more common than the larger cavernous haemangiomas and are often multiple. Small lesions are asymptomatic and an incidental finding; however, they may give rise to diagnostic difficulty in patients undergoing investigation. Once accurate diagnosis has been made no further therapy is needed. Haemangiomas are probably of congenital origin and do not undergo malignant transformation. The incidence of cavernous haemangioma in autopsy series varies considerably but has been reported to be as high as 8%. These lesions are the second most common hepatic tumour in the USA, exceeded only by hepatic metastases.[1] With the more widespread use of sensitive imaging studies of the upper abdomen, the identification of such lesions as an incidental finding will undoubtedly be more common. Cavernous haemangiomas may reach an enormous size, and lesions weighing up to 6 kg are well documented. There is poor agreement in the literature as to the exact definition of what constitutes a giant haemangioma. Some are defined as greater than 4 cm in diameter, others greater than 6 cm. Such haemangiomas are usually solitary, but multiple lesions have been described in about 10% of cases.[1] They may be associated with similar lesions in the skin and other organs. Lesions are usually evenly distributed throughout the liver and its substance but large lesions situated peripherally may form a pedicle.

Pathology

Cavernous haemangiomas are seen most frequently in patients in the third to fifth decades of life. They are more common and more likely to become clinically manifest at a younger age in women, are more common with increasing parity and may enlarge during pregnancy.[2–4] This indicates a possible role of female sex hormones in their development, although an association with the oral contraceptive pill has not been proven. The aetiology of liver haemangiomas is still unclear but they may represent benign congenital hamartomas. These lesions appear to grow by progressive ectasia rather than hyperplasia or hypertrophy. At operation,

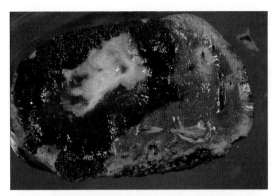

Figure 4.1 • A large haemangioma showing the characteristic honeycomb feature with a central scar.

or traumatic rupture of haemangioma is a very rare complication.[4] A past review of the literature included only 28 reports of spontaneous, life-threatening haemorrhage due to liver haemangiomas, a minimal figure considering the prevalence of the tumour.[7] Thrombocytopenia and hypofibrinogenaemia have also been associated with cavernous haemangiomas of the liver (Kasabach–Merritt syndrome), and this effect may be related to consumption of coagulation factors.[1]

A large haemangioma on the liver edge may be palpable on inspiration. It is difficult to differentiate the consistency of a haemangioma from normal liver through the abdominal wall unless it has calcified or undergone thrombosis or fibrosis. Occasionally, a bruit may be heard over a haemangioma, but this is a non-specific finding. Liver function tests are normal in the patient presenting without complication.

Such lesions are generally hyperechoic on ultrasound examination (**Fig. 4.2**). Farges et al.[5] found the diagnosis to be established by US alone in 80% of patients with haemangiomas smaller than 6 cm. However, this investigation alone cannot differentiate a haemangioma from hepatocellular carcinoma, liver cell adenoma, focal nodular hyperplasia or a solitary metastasis. CT has proven useful in the diagnosis of haemangiomas.[8] Prior to intravenous contrast infusion, CT shows the haemangioma to consist of a well-demarcated hypodense mass. After the intravenous injection of contrast medium, serial scans will reveal a zone of progressive enhancement peripherally that varies in thickness and often demonstrates an irregular margin (**Fig. 4.3**). The centre of the haemangioma remains hypodense and the overall lesion size does not change. Over the past decade MRI has emerged as a highly accurate technique for diagnosing and characterising liver haemangioma, with a reported 90% sensitivity, 95% specificity and 93% accuracy[9,10] (**Fig. 4.4**). Haemangiomas are typically very bright (light bulb sign) on T2-weighted images and show peripheral nodular enhancement on dynamic gadolinium-enhanced T1-weighted images.[11] Single-photon emission CT (SPECT) using technetium-99m-labelled red blood cells has been shown to increase the spatial resolution of planar scintigraphy and has been shown to have a sensitivity and accuracy close to that of MRI.[12] Fluorodeoxyglucose (FDG)-PET has been reported as useful to differentiate giant hepatic cavernous haemangiomas from malignant hepatic tumours.[13] In practice, a combination of these diagnostic modalities is preferred. Superficial lesions may be identified incidentally during abdominal laparoscopic procedures and should be recognised by their gross appearance and characteristic compressibility when gently palpated with a laparoscopic instrument. Needle biopsy of vascular liver lesions

they appear as well-circumscribed, reddish-purple, hypervascular lesions, which may be multilobulated or have a smooth surface. When sectioned, the lesion will partially collapse due to the escape of blood, and it has a honeycombed cut surface. There may be gross evidence of thrombosis, fibrosis or calcification (**Fig. 4.1**). Microscopically, haemangiomas are composed of cystically dilated vascular spaces, lined by endothelial cells and separated by fibrous septa of varying thickness. There is usually a clear plane between haemangioma and normal liver tissue as these lesions are usually encapsulated by a rim of fibrous tissue.

Clinical presentation

Most haemangiomas are asymptomatic but subcapsular lesions and larger lesions causing compression of adjacent organs may produce clinical features. Symptoms may include vague abdominal pain or fullness, early satiety, nausea, vomiting or fever. Rare presentations include obstructive jaundice, gastric outlet obstruction and spontaneous rupture. Although abdominal pain or discomfort is the most frequent indication for removing a liver haemangioma, it must be remembered that associated pathology may coexist and be the cause of the symptoms. Farges et al.[5] reported that 42% of the patients in their series had other pathology, such as gallbladder disease, liver cysts, gastroduodenal ulcers or hiatus hernia. The difficulty of attributing symptoms to the haemangioma is evidenced by the occasional persistence of symptoms after resection.[6]

Pain related to an uncomplicated haemangioma is likely due to stretching or inflammation of Glisson's capsule. Occasionally, large lesions located in the left lobe of the liver may cause pressure effects on adjacent structures and infarction or necrosis may account for the sudden onset of pain. Intra-abdominal haemorrhage due to spontaneous

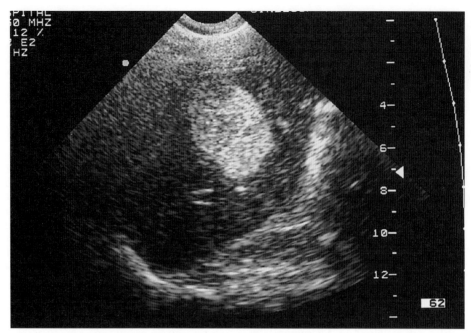

Figure 4.2 • Hyperechoic appearance of haemangioma on ultrasound examination.

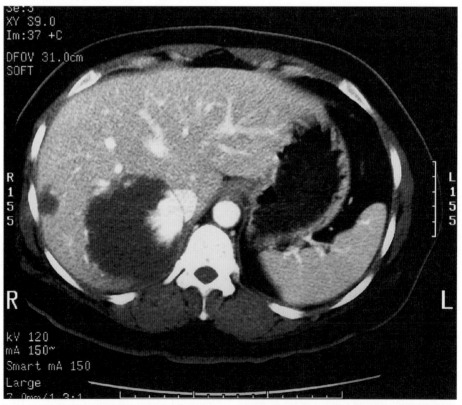

Figure 4.3 • CT scan demonstrating peripheral enhancement of a haemangioma after intravenous injection of contrast material.

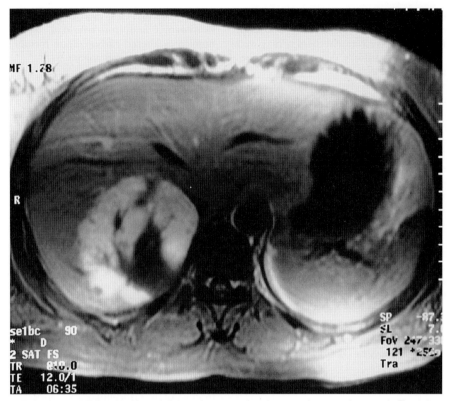

Figure 4.4 • T1-weighted MRI scan with gadolinium demonstrating the same haemangioma as in Fig. 4.3.

should not be performed. Diagnostic uncertainty is seldom a problem with cavernous haemangiomas, except in lesions not large enough to show cavernous characteristics.

Management

A wide range of management strategies from observation to resection has been advocated for such lesions. Simple reassurance should be given to patients in whom small lesions (i.e. <6 cm) have been detected as an incidental finding. For larger cavernous haemangiomas, consideration should be given to weighing the risk of operation against the natural history of untreated lesions. Trastek et al.[4] followed up 34 untreated patients over a maximum period of 15 years. No patient had a lesion that bled, none reported abdominal symptoms and no patient had compromise of quality of life. A further report from the same group, when the observation period had been extended to 21 years, reported two patients with large symptomatic lesions of questionable resectability at initial presentation who remained symptomatic but with little documented growth of the haemangioma. The remainder were asymptomatic and there was no instance of rupture.[14] Two more recent longitudinal

studies have supported the accepted view that asymptomatic giant haemangiomas of the liver can be managed safely by observation.[15,16]

Nichols et al.[14] reported no operative deaths and the single postoperative complication was a wound infection in 41 patients undergoing resection of such lesions. In a similar series of 69 patients, Weimann et al.[17] reported no postoperative deaths and a morbidity rate of 19%. Also in this series were 104 patients with haemangioma and 53 patients with focal nodular hyperplasia who were observed for a median of 32 months (range 7–132 months). There was no evidence of malignant transformation or tumour rupture. Therefore, safe resection is possible but there is no evidence that asymptomatic patients should undergo resection since the risk of rupture is minimal.[5,18]

When treatment is indicated, because of highly symptomatic or complicated lesions, surgical excision provides the only effective therapy. Reports of the effectiveness of hepatic arterial ligation are anecdotal. Arterial ligation or embolisation may, however, be considered for the temporary control of haemorrhage in exceptional circumstances in order to allow time for transfer of a patient for definitive management in a specialist centre. The benefits of radiation therapy and corticosteroids have not been well documented and are inconsistent. It is possible that the success of non-resectional therapy may well be largely due to the naturally occurring spontaneous involution of these lesions.

The choice of excision requires consideration of the size and anatomical location of the lesion. Haemangiomas can often be enucleated[19] to avoid loss of functional liver parenchyma, diminish blood loss and minimise postoperative bile leakage, although in some cases it may be wiser and safer to perform a formal anatomical liver resection. At enucleation, a plane between the lesion and the liver is easily found and this can be developed by blunt dissection. This can be facilitated by the use of the Cavitron ultrasonic surgical aspiration system (CUSA™) with concomitant control of the inflow vessels. Laparoscopic resection of liver haemangioma is increasingly reported,[20] and orthotopic liver transplantation has been used successfully to treat symptomatic patients with technically unresectable complicated giant haemangioma.[21]

> ✔ Liver haemangioma rarely causes complications and resection should only be considered for symptomatic lesions.

Liver cell adenoma

Although liver cell adenoma requires differentiation from any solid hepatic lesion, it is often considered alongside focal nodular hyperplasia.[22]

Hepatic adenomas arise in otherwise normal liver and present as a focal abnormality or mass. The true prevalence of the disease is difficult to assess but 90% develop in women in the third to fifth decades of life.[23] These tumours were rarely reported before 1960, but their apparent increase in incidence since then corresponded with the introduction of oral contraceptives at that time. The causal relationship between liver cell adenoma and oral contraceptives was first suggested by Baum et al.[24] in 1973. Ninety per cent of patients with liver cell adenomas have used oral contraceptives and the annual incidence among oral contraceptive users has been reported to be 3–4 per 100 000 if the contraceptives are taken for more than 2 years. The risk of developing a liver cell adenoma increases with the dose and duration of use of the contraceptive preparation.[23] Furthermore, pregnancy has been associated with increased symptoms and an increased risk of complications in patients with liver cell adenomas.[23,25] The introduction of low-oestrogen-containing contraceptive preparations may result in a reduction in incidence, although adenomas are also associated with non-contraceptive oestrogen use, androgenic

steroid use, diabetes, glycogen storage disease, galactosaemia and iron overload. This association implicates altered carbohydrate metabolism in the formation of liver cell adenomas.[26]

Pathology

Liver cell adenomas are usually solitary, round and occasionally encapsulated. Lesions are soft and smooth surfaced, but occasionally may be pedunculated. The cut surface has a pale yellow fleshy appearance unless haemorrhage and necrosis produce discoloration (**Fig. 4.5**). They are sharply demarcated from normal liver but without a fibrous capsule. Approximately 12–30% of these tumours are multiple, and if more than 10 adenomas are present, the condition is regarded as liver adenomatosis.[27] This may be a separate pathological entity from isolated liver cell adenoma as both sexes are equally affected and oral contraceptive usage is unusual. Microscopically, there are uniform masses of benign-appearing hepatocytes without ducts or portal triads. The hepatocytes appear paler than normal because of increased glycogen or fat content. Venous lakes (peliosis hepatis) are often seen.

Historically, liver cell adenomas have been considered precancerous. Rooks et al.[23] reported the finding of hepatocellular carcinoma 5 years after resection of a liver cell adenoma, and other authors have recognised unequivocal areas of hepatocellular carcinoma adjacent to or within liver cell adenomas.[23,28,29] Also reported is the development of hepatocellular carcinoma several years after diagnosis of biopsy-proven benign liver cell adenoma.[26,30,31] More recent studies have shown that there are different subtypes of liver cell adenoma and that the risk of malignant transformation varies. Liver cell adenoma occurring in men and large tumours are

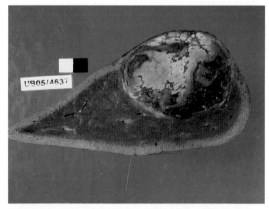

Figure 4.5 • Large liver cell adenoma showing the pale yellow fleshy appearance of its cut surface. There are areas of discoloration from haemorrhage.

at highest risk, but telangiectatic or unclassified liver cell adenomas have an increased risk whereas steatotic liver cell adenomas have a lower risk.[32] Recent innovations in molecular biology and immunohistochemistry have identified β-catenine mutation as a significant risk factor for malignant transformation.[33,34]

Clinical presentation

These lesions present frequently with abdominal pain from haemorrhage into the tumour or adjacent liver. Some patients develop severe acute abdominal pain due to intraperitoneal rupture and haemoperitoneum, which may present as hypovolaemic shock. The risk of bleeding is reported as 21–50% and is not related to tumour size.[32] Up to one-third of patients sense the presence of an abdominal mass. The remainder of adenomas are discovered incidentally at autopsy, laparotomy or during radiological assessment for another problem.

Although the clinical presentation may be suggestive of liver cell adenoma, definitive preoperative diagnosis may be difficult. Liver function tests are generally normal unless tumour necrosis or haemorrhage is present. Anaemia may therefore occur. US can detect small adenomas, which characteristically display a lesion of mixed echogeneity and heterogeneous texture. CT may show evidence of recent haemorrhage or necrosis. Lesions are generally hypodense prior to infusion of contrast medium and demonstrate a wide range of densities after intravenous contrast administration. They often appear as well-demarcated, fat-containing or haemorrhagic lesions on MRI. Conventional radiological imaging may not be able to differentiate between liver cell adenoma and hepatocellular carcinoma; however, promising results have been reported with the use of FDG-PET to differentiate benign from malignant lesions.[35]

Percutaneous needle biopsy or fine-needle aspiration cytology undertaken prior to referral is often misleading. Biopsy of these vascular tumours risks precipitating haemorrhage, and even an experienced histopathologist may experience difficulty in differentiating between liver cell adenoma and a well-differentiated hepatocellular carcinoma.

Management

In the symptomatic patient, surgical intervention will be required. A minority of patients will present with intraperitoneal bleeding, the cause of which might only be identified at laparotomy. Most deaths from liver cell adenomas are secondary to haemorrhage, with intraperitoneal bleeding carrying a 20% mortality rate in one series.[22] Hepatic arterial embolisation[36] or packing might be considered to facilitate transfer of the patient to a specialist centre. Definitive control of bleeding is best achieved by formal hepatic resection. In some patients, haemorrhage may be contained within the liver or subcapsularly. If the patient remains haemodynamically stable, it may be prudent to defer elective surgical intervention to enable resolution of the haematoma, thereby enabling a more limited hepatic resection (**Fig. 4.6**). Orthotopic liver transplantation has been described for unresectable benign liver tumours with severe symptoms and for patients with multiple adenomas.[17,37]

For the asymptomatic patient, surgical intervention should be considered; however, with new insights and understanding of the clinical–pathological and radiological features and recent innovations in molecular biology and immunohistochemistry, selected patients can now be managed conservatively.[32,38] Steatotic liver cell adenomas have a minimal risk of bleeding or malignant transformation. Furthermore, several case reports document regression of liver cell tumours following cessation of oral contraceptives,[39,40] although this is not a consistent finding, and development of hepatocellular carcinoma in the site of adenoma regression has been reported.[32] Non-operative discrimination between liver cell adenoma and hepatocellular carcinoma remains challenging.

Focal nodular hyperplasia

Focal nodular hyperplasia (FNH) is a hyperplastic process in which all the normal constituents of the liver are present but in a disorganised pattern. The incidence of FNH has been increasing, although this is more likely to be related to improvements in abdominal imaging. Many lesions are still found incidentally at laparotomy or autopsy. About 90% of cases occur in women, primarily in the second and third decades, although the condition may also afflict older women and a small number of men and children. The incidence of FNH does not appear to have increased since the introduction of oral contraceptives; however, some investigators have suggested that oral contraceptives may foster growth or increased vascularity of these lesions, and they have been implicated in the few cases that present with haemorrhage.

Pathology

FNH consists of a firm lobulated localised lesion in an otherwise normal liver. These nodules are generally several centimetres in size and occasionally can grow much larger. Lesions are well circumscribed

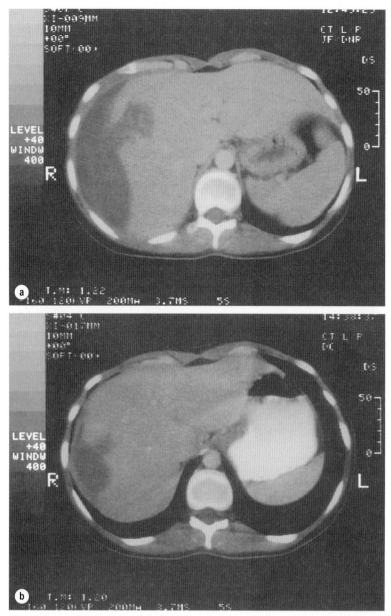

Figure 4.6 • (a) CT scan showing extensive subcapsular haematoma resulting from spontaneous haemorrhage into the liver. **(b)** CT scan taken 2 months later showing a reduction in the size of the haematoma. Contrast is now present within a small adenoma lying adjacent to the haematoma.

but have no capsule. On sectioning, there is generally a central scar with fibrous radiations which account for the nodular and sometimes umbilicated appearance. Lesions are usually similar or slightly lighter in colour than adjacent normal hepatic parenchyma (**Fig. 4.7**). FNH is multifocal in up to 20% of cases and may coexist with haemangiomas in 5–10% of patients.[1]

Microscopically, FNH looks similar to cirrhosis, with regenerating nodules and connective tissue septa. The lesions consist of many normal hepatic cells mixed with bile ducts or ductules and divided by fibrous septa. The septa contain numerous bile ducts and a moderate, predominantly lymphocytic, infiltration, and there is usually some evidence of mild cholestasis.

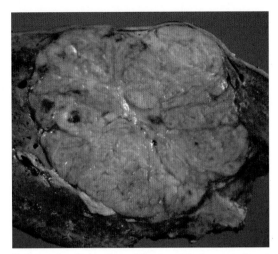

Figure 4.7 • Cut surface of focal nodular hyperplasia showing a central scar.

Clinical features

FNH is a benign process that rarely causes symptoms but the main difficulty lies in differentiating this process from other hepatic lesions. Less than 10% of patients with FNH have symptoms, the most common being mild, vague right upper quadrant abdominal pain. Acute symptoms due to haemorrhage are exceptional.

CT and MRI are important imaging modalities to characterise FNH. Classical CT appearance of FNH is of hyperattenuation during the arterial phase that becomes isoattenuating during the portal and delayed phase (**Fig. 4.8**). In approximately 40–60% of patients, the central scar will inially be hypoattenuating but becomes hyperintense in the delayed phase due to delayed washout of contrast. Typical MRI features of FNH are iso- or hypointensity on T1-weighted images, slight hyper- or isointensity on T2-weighted images and the presence of a central scar that appears hyperintense on T2-weighted imaging. After administration of gadolinium chelates, the appearance is similar to that seen on contrast-enhanced CT, i.e. dramatic enhancement in the arterial phase followed by isointensity during the portal venous phase with a high-intensity signal in the scar during the delayed phase. Cherqui et al.[41] reported a 70% sensitivity and 98% specificity for MRI in detecting FNH.

Management

Treatment of a patient with FNH depends essentially on the certainty of the diagnosis. In asymptomatic patients with the typical features of FNH unequivocally demonstrated by one or more radiological

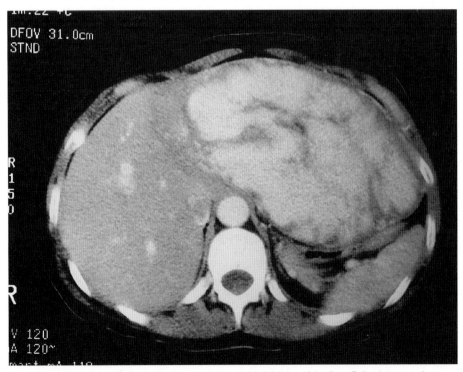

Figure 4.8 • CT scan demonstrating a large vascular lesion in the left lobe of the liver. Following resection, histopathology confirmed this to be a large area of focal nodular hyperplasia.

investigation, no further treatment is required. However, a malignant tumour will be found in up to 6% of patients with an undetermined, presumed benign lesion.[42] FNH on occasions may be difficult to differentiate from liver cell adenoma. If this is the case, it is advisable to proceed to biopsy of these lesions before committing to hepatic resection.

Data on the natural history of FNH have been gathered by Kerlin et al.[43] Of 41 patients studied, 11 had lesions found incidentally at autopsy. Sixteen patients had open surgical biopsies of clinically apparent lesions, with the majority of the lesions left in situ. These patients were observed for up to 15 years, during which time none of the lesions bled or increased in size. The vast majority of patients with FNH can be managed conservatively, with surgical excision (enucleation or resection) only rarely considered for large symptomatic or complicated lesions.

Nodular regenerative hyperplasia (macroregenerative nodules)

This is a benign proliferative process in which the normal hepatic architecture is entirely replaced by diffuse regenerative nodules of hepatocytes. Autopsy reports suggest the prevalence of nodular regenerative hyperplasia (NRH) is approximately 2%. It predominantly occurs in older patients, and is often associated with lymphoproliferative and rheumatological diseases or develops after organ transplantation.

The majority of patients are asymptomatic, are diagnosed incidentally and require no further treatment. The most common physical findings are splenomegaly and hepatomegaly. A small percentage of patients may develop portal hypertension due to compression of intrahepatic portal radicles by the regenerating nodules, and present with variceal bleeding or ascites. Rarely, patients may develop hepatic failure and in some instances have undergone liver transplantation. Liver function tests are usually normal or slightly elevated, and the radiological features are relatively non-specific. The diagnosis of NRH is confirmed on the gross and histological findings of the liver. Macroscopically, the hepatic parenchyma is entirely replaced by nodules varying in size from 0.1 to 4 cm. The histological findings of NRH are regenerating hepatocytes separated by atrophic parenchyma, curvilinear compression of the central lobule and absence of fibrous tissue or bands of scar tissue between the nodules. NRH may be suspected when a patient presents with symptoms of portal hypertension and a liver biopsy that fails to show cirrhosis or is interpreted as

being normal. Confirmation may require targeted liver biopsy. Liver cell dysplasia is a common finding in NRH and there are a small number of case reports of hepatocellular carcinoma developing in livers with NRH, leading some authors to suggest that NRH may represent a premalignant condition in some patients.

Bile duct adenoma (bile duct hamartoma)

Surgeons should be aware of bile duct adenomas since they are common and may be mistaken at operation as liver metastases. They do not manifest clinically but are incidental findings at laparotomy or autopsy.[44] They rarely exceed 1 cm in diameter and appear as raised greyish-white areas on the liver capsule. Histologically, they are composed of a mass of mature bile ducts surrounded by fibrous stroma, which blends indistinctly into the adjacent liver. They require to be distinguished from the nests of hyperplastic bile ducts that occur in focal nodular hyperplasia and also in undifferentiated adenocarcinoma of the biliary tract type.

The only clinical significance of bile duct adenoma is its possible confusion at laparoscopy or laparotomy with metastatic carcinoma, cholangiocarcinoma or other focal hepatic lesions. When encountered, excisional biopsy should be performed to confirm the diagnosis.

Hepatic pseudotumours

Hepatic pseudotumours may be considerable in size and can occur in any age group. These lesions are essentially overgrowths of chronic inflammatory tissue but may be mistaken for other neoplastic lesions of the liver.[45] The aetiology is not known but they may be secondary to thrombosis and infarction of a major vessel, represent a form of immune reaction, or result from resolution of an abscess. They may be either hyperechoic or hypoechoic on US and appear as a hypodense lesion on CT. Such pseudotumours may require resection to prevent reactivation of infection. The clinical history and presentation are likely to point towards a diagnosis of pseudotumour.

Miscellaneous benign tumours

Mesenchymal hamartomas are exceptional and probably of congenital origin. They are most commonly described in infants under 12 months; however, a few have been documented in adults.[46]

Although they are entirely benign, hamartomas can compromise the liver and the individual by progressive enlargement, and therefore these lesions should be resected. Microscopically, the tumour is characterised by a myxoid background of highly cellular embryonal mesenchyme, throughout which are found random groups of hepatic cells, bile ducts and multiple cysts, which may produce a honeycomb appearance. Recurrence following excision has not been reported.

Primary myxoma in the adult is exceptional. Primary lipomas are rarely described in life but have been identified incidentally at post-mortem.[1] Other solid tumours include leiomyoma, mesothelioma and fibroma. Benign teratoma of the liver has been reported but this generally occurs in children.

Liver abscess

The incidence of pyogenic liver abscess has remained relatively constant over the past century despite earlier diagnosis and treatment of underlying causes and more aggressive antibiotic therapies. In recent years, the decrease in cases resulting from haematogenous spread from infected foci has been mirrored by an increase in cases secondary to hepatobiliary pathology. In almost half the patients reviewed over a 5-year period, biliary sepsis was the major predisposing factor.[47] In 20% of patients, the presumed source of infection was from the portal route, but few cases were thought to have arisen from systemic infection. Hepatic abscesses secondary to ascending cholangitis are often multiple due to the distribution of the infecting organism along the biliary ductal system.[48] Early reports implicated choledocholithiasis as the main causative factor; however, more recent series document malignant biliary obstruction as a more common aetiological factor.[47,49]

Infections within organs drained by the portal vein are dependent on the underlying illness. In the early literature, portal vein pyelophlebitis secondary to appendicitis was often implicated, whereas diverticulitis, pancreatitis and diffuse peritonitis are now more frequently reported. Haematogenous spread from non-gastrointestinal sources accounts for 10–20% of liver abscesses and occurs most typically with bacterial endocarditis, other conditions associated with systemic bacteraemia such as urinary sepsis, pneumonia and osteomyelitis or following intravenous drug abuse. Abscesses may also occur from direct extension into the liver parenchyma from localised perforation of an adjacent viscus, such as the gallbladder, colon, stomach or duodenum. In a significant percentage of patients (approximately 15–35%), the aetiology of hepatic abscess remains obscure (cryptogenic abscess) despite extensive clinical and pathological investigation.

Clinical presentation

Patients present with a spectrum of symptoms and signs, the most consistent being fever associated with malaise, anorexia, weight loss and upper abdominal pain. Jaundice is a feature in approximately 50% of cases. Laboratory studies typically reflect a systemic bacterial infection. Commonly reported findings are of leucocytosis, anaemia, hyperbilirubinaemia, hypoalbuminaemia and raised levels of acute-phase proteins. US is invariably diagnostic and will often demonstrate a fluid-filled cavity. There may be a hyperechoic wall, the presence of which is dependent on the chronicity of the abscess. CT may be useful to exclude the presence of other abscesses and to identify a primary source within the abdomen (**Fig. 4.9**). Magnetic resonance cholangiography should be undertaken in patients with biliary symptoms, obstructive liver function tests or a dilated common bile duct, and can be combined with cross-sectional MRI to identify any hepatic parenchymal abnormality. Barium enema or colonoscopy may be indicated to exclude a colonic source of portal pyaemia.

Management

The key to successful management is drainage of the purulent collection combined with appropriate antibiotic therapy, which is determined by the results of culture of blood and aspirated pus. Although virtually all pathogenic organisms have been identified, enteric organisms predominate. Polymicrobial infection is seen frequently when hepatic abscess is secondary to infection arising from the portal venous system. Although antibiotic therapy as the sole treatment for hepatic abscess is rarely successful, prolonged systemic antibiotic administration may be the only option for patients with diffuse multiple microabscesses. In general, macroscopic hepatic collections require drainage of the purulent material. Over the past two decades, the introduction and refinement of percutaneous drainage techniques have dramatically altered the management of patients with pyogenic hepatic abscesses. Percutaneous drainage has become the first-line therapeutic option in most centres for patients with single or multiple liver abscesses.[48,50,51] Abscess communication with the intrahepatic biliary tree does not prevent pyogenic collections being successfully treated by percutaneous techniques, although the period of drainage may be prolonged. The use of percutaneous aspiration combined with systemic

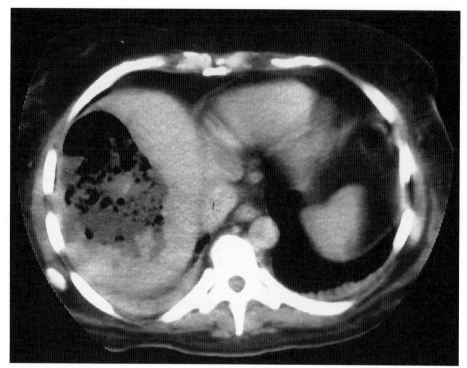

Figure 4.9 • Large liver abscess in right lobe of liver.

antibiotics without drainage has been advocated by some groups;[52] however, in the only randomised trial comparing the two techniques, aspiration was successful in only 60% of patients whereas percutaneous catheter drainage was successful in 100% of patients.[53]

Regular irrigation of drainage catheters reduces the risk of catheter blockage due to necrotic debris. Surgical drainage is rarely employed but is usually reserved for patients who have failed percutaneous drainage and those who require surgical management of the underlying problem. Liver resection is occasionally required for patients with liver abscess.[54] The indication is usually failed non-operative management, hepatolithiasis, intrahepatic biliary stricture or gross parenchymal destruction.

Effective decompression of the biliary tree is as important as abscess drainage where obstruction of the bile duct has contributed to the development of hepatic abscess. Following successful drainage of the abscess, antibiotic administration should be continued for a prolonged period (4–6 weeks) to assist in the complete eradication of infection.

Pyogenic liver abscess still carries a significant mortality. A significant number of patients will not survive admission to hospital, reflecting the high proportion of patients developing hepatic abscess related to underlying malignant biliary obstruction.

Amoebic abscess

This form of abscess is sufficiently common that it should be considered in the differential diagnosis of hepatic lesions. About 10% of the world's population is chronically infected with *Entamoeba histolytica*, although less than 10% of individuals are symptomatic. Liver abscess is the most common extraintestinal manifestation of amoebiasis and is reported in 3–10% of affected patients. Males are more commonly affected than females, and the highest incidence is in the 20- to 50-year-old age group.[55]

The diagnosis is likely to be straightforward in areas where amoebiasis is endemic but the liver abscess may present many years after previous intestinal infection. Some 75–90% of abscesses are in the right lobe, and involvement of the left lobe usually indicates more advanced disease. Rupture occurs in 2–17% of cases and usually occurs into the peritoneal cavity and rarely into the pleural cavity, the bronchial tree or pericardium. Signs and symptoms of amoebic infection are the same as for pyogenic abscess. On US and CT, the boundaries of the abscess are generally poorly defined (**Fig. 4.10**). Patients with amoebic liver abscess virtually always have serum antiamoebic antibodies, which can be detected by an indirect haemagglutination test or an enzyme-linked immunosorbent assay (ELISA) technique. Percutaneous aspiration produces a sterile

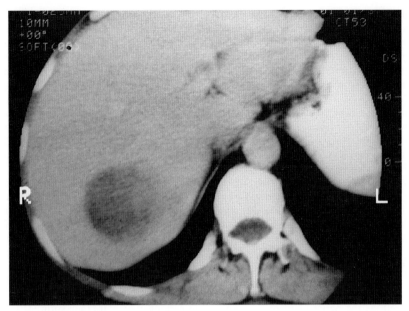

Figure 4.10 • Poorly defined boundaries of amoebic abscess shown on CT scan.

and odourless fluid, which is described as having the appearance of 'anchovy paste'. Routine percutaneous aspiration is now regarded as superfluous in the management of amoebic liver abscess unless serology is inconclusive, a therapeutic trial with antiamoebic drugs is deemed inappropriate (as in pregnancy), or rupture is suspected to be imminent. A preliminary diagnosis can be made on the basis of a dramatic clinical response to metronidazole, which should be commenced empirically in endemic areas.[55] If clinical symptoms do not resolve within 48–72 hours of treatment, an incorrect diagnosis or secondary bacterial infection should be suspected. Percutaneous aspiration may be beneficial for patients when medical treatment has failed. Percutaneous catheter drainage is indicated rarely as the abscess contents are viscous and bacterial superinfection may occur. Open surgical drainage is indicated in complicated cases and in those who fail to respond to conservative therapy. In a meta-analysis of 3081 patients with amoebic liver abscess the mortality rate was 4%, compared with a mortality rate of 46% in patients with pyogenic liver abscess.[56]

Hydatid cyst

Echinococcus infection is a zoonosis that can give rise to liver lesions. These collections are better classified as cysts rather than abscesses because the organism is almost entirely determined by the hepatic environment and little host inflammatory reaction is present. An intense fibrous reaction around the lesion is characteristic but there is no epithelial lining to the cyst. The incidence of *Echinococcus granulosus* is in decline but sporadic cases are reported in Europe, Australia, New Zealand, South America, Asia and Africa. The prevalence of human echinococciasis is directly related to contact with dogs and sheep. *Echinococcus multilocularis*, or alveolar hydatid disease, is rare, although it is a much more dangerous condition. It pursues a more invasive course than the more common form of the disease.

Hydatid cysts are most commonly unilocular and may grow as large as 20 cm. The cyst wall is about 5 mm thick and consists of an external laminated hilar membrane (ectocyst layer) and an internal enucleated germinal layer (endocyst layer), which is responsible for production of the colourless hydatid fluid, brood capsules and daughter cysts. Brood capsules are small cellular masses and together with calcareous bodies form 'hydatid sand'. About 70% of lesions are in the right lobe and 15% in the left, with both lobes involved in approximately 15% of cases.

Clinical presentation

Many infections are probably contracted during childhood and lie latent for many years, often until complications occur. Clinical symptoms of echinococcal cystic disease are often insidious but there is usually a history of contact with dogs or sheep. Distension of the liver capsule may produce right upper quadrant pain. Jaundice is infrequent but may be due to extrinsic biliary compression or due to rupture into the biliary tree leading to obstruction by cystic debris. Secondary bacterial infection of the cyst occurs in approximately 10% of cases. Liver function tests are generally abnormal and eosinophilia is present in up to one-third of patients.

Echinococcal disease may occasionally mimic a primary liver tumour or metastatic disease. Serology may be helpful in establishing a diagnosis. Plain abdominal radiographs may reveal a calcified cyst wall. US and CT may demonstrate septa, 'hydatid sand' or daughter cysts within the main cyst cavity, which are important signs for differentiating hydatid from other benign liver cysts (**Fig. 4.11**). Percutaneous aspiration and drainage should be avoided because of the risk of dissemination or anaphylaxis.

Management

Once the diagnosis has been established, surgery is generally required, as the natural history of viable hydatid cysts is one of growth and potential complications. Significant morbidity and mortality may result from rupture into the peritoneal or thoracic cavity or the development of a bronchobiliary fistula. Surgery might best be avoided in elderly frail patients with small, asymptomatic calcified cysts. Treatment with an oral anthelmintic agent, such as mebendazole or albendazole, to minimise the risks

of hydatid spread at surgery or reduce the incidence of postoperative recurrence, has been advocated by some authors, although there remains considerable doubt as to its efficacy. Aspiration of the hydatid cyst with instillation of scolicidal agents, such as hypertonic saline, silver nitrate, chlorhexidine, cetrimide, hydrogen peroxide, formalin or alcohol, has generally been abandoned because of the risk of anaphylaxis or the risk of developing sclerosing cholangitis if a bile duct communication is present. These have been generally replaced by perioperative cover with an anthelmintic agent.

The main principle of surgical treatment is to eradicate the parasite, prevent intraoperative spillage of cyst contents and obliterate the residual cavity.[57] At open operation, the operating field is generally packed off with swabs. After decompression, the cyst and contents are shelled out by peeling the endocyst off the host ectocyst layer. The fibrous host wall of the residual cavity should be carefully examined for any bile leakage from biliary–cyst communications, which are then sutured. The residual cyst cavity can be marsupialised, packed with omentum or plicated.[58] Pericystectomy is advocated by some but should preserve those portions of the cyst wall that come into contact with major blood vessels. For smaller, peripheral lesions, formal hepatic resection may be considered, particularly if a diagnostic dilemma remains. The mortality for surgery of hydatid disease should be low and confined to

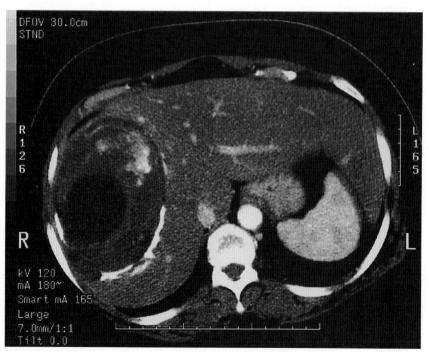

Figure 4.11 • Hydatid cyst with calcified cyst wall and a few peripheral daughter cysts.

complicated disease. In a series of 505 patients, Milicevic reported a mortality rate of 1.5% and a morbidity rate of 30%.[58]

Simple cysts of the liver

Non-parasitic cystic disease of the liver can result from a congenital malformation of the intrahepatic bile ducts. These cysts may be single, multiple or diffuse (polycystic liver disease). They contain serous fluid and do not communicate with the intrahepatic biliary tree. Small cysts are surrounded by normal liver tissue, although as these enlarge there is displacement and atrophy of adjacent hepatic tissue. A large cyst may occupy an entire lobe of the liver and result in compensatory hypertrophy of the residual liver. Such cysts have no vascularised septa and are unilocular. Microscopically, they are lined by a single layer of cuboidal or columnar epithelial cells, which resemble those of biliary epithelium. Simple cysts have a prevalence of about 3.6%. The female to male ratio is 4:1 in asymptomatic cases, but rises to 10:1 in symptomatic or complicated simple cysts.[59]

Clinical presentation

The vast majority of simple cysts are asymptomatic and are discovered incidentally. Large cysts may cause abdominal pain or discomfort, and a mass may be palpable in the right hypochondrium. Other symptoms may include anorexia, early satiety or vomiting. Rare complications include acute onset of pain from intracystic haemorrhage, rupture, torsion or infection. Jaundice is uncommon, but may be caused by external compression of the biliary tree. Likewise, portal hypertension has been reported as a consequence of portal vein compression.

Diagnosis can be made on the basis of abdominal US, which demonstrates a circular anechoic area that has a well-defined boundary with the liver. No wall is evident and there is posterior acoustic enhancement. Intracystic haemorrhage may cause internal acoustic shadowing; however, the presence of cyst wall nodules or solid intracystic components must be considered neoplastic. US examination of the kidneys is useful in patients with multiple liver cysts to exclude the presence of polycystic disease. Further diagnostic investigation is rarely required, although where intervention is contemplated, CT or MRI will provide more accurate anatomical localisation and exclude the presence of other cysts. Cysts appear as well-rounded, water-dense lesions without septa on CT (**Fig. 4.12**). Intravenous contrast enhancement will confirm the avascularity of these lesions. Where complications such as haemorrhage occur, the simple cyst may appear relatively thick-walled and may contain cystic debris. In such instances,

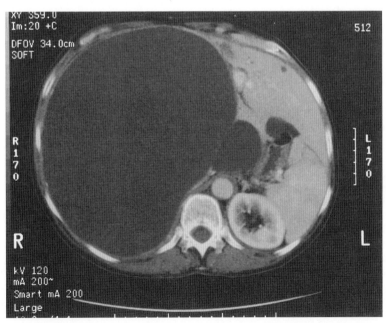

Figure 4.12 • CT scan demonstrating a large benign cyst occupying the entire right lobe of the liver. At least two further cysts are seen in the caudate and left lobes of the liver. Note the normal left kidney. This patient underwent successful laparoscopic deroofing of the cyst.

serological tests should be undertaken to exclude parasitic infection. It should be borne in mind that calcification is rarely present in simple cysts but may be present with hydatid cysts.

Management

Asymptomatic simple cysts require no treatment; however, symptomatic or complicated simple cysts may require intervention. Percutaneous aspiration risks introducing infection and does not provide definitive therapy; however, this technique may be useful as a diagnostic test for patients with questionable symptoms.[60] Aspiration followed by percutaneous instillation of sclerosant agents has shown promising results in reducing symptomatic and radiological cyst recurrence.[61] Open deroofing of simple liver cysts has, in the past, been the established conventional treatment. Total cystectomy is not required and may be hazardous since there is no plane of dissection between the cyst and the liver. In recent years, laparoscopic deroofing of such solitary cysts has been advocated. This technique was first described in 1991,[62] and is associated with higher patient acceptability and shorter postoperative stay compared with open surgical techniques. In a recent comprehensive review of 21 papers on the laparoscopic management of hepatic cysts, Klingler et al.[63] reported 61 laparoscopic deroofing procedures with an overall morbidity rate of 10%.

Even at open surgery, deroofing of large centrally placed cysts may not prevent reconstitution of the cyst with recurrence of symptoms. In such patients, more radical resection that does not generally involve substantial sacrifice of functioning hepatic parenchyma should be considered.

Polycystic liver disease (PCLD)

Adult polycystic kidney disease is frequently associated with multiple liver cysts, which are macroscopically and microscopically similar to simple cysts of the liver. However, in this condition the liver cysts are multiple when present and may extensively replace both lobes of the liver (**Fig. 4.13**). In addition to the macroscopic cysts, there are usually numerous microscopic cysts and clusters of multiple bile ductules, designated as von Meyenburg complexes. The condition is an autosomal dominant disorder and carries a much more sinister prognosis because of the risk of chronic renal failure. There is an increased prevalence associated with increasing age and the female sex.[64]

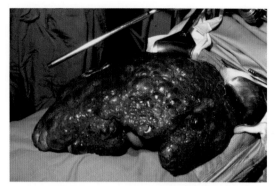

Figure 4.13 • Massive polycystic liver delivered from abdomen and pelvis before resection and deroofing.

Clinical presentation

In most patients with adult polycystic kidney disease, the polycystic hepatomegaly is clinically silent. The commonest symptoms are related to increase in liver size, and include abdominal and pelvic discomfort and respiratory compromise. An abdominal mass will be present in three-quarters of patients. There are rarely signs of cholestasis, liver failure or portal hypertension, and liver function tests are usually normal. Both US and CT will demonstrate multiple fluid-filled cysts with well-defined margins in the liver and the kidneys (**Fig. 4.14**). Liver cysts increase in size slowly and complications are uncommon. Rupture and bacterial infection are reported to be more common with immunosuppression following kidney transplantation.[65]

Management

Asymptomatic patients require no treatment. Percutaneous aspiration of cysts and instillation of sclerosant rarely produce satisfactory long-term relief of symptoms. Surgical deroofing or fenestration according to the technique described by Lin et al.[66] is the most widely used treatment modality for symptomatic patients but must be extensive and radical to achieve satisfactory results. Some have suggested that laparoscopic deroofing may provide good relief of symptoms.[67] However, in our own series this technique was associated with a high recurrence rate.[59] Recent evidence suggests that a more aggressive open surgical approach involving resection of the liver may provide longer-lasting relief of symptoms,[68,69] but it should be appreciated that hepatic resection is difficult in such patients and is associated with significant morbidity. Nonetheless, extensive resection and

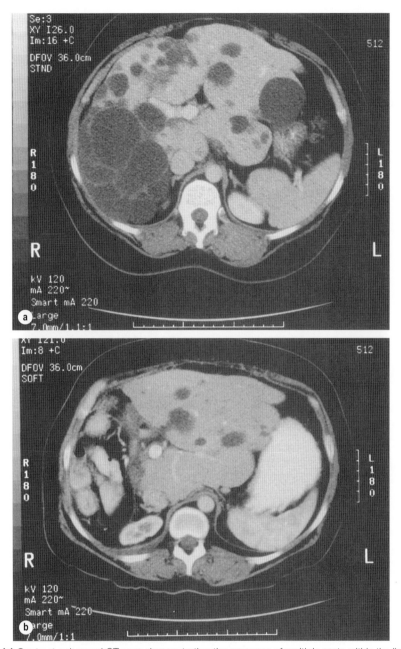

Figure 4.14 • (a) Contrast-enhanced CT scan demonstrating the presence of multiple cysts within the liver and kidneys. Note the predominance of large cysts within the right lobe of the liver. **(b)** CT scan taken 1 month following right hepatectomy and deroofing of the residual cyst in the same patient.

cyst deroofing may allow the abdomen to better accommodate the enlarged residual liver. Surgical intervention is often associated with transient but massive ascites in the postoperative period.[70] Liver transplantation may be indicated in selected patients with hepatic failure.[71]

Cystadenoma

Cystadenoma of the liver is rare, but it has a strong tendency to recur and has a malignant potential. It is usually solitary and mainly affects women over 40 years of age. Cystadenomas are often multiloculated and may measure up to 20cm in diameter. Histologically, the locules are mostly lined by a single layer of cuboidal or columnar cells; however, in areas the epithelium may form papillary projections. The presenting features are similar to other mass-forming hepatic pathologies, namely abdominal discomfort, anorexia, nausea and abdominal swelling. A large hepatic mass may be palpable. Liver function tests are usually normal. Diagnosis is based on US, MRI or CT (**Fig. 4.15**). US characteristics are of a large, anechoic, fluid-filled area with irregular margins. Internal echoes may be seen due to septa or papillary projections from the cyst wall. CT provides more accurate localisation, but may be less sensitive than US for demonstrating the thin septations. Cystadenomas grow very slowly and complications include biliary obstruction, intracystic haemorrhage, bacterial infection, rupture, recurrence after partial excision and transformation into cystadenocarcinoma. This may be suspected radiologically by the presence of large projections into the cyst lobules and septal calcification.[72] Cystadenoma of the liver, even if asymptomatic, must be treated by complete excision.

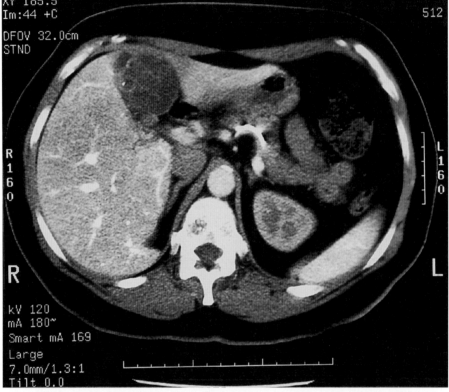

Figure 4.15 • CT scan demonstrating septa within a cystadenoma in segment 4 of the liver.

Key points

- Successful management of patients with benign solid or cystic lesions of the liver requires accurate diagnosis and thorough knowledge of the natural history.
- Inappropriate investigation may give rise to morbidity and compromise definitive management.
- Modern liver resection for benign lesions can now be undertaken with minimal morbidity and mortality because of increasing centralisation of expertise and improved operative techniques.
- A better understanding of the prognosis of unresected haemangioma, focal nodular hyperplasia and liver cell adenoma has made it possible to consider a more conservative approach in management.
- Patients with symptomatic lesions or lesions that have the potential for further growth, complications or malignant transformation should undergo surgical treatment.
- Careful consideration must be given to the risk of hepatic resection against the possible morbidity or mortality from observation.

References

1. Ishak KG, Rabin L. Benign tumors of the liver. Med Clin North Am 1975;59:995–1013.

2. Schwartz SI, Husser WC. Cavernous hemangioma of the liver: a single institution report of 16 resections. Ann Surg 1987;205:456–65.

3. Sewell JH, Weiss K. Spontaneous rupture of hemangioma of the liver. Arch Surg 1961;83:105–9.

4. Trastek VF, van Heerden JA, Sheedy PF, et al. Cavernous hemangiomas of the liver: resect or observe? Am J Surg 1983;145:49–53.

5. Farges O, Daradkeh S, Bismuth H. Cavernous hemangiomas of the liver: are there any indications for resection? World J Surg 1995;19:19–24.

6. Bornman PC, Terblanche J, Blumgart RL, et al. Giant hemangiomas: diagnostic and therapeutic dilemmas. Surgery 1987;101:445–9.

7. Yamamoto T, Kawarada Y, Yano T, et al. Spontaneous rupture of haemangioma of the liver: treatment with transcatheter hepatic arterial embolisation. Am J Gastroenterol 1991;86:1645–9.

8. Johnson CM, Sheedy PF, Stanson AW, et al. Computed tomography and angiography of cavernous hemangiomas of the liver. Radiology 1985;138:115–21.

9. Birnbaum BA, Weinreb JC, Mengibow AJ, et al. Definitive diagnosis of hepatic hemangiomas: MR imaging versus Tc-99m labelled red blood cell SPECT. Radiology 1990;176:95–102.

10. Choi BI, Shin YM, Chung JW, et al. MR findings of hepatic cavernous hemangioma after intra-arterial infusion of iodized oil. Abdom Imaging 1994;16:507–11.

11. Mahfouz AE, Hamm B, Taupitz M, et al. Hypervascular liver lesions: differentiation of focal nodular hyperplasia from malignant tumours with dynamic gadolinium-enhanced MR imaging. Radiology 1993;186:133–42.

12. Krause T, Hauenstein K, Studier-Fischer B, et al. Improved evaluation of technetium-99m-red blood cell SPECT in haemangioma of the liver. J Nucl Med 1993;34:375–80.

13. Shimada K, Nakamoto Y, Isoda H, et al. FDG PET for giant cavernous haemangioma: important clue to differentiate from a malignant vascular tumour in the liver. Clin Nucl Med 2010;35:924–6.

14. Nichols FC, van Heerden JA, Weiland LH. Benign liver tumors. Surg Clin North Am 1989;69:297–314.

15. Pietrabissa A, Giulianotti P, Campatelli A, et al. Management and follow-up of 78 giant haemangiomas of the liver. Br J Surg 1996;83:915–8.

16. Terkivatan T, Vrijland WW, Den Hoed PT, et al. Size of lesion is not a criterion for resection during management of giant liver haemangioma. Br J Surg 2002;89:1240–4.

17. Weimann A, Ringe B, Klempnauer J, et al. Benign liver tumours: differential diagnosis and indications for surgery. World J Surg 1997;21:983–91.

18. Foster JH, Adson MA, Schwartz SI, et al. Symposium: benign liver tumours. Contemp Surg 1982;21:67–102.

19. Baer HU, Dennison AR, Mouton W, et al. Enucleation of giant hemangiomas of the liver. Ann Surg 1992;216:673–6.

20. Descottes B, Glineur D, Lachachi F, et al. Laparoscopic liver resection of benign liver tumors. Surg Endosc 2003;17:23–30.

21. Longeville JH, de-la-Hall P, Dolan P, et al. Treatment of a giant haemangioma of the liver with Kasabach–Merritt syndrome by orthotopic liver transplant, a case report. HPB Surg 1997;10:159–62.

22. Nagorney DM. Benign hepatic tumors: focal nodular hyperplasia and hepatocellular adenoma. World J Surg 1995;19:13–8.

23. Rooks JB, Ory HW, Ishak KG, et al. Epidemiology of hepatocellular adenoma: the role of oral contraceptive use. JAMA 1979;242:644–8.

24. Baum JK, Bookstein JJ, Holtz F, et al. Possible association between benign hepatomas and oral contraceptives. Lancet 1973;2:926–9.

25. Kent DR, Nissen ED, Nissen SE, et al. Effect of pregnancy on liver tumour associated with oral contraceptives. Obstet Gynecol 1978;51:148–51.

26. Leese T, Farges O, Bismuth H. Liver cell adenomas: a 12 year surgical experience in a specialist hepatobiliary unit. Ann Surg 1988;208:558–64.

27. Chiche L, Dao T, Salame E, et al. Liver adenomatosis: reappraisal, diagnosis, and surgical management: eight new cases and review of the literature. Ann Surg 2000;231:74–81.

28. Ferrell LD. Hepatocellular carcinoma arising in a focus of multilobular adenoma. Am J Surg Pathol 1993;17:525–9.

29. Scott FR, El-Rafaie A, More L, et al. Hepatocellular carcinoma arising in an adenoma: value of Qbend 10 immunostaining in diagnosis of liver cell carcinoma. Histopathology 1996;28:472–4.

30. Gordon SC, Reddy KR, Livingstone AS, et al. Resolution of a contraceptive steroid-induced hepatic adenoma with subsequent evolution into hepatocellular carcinoma. Ann Intern Med 1986;105:547–9.

31. Gyorffy EJ, Bredfeldt JE, Black WC. Transformation of hepatic cell adenoma to hepatocellular carcinoma due to oral contraceptive use. Ann Intern Med 1989;110:489–90.

32. Dardenne S, Hubert C, Sempoux C, et al. Conservative and operative management of benign solid hepatic tumours: a successful stratified algorithm. Eur J Gastroenterol Hepatol 2010;22:1337–44.

33. Zucman-Rossi J, Jeannot E, Nhieu JT, et al. Genotype–phenotype correlation in hepatocellular adenoma: new classification and relationship with HCC. Hepatology 2006;43:515–24.

34. Bioulac-Sage P, Balabaud C, Bedossa P, et al. Pathological diagnosis of liver cell adenoma and focal nodular hyperplasia: Bordeaux update. J Hepatol 2007;46:521–7.

35. Delbeke D, Martin WH, Sandler MP, et al. Evaluation of benign vs malignant hepatic lesions with positron emission tomography. Arch Surg 1998;133:510–6.

36. Stoot JHMB, van der Linden E, Terpstra OT, et al. Life-saving therapy for haemorrhaging liver adenomas using selective arterial embolisation. Br J Surg 2007;94:1249–53.

37. Tepetes K, Selby R, Webb M, et al. Orthoptic liver transplantation for benign hepatic neoplasms. Arch Surg 1995;130:153–6.

38. Laumonier H, Biolac-Sage P, Laurent C, et al. Hepatocellular adenomas: magnetic resonance features as a function of molecular pathological calssification. Hepatology 2008;48:808–18.

39. Buhler H, Pirovino M, Akobiantz A, et al. Regression of liver cell adenoma. A follow-up study of three consecutive cases after discontinuation of oral contraceptive use. Gastroenterology 1982;82:775–82.

40. Aseni P, Sansalone CV, Sammartino C, et al. Rapid disappearance of hepatic adenoma after contraceptive withdrawal. J Clin Gastroenterol 2001;33:234–6.

41. Cherqui D, Rahmouni A, Charlotte F, et al. Management of focal nodular hyperplasia and hepatocellular adenoma in young women: a series of 41 patients with clinical, radiological, pathological correlations. Hepatology 1995;22:1674–81.

42. Belghiti J, Pateron D, Panis Y, et al. Resection of presumed benign liver tumours. Br J Surg 1993;80:380–3.

43. Kerlin P, Davis GL, McGill DB, et al. Hepatic adenoma and focal nodular hyperplasia: clinical, pathologic and radiologic features. Gastroenterology 1983;84:994–1002.

44. Allaire GS, Rabin L, Ishak KG. Bile duct adenoma: a study of 152 cases. Am J Surg Pathol 1988;12:708–15.

45. Shek TW, Ng IO, Chan KW. Inflammatory pseudotumor of the liver: report of four cases and review of the literature. Am J Surg Pathol 1993;17:231–8.

46. Grases PJ, Matos-Villalobos M, Arcia-Romero F, et al. Mesenchymal hamartoma of the liver. Gastroenterology 1979;76:1466–9.

47. Rintoul R, O'Riordain MG, Laurenson IF, et al. The changing management of pyogenic liver abscess. Br J Surg 1996;83:215–8.

48. Chou FF, Sheen-Chen SM, Chen YS, et al. Single and multiple pyogenic liver abscesses: clinical course, etiology and results of treatment. World J Surg 1997;21:384–9.

49. Huang CJ, Pitt HA, Lipsett PA, et al. Pyogenic hepatic abscess: changing trends over 42 years. Ann Surg 1996;223:600–9.

50. Chu KM, Fan ST, Lai EC, et al. Pyogenic liver abscess: an audit of experience over the past decade. Arch Surg 1996;131:148–52.

51. Pearce NW, Knight R, Irving H, et al. Non-operative management of pyogenic liver abscess. HPB (Oxford) 2003;5:91–5.

52. Giorgio A, Tarantino L, Mariniello N, et al. Pyogenic liver abscesses: 13 years of experience in percutaneous needle aspiration with US guidance. Radiology 1995;195:122–4.

53. Rajak CL, Gupta S, Jain S, et al. Percutaneous treatment of liver abscess: needle aspiration versus catheter drainage. AJR Am J Roentgenol 1998;170:1035–9.

54. Strong RW, Fawcett J, Lynch SV, et al. Hepatectomy for pyogenic liver abscess. HPB (Oxford) 2003;5:86–90.

55. Akgun Y, Tacyilmaz IH, Celik Y. Amebic liver abscess: changing trends over 20 years. World J Surg 1999;23:102–6.

56. Pitt HA. Surgical management of hepatic abscesses. World J Surg 1990;14:498–504.

57. Agaoglu N, Turkyilmaz S, Arslan MK. Surgical treatment of hydatid cysts of the liver. Br J Surg 2003;90:1536–41.

58. Milicevic M. Hydatid disease. In: Blumgart LH, editor. Surgery of the liver and biliary tract. 3rd ed. London: WB Saunders; 2000. p. 1167–204.

59. Martin IJ, McKinley AJ, Currie EJ, et al. Tailoring the management of nonparasitic liver cysts. Ann Surg 1998;228:167–72.

60. Gigot JF, Legrand M, Hubens G, et al. Laparoscopic treatment of nonparasitic liver cysts: adequate selection of patients and surgical technique. World J Surg 1996;20:556–61.

61. Montorsi M, Torzilli G, Fumagalli U, et al. Percutaneous alcohol sclerotherapy of simple hepatic cysts. Results from a multicentre survey in Italy. HPB Surg 1994;8:89–94.

62. Paterson-Brown S, Garden OJ. Laser assisted laparoscopic excision of liver cyst. Br J Surg 1991;78:1047.

63. Klingler PJ, Gadenstatter M, Schmid T, et al. Treatment of hepatic cysts in the laparoscopic era. Br J Surg 1997;84:438–44.

64. Milutinovic J, Failkow PJ, Rudd TG, et al. Liver cysts in patients with autosomal dominant polycystic kidney disease. Am J Med 1980;68:741–4.

65. Bourgeois N, Kinnaert P, Vereerstraeten P, et al. Infection of hepatic cysts following kidney transplantation in polycystic disease. World J Surg 1983;7:629–31.

66. Lin TY, Chen CC, Wang SM. Treatment of nonparasitic disease of the liver: a new approach to therapy of the polycystic liver. Ann Surg 1968;168:921–7.

67. Morino M, De Giuli M, Festa V, et al. Laparoscopic management of symptomatic non-parasitic cysts of the liver: indications and results. Ann Surg 1994;219:157–64.

68. Que F, Nagorney DM, Gross Jr JB, et al. Liver resection and cyst fenestration in the treatment of severe polycystic liver disease. Gastroenterology 1995;108:487–94.

69. Gigot JF, Jadoul P, Que F, et al. Adult polycystic liver disease: is fenestration the most adequate opeariton for long-term management ? Ann Surg 1997;225:286–94.

70. Farges O, Bismuth H. Fenestration in the management of polycystic liver disease. World J Surg 1995;19:25–30.

71. Starzl TE, Reyes J, Tzakis A, et al. Liver transplantation for polycystic liver disease. Arch Surg 1990;125:575–7.

72. Korobkin M, Stephens DH, Lee JKT, et al. Biliary cystadenoma and cystadenocarcinoma: CT and sonographic findings. AJR Am J Roentgenol 1989;153:507–11.

5

Primary malignant tumours of the liver

Chetana Lim
Olivier Farges

Introduction

With the exception of hepatocellular carcinoma (HCC), which is one of the most common malignancies, primary tumours of the liver are relatively rare in adults. HCC arises from hepatocytes, and cirrhosis is its main aetiological factor. This tumour remains a subject of considerable interest due to its rising incidence and the development of innovative treatments. Intrahepatic cholangiocarcinoma (ICCA) arises from the peripheral intrahepatic biliary radicles and other rare primary tumours arise from mesodermal cells, and include angiosarcoma, epithelioid haemangio-endothelioma and sarcoma.

Hepatocellular carcinoma

HCC accounts for 90% of all primary liver malignancy and its incidence continues to increase. It is the sixth most common neoplasm, accounting for more than 5% of all cancers, and is the third most common cause of cancer-related death. The International Agency for Research on Cancer has estimated in 2008 through its GLOBOCAN series that primary liver cancer caused more than 690 000 deaths worldwide, similar to colon or rectal cancer.[1]

HCC usually occurs in male patients, and cirrhosis precedes its development in most cases. Due to better medical management of cirrhosis, survival of cirrhotic patients has steadily increased in recent years, resulting in a greater risk of developing HCC. Cohort studies have reported that in patients with HCC, the death rate due to cancer is 50–60%, while hepatic failure and gastrointestinal bleeding are responsible for approximately 30% and 10% of the deaths, respectively. HCC may now be identified at an early stage, particularly through the screening of high-risk patients.

Control of HCC nodules may be achieved successfully by surgical resection and by percutaneous treatment. The indications for these therapies depend on the morphological features of the tumour and the functional status of the non-tumorous liver. Unfortunately, these treatments are associated with a high incidence of tumour recurrence due to the persistence of the underlying cirrhosis, which represents a preneoplastic condition. Liver transplantation may seem a logical alternative treatment but has its own limitations, including tumour recurrence, the limited availability of grafts, and cost. The most exciting areas of progress are the control of hepatitis B virus (HBV) or hepatitis C virus (HCV), the prevention of carcinogenesis in patients with chronic liver disease, early radiological screening and the development of medical therapies. In the setting of liver surgery, better liver function assessment and understanding of the segmental liver anatomy with more accurate imaging evaluation are the most important factors that have led to a decrease in postoperative mortality. Active follow-up and treatment of recurrence have also contributed to increased 5-year survival rates as high as 70%.[2]

Incidence of HCC

The world age-adjusted incidence of HCC in men is 14.9 per 100 000, but has geographical variation related to the prevalence of HBV and HCV infections,

Table 5.1 • Age and prevalence of HBV and HCV among patients with HCC in different geographical areas

Area	Age (years)	HBV (%)	HCV (%)	Combined (%)
Africa	47	47	18	65
USA	63	16	48	64
South America	55	43	21	64
Western Europe	65	18	44	62
Eastern Europe	60	51	15	66
South-western Asia	52	42	27	69
Japan	65	15	75	91
China, Korea	52	70	18	88
World		53	25	78

which are the two main risk factors worldwide and account for more than three-quarters of all cases (Table 5.1). The incidence may be as high as 99 cases per 100 000 in Mongolian men; other high-rate areas include Senegal, Gambia, South Korea, Hong Kong and Japan. By contrast, North and South America, Northern Europe and Oceania are areas with low incidences (less than 5 cases per 100 000); in these areas, HCV is the main risk factor, together with alcohol abuse, non-alcoholic fatty liver disease and obesity. Southern European countries have intermediate rates.

The rising incidence of HCC was first documented in the USA, where this doubled between the late 1970s and the early 1990s, reaching 3 cases per 100 000. The recent epidemic of HCV infection probably accounts for a large part of this increase. Alternative explanations include ageing of the population, increased detection, improved survival of cirrhotic patients, and the recent epidemic of obesity and type II diabetes.

It has been estimated that HCV began to infect large numbers of young adults in North America and South and Central Europe in the 1960s and 1970s as a result of intravenous drug use. The virus moved into national blood supplies and circulated until a screening test was developed in 1990, after which rates of new infection decreased dramatically. In Canada, Australia, Japan and various European countries, where HCV infection spread earlier than in the USA, a similar trend was observed but in some countries the incidence of HCC is now decreasing. In the USA, the incidence of HCV-related HCC is still increasing and is projected to peak in 2019 if the risk in HCV-infected persons with fibrosis remains stable.

Risk factors for HCC

The main risk factor for HCC is liver cirrhosis. Once present, male gender, age (as a marker of the duration of exposure to a given aetiological agent), stage of cirrhosis and diabetes are additional independent risk factors.

Cirrhosis

Up to 80–90% of all HCC arises in patients with underlying liver disease. The risk of tumour development varies with the type of cirrhosis; the highest risk is reported for chronic viral hepatitis (78% of HCC worldwide), whereas lower risks are associated with other forms of cirrhosis such as primary biliary cirrhosis.

HCC developing in the absence of cirrhosis is found in 10–20% of patients. The term 'absence of cirrhosis' appears more appropriate than 'normal liver' as these patients frequently have some degree of mild fibrosis, necroinflammation, steatosis or liver cell dysplasia. HCC in the absence of cirrhosis may be related to some of the same aetiological factors as those responsible for HCC in cirrhotic livers, such as HBV infection or alcohol abuse. Alternatively, HCC may occur as a result of conditions that infrequently lead to cirrhosis such as α_1-antitrypsin deficiency, haemochromatosis, or in the setting of specific aetiological factors that do not result in cirrhosis such as hormonal exposure or glycogenosis.

HBV infection

Chronic HBV infection is the most frequent risk factor for HCC worldwide, and accounts for more than 50% of all cases. It is estimated that 40 million people are currently affected by HBV, particularly in developing countries; HBV infection should, however, begin to decline as a result of increased utilisation of HBV immunisation.

There is evidence that HBV-DNA sequences integrate into the genome of malignant hepatocytes and can be detected in the liver tissues of patients with HCC despite the absence of classical HBV serological markers. HBV-specific protein may also interact with liver genes. HBV is therefore a direct risk factor for HCC and can occur in patients without cirrhosis.

The risk of HBV-associated HCC increases with the severity of the underlying hepatitis, age at infection and duration of infection, as well as level of viral replication. An Asian patient with HBV-related cirrhosis has a 17% cumulative risk of developing HCC over a 5-year period. In the West, this cumulative risk is 10%. This may be explained by the earlier acquisition of HBV in Asia through vertical transmission (rather than horizontal transmission in the West through sexual or parenteral routes), longer duration of disease, or additional exposure to environmental factors. Ongoing HBV replication or hepatitis B e-antigen (HBeAg) infection accelerates the progression to cirrhosis and also to HCC. A study conducted in Taiwanese men reported that the risk of HCC increased 10-fold when HBsAg was present and 60-fold when HBeAg was present. Similarly, HBV-DNA levels greater than 10^4 or 10^6 copies/mL are associated with a 2.3 and 6.1 hazard risk, respectively, compared to patients with lower levels of replication.[3] Additional cofactors that increase the risk of HCC are male gender (three- to sixfold), age >40 years, concurrent HCV infection (twofold), HDV co-infection (threefold), heavy alcohol consumption (two- to threefold) and, in endemic regions, aflatoxin ingestion.

HCV infection

The expansion of HCV infection probably accounts for a significant proportion of the increased incidence of HCC observed over the past 10 years. In Western countries, up to 70% of HCC patients have anti-HCV antibodies in their serum and the mean time for developing HCC following HCV infection is approximately 30 years.

In HCV-positive patients with initially compensated viral cirrhosis, HCC is both the most frequent and first complication. The annual incidence of HCC is 0–2% in patients with chronic hepatitis and 1–4% in those with compensated cirrhosis, although rates as high as 7% have been reported in Japan. In patients with cirrhosis, additional independent risk factors increasing the risk of HCC are age >55 years (two- to fourfold), male gender (two- to threefold), diabetes (twofold), alcohol intake greater than 60–80 g/day (two- to fourfold) and HBV co-infection (two- to six fold). Obesity is also a likely cofactor. In contrast, the viral genotype or viral concentration has no impact on the risk of HCC.

The mechanism of HCV-related HCC is still not very clear. The great majority of patients with HCV-related HCC have cirrhosis, suggesting that it is the presence of cirrhosis that is crucial for the development of this tumour.

> ✓ Because anti-HCV vaccination is not available, prevention of HCV infection and minimising the risk of progression of chronic HCV infection to cirrhosis using antiviral treatment is the only means to reduce the incidence of HCV-related HCC. Sustained virological response in HCV-infected patients is associated with a significantly decreased risk of developing HCC.[4]

Human immunodeficiency virus (HIV) infection

The incidence of HCC is expected to rise in HIV-positive persons predominantly because of the higher prevalence of associated well-known risk factors: not only co-infection with HCV and HBV, but also alcohol abuse, non-alcoholic steatohepatitis (NASH) and diabetes. HIV-positive patients who are co-infected with HBV or HCV may have more rapidly progressive liver disease, and when they develop cirrhosis they also have an increased risk of HCC. The Mortavic study indicated that HCC caused 25% of all liver-related deaths among HIV patients.[5]

Cirrhosis and HCC occur 15–20 years earlier in HIV–HCV co-infected patients than in patients infected by HCV alone. The course of the disease is also considered more aggressive.[6] Screening for HCC should, however, be the same as in HIV-negative patients.

Other viral infections

Infection with the hepatitis delta virus (HDV) is found in patients who are also infected with HBV (see above). Hepatitis A virus (HAV) and hepatitis E virus (HEV) infection cause neither chronic hepatitis nor HCC.

Alcohol

Heavy (>50–70 g/day) and prolonged alcohol ingestion is a classical risk factor for cirrhosis and therefore HCC. Data available from cohort studies of European or US patients with alcohol-related cirrhosis suggest an annual incidence of HCC of 1.7% (as compared with 2.2% and 3.7% in patients of the same geographical area with HBV- or HCV-associated cirrhosis). Alcohol is also a very frequent additional risk factor in patients with HBV or HCV cirrhosis, as well as in those patients with chronic liver disease associated with the metabolic syndrome.

Non-alcoholic fatty liver disease (NAFLD)

NAFLD has been recognised as being one of the most common causes of liver disease in the USA (and other Western countries). Histological changes in the liver range from simple steatosis to more severe forms of non-alcoholic steatohepatitis (NASH), including cirrhosis. It is closely associated with type II diabetes, central obesity and dyslipidaemia as part of the metabolic syndrome, the prevalence of which has increased as an epidemic.

✅ NAFLD (and the metabolic syndrome) accounts for a substantial portion of what was considered in the past as cryptogenic cirrhosis and carries an inherent risk for the development of HCC. Obesity has definitely been established as a risk factor for the development of HCC, with a 1.5–4 times increased risk.[7]

An association between NAFLD and HCC was first identified in 2002 by several studies focusing on HCC patients with chronic liver disease in the absence of HBV/HCV infection or alcohol abuse. In this population, there was a much higher prevalence of obesity, diabetes, hypertriglyceridaemia and pathological features of NAFLD. At the same time, evidence was accumulating linking common features of the metabolic syndrome/NASH with HCC. In particular, obesity was noted to increase the mortality from liver cancer far more than for any other cancer.[7] Similarly, diabetes was found to increase the risk of HCC with and without acute or chronic liver disease.[8]

Precise figures on the incidence of HCC in patients with NAFLD are still lacking. It increases with male gender, increasing age, sinusoidal iron deposition and severity of underlying liver disease. In surgical series, overt cirrhosis is present in only one-third of patients while the others have less severe liver damage.[9] In addition, there is also evidence that NAFLD may act synergistically with other risk factors, such as chronic HCV or alcoholic consumption, in the development of HCC.

Hereditary haemochromatosis

Hereditary haemochromatosis (HH) is an autosomal recessive disorder associated with homozygosity for the C282Y mutation in the haemochromatosis gene and characterised by excessive gastrointestinal absorption of iron. HH is a long-known risk factor for HCC, and the risk increases in patients with cirrhosis. Other risk factors include male gender and diabetes. Several additional risk factors such as HBV infection (4.9-fold), age greater than 55 years (13.3-fold) and alcohol abuse (2.3-fold) may act synergistically with iron overload to increase the risk of HCC in patients with cirrhosis caused by hereditary haemochromatosis. In a recent meta-analysis of nine studies including 1102 HCC cases, mainly from European populations, it has been reported that C282Y mutation was associated with increased risk of HCC (fourfold) in

patients with alcoholic liver cirrhosis, but not in those with viral liver cirrhosis.[10] Interestingly, pathological conditions other than haemochromatosis that are associated with iron overload, such as homozygous β-thalassaemia or the so-called African overload syndrome, are also associated with an increased risk of HCC. Similarly, there is evidence of a link between iron deposits within the liver and HCC in patients with and without cirrhosis.

Cirrhosis of other aetiologies

Primary biliary cirrhosis (PBC) has been considered as a low-risk factor for HCC, not only because of its rare incidence but also because it predominantly affects women (with a sex ratio of 9:1). A recent meta-analysis of 12 studies has reported that PBC is significantly associated with an increased risk of HCC (18.8-fold) compared to the general population.[11] However, there were several confounding factors in this meta-analysis, such as advanced histological stage of PBC, history of blood transfusion, and smoking or drinking habits that might be associated with an increased probability for HCC development in PBC patients, or may be directly associated with PBC development. In contrast, HCC development in patients with secondary biliary cirrhosis is exceptional if it even exists.

Autoimmune hepatitis has a low risk of HCC development. Potential reasons are the female predominance and the delayed development of cirrhosis through corticosteroid therapy. HCV infection needs to be ruled out as it may induce autoantibodies. Recent data reported that cirrhosis at presentation is an important prognostic risk factor for HCC. In a prospective multicentre cohort study evaluating 193 Japanese patients with autoimmune hepatitis, seven (3.6%) developed HCC during an 8-year period, all of whom had underlying cirrhosis.[12]

Aflatoxin

Aflatoxin B1 has also long been associated with the development of HCC because areas with a large consumption of this toxin coincide with areas with a high incidence of HCC (Asia and sub-Saharan Africa). Aflatoxin is ingested in food as a result of contamination of imperfectly stored staple crops by *Aspergillus flavus*. It is thought to induce HCC through mutation of the tumour suppressor gene p53. Although some studies suggest that it is an independent risk factor, others suggest that it could be a co-carcinogen only in patients with HBV infection. HCC in this setting frequently develops in a non-cirrhotic liver.

Metabolic liver diseases

An increased risk of HCC is recognised in some other forms of metabolic liver diseases such as α_1-antitrypsin deficiency, porphyria cutanea tarda, tyrosinaemia and hypercitrullinaemia. Patients with glycogenosis type IV, hereditary fructose intolerance and Wilson disease may also develop HCC, but with a lower risk. There is evidence that iron and copper overload in haemochromatosis and Wilson disease generate, respectively, oxygen/nitrogen species and unsaturated aldehydes that cause mutations in the p53 tumour suppressor gene.

Adenoma, contraceptives and androgens

Like adenoma in other locations, hepatocellular adenomas (HCAs) have a risk of malignant transformation and hepatocyte dysplasia is the intermediate step between HCAs and HCC. A recent systematic review estimated the risk to be 4.2%.[13] This risk and the treatment strategy to prevent it may, however, be refined.

HCAs are most classical in women of childbearing age and are associated with the prolonged use of contraceptives and oestrogen treatments. Discontinuation of oral contraceptives does not completely avoid the risk of malignant transformation. Malignancy within HCAs measuring less than 4 cm in diameter is exceptional. There is also recent evidence that HCAs may develop in men, especially if there is a background of a metabolic syndrome. The risk of malignant transformation in men is 50% (10 times higher than in women) and malignancy can occur in HCAs as small as 1 cm.[14] Therefore, whereas resection of HCAs larger than 4 cm is recommended in women, all HCAs irrespective of size should be resected (or ablated) in men.

The number of HCAs does not appear to increase the risk of malignant transformation and, in particular, patients with polyadenomatosis are not at increased risk.[14–16]

Malignant transformation of HCAs has also been linked to the genotype and phenotype of HCAs. It is more prevalent in telangiectatic or atypical HCAs than in steatotic HCAs. Most importantly, the presence of a β-catenin mutation (observed in approximately 10–15% of HCAs) confers a particularly high risk of malignancy.[17]

Malignant transformation of HCAs may also occur within known specific aetiologies, such as with type I glycogenosis, anabolic steroid use, androgen treatments and Fanconi disease. Recreational anabolic steroid use is also known to potentially result in the development of adenoma, and malignant transformation to HCC has been reported.

Pathology of HCC and nodular lesions in chronic liver disease

Preneoplastic lesions are morphologically characterised by dysplastic lesions in the form of microscopic dysplastic foci and macroscopic dysplastic nodules (DNs).

Dysplastic foci are microscopic lesions composed of dysplastic hepatocytes of less than 1 mm in size, and occur in chronic liver disease, particularly in cirrhosis. DNs are defined as a nodular region of less than 2 cm in diameter with dysplasia but without definite histological criteria of malignancy. They are divided into low and high grade depending on the degree of cytological or architectural atypia. Low-grade DNs are approximately 1 cm in diameter, slightly yellowish, and have a very low probability of becoming malignant. High-grade DNs are less common but are typically slightly larger nodules (up to 2 cm) characterised by increased cell density with an irregular thin-trabecular pattern and occasionally unpaired arteries. These are often difficult to differentiate from highly differentiated HCCs. They may contain distinct foci of well-differentiated HCC and are therefore considered as precancerous lesions and become malignant in a third of cases. It must, however, be appreciated that lesions smaller than 2 cm may also represent HCC.

HCCs can be subdivided according to their gross morphology, degree of differentiation, vascularity, presence of a surrounding capsule and presence of vascular invasion. All of these criteria have practical implications.

On gross morphology, HCCs can be solitary or multinodular, consisting of either a collection of discrete lesions in different segments that develop synchronously (multicentric HCC), or as one dominant mass and a number of 'daughter' nodules (intrahepatic metastases) located in the adjacent segments. Diffuse HCCs are relatively rare at presentation and consist of poorly defined, widely infiltrative masses that present particular diagnostic challenges on imaging. A third type is the infiltrating HCC, which typically is less differentiated with ill-defined margins.

Microscopically, HCCs exhibit variable degrees of differentiation that are usually stratified into four different histological grades, known as Edmondson grades 1–4, which correspond to well-differentiated, moderately differentiated, poorly differentiated and undifferentiated types. The degree of differentiation typically decreases as the tumour increases in diameter. Very-well-differentiated HCCs can resemble normal hepatocytes and the trabecular structure may reproduce a near normal lobar architecture so that histological diagnosis by biopsy or following resection may be difficult. A number of immunomarkers have been described to selectively identify the malignant nature of these HCCs, not only in resected specimens but also in liver biopsies: glypican 3 (GPC3), heat shock protein 70 (HSP70) and glutamine synthetase (GS). Positive immunomarker staining for any two markers can detect early and well-differentiated HCC in 50–73% of cases, with 100% specificity when the analysis is performed on resected specimens.[18]

Vascularisation is a key parameter in differentiating HCC from regenerating nodules. Progression from macroregenerative nodule to low-grade DN, high-grade DN and frank HCC is characterised by loss of visualisation of portal tracts and development of new non-triadal arterial vessels, which become the dominant blood supply in overt HCC lesions. This arterial neoangiogenesis is the landmark pathological feature of HCC diagnosis, and the rationale for chemoembolisation and anti-angiogenic treatment.

A distinct fibrous capsule may surround tumour nodules. This capsule, present in 80% of resected HCCs, has a variable thickness, which may not be complete, and is frequently infiltrated by tumour cells. Capsular microscopic invasion by tumour cells is present in almost one-third of tumours smaller than 2 cm in diameter, as compared with two-thirds of those with a larger diameter.

HCC has a great tendency to spread locally and to invade blood vessels. The rate of portal invasion is higher in the expansive type, in poorly differentiated HCCs and in large tumours. Characteristically, microscopic vascular invasion is seen in 20% of tumours measuring 2 cm in diameter, in 30–60% of cases with nodules measuring 2–5 cm and in up to 60–90% when nodules are more than 5 cm in size. The presence of portal invasion is the most important predictive factor associated with recurrence. The tumour thrombus has its own arterial supply, mainly from the site of the original venous invasion. Once HCC invades the portal vein, tumour thrombi grow rapidly in both directions, and in particular towards the main portal vein. As a consequence, tumour fragments spread throughout the liver as the thrombus crosses segmental branches. Once the tumour thrombus has extended into the main portal vein, there is a high risk of complete thrombosis and increased portal hypertension. This accounts for the frequent presentation with fatal rupture of oesophageal varices, or liver decompensation including ascites (**Fig. 5.1**), jaundice and encephalopathy. Invasion of hepatic veins is possible, although less frequent. The thrombus eventually extends into the suprahepatic vena cava or the right atrium and is associated with a high risk of lung metastases. Rarely, HCC may invade the biliary tract and give rise to jaundice or haemobilia. Mechanisms of HCC-induced biliary obstruction include:

- intraductal tumour extension;
- obstruction by a fragment of necrotic tumour debris;

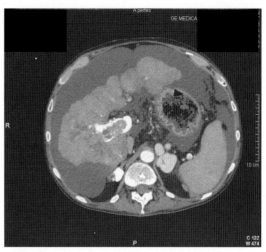

Figure 5.1 • CT scan of a patient with a tumour thrombus originating from an HCC located in the right liver. The thrombus extends in to the main portal vein. Ascites is present.

- haemorrhage of the tumour resulting in haemobilia;
- metastatic lymph node compression of major bile ducts in the porta hepatis.

The rate of invasion of the portal vein, hepatic vein and bile duct at the time of diagnosis is 15%, 5% and 3%, respectively. However, it is estimated that during the natural history of HCC, approximately 1 in 3 patients will develop portal vein thrombosis.

When present, metastases are most frequently found in the lung. Other locations, in decreasing order of frequency, are: adrenal glands, bones, lymph nodes, meninges, pancreas, brain and kidney. Large tumour size, bilobar disease and poor differentiation are risk factors for metastatic disease.

Clinical presentation

HCC rarely occurs before the age of 40 years and reaches a peak at around 70 years of age. The age-adjusted incidence in women is two to four times less than in men and the difference is most pronounced in medium-risk south European populations and premenopausal women. Reasons for this higher rate in men include differences in exposure to risk factors, higher body mass index and higher levels of androgenic hormones.

There are basically three circumstances of diagnosis: (1) incidental finding during routine screening; (2) incidental finding during investigation of abnormal liver function tests or of another pathological condition; and (3) presence of liver- or cancer-related symptoms, the severity of which depend on the stage of the tumour and the functional status of the non-tumorous liver. In developed countries, a growing number of tumours are discovered incidentally at an asymptomatic stage. As tumours increase in size, they may cause abdominal pain, malaise, weight loss, asthenia, anorexia and fever. These symptoms may be acute as a result of tumour extension or complication.

Spontaneous rupture occurs in 5–15% of patients and is observed particularly in patients with superficial or protruding tumours. The diagnosis should be suspected in patients with known HCC or cirrhosis presenting with acute epigastric pain, as well as in Asian or African men who develop an acute abdomen (**Fig. 5.2**). Minor rupture manifests as abdominal pain or haemorrhagic ascites, and hypovolaemic shock is only present in about half of the patients. Portal vein invasion may manifest as upper gastrointestinal bleeding or acute ascites, and invasion of hepatic veins or the inferior vena cava may result in pulmonary embolism or sudden death.

Clinical symptoms resulting from biliary invasion or haemobilia are present in 2% of patients. Possible paraneoplastic syndromes associated with HCC include polyglobulia, hypercalcaemia and hypoglycaemia. Finally, in patients with underlying liver disease, a sudden onset or worsening ascites or liver decompensation may be the first evidence of HCC formation.

Clinical examination may only reveal large or superficial tumours. There may be clinical signs of cirrhosis, in particular ascites, a collateral circulation, umbilical hernia, hepatomegaly and splenomegaly.

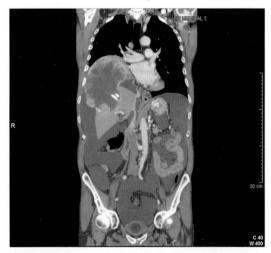

Figure 5.2 • CT scan of a patient with a ruptured HCC. Note that the rupture is limited at the upper part of the liver. This patient had haemorrhagic ascites.

Liver function tests and tumour markers

Liver function tests

Abnormal liver function tests are a non-specific finding and reflect an underlying liver pathology or the presence of a space-occupying lesion. Because most HCCs develop within a cirrhotic liver and since HCCs in normal livers are usually large, entirely normal liver function tests are exceptional. Jaundice is most frequently the result of liver decompensation.

Serum tumour markers

α-Fetoprotein

Serum α-fetoprotein (AFP) is the most widely recognised serum marker of HCC. It is secreted during foetal life but residual levels are very low in adults (0–20 ng/mL). It may increase in patients with an HCC, and serum levels greater than 400 ng/mL can be considered as diagnostic of HCC with 95% confidence. Levels may exceed 10 000 ng/mL in 5–10% of patients with HCC. Very high levels usually correlate with poor differentiation, tumour aggressiveness and vascular invasion. An AFP >20 ng/mL has a sensitivity of 60% and therefore a surveillance programme using this cut-off value would miss 40% of tumours. If a value of >200 ng/mL is used, 22% of tumours would be missed. Only 10% of small tumours are associated with raised AFP levels, whereas 30% of patients with chronic active hepatitis without an HCC have a moderately increased AFP. This usually correlates with the degree of histological activity and raised levels of transaminase, and it may therefore fluctuate. Tumours other than HCC can also be associated with increased AFP levels, but these are rare (non-seminal germinal tumours, hepatoid gastric tumours, neuroendocrine tumours).

Others serum tumour markers

Alternative serum markers for HCC, such as des-γ-carboxy prothrombin (DCP) or prothrombin induced by vitamin K absence (PIVKA-II; >40 mAU/mL) and AFP-L3 (>15%) have not come into common practice except in Japan, where they are covered under the national health insurance. A prospective study of at-risk patients comparing the accuracy of AFP and DCP in the early detection of HCC showed that the combination of both markers increased the sensitivity from 61% and 74%, for each marker alone, to 91% for both markers combined.[19]

Radiological studies

The aims of imaging in the context of HCC are to screen high-risk patients, differentiate HCC from other space-occupying lesions and select the most appropriate treatment.

Differentiation of HCC from other tumours relies on its vascularisation. The most reliable imaging features of an HCC are the presence of hyperarterialisation of the nodule in the early (arterial) phase and washout during the portal or late phase following injection (the tumour becomes hypovascular compared to the adjacent parenchyma). By definition, the term 'washout' can only be applied to tumours that are hypervascular in the arterial phase (although this may be very transient).

Critical in choosing the most appropriate treatment are the number of lesions, their size and extent, and the presence of daughter nodules, vascular invasion, extrahepatic spread and underlying liver disease.

These aims may be achieved by ultrasound (US), contrast-enhanced US, computed tomography (CT), magnetic resonance imaging (MRI), angiography or a combination of these.

✅ Imaging aims to:
- screen patients for the development of HCC, and this is best achieved by US;
- differentiate potential HCC from other tumours, and this is best achieved by demonstrating the presence of hypervascularisation during the arterial phase and washout during the portal or late phase.

Ultrasound

US is the first-line investigation for screening because of its low cost, widespread availability and high sensitivity in identifying a focal liver mass. In experienced hands, US may identify 85–95% of lesions measuring 3–5 cm in diameter and 60–80% of lesions measuring 1 cm. Differences in accuracy worldwide may be explained by steatosis rates, heterogeneity of the liver disease and in operator variability. Typically, small HCCs are hypoechoic and homogeneous and cannot be differentiated from regenerating or dysplastic nodules. With increasing size, they may become hypo- or hyperechoic but most importantly heterogeneous. A hypoechoic peripheral rim corresponds to the capsule. The infiltrating type is usually very difficult to identify in a grossly heterogeneous cirrhotic liver. Besides echogenicity, the accuracy of US depends on the dimension and location of the tumour, as well as operator experience. A 1-cm-diameter tumour can be visualised if it is deeply located, whereas the same lesion located on the surface of the liver can be missed. Similarly, tumours located in the upper liver segments or on the edge of the left lateral segment may be missed. Tumours detected at an advanced stage despite surveillance are frequently located at one of these two sites. Obesity may also prevent accurate assessment of the liver (thickened abdominal wall or steatotic liver). Doppler US may demonstrate a feeding artery and/or draining veins. US is also accurate in identifying vascular or biliary invasion and indirect evidence of cirrhosis such as segmental atrophy, splenomegaly, ascites or collateral veins. Tumour thrombosis is associated with enlargement of the vascular lumen, and duplex Doppler may detect an arterial signal. Contrast US is addressed below.

Computed tomography

CT is more accurate than US in identifying HCCs and their lobar or segmental distribution, particularly with the development of helical and multislice spiral scanners. Spiral CT is undertaken without contrast and during arterial (25–50 s), portal (60–65 s) and equilibrium (130–180 s) phases after contrast administration. In addition, it is useful for identifying features of underlying cirrhosis, accurately measuring liver and tumour volumes, and assessing extrahepatic tumour spread. HCCs are usually hypodense and spontaneous hyperdensity is usually associated with iron overload or fatty infiltration, which is seen in 2–20% of patients. Specific features are early uptake of contrast and a mosaic shape pattern. During the portal phase, the density diminishes sharply and results in washout (tumour is hypodense compared to adjacent parenchyma) during the late phase (**Fig. 5.3**). HCCs may show variable vascularity depending on tumour grade and some are poorly vascularised. The capsule, when present, is best seen during the portal or late phase as an enhanced thickening at the periphery (delayed vascular enhancement is characteristic of fibrosis). Vascular invasion of segmental branches may also be identified. Intratumoral arterioportal fistula may develop and present as early enhancement of portal branches or as a triangular area distal to the tumour with contrast enhancement different from the adjacent parenchyma. Nonetheless, such fistulas are seen frequently in cirrhotic patients without HCC as infracentimetric hypervascular subcapsular lesions.

Magnetic resonance imaging

MRI tends to be more accurate than other imaging techniques in differentiating HCC from other liver tumours, especially those >2 cm in diameter. As for CT, the technique of MRI should be accurate with T1- and T2-weighted images and with early, intermediate and late phases following contrast injection of gadolinium. The characteristics of an HCC are the mosaic shape structure and the presence of a capsule. Tumours are hypointense on T1-weighted

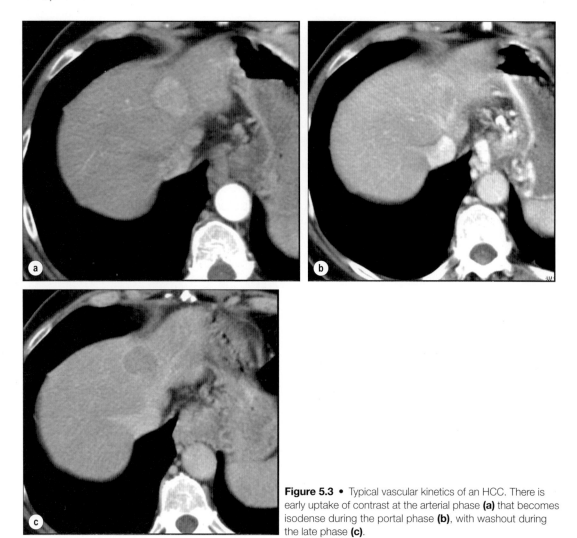

Figure 5.3 • Typical vascular kinetics of an HCC. There is early uptake of contrast at the arterial phase **(a)** that becomes isodense during the portal phase **(b)**, with washout during the late phase **(c)**.

images and hyperintense on T2-weighted images, but these characteristics are present in only 54% of patients; 16% of HCCs demonstrate hypointensity on both T1 and T2 images. Hyperintensity on T1-weighted images is also possible, and associated with fatty, copper or glycogen infiltration of the tumour. The kinetics of vascular enhancement following injection of contrast are the same as during CT, with early uptake and late washout. Recently, liver-specific magnetic resonance contrast medium such as Gd-EOB-DTPA that accumulates in Kuppfer cells (due to phagocytosis) or in hepatic cells has increased the accuracy of MRI, but has not yet come into common practice except in Eastern countries.

Contrast-enhanced ultrasound

Contrast-enhanced US (CEUS) is the most recent technique to assess vascularisation of tumours.

A contrast agent (stabilised microbubbles) is administered intravenously via a bolus injection followed by saline flush. Enhancement patterns are typically described during the arterial (10–20 s postinjection), portal venous (30–80 s) and late phase (120–360 s). Whereas US microbubbles are confined to the vascular spaces, contrast agents for CT and MRI are rapidly cleared from the blood into the extracellular space. The sensitivity of CEUS to detect arterial enhancement is greater than that of CT or MRI because of the continuous monitoring of the images. Washout is slower for well-differentiated than for poorly differentiated tumours. However, it is subject to the same limitations as other US modes: if the baseline scan is unsatisfactory, the CEUS study will also be unsatisfactory. The advent of the second-generation US contrast agent Sonazoid, approved exclusively in Japan in 2007, has made

Sonazoid-CEUS more effective for screening and staging than CEUS using other vascular agents such as SonoVue. Sonazoid contrast agent is taken up by Kupffer cells in the postvascular phase or Kupffer phase (starting 10 min postinjection) and provides extremely stable Kupffer images suitable for repeated scanning from 10 to about 120 min after injection.[20]

Other imaging

Angiography

Although the diagnostic usefulness of angiography has been considerably reduced, it is still widely used as part of arterial chemoembolisation. Arteriography shows early vascular uptake (blush) and, if used, lipiodol injection is retained selectively for a prolonged period by the tumour. On subsequent CT, the retained radiodense lipiodol reveals the tumour as a high-density area. Uptake within the liver is not specific for HCC, since all hypervascular liver tumours, including focal nodular hyperplasia, adenoma, angioma and metastases, will retain Lipiodol. False-negative results may be observed with an avascular, necrotic or fibrotic HCC.

Positron emission tomography

The contribution of fluorodeoxyglucose (FDG)-positron emission tomography (PET) in the diagnosis of HCC remains limited because of low sensitivity (60%). FDG-PET can detect poorly differentiated but not-well differentiated HCC due to similarities between the metabolism of FDG in normal hepatocytes and hepatocellular cells. Recently, [^{18}F]fluorocholine (FCH), a PET tracer of lipid metabolism, has been shown to be significantly more sensitive than [^{18}F]FDG at detecting HCC, particularly in well-differentiated tumours.[21] Interestingly, in metastatic HCC, FDG-PET has a high sensitivity and is more suitable for the detection of bone metastases than CT or bone scintigraphy.[22]

Accuracy of imaging techniques

CT and MRI with contrast enhancement have the highest diagnostic accuracy (>80%) and the techniques can be combined. However, pathological analysis of explanted livers from transplant patients shows that both techniques lose accuracy in assessing extension of the disease. For any technique, additional intrahepatic tumours, especially those less than 1 cm, are not diagnosed preoperatively in 30% of cases. MRI angiography with 2-mm sections is currently considered the most accurate technique, with a sensitivity of 100% for nodules more than 20 mm, 89% for nodules 10–20 mm and 34% for nodules <10 mm.

Requirement for and reliability of histological assessment

Pathological confirmation of HCC can be obtained by cytology, histology or a combination of these with increasing accuracy. The accuracy of pathological assessment is increased if a sample of non-tumorous tissue is available for comparison. Liver biopsy is limited by the potential for haemorrhage and pain, and may occasionally be responsible for neoplastic seeding and vascular spread. The reported incidence of needle tract seeding is 1–5%. Tumour involvement is generally limited to subcutaneous tissues, has a slow progression and it is possible to perform local excision without apparent impact on survival. Even if the false-positive rate is low, the risk of needle tract seeding is balanced by the risk of pursuing an aggressive treatment such as resection or transplantation in a patient without malignancy. Every attempt should be made not to puncture the nodule directly but to access the nodule through a thick area of normal liver. As described below, several studies have shown that expert pathological diagnosis of HCC can be reinforced by staining for GPC3, HSP70 and GS, particularly in biopsies of small lesions that are not clearly HCC.

✔ There is a significant false-negative rate for fine-needle biopsy, especially in small lesions, lesions that are difficult to access or those developing on the background of a multinodular parenchyma. A negative result should therefore never rule out malignancy.

Diagnosis of HCC

The standard for the diagnosis of HCC is histology. This is particularly true for tumours measuring 3 cm or less or when active treatment is required. Ideally, these samples should be associated with a biopsy of the non-tumorous liver and be made available for research, with patient consent. Non-invasive diagnosis (using radiological imaging alone) requires rigorous technique and interpretation.

The first attempt to standardise the diagnostic criteria was in 2000 by the European Association for the Study of Liver Disease (EASLD). Since the last publication of the AASLD practice guidelines for the management of HCC in 2005, several studies have reported that AFP determination lacks adequate sensitivity and specificity for effective surveillance and diagnosis.[19] The advocated strategy in the

2011 updated version of the diagnostic criteria[23] was based on imaging techniques and/or biopsy as follows:

- For nodules less than 1 cm found on US, it was considered that other imaging techniques would be unlikely to reliably confirm the diagnosis. Since the accuracy of liver biopsy for such small lesions and the likelihood of HCC are low, it was felt reasonable to repeat an US at 3- to 6-month intervals until the lesion disappeared, enlarged or displayed characteristics of HCC. If there has been no growth over a period of up to 2 years, routine surveillance can be resumed.
- For nodules larger than 1 cm found on US screening of a cirrhotic liver, diagnosis of HCC can be established by one contrast-enhanced imaging technique (multidetector CT or dynamic contrast-enhanced MRI). The specific imaging pattern of HCC is defined by intense contrast uptake during the arterial phase followed by contrast washout during the venous or delayed phases. The value of these non-invasive criteria for HCC in cirrhosis has been confirmed prospectively.[24-26] These typical imaging features have a specificity and predictive positive value of approximately 100% and sensitivity of 71%.
- If the findings are not characteristic or the vascular features are not typical, and in other clinical settings (e.g. absence of cirrhosis), a diagnostic biopsy was recommended, although it was acknowledged that a negative biopsy did not exclude the diagnosis.

Subsequent to these recommendations, several studies have reported that CEUS may give a false-positive HCC diagnosis and cannot selectively differentiate intrahepatic cholangiocarcinoma from HCC. This technique has therefore been withdrawn from the diagnostic algorithm proposed by the AASLD.

✅ Current guidelines[23] for the positive diagnosis of HCC are:
- For nodules >1 cm with cirrhosis, early uptake and delayed washout on a single dynamic imaging study (triphasic CT or MRI with gadolinium) is considered characteristic of HCC.
- For nodules >1 cm without cirrhosis or if the vascular features are not typical, a diagnostic biopsy is recommended.

- Biopsy of small lesions should be evaluated by expert pathologists. Tissue that is not clearly an HCC should be stained with CD34, CK7, GPC3, HSP70 and GS to improve diagnostic accuracy.
- If the biopsy is negative for HCC, it is recommended that the lesion should be re-evaluated using US at 3- to 6-month intervals. If the lesion enlarges but remains atypical for HCC, a repeat biopsy is recommended.

Natural history of HCC and staging systems

Traditionally, the natural history of HCC is considered to be particularly grim, with a median survival of 6 months in symptomatic patients. However, the 3-year survival of asymptomatic untreated patients who are not end-stage at the time of presentation may be as high as 50%. These observations have important implications for patients with an HCC diagnosed at an early stage, particularly in patients with preserved liver function.

The aim of staging systems is to predict outcome. This can either be used to anticipate prognosis or, more recently, for selection of treatment. Survival of patients with HCC is mainly influenced by the morphological spread of tumour, the presence and severity of cancer-related symptoms, and the severity and evolution of the underlying cirrhosis. The most recent systems attempt to integrate all three groups of parameters.

- Although staging was assessed initially by the TNM classification, the pathological staging of HCC has evolved in Eastern (Liver Cancer Study Group of Japan) and Western (American Joint Committee on Cancer, International Union Against Cancer) countries. These take into account the number of tumours, vascular invasion and tumour size (Table 5.2). A limitation is that they are based on pathological findings and can only be applied accurately (retrospectively) in operated patients.
- Cancer-related symptoms have a detrimental impact on outcome that is assessed by the WHO performance status or the Karnofsky index. The presence of pain is a poor indicator of outcome.
- Liver damage induced by underlying liver disease has traditionally been assessed by the Child–Pugh score. This was, however, designed to assess the functional reserve of cirrhotic patients undergoing portocaval shunt surgery and is not entirely appropriate for HCC patients in whom therapeutic options may include liver transplantation and liver resection.

Table 5.2 • Comparison of the tumour (T) staging in the Liver Cancer Study Group of Japan (LCSGJ) and American Joint Committee on Cancer (AJCC) staging systems

LCSGJ

T1	Tumour <2 cm, unique *and* without vascular invasion
T2	Tumour <2 cm, multiple *or* with vascular invasion
	Tumour >2 cm single *and* without vascular invasion
T3	Tumour <2 cm, multiple *and* with vascular invasion
	Tumour >2 cm, multiple *or* with vascular invasion
T4	Tumour >2 cm, multiple *and* with vascular invasion

AJCC

T1	Single tumour without vascular invasion
T2	Tumour <5 cm, multiple *or* with vascular invasion
T3A	Multiple tumours, any >5 cm *or* tumour(s) involving major branch of portal or hepatic vein(s)
T3B	Any tumour N1
T4	Any tumour M1

AJCC/UICC and LCSGJ TNM classification of HCC.

Several groups have attempted to combine these features within integrated staging systems. There are currently six such systems, designated as the CLIP (from Italy), GRETCH (from France), BCLC (from Spain), CUPI (from China), JSS and JIS (from Japan) scores. It is beyond the scope of this chapter to detail all of them (Table 5.3). It should be appreciated that these scores have been computed retrospectively by multivariate analysis of a specific patient population and not all have been externally validated.

Currently, the BCLC system is widely accepted, as it includes variables linked to tumour stage and function, physical status and cancer-related symptoms, and it combines each stage (very early stage: 0; early stage: A; intermediate stage: B; advanced stage: C; and end stage: D) with a treatment algorithm. It has been externally validated and has been recently supported by both the AASLD and EASL. However, validation in Eastern countries has not been achieved to date. One area of concern regards the definition of intermediate and advanced HCC; most Asian experts agree that early stage means that HCC can be controlled by curative treatment, but advanced stage (which includes portal vein invasion and distant metastatis) is hard to define in the BCLC system as it can be divided into two other different groups: locally advanced with portal vein invasion and advanced with extrahepatic metastasis. At present, most Asian countries have their own HCC staging system with different constituent variables.

Screening for HCC

Screening is used routinely in countries where effective therapeutic interventions are available. HCC fulfils most of the criteria required for a surveillance or screening programme to be justified.

Table 5.3 • Main variables retained in prognostic models

	GRETCH		CLIP		CUPI	
Tumour morphology			Multinodular extension <50%	1	TNM I and II	−3
			Multinodular extension >50%	2	TNM III	−1
					TNM IV	0
	Portal thrombosis	1	Portal thrombosis	1		
Tumour biology	AFP >35 ng/mL	2	AFP >400 ng/mL	1	AFP >500 ng/mL	3
Liver function	Bilirubin >50 μmol/L	3	Child–Pugh A	0	Bilirubin <34 μmol/mL	0
	Alk. phosph. >2N*	2	Child–Pugh B	1	Bilirubin 34–51 μmol/mL	3
			Child–Pugh C	2	Bilirubin >51 μmol/mL	4
					Alk. phosph. >200 IU/L	3
General status	Karnofsky index <80	3			Asymptomatic	−4
Score range		0–11		0–6		−7 to 12

The numbers refer to the score given to each variable. A total score is obtained by adding each individual score. In the CLIP score, the median survivals according to the score in the initial[30] and prospective validations[32] were: score 0, 36–42 months; score 1, 22–32 months; score 2, 8–16 months; score 3, 4–7 months, score 4 or above, 1–3 months.
*2N = twice normal.

HCC is common in highly endemic areas (and its incidence is growing in others) and it is associated with a high mortality. Furthermore, survival is extremely poor by the time patients present with symptoms related to the tumour, and the population at risk is clearly defined (in particular – but not exclusively – patients with HCV- and HBV-related cirrhosis, especially when they are male and over 60 years of age). Acceptable screening tests with low morbidity and high efficacy exist that allow the tumour to be recognised in the latent/early stage. Finally, effective treatments exist in selected patients.

The two most common tests used for screening of HCC are US and serum AFP measurements, although many clinicians consider the latter investigation to be of little value for screening. However, a progressive increase of AFP in patients who have a normal AFP at baseline should prompt a CT or MRI scan if US is negative. It should be underlined that US is most difficult in obese patients with fatty liver disease and cirrhosis, but no alternative strategy for surveillance has been adequately tested.

No clear evidence is available to determine the optimal interval for periodic screening. Tumour doubling times vary widely, with an average of 200 days. It has been estimated that the time taken for an undetectable lesion to grow to 2 cm is about 4–12 months, and that it takes 5 months for the most rapidly growing HCC to reach 3 cm. Because treatments are most effective for tumours <3 cm, screening programmes are usually performed at 6-monthly intervals. The efficacy of screening to improve the prognosis of HCC has mainly been demonstrated in China on HBV carriers.[27] These results need to be validated in other geographical areas. Until then, most rely on a 6-month interval (3–4 months in Japan) in high-risk patients. It has been reported that surveillance is cost-effective if the expected HCC risks exceeds 1.5% per year in patients with HCV and 0.2% per year in patients with HBV.[28]

There are limitations to screening programmes. Of patients presenting with HCC, 20–50% have previously undiagnosed cirrhosis and therefore escape surveillance. Access to medical care and compliance is a limitation in highly endemic areas, with 50% of patients with alcoholic cirrhosis defaulting from surveillance over 5 years. US is highly operator dependent, and the cost and invasiveness of CT and MRI make them unsuitable for screening. However, these latter modalities are particularly suited in patients with irregular background liver parenchyma or obesity. Physicians should also take into account the presence of comorbid disease, severity of liver disease and available treatment options when deciding whether or not to screen a cirrhotic patient.

Screening of Child C patients in particular is inappropriate if they are not potential liver transplant candidates.

✔ Surveillance of at-risk patients is being used increasingly at 6-monthly intervals with US to detect HCC at an early stage.

✔ High-risk groups consist of those with established cirrhosis due to HBV, HCV and haemochromatosis. Male patients with alcohol-related cirrhosis abstaining from alcohol or likely to comply with treatment should also be considered. US is recommended as a screening tool, whereas CT and MRI are most useful in confirming the diagnosis.

Treatment options

There is a wide range of treatment options for HCC (liver transplantation, liver resection, ablation, chemoembolisation, systemic treatments) and the decision should therefore be taken in a multidisciplinary team meeting involving a hepatic–pancreatic–biliary surgeon, interventional radiologist, oncologist and hepatologist, using predefined guidelines.

Liver transplantation, liver resection and ablation are traditionally defined as curative treatments. However, when underlying liver disease is present (typically cirrhosis), only transplantation is curative by simultaneously treating the aetiology of HCC. Recurrence is essentially invariable with all other treatments.

In patients without cirrhosis, liver resection is the ideal treatment but this group accounts for only a small proportion of patients with HCC. In cirrhotic patients, management is more challenging and should take into account tumour extension, status of the non-tumoral liver and general condition of the patient.

HCC in normal livers

The treatment of choice in patients with no or minimal coexisting fibrosis is partial liver resection. The non-tumorous liver has a high regenerating capacity, allowing even major hepatectomies to be performed. Perioperative mortality and morbidity are less than 1% and 15%, respectively. Five-year survival is greater than 50%.[29] These results may, however, vary according to the population studied. Patients with a metabolic syndrome in particular are at increased risk of postoperative mortality. Lymphadenectomy is recommended as the prevalence of lymph node metastases is approximately 15%, compared to less than 5% in cirrhotic patients. Adjuvant chemotherapy is not recommended.

Regular follow-up with throraco-abdominal CT at 6-monthly intervals is recommended, as early detection and treatment of recurrence may improve survival.

There is very little place for other invasive treatments. Percutaneous ablation, as a rule, has no role due to the usually large tumour size at diagnosis. Liver transplantation is associated with a perioperative mortality of 10%, a need for long-term immunosuppression and long-term results not significantly different from those of resection. In a recent multicentre study based on a collaboration of 38 European transplant centres, only 105 patients transplanted for an HCC occurring in a normal liver were identified.[30] Transplantation had been performed as the primary treatment because partial liver resection was precluded by anatomical factors or the need to preserve a sufficient volume of liver remnant, or as rescue treatment for intrahepatic tumour recurrence not amenable to repeat resection. The 5-year survival rate was 59% in patients without macrovascular or lymph node invasion, irrespective of tumour size and differentiation.

Liver resection of HCC in cirrhotic patients

Liver resection

Main limitations

Resection of HCC has four limitations in cirrhotic patients: (i) the tumour is multifocal in 20–60% of patients at the time of diagnosis and liver resection can normally only be considered in patients with unifocal tumours; (ii) cirrhosis is an important risk factor for the development of postoperative complications; (iii) oncological resections dictate wide margins whereas the diseased underlying liver usually requires parenchymal sparing; (iv) recurrence is invariable as cirrhosis persists.

Risk of surgery and patient selection

The risk of hepatectomy is increased in cirrhotic patients due to coagulation defects, portal hypertension, liver failure and impaired regeneration. In-hospital death was 10% in the 1990s (even higher in some subgroups) but has decreased since then as a result of improved patient selection, operative technique and perioperative management. Although some very large series report no mortality, the average mortality rates in national surveys or registries are 4–6% and are therefore higher than in non-cirrhotic patients or after resection of other malignancies.

Hepatectomy, as a rule, should only be performed in Child–Pugh A cirrhotic patients. Child–Pugh B or C patients are at a prohibitive risk of early liver failure even after a minor hepatectomy or mere laparotomy. Child–Pugh A patients may, however, still be at increased risk of postoperative liver failure, in particular after major resections, due to impaired ability to regenerate. This correlates with the fibrosis grade, although it is only in patients with extensive fibrosis or cirrhosis that this impairment has clinical impact. Typically, following a major liver resection, there is an increase in prothrombin time (peak on postoperative day 1) and an increase in serum bilirubin (peak on postoperative days 3–5) that tend to normalise within 5–7 days. Recovery of both tests is, in contrast, delayed or absent in cirrhotic patients. When the prothrombin time is less than 50% of normal and serum bilirubin is greater than 50 μmol/L on postoperative day 5, the risk of postoperative mortality is close to 50%.

Additional selection criteria for surgery have therefore been proposed for Child–Pugh A patients. In Japan, the indocyanine green (ICG) test is usually used. After injection of 0.5 mg ICG/kg body weight, retention of ICG is measured in peripheral blood, in particular 15 min after the injection (ICG-R15). Normal values of ICG-R15 are 10%. In cirrhotic patients, minor resections can be performed when it is 22% or less, but major resections only if it less than 14–17%. In contrast, in Europe and the USA, selection mainly relies on the absence of significant portal hypertension or cytolysis. This requires that patients have no evidence of oesophageal varices, splenomegaly, portosystemic shunts (including a patent umbilical vein) or ascites (even on imaging studies), and that they have a platelet count greater than 100×10^9/L. Some groups even advocate that invasive measurement of the hepatic vein–portal vein gradient should be less than 10 mmHg. Several studies have shown that a normal serum bilirubin and the absence of clinically significant portal hypertension are the best predictors of good outcomes after resection.[31] Recently, the MELD score and thrombocytopenia, irrespective of Child–Pugh grade and tumour features, have been shown to be associated not only with postoperative mortality and morbidity but also with long-term survival.[32,33]

✔ In cirrhotic patients who have a single resectable lesion, hepatectomy should only be performed if patients have well-preserved liver function, normal bilirubin and hepatic vein pressure <10 mmHg.

There has been considerable interest during the past 5 years in the optimal management of the remnant liver. This includes: (i) more selective use of inflow occlusion; (ii) avoiding excessive mobilisation of the liver; and (iii) measuring the future remnant liver volume (RLV) using CT reconstruction. In patients with chronic liver disease, an RLV of approximately 40% of the total liver volume is required before a major hepatectomy is performed. When this is not the case, preoperative portal vein embolisation (PVE) is indicated as a means of increasing the RLV and, perhaps more importantly, preoperatively testing the ability of the liver to regenerate. When right hepatectomy is contemplated (the most frequent circumstance when there is a risk of small RLV), the right portal vein is percutaneously injected, under ultrasound guidance, with glue or ethanol. This should induce atrophy of the right liver within 2–6 weeks and a compensatory hypertrophy of the left RLV. Due to its efficacy, PVE (alone or in association with transarterial chemoembolisation) has become almost routine before a right hepatectomy in cirrhotic patients.[34] The absence of hypertrophy of the left liver following a successful right PVE means that the liver is unable to regenerate and that hepatectomy is contraindicated. There is also increasing evidence that parenchymal size alone does not necessarily reflect function and there is therefore interest in the functional evaluation of the remnant liver volume.

> ✅ When major hepatectomy is contemplated, preoperative portal vein embolisation (PVE) of the lobe to be resected should be performed to test the ability of the future remnant liver to regenerate.

Technique

There is increasing evidence that both anatomical resections (as opposed to tumorectomies) and wide (as opposed to limited) margins may improve long-term survival without increasing the perioperative risk. The rationale is tumour spread through microvascular invasion, the incidence and extent of which is related to tumour diameter and degree of tumour differentiation. Several retrospective studies have reported an approximately 20% improvement in overall and disease-free survival following anatomical compared to limited resections.[35] The impact of the margin width has been evaluated in a prospective controlled trial.[36] A 2-cm margin was associated with a 75% 5-year survival as compared to 49% for 1-cm margins. Both concepts are not exclusive and should be taken into account, especially in tumours with diameters between 2 and 5 cm.

> ✅ The concept of anatomical resections is to remove both the tumour and the adjacent segments that have the same portal tributaries and to achieve wide margins. Margins greater than 1–2 cm should be achieved to ensure that potential satellite nodules are also resected.

There is increasing interest in laparoscopic resections for HCC.[37] Although not formally proven yet, it may have the advantage of less intraoperative bleeding, postoperative complications, postoperative analgesic drug consumption and a shorter hospitalisation time. More specifically in the context of cirrhotic patients, it may also reduce the risk of postoperative ascites and its consequences, as well as facilitate subsequent liver transplantation if required, because of fewer adhesions.[38]

Outcome after resection

The largest series from the Liver Cancer Study Group in Japan has reported 1-, 3-, 5- and 10-year survival rates of 87%, 66%, 48% and 21%, respectively in 11631 cirrhotic patients treated by hepatic resection between 1992 and 2003. Comparable results have been reported by other groups worldwide, with no differences between Western and Asian studies. Independent predictors of survival are age, degree of liver damage, AFP level, tumour diameter, number of nodules, vascular invasion and surgical margins. Survival rates as high as 68% at 5 years have been reported in Child grade A patients with well-encapsulated tumours of 2 cm diameter or less. These figures continue to improve, even when patients with larger tumours are included. Active treatment of recurrences has been a major reason for this improvement.

Treatment of recurrence

Tumour recurrence is the major cause of death following resection of HCC in the cirrhotic patient. Its incidence is 40% within the first year, 60% at 3 years and approximately 80% at 5 years. However, it is invariable if follow-up is extended beyond 10 years as the precursor condition (cirrhosis) persists after surgery. It is frequently difficult to differentiate true recurrence from de novo tumours. The former tend to occur within the first 2 years and their main risk factors are vascular invasion, poor histological differentiation, presence of satellites and number of nodules. De novo recurrent tumours occur later and the main risk factors are the same as those of a primary HCC. Molecular analysis suggests that their respective proportions are 60–70% and 30–40%. Recurrence within the liver is multifocal in 50% of patients and is associated with distant metastasis in 15%, especially in the lungs, adrenal gland or bones. Extrahepatic recurrence without simultaneous intrahepatic recurrence is infrequent in cirrhotic livers. Anatomical resection and a tumour-free margin of 2 cm are associated with improved survival.

Evidence that neoadjuvant or adjuvant treatments reduce the risk of recurrence is currently lacking and these treatments are therefore not recommended.

This applies to preoperative chemoembolisation, neoadjuvant or adjuvant chemotherapy, internal radiation with ^{131}I-labelled Lipiodol, adoptive immunotherapy, retinoic acid or interferon, although some of these strategies initially showed promising results. An updated follow-up of the only randomised trial of adjuvant ^{131}I-labelled Lipiodol has shown that the improved overall and disease-free survivals in the treatment group persisted until the seventh postoperative year.[39] This study was characterised by a very high proportion of HBV-related HCC (88%). Three recent meta-analyses of published studies[40–42] favour the use of interferon to reduce the risk of HCC recurrence; however, the quality of the studies was low due to heterogeneity of the patient populations, interferon used, duration of the treatment regimen and whether results were independent of the effect of viral suppression. No study has confirmed the potential efficacy of retinoic acid. Anti-angiogenic treatments are currently being evaluated.

The most effective strategy to prevent HCC recurrence is liver transplantation in selected patients (see below). However, there are two other important strategies. The first is management of the underlying chronic liver disease, as this improves prognosis and it is possible that it also reduces tumour recurrence. The second is to actively screen operated patients and actively treat recurrences if they are confined to the liver, by repeat surgery, ablation, chemoembolisation or liver transplantation.

> ✔ At present, the best way to improve survival is to monitor resected patients regularly, as some may benefit from treatment of the recurrence if it is confined to the liver.

Liver transplantation (LT)

Rationale

HCC is the only tumour for which transplantation plays a significant role, and this is the most attractive therapeutic option because it removes both detectable and undetectable tumour nodules together with all the preneoplastic lesions that are present in the cirrhotic liver. In addition, it simultaneously treats the underlying cirrhosis and prevents the development of postoperative or distant complications associated with portal hypertension and liver failure.

Patient selection

LT is not readily available in most high endemic areas of HCC. Even when available, there is donor shortage; LT can therefore only be performed in a fraction (less than 5% in most Western countries) of

HCC patients. HCC patients are considered potential candidates for LT if their anticipated survival is approximately the same as those patients transplanted for other indications. This may be achieved if strict selection criteria are applied; otherwise, HCC patients are at high risk of death from tumour recurrence. These include an HCC: (i) confined to the liver (i.e. no extrahepatic disease, including lymph nodes); (ii) without vascular extension; and (iii) with limited tumour burden.

Tumour burden was initially defined as a single tumour less than 5 cm in diameter or the presence of two or three tumours less than 3 cm in diameter (the so-called Milan criteria).[43] With the adoption of these criteria, the 5-year survival after LT ranges between 60% and 75%. There have subsequently been concerns that these criteria were too restrictive, which led to the proposal of expanded criteria. The best known and validated of these are the UCSF criteria – a single tumour less than 6.5 cm in diameter, or three or fewer tumours, the largest of which is less than 4.5 cm with the sum of the tumour diameters being less than 8 cm.[44] Others take into account poor tumour differentiation or a high (or rapidly increasing) AFP serum concentration. An international consensus conference held in 2012 recommended a limited expansion of the listing criteria beyond the standard Milan criteria.[45] Predicting tumour biology through molecular profiling rather than tumour morphology is the aim of current research in this field.

Treatment on the waiting list

The average time from listing to transplantation in Europe and the USA is usually greater than 12 months. Up to 25% of patients may be excluded from the waiting list due to disease progression. Three approaches have been developed to avoid these drop-outs:

- Living-donor liver transplantation (LDLT) is an alternative source of grafts but has its own drawbacks, including the inherent risk for the donor, the risk of small-for-size grafts and the fact that only 25–30% of transplant candidates have a potential donor. It has the advantage of being performed rapidly, so avoiding drop-out on the waiting lists. The number of LDLT in Western countries has, however, decreased recently and the trend is to favour cadaveric transplantation through changes in allocation policies.

- New rules of graft allocation have been implemented, initially in the USA and subsequently in Europe. In the USA, the Model of End-stage Liver Disease (MELD) organ allocation policy implemented in 2002 has given priority to candidates with HCC within the Milan criteria. Waiting times have shortened, obviating the need for LDLT. Similar policies have been applied in other countries such as France and the UK.

• Treatment of the tumour by resection, ablation or chemoembolisation is widely used while the patient is on the waiting list to avoid tumour progression beyond the oncological criteria. There is some evidence that these treatments may reduce drop-out rates on the waiting lists, but it is not clear if the outcome is the same for patients within or beyond the Milan criteria. The impact of these treatments on downstaging and post-transplantation survival is similarly uncertain. A specific advantage of resection over ablation or chemoembolisation is that it provides pathological details of the tumours. However, it is still unclear if the presence of poor prognostic factors should encourage or discourage transplantation.

✓ • Liver transplantation is an effective option for HCC patients who fulfil the Milan criteria.
• Decreasing drop-out rates on the waiting list rely on changes in graft allocation policies and on treatment of the HCC while the patient is on the waiting list if this time exceeds 6 months.
• Living donor transplantation can be proposed for HCC if the waiting list is expected to be so long that there is a high risk of drop-out because of tumour progression.

Transarterial chemoembolisation (TACE)

Technique

HCC, in contrast to the liver parenchyma, receives almost 100% of its blood supply from the artery. When the feeding artery is obstructed, the tumour experiences an ischaemic insult that results in extensive necrosis. With the development of more supraselective embolisations, greater attention is paid to accessory arteries that may contribute to tumour vascularity, such as the diaphragmatic or mammary arteries, that should also be embolised to achieve adequate control. Injection of iodised oil has been combined to improve the efficacy of embolisation. Iodised oil (Lipiodol), which is hyperdense on CT, is cleared from the normal hepatic parenchyma but retained in malignant tumours for periods ranging from several weeks to over a year.

This accumulation, which is not associated with significant adverse effects, may be used for targeting cytotoxic drugs and increasing their concentration in tumour cells. Recently drug-eluting beads (DC-Beads) loaded with doxorubicin have been developed. This technique is much more expensive than conventional TACE, but preliminary results show superior treatment response and delayed tumour progression.[46] Combination of TACE and anti-angiogenic treatments is under evaluation.[47]

Contraindications

TACE should not be performed in patients with liver decompensation, biliary obstruction, bilioenteric anastomosis and impaired kidney function. Portal vein thrombosis is also a contraindication unless it is limited to a liver section only and TACE can be performed in a highly selective manner on a limited tumour volume.

Morbidity and mortality

Mortality is less than 1% if these contraindications are applied. Overall, more than 75% of patients develop a postembolisation syndrome characterised by fever, abdominal pain, nausea and raised serum transaminase levels. These symptoms, which are not prevented by antibiotics or anti-inflammatory drugs, are self-limiting and last for less than 1 week. More severe complications occur in less than 5% of patients and include, in decreasing order of frequency: cholecystitis or gallbladder infarction, gastric or duodenal wall necrosis, and acute pancreatitis. These, along with the postembolisation syndrome, have become less frequent with the use of supraselective embolisation. Hepatic abscess formation is rare, occurring in 0.3%, but is associated with a high mortality. The main risk factors are a previous history of bilioenteric anastomosis, large tumours and portal vein thrombosis.

Monitoring

The efficacy of TACE is assessed by CT (usually at 1 month) as the disappearance of the arterial vascular supply to the tumour and a decrease in its diameter. These features do not necessarily evolve in parallel. A decrease in tumour size may, for example, be associated with persistent vascularisation (i.e. residual tumour), whereas compact Lipiodol uptake without residual vascularisation may indicate complete tumour necrosis despite no significant decrease in size (**Fig. 5.4**).

Efficacy

There is grade A evidence that TACE improves survival.[48] One of the largest studies is a prospective Japanese nationwide survey reporting median and 1-, 3-, 5- and 7-year survivals of 34 months, 82%,

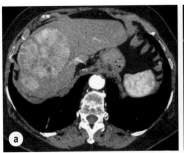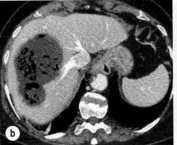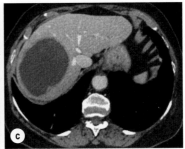

Figure 5.4 • HCC treated with microbead chemoembolisation. **(a)** Before treatment. **(b)** Two weeks after chemoembolisation: note the presence of necrosis. **(c)** Two years after chemoembolisation: the image of the tumour remains, but it is avascular, indicating complete local control.

47%, 26% and 16%, respectively, with a TACE-related mortality of 0.5%. Independent predictors of survival were, in decreasing order of influence: the degree of liver damage, portal vein invasion, maximum tumour size and number of lesions, and AFP levels.

> ✓✓ • TACE is one of the two non-curative treatments options (with sorafenib, as described above) that improves survival.
> • TACE should be recommended as first-line palliative treatment for non-surgical patients with compensated Child–Pugh A and with large or multifocal HCC, without portal vein thrombosis or extrahepatic metastasis.

Percutaneous local ablative therapy

Technique

Locoregional therapies are percutaneous treatment modalities that allow the injection of a damaging agent or the application of an energy source directly into the tumour. Damaging agents include chemicals such as ethanol (percutanenous ethanol injection, PEI) or acetic acid. Energy sources either aim at increasing temperature by radiofrequency, microwave or interstitial laser photocoagulation or, alternatively, at decreasing temperature (cryo-ablation). Irreversible electroporation is a new non-thermal ablation therapy that uses a high-voltage direct electrical current to create nanopores in the cellular membrane and results in cell death via apoptosis. Radiofrequency ablation (RFA) has emerged as the most effective of these techniques. It exploits the conversion of electromagnetic energy into heat via a needle electrode (15–18 G) positioned in the tumour, while patients are made into an electric circuit by grounding pads applied to their thighs. The radiofrequency emitted from the tip causes ionic agitation and frictional heat, which leads to cell death from coagulation necrosis. The objective is to maintain a temperature of 55–100 °C

throughout the entire target volume for a sufficient period of time. Monitoring the impedance is important because excessive heating results in tissue charring, increased tissue impedance and decreased energy absorption.

> ✓✓ The most widely used ablative techniques are PEI and RFA. All randomised controlled trials comparing PEI and RFA have suggested that the actuarial probability of local recurrence was significantly lower with RFA compared to PEI, and that RFA required fewer treatment sessions to achieve comparable antitumoral effects.[49,50]

Advantages and drawbacks

These ablative methods are minimally invasive, preserve the uninvolved liver parenchyma, have no systemic side-effects, and avoid the mortality and morbidity of major hepatic surgery. On the other hand, only tumours less than 5 cm are likely to be treated successfully but the smaller the diameter, the greater the probability of complete local control. The presence of multiple tumours (more than three) is also a limitation because of the need for repeated punctures. In addition, multiple tumours are either the result of multifocal carcinogenesis or vascular extension, and therefore a focal treatment is unlikely to be very effective. Obviously, a common requirement is also the need to clearly visualise the tumour by US and access it safely. Hence, isoechoic HCC or tumours located in the upper part of segments 4, 7 and 8 or at the edge of the left lateral section if it extends behind the spleen may occasionally be unsuitable for treatment. Finally, whichever technique is used, the needle should not enter the tumour directly but pass through the hepatic parenchyma so as to prevent intraperitoneal bleeding or seeding of tumour cells. This may prove impossible for some superficial or protruding tumours. Recently, an experienced group reported that up to one-third of patients who were theoretically good candidates for ablation could not be treated due to non-visibility of the HCC on US, risk of thermal injury or absence of a safe path.[51]

Contraindications and limitations

Contraindications to ablation procedures include gross ascites that favours intraperitoneal bleeding, coagulopathy that cannot be corrected, previous history of bilioenteric anastomosis or endoscopic sphincterotomy associated with bile bacterial contamination and therefore a risk of abscess formation. Additional contraindications (more specific to radiofrequency or microwave rather than ethanol injection) come from the proximity of the tumour to the colon, duodenum, stomach or biliary confluence, which may be injured or perforated by the heating process. RFA, unlike microwave ablation, is as a rule contraindicated in patients with a pacemaker. The efficacy of RFA also seems to be more impacted by the proximity of a vascular pedicle (the so-called cooling effect) than microwave ablation. Whereas PEI is a quick and very cheap procedure performed under light sedation, RFA is more costly, prolonged (20–90 minutes) and painful, and therefore generally performed under general anaesthesia. Microwave ablation is also performed under general anaesthesia but the procedure is quicker.

Mortality following ablation is less than 1% and morbidity less than 10%. The most frequent complications are pleural effusion and segmental intrahepatic dilatation, which have no or limited impact. Severe complications include abscess formation, perforation of adjacent organs and intraperitoneal bleeding. Tumour seeding is 5% or less. Risk factors include subcapsular location and poor histological differentiation of the tumour. Coagulating the needle tract while removing the needle may reduce this risk.

Methods and margins

Ablation should not only target the tumour but also aim to achieve a safety margin so as to control satellite nodules. The incidence of these satellite nodules, as well as their distance from the main tumour, increases as the main tumour enlarges. Both incidence and distance also increase for poorly, compared to well differentiated, tumours. This safety margin should be 5 mm at least; hence, for an HCC measuring 3 cm in diameter, the diameter of the ablation should be 4 cm. This is best achieved with thermal rather than chemical ablation. Methods to further improve tumour and margin control include multipolar ablation (several probes are placed around the tumour) and combining ablation with TACE.[52] Treatment response is assessed by CT or MRI no earlier than 1 month after the procedure. RFA may result in a rim of fibrotic tissue (hypervascular on late-phase MRI or CT) at the periphery of the tumour and should not be mistaken for residual tumour tissue. Follow-up thereafter relies on imaging studies at 3-monthly intervals to ensure that there is no recurrence of contrast enhancement.

Indication

Percutaneous ablative therapies have initially been performed in patients who were unsuitable for resectional surgery and both the EASLD and AASLD have recommended this strategy. It has thereafter been used as neoadjuvant treatment in liver transplant candidates and for treatment of recurrences after liver resection.

As the results of ablation improve, due to improved technology and patient selection, it may also be considered as an alternative to surgery or even as a first-line treatment in selected situations. A large multicentre phase 2 trial reported a 97% sustained complete response and a 68% actuarial 5-year survival following ablation in patients with HCC of 2 cm or less.[53] The results of two randomised controlled trials comparing ablation and resection in patients with early HCC demonstrated no difference.[54,55]

✅ RFA has now demonstrated its effectiveness to a point where it is considered by some centres as the first-line treatment for single nodules less than 2 cm in diameter.

However, meta-analyses still favour surgery compared to ablation in terms of 3-year survival and local control.[56,57] One additional concern is that both in the USA[58] and in Italy[59] there has been a recent temporal trend of increased use of ablation as a treatment for HCC with a simultaneous decrease in survival following this treatment, unlike what has been observed for other treatments. These observations suggest that the extension of indications for ablation should be strictly evaluated.

Other palliative treatments

Conventional systemic chemotherapy

Systemic chemotherapy has had very limited value in the past as only a very small number of patients obtained partial response or meaningful palliation using conventional drugs. Therefore, there is no rationale for using chemotherapy in patients with unresectable HCC outside of clinical trials.

Anti-angiogenic targeted therapies

✔✔ • A recent trial using molecularly targeted agents has, for the first time, demonstrated an improved overall survival in this disease and sets a new standard for the first-line treatment of advanced HCC. These new agents target angiogenesis and epidermal growth factor (EGF) receptor pathways.

• Sorafenib is therefore recommended as a first-line palliative option in patients not eligible for resection, liver transplantation, percutaneous ablation or TACE, if they still have preserved liver function.

Sorafenib (Nexavar®) exerts an anti-angiogenic effect by targeting the tyrosine kinases vascular endothelial growth factor (VEGF) receptors 2 and 3, and the platelet-derived growth factor receptor β. In an initial phase 3 trial, the median overall survival of Child–Pugh A cirrhotic patients with histologically proven and advanced HCC was 10.7 months in the treated group versus 7.9 months in the placebo double-blinded controlled arm of the study ($P=0.00058$), and the median times to tumour progression were 24 weeks and 12 weeks, respectively ($P=0.000007$).[60] This efficacy in advanced HCC (unresectable or metastatic) has been confirmed in an Asian randomised placebo-controlled trial that included mostly patients with HBV-related HCC[61] and in a large phase 4 study with more than 3000 patients.[62] Side-effects included diarrhoea (39%), hand–foot syndrome (21%), anorexia (14%) and alopecia (14%). The antitumour effect, the pharmacokinetic profile and safety profile were similar in Child–Pugh A and B. These results have established sorafenib as the standard of treatment for advanced HCC in Child A (or B) patients.[23] Several trials assessing strategies such as combination or sequential treatments are under way.

Other agents with comparable action pathways that have been evaluated in phase 2 trials include bevacizumab and sunitinib. Anti-EGF receptor agents such as tarceva and cetuximab also show promising results. Contraindications to these treatments include coronary artery disease, cardiac failure, systemic hypertension and Child B or C cirrhosis.

Radioembolisation

External beam radiation therapy has been of limited value in treating HCC because the normal liver parenchyma is very radiosensitive. Greater interest has therefore been given to injecting radioisotopes such as ^{131}I-iodised oil or ^{90}Y-labelled microspheres directly into the hepatic artery (radioembolisation), which offers the advantage of increased delivery within the tumour and decreased toxicity. The former agent has an efficacy comparable to that of chemoembolisation in patients with HCC not complicated by portal thrombosis but is superior in patients with tumour portal extension. The use of ^{90}Y microspheres is more recent and has been shown in a phase 2 trial to be safe and effective, in particular in patients with portal vein thrombosis.[63] These results have been reproduced in three recent studies, but without randomised controlled trials comparing ^{90}Y-labelled microspheres, TACE or other established treatments, defining the role of this expensive treatment in clinical practice is not possible.

Other treatments

Anti-androgenic, anti-oestrogenic and somatostatin analogues, once proposed, are currently considered ineffective.[23]

✔ New treatments such as radioembolisation and antiangiogenics are promising, but costly. The additional efficacy of radioembolisation over TACE, or of anti-angiogenics over no treatment, is required in a context of limited financial resources.

Defining a treatment strategy

Uncomplicated HCC associated with chronic liver disease

Treatment algorithms need to take account of availability of treatments.

• Liver transplantation, when available, is considered first and attention is therefore paid to the extent of liver disease, patient age and presence or absence of associated conditions. If a long waiting time (> 6 months) is expected, resection, ablation or TACE are considered prior to liver transplantation.

• If transplantation is not available or not indicated, resection should be considered. Limiting factors are the number of nodules (ideally there should be only one) and the severity of underlying liver disease (patients should be Child–Pugh A and have neither cytolysis, portal hypertension nor impaired ICG tests). If a right hepatectomy is considered it should be preceded by PVE (with or without TACE).

• If resection is not considered due to the severity of the underlying liver disease and the nodule is single (or if there are less than three nodules), ablation is the treatment of choice provided the tumour is less than 3–5 cm. For single tumours 2 cm or less, RFA is becoming a first-line treatment, as an alternative to resection.

- If neither resection nor RFA is considered, TACE is performed provided there is no ascites or liver failure (and in particular that the serum bilirubin is less than 50 μmol/L) and that the tumour burden is not too extensive (no vascular invasion or extrahepatic metastases).
- Remaining patients are currently considered for anti-angiogenic treatments provided there is neither liver failure nor vascular disease.

According to this algorithm, it may be considered that the proportion of HCC patients who are candidates for transplantation is less than 5%, for resection 10–15%, for ablation 15–20% and for TACE 30–40%.

Treatment of complicated HCC

HCC with macroscopic portal vein invasion

This is a contraindication for liver transplantation and ablative treatments. Traditionally, TACE was also contraindicated (because of the risk of liver necrosis); today it is occasionally performed provided the thrombus is limited to a liver section or less and that embolisation is highly selective, with reduced doses and partial (rather than total) arterial occlusion as the end-point. If thrombus does not extend into the main portal vein, surgical resection can be considered. Radioembolisation and anti-angiogenic therapy is otherwise indicated.

HCC with macroscopic invasion of hepatic veins

This seems to carry an even worse prognosis as the tumour thrombus will extend into the inferior vena cava. When the thrombus is confined to the hepatic vein, resection if possible can be proposed. There is, however, a very high risk of pulmonary metastases developing within 6–12 months of surgery. Extension into the inferior vena cava or the right atrium is usually beyond any treatment.

Ruptured HCC

This should be actively treated unless it occurs as a terminal presentation in patients with multiple tumours, portal thrombosis and end-stage liver failure. The primary aim of treatment is to stop bleeding, ideally by arterial embolisation. Subsequent hepatectomy can be associated with long-term survival. Indeed, (i) bleeding is not necessarily due to tumour rupture, but occasionally due to rupture of an artery at the junction of the tumour and the adjacent parenchyma, and (ii) even if the tumour has ruptured, this is not always associated with peritoneal seeding of tumour cells.

Fibrolamellar carcinoma (FLC)

FLC is a rare variant of HCC, defined as well-differentiated polygonal hepatic tumour cells with an eosinophilic granular cytoplasm surrounded by a fibrous lamellar stroma. It is most frequently observed in the Western hemisphere, where it accounts for approximately 1% of all HCCs. These tumours occur at a younger age than HCC (20–35 years), preferentially in women, and classically do not arise on a background of chronic liver disease.

- FLCs are usually large at the time of diagnosis (8–10 cm), and the common revealing symptoms are a palpable mass, abdominal pain, weight loss, malaise and anorexia.
- The prognosis is better than that of HCC overall. Five-year survival following resection is 50–75%.[64]
- Resection is preferred to transplantation as the latter has very little or no place.

On imaging, FLC presents as a large solitary hypervascular heterogeneous liver mass with a central hypodense region due to central necrosis or fibrosis. On MRI, the central scar has low attenuation on T2 images, whereas the central scar of focal nodular hyperplasia has high attenuation. They have well-defined margins and calcification is present in 68%. Histology demonstrates deeply eosinophilic, polygonal neoplastic cells surrounded by a dense, layered fibrous stroma.

AFP levels are raised in less than 10% of patients.[64] Lymph node invasion within the hepatic pedicle is frequent (60%) and if resection is considered, simultaneous lymphadenectomy is recommended. There is a significant risk of recurrence, not only within the liver but also as lymph node or distant metastases. Close long-term follow-up is mandatory since recurrence and death beyond 5 years are common. Repeat surgery is a reasonable option in this younger patient population due to the relatively indolent course of the disease and the relative inefficacy of non-surgical treatments.

A recent study has suggested that true FLC should be differentiated from mixed FLC–HCC, defined as conventional HCC displaying some distinct area with FLC features.[65]

Intrahepatic cholangiocarcinoma (ICCA)

ICCA, also known as peripheral cholangiocarcinoma, is the second most frequent primary tumour of the liver after HCC. Tumours arise from the peripheral intrahepatic biliary radicles, which differentiates them from hilar (Klatskin) tumours and common bile duct cholangiocarcinoma.

Until the very end of the 1980s, there was no immunohistological marker that could pinpoint the biliary origin of adenocarcinoma, and ICCAs were therefore probably frequently considered as being liver metastases of an adenocarcinoma of unknown origin. The diagnosis is currently ascertained through immunostaining that shows that they are CK7 positive and CK20 negative (colorectal metastases are CK7 negative and CK20 positive).

This tumour has a poor prognosis overall and resection, sometimes at any cost, was the only therapeutic option. However, the recent implementation of a specific staging system and evidence that chemotherapy is effective pave the way for improved management.

Incidence

In the Western world, the incidence of ICCA is 0.3–3 per 100 000, 10 times less than HCC. Recent reports suggest the incidence is increasing, particularly in the USA, UK, France, Italy, Japan and Australia. Although this increase may be real, it is probably mainly explained by improved identification of this tumour and changing rules on how they should be coded according to the International Classification of Diseases for Oncology (ICD).[66]

Risk factors

The traditional risk factors for cholangiocarcinoma include chronic biliary inflammation such as primary sclerosing cholangitis, chronic choledocholithiasis, hepatolithiasis, parasitic biliary infestation, Caroli's disease and choledochal cyst. However, in most patients with ICCA (more than 95%) none of these risk factors can be identified. The exception occurs in some areas of Asia and in particular northeastern Thailand, where the parasite *Opisthorcis viverrini* is particularly prevalent.

New risk factors are emerging, including chronic non-alcoholic liver disease, HBV infection, HCV infection, diabetes and the metabolic syndrome.[67] However, in contrast to HCC, most ICCAs develop without a background of liver disease. In surgical series, 75% of patients have normal livers, 16% have chronic hepatitis/liver fibrosis and 9% have cirrhosis.

Classification and staging

The Liver Cancer Study Group of Japan proposed a gross classification of ICCAs into three types based on macroscopic findings: mass forming, which is by far the commonest type (75% in Asian series and probably more in the West); periductal infiltrating, which spreads along the bile ducts; and intraductal growth type with intraluminal spread. However, tumours may have mixed components, in particular a combination of mass forming and periductal infiltrating.

Whereas previously ICCAs were staged using a similar system as HCCs, the AJCC implemented a specific classification for ICCAs in 2010.[68] The T staging takes into account number of tumours and vascular invasion (the presence of either defines T2), rather than tumour size. The reason for this is that it is very unusual to diagnose ICCA early and size does not independently impact survival in published surgical series. T3 tumours are those perforating the visceral peritoneum or involving local extrahepatic structures by direct invasion, although this is fairly rare. The T staging also aims to take into account the periductal-infiltrating pattern of ICCA and, when present, defines T4. However, this infiltrating pattern may be difficult to identify on imaging studies or even on pathological specimens and there is no standardised definition yet. Lymph node involvement has a major impact on survival and, when present, defines TNM stage III. Prevalence of lymph node extension is high and therefore lymphadenectomy should be routinely performed to achieve accurate staging. Median survival of patients with stage I is greater than 5 years (but these patients are very rare), whereas that of patients with stage II is 53 months and that of patients with stage III is 16 months.[69]

Pathology and progression analysis

Two distinct conditions that precede invasive cholangiocarcinoma have been identified. The first is a flat or micropapillary growth of atypical biliary epithelium, which has been called biliary dysplasia or biliary intraepithelial neoplasia. The second is an intraductal papillary neoplasm of the bile duct characterised by the prominent papillary growth of atypical biliary epithelium with distinct fibrovascular cores and frequent mucin over-production. These preneoplastic conditions have mainly been analysed in hepatolithiasis and are observed more frequently in large bile ducts as hilar tumours than in small septal–interlobular bile ducts such as with ICCA.[70] The dysplasia–carcinoma sequence therefore appears more obvious for hilar lesions than peripheral lesions. This suggests that an alternative source of ICCA could be the canals of Hering or hepatic progenitor cells, which are a target cell population for carcinogenesis in chronic liver disease.

Clinical presentation and laboratory tests

As a rule, ICCA tends to be diagnosed at an advanced stage because the tumour remains clinically silent for a long time. Symptoms, when present, include abdominal pain, malaise, night sweats, asthenia, nausea and weight loss. When they appear, the tumour is frequently unresectable.

ICCAs typically appear with equal frequency in men or women aged 55–75 years. Liver function tests are non-specific even though an increase in liver enzymes (in particular γ-glutamyl transferase) may be the only initial finding in some patients. Although ICCA by definition excludes tumours arising from the biliary confluence or first-order branches, jaundice may be present if the tumour compresses or invades the biliary confluence.

Serum markers lack sensitivity and specificity. Carcinoembryonic antigen (CEA) exceeds 20 ng/mL in 15% and carbohydrate antigen (CA) 19-9 is greater than 300 U/mL in 40% of cases. AFP exceeds 200 ng/mL in only 6% of patients.

Imaging studies

The main characteristic of mass-forming ICCA is that it is a fibrous tumour and therefore displays no enhancement on the arterial phase and delayed enhancement during the late phase. This may be seen both on CT and MRI. On MRI, lesions are hypointense on T1-weighted images and moderately to markedly hyperintense on T2-weighted images (**Fig. 5.5**). They are typically large,

non-encapsulated, heterogeneous, associated with narrowing of adjacent portal veins and retraction of the liver capsule. As the tumour grows, satellite nodules frequently develop in the vicinity of the tumour, and subsequently in the contralateral lobe (**Fig. 5.6**). When superficial, these satellite nodules may not be visible on imaging. There is a high propensity for lymph node invasion (present in 40% of resected patients if lymphadenectomy is performed routinely), but imaging studies only have a sensitivity of 50% and a specificity of 75% to predict this.

Diagnosis

The main differential diagnoses of ICCA are other fibrous tumours and in particular metastases from colorectal cancer. Both tumours may easily be confused on imaging studies. The diagnosis relies on a biopsy that shows an adenocarcinoma of biliary phenotype (CK7 positive, CK20 negative). Colorectal metastases are, in contrast, CK7 negative and CK20 positive.

Treatment

Surgical resection is the only curative treatment. Unlike HCC, there is currently no place for liver transplantation.

As the tumour is usually diagnosed at an advanced stage, has ill-defined borders and occasionally extends to major portal branches or hepatic veins, surgery is frequently extensive. A major hepatectomy is required in 75–80%, extended to segment 1 in 30% of cases and including the common bile duct in 20% of cases to achieve a complete resection. This surgery is therefore associated with significant postoperative mortality. This is estimated to be 6%, higher than following surgery

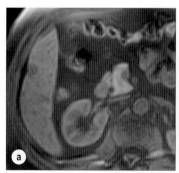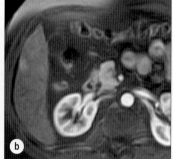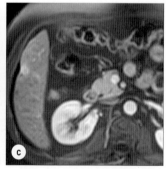

Figure 5.5 • Vascular kinetics of a small cholangiocarcinoma on MRI (arrowed). Note that the lesion is spontaneously hypointense **(a)**, that the uptake of vascular contrast is more pronounced at the late phase **(b)** than at the arterial phase **(c)**, and that there is a retraction of the capsule.

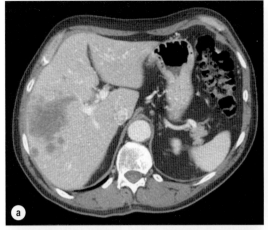
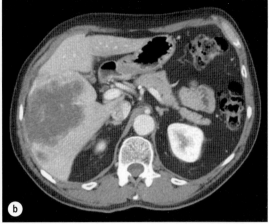
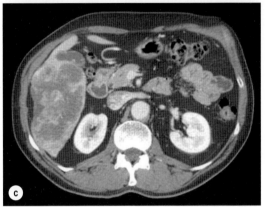

Figure 5.6 • CT scan of a patient with an intrahepatic/peripheral cholangiocarcinoma. Note the presence of typical satellite nodules at the periphery of the tumour **(a)**, the absence of vascular uptake **(b)** and the retraction of the capsule **(c)**.

for colorectal metastases and almost comparable to that of surgery for HCC despite the usual absence of chronic liver disease.

There is a significant risk (20–30%) that, despite adequate preoperative imaging, contraindications to a curative resection are identified at laparotomy. Staging laparoscopy has been advocated, but is also associated with high false-negative rates and, as a consequence, patients should be warned preoperatively about this possibility. Furthermore, approximately 25% of resected patients will have an R1 or R2 resection. Survival following an R2 resection is usually comparable to, and occasionally worse than, that of non-resected patients. Median survival following an R1 resection is typically 12 months and the 3-year survival is nil.

According to the series published over the past decade, the 1-, 3- and 5-year survival rates following resection of ICCA are 67%, 38% and 27%, respectively. There are few data on survival beyond 5 years. Variables that influence postoperative survival most are the presence of lymph node invasion and an R1 resection.[71] Intraductal growth-type ICCAs are rare but have a better long-term prognosis. Infiltrating-type ICCAs have a worse prognosis than the mass-forming type due to spread along Glisson's capsule and high incidence of lymph node involvement.

There is little evidence that these figures have improved over the past 10 years. However, the recent demonstration that systemic chemotherapy may be effective in unresectable patients opens the possibility of combining surgery with either adjuvant and/or neoadjuvant chemotherapy.[72]

> ✔ There is growing interest in the management of ICCA. Improvement in outcome will require that additional treatments other than surgery are evaluated.

Epithelioid haemangio-endothelioma (EHE)

EHEs are neoplasms of vascular origin that arise predominantly from soft tissues, bones and visceral organs, in particular the lung and the liver. Hepatic EHE develops from the endothelial cells lining the sinusoids and progresses along the sinusoids and vascular pedicles. It is extremely rare (no more than 200 cases have been reported), with an incidence of less than 1 per million population. It does not arise on a background of liver disease and there is no identified causative factor. Mean age at presentation is 42 years, with a female to male ratio of 3:2.[73] Half present with right upper quadrant pain, a quarter incidentally, and the remainder with severe symptoms such as ascites, jaundice, weakness and weight loss. Liver failure as a result of massive infiltration has been described.

These tumours are usually discovered at an advanced stage; almost 90% are multifocal and then usually involve both lobes. Approximately one-third of patients have extrahepatic spread to regional lymph nodes, peritoneum, lung and spleen.

Although the diagnosis is obvious when appropriate immunohistochemical staining is performed on tumour samples, it is frequently misdiagnosed on other investigations. Laboratory parameters are non-specific and tumour markers are normal. On imaging studies, the lesions are frequently confused with cholangiocarcinoma, metastatic carcinoma, sclerosing angioma or inflammatory pseudotumours. They are usually hypoechoic or heterogeneous on US, hypodense on CT with peripheral and/or central marginal enhancement on the arterial phase becoming isodense during the later phase, and may display a halo or target pattern of enhancement. On MRI, they are hypointense on T1-weighted images and heterogeneously hyperintense on T2-weighted images, with similar contrast enhancement to that seen on CT. Multiplicity of lesions (especially if coalescent), their subcapsular location with liver capsule retraction, and the presence of calcification (10–30%) or central necrotic and haemorrhagic areas should raise the suspicion of the diagnosis, especially in young patients. Histology shows a tumour composed of epithelioid and dendritic cells in variable proportions, with a propensity for invasion of hepatic and portal veins, an overall ill-defined growth pattern and infiltrative margins. These features are difficult to identify or differentiate from other tumours on a percutaneous biopsy sample, but immunostaining for factor VIII-related antigens is highly specific, demonstrating endothelial differentiation. Most tumours also stain positive for CD34 and CD31 endothelial markers. Epithelial markers including cytokeratins are negative.

The natural history of this tumour is highly variable. Although exceptional, prolonged survival of more than 10 years has been reported without treatment, and both partial and complete spontaneous tumour regression has even been described. On the other hand, some patients die within 2 weeks of diagnosis and 20% are dead within 1 year. Overall, only 20–40% survive more than 5 years.[73] Because of the rarity of this tumour and its highly variable course, there is no widely accepted therapeutic strategy.

Partial hepatectomy is rarely feasible due to the invariable multifocal involvement of the liver. Palliative resection is not advocated as some have raised concerns that liver regeneration could promote a flare-up of residual tumours. Reports of favourable outcome with an estimated 5-year survival of 75% probably represent a highly selected subgroup.[73]

The place of liver transplantation has recently been clarified by a multi-institutional analysis.[74] In 59 patients reported to the European Liver Transplant Registry, impressive 5- and 10-year survival rates of 83% and 74%, respectively, were reported. Invasion of lymph nodes and presence of restricted extrahepatic involvement had limited impact on survival and should therefore not be considered as contra-indications to transplantation. The current shortage of liver grafts and the prolonged waiting time may dictate that liver transplantation is only indicated in highly selected patients. Experience with locoregional or systemic chemotherapy is small and of limited value, especially as first-line therapy. Neoadjuvant combination therapies using anti-VEGF antibodies, however, deserve investigation.

Angiosarcoma

Angiosarcomas of the liver are rare tumours with a dismal prognosis. A recent European survey estimated its incidence as being 0.1 per million/year, being less than 1% of primary liver tumours. The 1-, 3- and 5-year survival rates were 20%, 8% and 5%, respectively. Despite its rarity, it has received attention because of its frequent association with environmental carcinogens. There is clear association with prior exposure to thorium dioxide (Thorotrast), arsenicals and vinyl chloride. Association with androgenic anabolic steroids, oestrogens, oral contraceptives, phenelzine and cupric acid has also been reported. Overall, up to 50% of angiosarcomas are associated with previous exposure to a chemical carcinogenic agent.

These environmental risk factors may account for the male predominance (gender ratio of 3:1) and age at the time of diagnosis (50–70 years). Patients usually experience non-specific symptoms such as abdominal pain, weakness, fatigue, anorexia and weight loss, but an acute abdomen related to tumour rupture is a classical presentation. Biological abnormalities may include haemolytic anaemia and thrombocytopenia, which are related to microangiopathic haemolysis and intravascular coagulation, respectively.

Morphologically, angiosarcoma may present as a large solitary mass or as multinodular lesions. On CT, they are usually hypodense and remain so after contrast injection, except for occasional focal areas of central or peripheral ring-shaped enhancement. On delayed imaging, the lesion continues to enhance compared with that of the early-phase images. On MRI, the lesions tend to be hyperintense on T2-weighted images and heterogeneous on T1-weighted images, with focal hyperintensity on a background of hypointensity. Enhancement on the arterial and portal phases is heterogeneous. Although the progressive enhancement could mimic that of angioma, angiosarcomas clearly differ in that they are usually multiple and more heterogeneous, and enhancement is of lower intensity compared to the aorta, whereas it is the same for angioma.

The tumour develops from endothelial cells lining the hepatic sinusoids, and grows along these and the blood vessels. Disruption of hepatic plates may result in the development of cavities filled with tumour debris or haematoma, which favours the invasion of hepatic and portal veins. These tumours have ill-defined borders and typically involve the entire liver.

Angiosarcomas are rapidly growing and median survival is 6 months. Most patients have metastases at presentation, most notably in the lung and spleen. The latter may be involved in up to half of patients. Death may also result from liver failure or intraperitoneal bleeding due to tumour rupture.

It is considered reasonable to attempt resection when possible and to administer chemotherapy, although it is still poorly effective. Radiation therapy may have some value in this particular tumour. Transplantation has not been associated with survival beyond 3 years due to tumour recurrence, and is therefore not indicated.

Other sarcomas, including leiomyosarcoma, tend to have a better prognosis and should be resected if feasible.[75]

Primary hepatic lymphoma

Although malignant lymphoma frequently involves the liver, primary hepatic lymphomas are rare. Gross examination reveals a single large tumour mass, multiple masses or diffuse infiltration in approximately a third of cases each. Most primary hepatic lymphomas are classified as diffuse large-cell lymphomas of B-cell lineage. Some cases of primary hepatic lymphomas have been reported in association with AIDS or with chronic liver disease. On imaging, they appear as hypodense lesions, not always homogeneous. Rim enhancement and calcifications may be present. They are hypointense on T1-MRI and are slightly enhanced on T2 sequences. The primary treatment is chemotherapy. However, some solitary lesions are resected without a preoperative diagnosis and chemotherapy is then administered postoperatively.

Key points

- The incidence of HCC is still rising.
- Its development is linked to the presence of an underlying liver disease. Major risk factors for HCC include viral infection, alcohol ingestion and metabolic syndrome.
- Surveillance of cirrhotic patients and at-risk populations is recommended to detect HCC at an early stage provided treatment is feasible.
- US is recommended as a screening tool, while CT and MRI are useful to confirm the diagnosis. Liver biopsy is recommended in selected cases.
- Patients with HCC should be managed by a multidisciplinary team including hepatologists, liver surgeons, liver transplant teams, oncologists, pathologists and interventional radiologists.
- The level of evidence for most treatment options for HCC is limited to cohort investigations with a few randomised controlled trials, most of which deal with treatment of advanced disease.
- Liver transplantation is the treatment of choice in cirrhotic patients with limited tumour involvement, as it removes both tumour and preneoplastic underlying liver.
- Liver resection is the treatment of choice in patients with normal livers and is indicated in cirrhotic patients with preserved liver function, no severe portal hypertension and no associated active hepatitis.
- Percutaneous treatments are effective in patients with small tumours.
- Transarterial chemoembolisation (TACE) is effective in selected non-surgical patients with preserved liver function.
- Sorafenib is effective in selected palliative patients who still have preserved liver function.

References

1. Ferlay J, Shin HR, Bray F, et al. Estimates of world-wide burden of cancer in 2008: GLOBOCAN 2008. Int J Cancer 2010;127(12):2893–917.

2. Eguchi S, Kanematsu T, Arii S, et al. Recurrence-free survival more than 10 years after liver resection for hepatocellular carcinoma. Br J Surg 2011;98(4):552–7.

3. Chen CJ, Yang HI, Su J, et al. Risk of hepatocellular carcinoma across a biological gradient of serum hepatitis B virus DNA level. JAMA 2006;295(1):65–73.

4. Braks RE, Ganne-Carrie N, Fontaine H, et al. Effect of sustained virological response on long-term clinical outcome in 113 patients with compensated hepatitis C-related cirrhosis treated by interferon alpha and ribavirin. World J Gastroenterol 2007;13(42):5648–53.

5. Lewden C, May T, Rosenthal E, et al. Changes in causes of death among adults infected by HIV between 2000 and 2005: the "Mortalité 2000 and 2005" surveys (ANRS EN19 and Mortavic). J Acquir Immune Defic Syndr 2008;48(5):590–8.

6. Berretta M, Garlassi E, Cacopardo B, et al. Hepatocellular carcinoma in HIV-infected patients: check early, treat hard. Oncologist 2011;16(9):1258–69.

7. Calle EE, Rodriguez C, Walker-Thurmond K, et al. Overweight, obesity, and mortality from cancer in a prospectively studied cohort of U.S. adults. N Engl J Med 2003;348(17):1625–38.

8. El-Serag HB, Tran T, Everhart JE. Diabetes increases the risk of chronic liver disease and hepatocellular carcinoma. Gastroenterology 2004;126(2):460–8.

9. Paradis V, Zalinski S, Chelbi E, et al. Hepatocellular carcinomas in patients with metabolic syndrome often develop without significant liver fibrosis: a pathological analysis. Hepatology 2009;49(3):851–9.

10. Jin F, Qu LS, Shen XZ. Association between C282Y and H63D mutations of the HFE gene with hepatocellular carcinoma in European populations: a meta-analysis. J Exp Clin Cancer Res 2010;29:18.

11. Liang Y, Yang Z, Zhong R. Primary biliary cirrhosis and cancer risk: a systematic review and meta-analysis. Hepatology 2012;56(4):1409–17.

12. Migita K, Watanabe Y, Jiuchi Y, et al. Hepatocellular carcinoma and survival in patients with autoimmune hepatitis (Japanese National Hospital Organization – autoimmune hepatitis prospective study). Liver Int 2012;32(5):837–44.

13. Stoot JH, Coelen RJ, De Jong MC, et al. Malignant transformation of hepatocellular adenomas into hepatocellular carcinomas: a systematic review including more than 1600 adenoma cases. HPB (Oxford) 2010;12(8):509–22.

14. Farges O, Ferreira N, Dokmak S, et al. Changing trends in malignant transformation of hepatocellular adenoma. Gut 2011;60(1):85–9.

15. Bioulac-Sage P, Laumonier H, Couchy G, et al. Hepatocellular adenoma management and phenotypic classification: the Bordeaux experience. Hepatology 2009;50(2):481–9.

16. Dokmak S, Paradis V, Vilgrain V, et al. A single-center surgical experience of 122 patients with single and multiple hepatocellular adenomas. Gastroenterology 2009;137(5):1698–705.

17. Bioulac-Sage P, Rebouissou S, Thomas C, et al. Hepatocellular adenoma subtype classification using molecular markers and immunohistochemistry. Hepatology 2007;46(3):740–8.

18. Di Tommaso L, Destro A, Seok JY, et al. The application of markers (HSP70, GPC3 and GS) in liver biopsies is useful for detection of hepatocellular carcinoma. J Hepatol 2009;50(4):746–54.

19. Lok AS, Sterling RK, Everhart JE, et al. Des-gamma-carboxy prothrombin and alpha-fetoprotein as biomarkers for the early detection of hepatocellular carcinoma. Gastroenterology 2010;138(2):493–502.

20. Kudo M, Hatanaka K, Kumada T, et al. Double-contrast ultrasound: a novel surveillance tool for hepatocellular carcinoma. Am J Gastroenterol 2011;106(2):368–70.

21. Talbot JN, Fartoux L, Balogova S, et al. Detection of hepatocellular carcinoma with PET/CT: a prospective comparison of ^{18}F-fluorocholine and ^{18}F-FDG in patients with cirrhosis or chronic liver disease. J Nucl Med 2010;51(11):1699–706.

22. Kawaoka T, Aikata H, Takaki S, et al. FDG positron emission tomography/computed tomography for the detection of extrahepatic metastases from hepatocellular carcinoma. Hepatol Res 2009;39(2):134–42.

23. Bruix J, Sherman M. Management of hepatocellular carcinoma: an update. Hepatology 2011;53(3):1020–2.

24. Forner A, Vilana R, Ayuso C, et al. Diagnosis of hepatic nodules 20 mm or smaller in cirrhosis: prospective validation of the noninvasive diagnostic criteria for hepatocellular carcinoma. Hepatology 2008;47(1):97–104.

25. Sangiovanni A, Manini MA, Iavarone M, et al. The diagnostic and economic impact of contrast imaging techniques in the diagnosis of small hepatocellular carcinoma in cirrhosis. Gut 2010;59(5):638–44.

26. Khalili K, Kim TK, Jang HJ, et al. Optimization of imaging diagnosis of 1–2 cm hepatocellular carcinoma: an analysis of diagnostic performance and resource utilization. J Hepatol 2011;54(4):723–8.

27. Zhang BH, Yang BH, Tang ZY. Randomized controlled trial of screening for hepatocellular carcinoma. J Cancer Res Clin Oncol 2004;130(7):417–22.

28. Thompson Coon J, Rogers G, Hewson P, et al. Surveillance of cirrhosis for hepatocellular carcinoma: a cost–utility analysis. Br J Cancer 2008;98(7):1166–75.

29. Smoot RL, Nagorney DM, Chandan VS, et al. Resection of hepatocellular carcinoma in patients without cirrhosis. Br J Surg 2011;98(5):697–703.

30. Mergental H, Adam R, Ericzon BG, et al. Liver transplantation for unresectable hepatocellular carcinoma in normal livers. J Hepatol 2012;57(2):297–305.

31. Ishizawa T, Hasegawa K, Aoki T, et al. Neither multiple tumors nor portal hypertension are surgical contraindications for hepatocellular carcinoma. Gastroenterology 2008;134(7):1908–16.

32. Delis SG, Bakoyiannis A, Biliatis I, et al. Model for end-stage liver disease (MELD) score, as a prognostic factor for post-operative morbidity and mortality in cirrhotic patients, undergoing hepatectomy for hepatocellular carcinoma. HPB (Oxford) 2009;11(4):351–7.

33. Maithel SK, Kneuertz PJ, Kooby DA, et al. Importance of low preoperative platelet count in selecting patients for resection of hepatocellular carcinoma: a multi-institutional analysis. J Am Coll Surg 2011;212(4):638–50.

34. Ogata S, Belghiti J, Farges O, et al. Sequential arterial and portal vein embolizations before right hepatectomy in patients with cirrhosis and hepatocellular carcinoma. Br J Surg 2006;93(9):1091–8.

35. Wakai T, Shirai Y, Sakata J, et al. Anatomic resection independently improves long-term survival in patients with T1–T2 hepatocellular carcinoma. Ann Surg Oncol 2007;14(4):1356–65.

36. Shi M, Guo RP, Lin XJ, et al. Partial hepatectomy with wide versus narrow resection margin for solitary hepatocellular carcinoma: a prospective randomized trial. Ann Surg 2007;245(1):36–43.

37. Dagher I, Belli G, Fantini C, et al. Laparoscopic hepatectomy for hepatocellular carcinoma: a European experience. J Am Coll Surg 2010;211(1):16–23.

38. Laurent A, Tayar C, Andreoletti M, et al. Laparoscopic liver resection facilitates salvage liver transplantation for hepatocellular carcinoma. J Hepatobiliary Pancreat Surg 2009;16(3):310–4.

39. Lau WY, Lai EC, Leung TW, et al. Adjuvant intra-arterial iodine-131-labeled lipiodol for resectable hepatocellular carcinoma: a prospective randomized trial – update on 5-year and 10-year survival. Ann Surg 2008;247(1):43–8.

40. Breitenstein S, Dimitroulis D, Petrowsky H, et al. Systematic review and meta-analysis of interferon after curative treatment of hepatocellular carcinoma in patients with viral hepatitis. Br J Surg 2009;96(9):975–81.

41. Miyake Y, Takaki A, Iwasaki Y, et al. Meta-analysis: interferon-alpha prevents the recurrence after curative treatment of hepatitis C virus-related hepatocellular carcinoma. J Viral Hepat 2010;17(4):287–92.

42. Shen YC, Hsu C, Chen LT, et al. Adjuvant interferon therapy after curative therapy for hepatocellular carcinoma (HCC): a meta-regression approach. J Hepatol 2010;52(6):889–94.

43. Mazzaferro V, Regalia E, Doci R, et al. Liver transplantation for the treatment of small hepatocellular carcinomas in patients with cirrhosis. N Engl J Med 1996;334(11):693–9.

44. Yao FY. Liver transplantation for hepatocellular carcinoma: beyond the Milan criteria. Am J Transplant 2008;8(10):1982–9.

45. Clavien PA, Lesurtel M, Bossuyt PM, et al. Recommendations for liver transplantation for hepatocellular carcinoma: an international consensus conference report. Lancet Oncol 2012;13(1): e11–22.

46. Song MJ, Chun HJ, Song DS, et al. Comparative study between Doxorubicin-eluting beads and conventional transarterial chemoembolization for treatment of hepatocellular carcinoma. J Hepatol 2012;57(6):1244–50.

47. Qu X, Chen C, Wang J, et al. The efficacy of TACE combined sorafenib in advanced stages hepatocellular carcinoma. BMC Cancer 2012;12(1):263.

48. Llovet JM, Bruix J. Systematic review of randomized trials for unresectable hepatocellular carcinoma: chemoembolization improves survival. Hepatology 2003;37(2):429–42.
   This meta-analysis of randomised controlled trials demonstrates that TACE should be recommended as first-line non-curative option for intermediate HCC (as defined by the BCLC stagin system) as it improved survival.

49. Lopez PM, Villanueva A, Llovet JM. Systematic review: evidence-based management of hepatocellular carcinoma – an updated analysis of randomized controlled trials. Aliment Pharmacol Ther 2006;23(11):1535–47.
   This meta-analysis of four randomised controlled trials shows the efficacy of RFA in terms of local better control in HCC >2 cm, as compared to PEI.

50. Cho YK, Kim JK, Kim MY, et al. Systematic review of randomized trials for hepatocellular carcinoma treated with percutaneous ablation therapies. Hepatology 2009;49(2):453–9.
   This meta-analysis of four randomised controlled trials demonstrates that RFA significantly improved survival for patients with HCC, as compared to PEI.

51. Kim JE, Kim YS, Rhim H, et al. Outcomes of patients with hepatocellular carcinoma referred for percutaneous radiofrequency ablation at a tertiary center: analysis focused on the feasibility with the use of ultrasonography guidance. Eur J Radiol 2011;79(2):e80–4.

52. Wang W, Shi J, Xie WF. Transarterial chemoembolization in combination with percutaneous ablation therapy in unresectable hepatocellular carcinoma: a meta-analysis. Liver Int 2010;30(5):741–9.

53. Livraghi T, Meloni F, Di Stasi M, et al. Sustained complete response and complications rates after radiofrequency ablation of very early hepatocellular carcinoma in cirrhosis: is resection still the treatment of choice? Hepatology 2008;47(1):82–9.

54. Chen MS, Li JQ, Zheng Y, et al. A prospective randomized trial comparing percutaneous local ablative therapy and partial hepatectomy for small hepatocellular carcinoma. Ann Surg 2006;243(3):321–8.

55. Lu MD, Kuang M, Liang LJ, et al. Surgical resection versus percutaneous thermal ablation for early-stage hepatocellular carcinoma: a randomized clinical trial. Zhonghua Yi Xue Za Zhi 2006;86(12):801–5.

56. Bouza C, Lopez-Cuadrado T, Alcazar R, et al. Meta-analysis of percutaneous radiofrequency ablation versus ethanol injection in hepatocellular carcinoma. BMC Gastroenterol 2009;9:31.

57. Zhou Y, Zhao Y, Li B, et al. Meta-analysis of radiofrequency ablation versus hepatic resection for small hepatocellular carcinoma. BMC Gastroenterol 2010;10:78.

58. Massarweh NN, Park JO, Farjah F, et al. Trends in the utilization and impact of radiofrequency ablation for hepatocellular carcinoma. J Am Coll Surg 2010;210(4):441–8.

59. Santi V, Buccione D, Di Micoli A, et al. The changing scenario of hepatocellular carcinoma over the last two decades in Italy. J Hepatol 2012;56(2):397–405.

60. Llovet JM, Ricci S, Mazzaferro V, et al. Sorafenib in advanced hepatocellular carcinoma. N Engl J Med 2008;359(4):378–90.

This is a randomised controlled trial demonstrating an improved survival benefit of sorafenib in patients with advanced HCC.

61. Cheng AL, Kang YK, Chen Z, et al. Efficacy and safety of sorafenib in patients in the Asia-Pacific region with advanced hepatocellular carcinoma: a phase III randomised, double-blind, placebo-controlled trial. Lancet Oncol 2009;10(1):25–34.

62. Lencioni R, Kudo M, Ye SL, et al. First interim analysis of the GIDEON (Global Investigation of therapeutic DEcisions in hepatocellular carcinoma and Of its treatment with sorafeNib) non-interventional study. Int J Clin Pract 2012;66(7):675–83.

63. Kulik LM, Carr BI, Mulcahy MF, et al. Safety and efficacy of ^{90}Y radiotherapy for hepatocellular carcinoma with and without portal vein thrombosis. Hepatology 2008;47(1):71–81.

64. Stipa F, Yoon SS, Liau KH, et al. Outcome of patients with fibrolamellar hepatocellular carcinoma. Cancer 2006;106(6):1331–8.

65. Malouf GG, Brugières L, Le Deley MC, et al. Pure and mixed fibrolamellar hepatocellular carcinomas differ in natural history and prognosis after complete surgical resection. Cancer 2012;118(20):4981–90.

66. Khan SA, Emadossadaty S, Ladep NG, et al. Rising trends in cholangiocarcinoma: is the ICD classification system misleading us? J Hepatol 2012;56(4):848–54.

67. Welzel TM, Graubard BI, Zeuzem S, et al. Metabolic syndrome increases the risk of primary liver cancer in the United States: a study in the SEER-Medicare database. Hepatology 2011;54(2):463–71.

68. Edge SB, Compton CC. The American Joint Committee on Cancer: the 7th edition of the AJCC cancer staging manual and the future of TNM. Ann Surg Oncol 2010;17(6):1471–4.

69. Farges O, Fuks D, Le Treut YP, et al. AJCC 7th edition of TNM staging accurately discriminates outcomes of patients with resectable intrahepatic cholangiocarcinoma: by the AFC-IHCC-2009 study group. Cancer 2011;117(10):2170–7.

70. Aishima S, Kuroda Y, Nishihara Y, et al. Proposal of progression model for intrahepatic cholangiocarcinoma: clinicopathologic differences between hilar type and peripheral type. Am J Surg Pathol 2007;31(7):1059–67.

71. Farges O, Fuks D, Boleslawski E, et al. Influence of surgical margins on outcome in patients with intrahepatic cholangiocarcinoma: a multicenter study by the AFC-IHCC-2009 study group. Ann Surg 2011;254(5):824–30.

72. Valle J, Wasan H, Palmer DH, et al. Cisplatin plus gemcitabine versus gemcitabine for biliary tract cancer. N Engl J Med 2010;362(14):1273–81.

73. Mehrabi A, Kashfi A, Fonouni H, et al. Primary malignant hepatic epithelioid hemangioendothelioma: a comprehensive review of the literature with emphasis on the surgical therapy. Cancer 2006;107(9):2108–21.

74. Lerut JP, Orlando G, Adam R, et al. The place of liver transplantation in the treatment of hepatic epitheloid hemangioendothelioma: report of the European liver transplant registry. Ann Surg 2007;246(6):949–57.

75. Matthaei H, Krieg A, Schmelzle M, et al. Long-term survival after surgery for primary hepatic sarcoma in adults. Arch Surg 2009;144(4):339–44.

6

Colorectal liver metastases

Declan F.J. Dunne
Robert P. Jones
René Adam
Graeme J. Poston

Introduction

Colorectal cancer is the commonest gastrointestinal malignancy and the second commonest cause of cancer death in Western society. Worldwide there are 1.2 million new cases and 608 000 deaths annually.[1] The liver is usually the first site of metastatic disease and may be the only site in 30–40% of patients with advanced disease.[2] At the time of initial diagnosis of colorectal cancer, 20–25% of patients will have detectable liver metastases. A further 40–50% will develop liver metastases, usually within the first 3 years of follow-up after successful resection of the primary tumour.[3]

Without treatment, the median survival for colorectal liver metastases (CRLMs) is just 6–8 months, varying with the extent of disease at presentation. The prognosis is best for those whose metastases are isolated to a single lobe of the liver or are limited in number.[3] However, even for the best prognostic groups, very few survive 5 years without treatment. Surgery is the only treatment that offers the prospect of cure for CRLMs. Traditionally, only 10–20% of patients were considered suitable for attempted curative resection; the remaining patients were offered palliative and symptomatic treatment.

This review focuses on a variety of recent strategies that have led to an increase in the number of patients for whom curative treatment is possible. These include improved preoperative staging and patient selection, new standards for surgical resection, novel surgical strategies, the application of modern systemic chemotherapy, use of ablative therapies and an emphasis on the collaborative, multidisciplinary management of this disease.

Preoperative staging: the key to selection of candidates for curative treatment

On the detection of colorectal liver metastases it is recommended that patients should be fully staged prior to any planned chemotherapy, and the staging and management plan should be coordinated by a specialist multidisciplinary team.[4] Individual imaging techniques used in preoperative staging have different strengths and weaknesses, but consensus is now emerging on the optimal choice of technique and the sequence with which it should be employed.[5,6] Imaging techniques are often complementary in the management of colorectal liver metastases, and multiple imaging modalities are often employed.

Computed tomography (CT)

CT is considered a standard of care for all patients identified to have hepatic metastasis.[4] Intravenous iodinated contrast media should be used routinely. This helps characterise liver lesions based on their enhancement patterns during the various phases of contrast circulation in the liver.[7] During the portal venous phase, normal liver parenchyma usually enhances intensely while liver metastases (with their dominant arterial supply) appear as relatively hypodense hypovascular lesions. In small-sized liver metastases, arterial dominant phase imaging may be useful to detect faint peripheral rim enhancement. Delayed images should be obtained 4–5 minutes after contrast injection. This is helpful in differentiating metastases from benign liver lesions, particularly a haemangioma.[8] Whilst CT is considered a standard of care, it has limitations, including the need for a high radiation dose and low sensitivity for the detection and characterisation of lesions smaller than 1 cm (**Figs 6.1–6.6**).

Magnetic resonance imaging (MRI)

MRI is a highly effective imaging modality for detecting and characterising liver lesions and provides high lesion-to-liver contrast without using ionising radiation. Typically, CRLMs show low signal intensity on T1-weighted images and moderately high signal intensity on T2-weighted images with fat suppression. Gadolinium, the most commonly used MRI contrast agent, behaves similarly to the iodinated contrast agents used in CT. Liver-specific contrast media such as superparamagnetic iron oxide (SPIO), gadoxetic acid (Primovist®) and Mangafodipir trisodium (Mn DPDP, Teslascan) are not taken up by colorectal hepatic metastases, so may aid in the detection of CRLMs.[9,10] These agents are of particular value in the characterisation of liver lesions that are either small or indeterminate on other imaging modalities.[8,10]

Whilst the benefits of MRI are evident, it does have a number of limitations. MRI has a low sensitivity for detecting extrahepatic disease in the peritoneum and chest, and takes longer to perform than

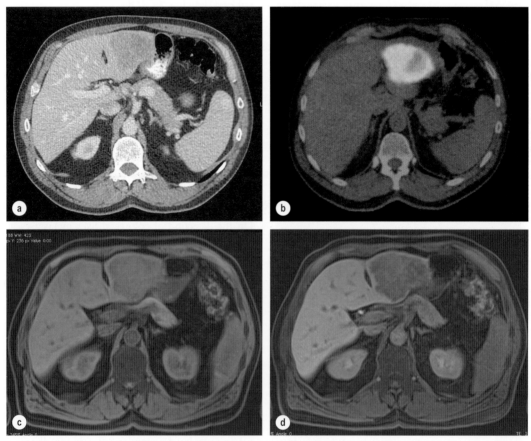

Figure 6.1 • (a) CT image in the portal-venous phase demonstrating a hypodense colorectal liver metastasis occupying segments 2 and 3. **(b)** PET-CT image of the same metastasis demonstrating high uptake of FDG. **(c)** T1-weighted MRI image of the same metastasis demonstrating a typical hypodense colorectal metastasis. **(d)** T1-weighted MRI image following primovist contrast administration. Evidence of contrast take-up within the liver and excretion within the common bile duct is observed. No evidence of contrast take-up within the metastasis can be seen.

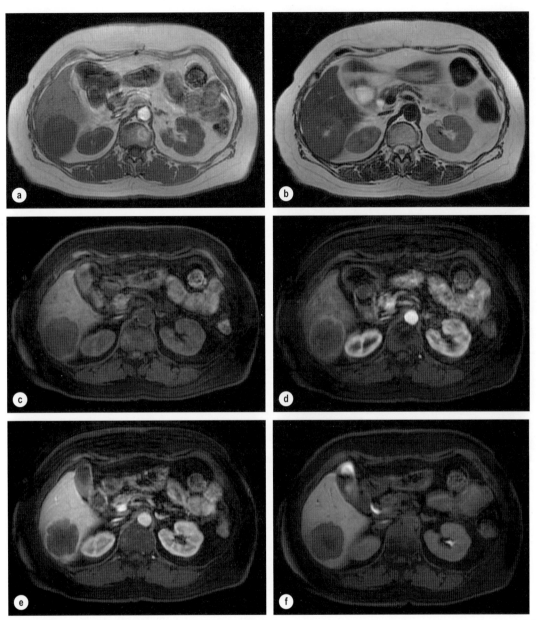

Figure 6.2 • (a) T1-weighted MRI image without contrast demonstrating a typical hypodense metastasis in segment 6. **(b)** T2-weighted MRI image of the same metastasis, where the metastasis is brighter than the surrounding liver. Evidence of central necrosis is seen as a brighter central area of the metastasis. **(c)** T1-weighted MRI image with fat suppression before contrast administration. **(d)** T1-weighted MRI image with fat suppression in the arterial phase following primovist contrast administration. The metastasis demonstrates typical rim enhancement. **(e)** T1-weighted MRI image with fat suppression following primovist contrast administration in the portal venous phase. Good contrast take-up within the liver is observed. **(f)** T1-weighted MRI image with fat suppression 20 minutes following primovist contrast administration. No evidence of contrast take-up within the metastasis is seen. Evidence of contrast excretion within the gallbladder, common bile duct and kidney can be observed.

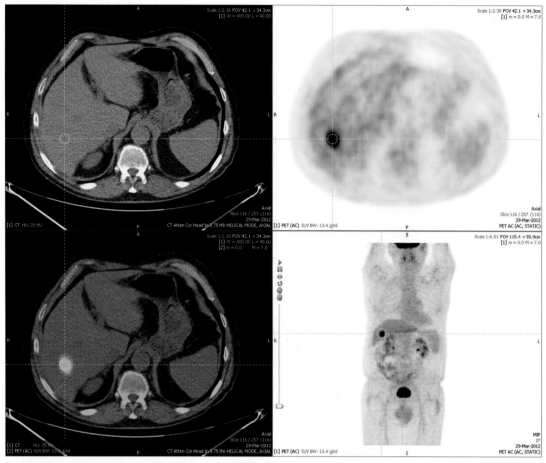

Figure 6.3 • Images extracted from a PET-CT scan demonstrating CT, PET and fused PET-CT images of a liver metastasis in the right liver.

contrast-enhanced CT. There are also a number of contraindications to MRI, including patients with pacemakers, implantable cardiac defibrillators, cochlear implants and metallic orbital foreign bodies.[10] However, it can be used safely in patients with allergies to iodinated contrast agents (Figs 6.1 and 6.2).

Positron emission tomography (PET)

PET has emerged as an important diagnostic tool in the evaluation of CRLMs. Colorectal malignancies are often metabolically active and therefore have a greater glucose uptake relative to that of surrounding normal tissues. This can be identified with [^{18}F]fluoro-2-D-glucose (FDG-PET). This modality is highly sensitive, especially when combined with CT.[11] PET-CT is often used in the preoperative assessment of CRLMs, often with the aim of identifying irresectable extrahepatic

disease that would make liver resection futile.[12] It can sometimes be difficult to differentiate between malignant tissue and other metabolically active tissue, e.g. inflammatory tissue due to infective or postsurgical causes.[12] Mucinous colorectal metastases may also prove difficult to detect due to reduced glucose uptake.[13] Other disadvantages of PET include high cost and limited sensitivity for lesions smaller than 1 cm (Figs 6.1 and 6.3–6.6).

Staging laparoscopy

The role of staging laparoscopy has evolved as radiology has improved and criteria for resection have changed. However, staging laparoscopy may be useful for the detection of unresectable peritoneal disease not detected by conventional radiology.

The yield of laparoscopy for detecting unresectable disease varies from 6% to 36%.[13–19] Staging

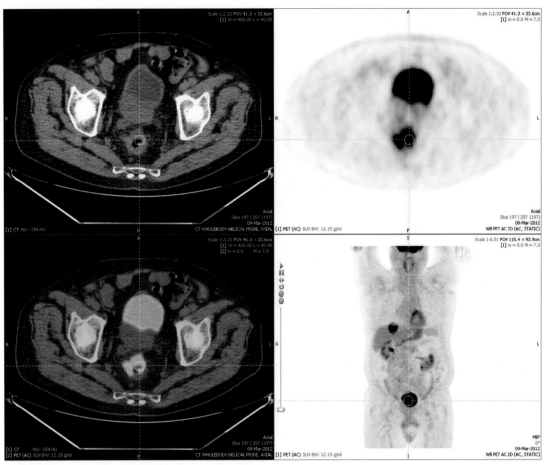

Figure 6.4 • Images extracted from a PET-CT scan demonstrating CT, PET and fused PET-CT images of a PET-positive primary rectal cancer. Evidence of a left lobe liver metastasis can be seen in the bottom right image.

laparoscopy cannot be performed in 6–16% of patients due to adhesions from previous surgery.[13–19] One study suggested that staging laparoscopy had greater value in those patients with a higher clinical risk score (CRS).[20] The CRS ranges from 0 to 5 based on the presence of the following characteristics: node-positive primary tumour, prehepatectomy carcinoembryonic antigen (CEA) greater than 200 ng/mL, more than one liver tumour, liver tumour size greater than 5 cm and disease-free interval of less than 1 year. In a Memorial Sloan Kettering Cancer Center study,[20] only 4% of patients with CRS of 0–1 were irresectable and none were identified as unresectable at preoperative laparoscopy. At scores of 2–3, 21% of lesions were unresectable and only one-half were found at laparoscopy (yield of 11%). The highest yield was at scores of 4–5, where the yield of laparoscopy was 24%.

The value of staging laparoscopy is likely to have diminished with recent advances in imaging and an expanding view of what is resectable disease, so whilst there may be a role for staging laparoscopy in selected high-risk individuals, its routine use for all patients cannot be justified.

Cardiopulmonary exercise testing

Traditionally, selection of patients for resection has been centred on identifying patients with resectable disease. Recently interest has grown in identifying patients who have a higher operative risk, either from reduced fitness or previously unknown cardiorespiratory comorbidities. Cardiopulmonary exercise testing (CPET) has been shown to be useful in quantifying surgical risk in patients undergoing major hepatobiliary surgery.[21] Given that patients over the age of 70 are known to have significantly higher operative risk[22,23] and that 50% of patients diagnosed with colorectal cancer are over 70, this technique may have a role to play in the appropriate selection and management of patients undergoing liver resection.

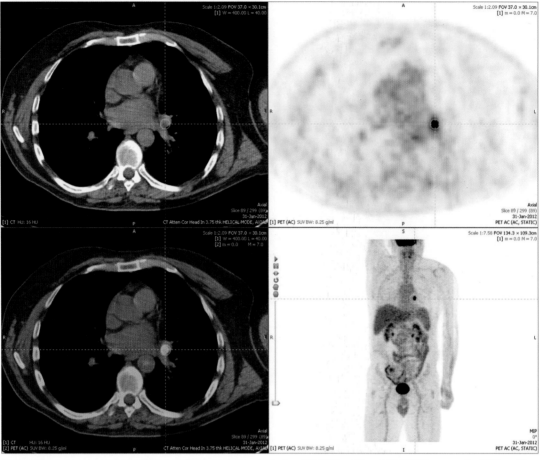

Figure 6.5 • Images extracted from a PET-CT scan demonstrating CT, PET and fused PET-CT images of a PET-positive nodal mass in the left superior mediastinum.

✔✔ Contrast-enhanced CT should be performed in the assessment of all patients with colorectal liver metastasis. Further assessment of liver metastases varies depending on local expertise and availability of other modalities. MRI and PET-CT are useful to characterise hepatic lesions and assess the extent of extrahepatic disease.[4]

Surgery: the old and the new standards for resection

Criteria for resection

If CRLMs are resectable, patients can look forward to a 5-year survival of 40–50% and a 10-year survival of 24%, with age being no barrier to resection if fit (**Fig. 6.7**). In the past, liver resection was attempted only in patients who had one to three unilobar metastases, preferably presenting at least 12 months after resection of the primary tumour, whose disease was resectable with at least a 1-cm margin of healthy liver tissue and who had no hilar lymphadenopathy or extrahepatic disease.

Recent experience has demonstrated that patients outside these narrow parameters can experience long-term survival following liver resection.[24,25] Modern criteria for resection are now based on whether a macroscopically complete resection of the disease can be achieved. Instead of resectability being defined by what is removed, resectability is now being determined by what will remain.

In 2006, consensus statements from the American Hepato-Pancreato-Biliary Association (AHPBA) and a pan-European group changed the criteria for resection.[5,26] The American consensus suggested CRLMs should be considered resectable if (i) the disease can be completely resected (regardless of

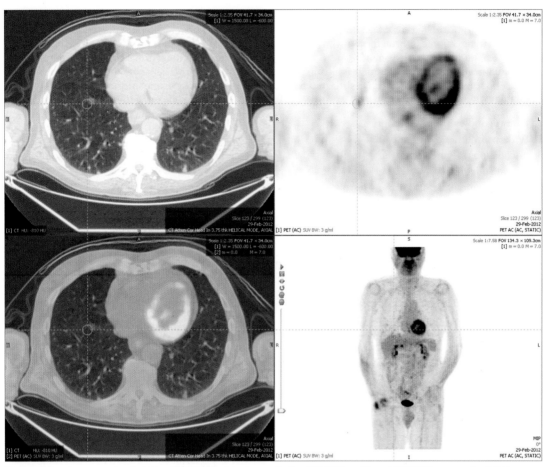

Figure 6.6 • Images extracted from a PET-CT scan demonstrating CT, PET and fused PET-CT images of a right lower lobe PET-positive lung metastasis.

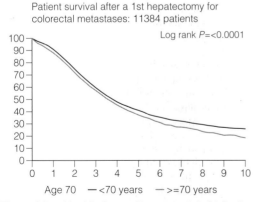

Figure 6.7 • LiverMetSurvey. Ten-year survival following hepatectomy for CRLMs comparing patients <70 years of age with those >70 years of age. Reproduced with permission.

margin), (ii) two adjacent liver segments can be spared with adequate vascular inflow and outflow and biliary drainage, and (iii) the volume of the liver remaining after resection, i.e. the 'future liver remnant' (FLR), will be adequate.[5] The European group concluded that criteria rendering patients irresectable included invasion of one branch of the liver pedicle and contact with the contralateral branch, contact with the inferior vena cava, invasion of all three hepatic veins, the presence of coeliac lymph nodes and the presence of non-resectable extrahepatic disease.[26] These criteria have already been challenged with long-term survival in patients undergoing nodal resection and resection of metastasis involving the inferior vena cava (IVC).[27,28] Resection has also been performed for lesions involving all three hepatic veins, though long-term survival data are not available.[29]

The 2011 UK national guidance recommended that resection should be offered if a patient is fit enough, and complete resection can be achieved whilst leaving an adequate future liver remnant.[4] There are no absolute contraindications to resection issued in this guidance, but in normal circumstances they recommend that contraindications to liver resection are:

1. Non-treatable primary tumour
2. Widespread pulmonary disease
3. Locoregional recurrence
4. Uncontrollable peritoneal disease
5. Extensive nodal disease, such as retroperitoneal or mediastinal lymph nodes
6. Bone or CNS metastases.

> ✔✔ Without resection very few patients with colorectal liver metastases are alive 5 years after their detection.[3]

Surgical strategies to improve resectability

A variety of strategies have been employed to bring patients with unresectable disease to surgical resection.

Portal vein embolisation

Portal vein embolisation (PVE) induces atrophy of the liver to be resected and hypertrophy of the liver that will remain (i.e. increases the future liver remnant), with the aim of avoiding post-resection hepatic insufficiency, liver failure and death. A meta-analysis of 1088 patients confirmed that this technique significantly increased the FLR, making more patients suitable for liver resection.[30] The overall morbidity rate was 2.2% without mortality. Following PVE, 930 patients (85%) proceeded to laparotomy. Resection was not performed in 158 patients (17%): in 131 because of inadequate hypertrophy of the FLR and in 27 because of disease progression.

Although there is no consensus on what constitutes a safe volume of remnant liver, minimum values of 20–25% for patients with normal livers, 30% following neoadjuvant chemotherapy and 40% in the presence of chronic liver disease have been suggested.[5,31,32] PVE also appears to be safe when combined with neoadjuvant chemotherapy.[33]

Two-stage hepatectomy

Two-stage hepatectomy involves delayed re-hepatectomy after hypertrophy of the residual liver and may be used for large bilateral lesions in which a one-stage resection of all the involved segments would lead to liver failure.[34] The first stage involves resection of metastases from the FLR and PVE (or portal vein ligation during surgery), followed by a period of liver regeneration and hypertrophy of the FLR alongside systemic chemotherapy. The second stage is performed 2–3 months later and consists of the major hepatectomy to remove the residual disease. A large series reported 1- and 3-year survival of 70.0% and 54.4%, respectively, in 25 of 33 patients in whom a two-stage hepatectomy could be completed.[35] There was no operative mortality; postoperative morbidity was 15.1% and 56.0% after first- and second-stage hepatectomy, respectively.

Repeat hepatectomy

Repeat hepatectomy for patients with colorectal liver metastases is safe and provides survival benefit. A meta-analysis of 21 studies, comprising 3741 patients, showed that there was no difference in perioperative morbidity, mortality or long-term survival between patients undergoing a first or repeat hepatectomy.[36] A study looking at 1706 patients undergoing repeat hepatectomy for CRLMs demonstrated similar morbidity and mortality after third and fourth hepatectomies, though 5-year survival decreased from 47.1% for a first resection to 23.8% for a third or fourth resection.[37]

Extreme liver surgery

Resection of tumours involving the hepatic vascular inflow has been described, including portal vein resection and reconstruction, hepatic artery resection and reconstruction (or arterialisation of the portal vein as an alternative).[38] Resections of tumours with involvement of the IVC or the three major hepatic veins have also been performed, using techniques such as total hepatic vascular exclusion, in situ hypothermic perfusion and ex vivo (bench) hepatic resection.[39–41] These techniques are at the frontier of what is currently feasible and are associated with significant morbidity and mortality. Nonetheless, this aggressive surgical approach may offer hope for patients with hepatic tumours involving the IVC, who would otherwise have a poor prognosis.

Extrahepatic colorectal disease

Extrahepatic colorectal metastases, such as direct diaphragmatic invasion, adrenal metastases and lung metastases, may be resected with curative intent. Reported long-term survival after pneumonectomy for colorectal metastases mirrors very closely that seen after hepatectomy, with most series quoting a 5-year survival of the order of 40–50%, with similar low operative morbidity and mortality.[42–45] More recent series have identified 5-year survival approaching 70%[46] and showed that repeat resection of pulmonary metastases is also of benefit, with 5-year survival of 42% following second pneumonectomy.[47]

Other series looking at liver resection in the presence of extrahepatic disease have demonstrated that there is a role for resection of other limited extraheptic disease, including peritoneal, hepatic pedicle nodal disease, aortocaval nodal disease, ovarian and bone metastases.[28,48,49] Five-year survival following limited peritoneal and hepatic pedicle nodal disease is quoted at 27% and 26%, respectively.[48] Aortocaval nodal disease is associated with worse long-term survival, with a 5-year survival of just 7%.[49]

✔✔ There are no absolute contraindications to surgical resection of colorectal liver metastases as long as the disease can be fully resected (including extrahepatic disease). The use of advanced surgical techniques may bring patients previously considered irresectable to surgery with curative intent.[4,30–41]

Techniques of surgical resection

Transection techniques

Technological innovations in liver surgery have mainly focused on minimising blood loss during transection of the hepatic parenchyma, as blood transfusion is associated with increased postoperative morbidity and mortality, as well as reduced long-term survival.[50] Inflow occlusion (Pringle manoeuvre) and low central venous pressure (CVP) anaesthesia minimise blood loss but may cause liver damage by ischaemia and reperfusion injury. Consequently, there has been an interest in devices that facilitate a more bloodless liver transection, obviating the need for inflow occlusion associated with the traditional clamp-crushing technique.

The most popular of these techniques include the ultrasonic aspirating dissector (CUSA) using ultrasonic energy, the Hydrojet using a pressurised jet of water and the dissecting sealer (TissueLink) using radiofrequency energy. These techniques were compared in a randomised controlled trial[51] and in a subsequent Cochrane review.[52] There was little difference demonstrated between the four techniques, though the clamp-crushing technique was found to be associated with faster tissue transection and lower transfusion requirements. The Cochrane review also found an association with fewer infective

complications. Both studies highlighted the significantly reduced cost associated with the clamp-crushing technique, and therefore could not advocate the use of newer techniques in standard practice. A further randomised control trial of radiofrequency-assisted versus clamp-crushing transection in 50 patients showed a higher rate of postoperative complications in the radiofrequency group (20%), compared to none in the clamp-crushing group.[53]

Fibrin sealants

Fibrin sealants have become popular as a means of improving perioperative haemostasis and reducing biliary leakage after liver surgery. However, a randomised study of 300 patients showed no differences in transfusion requirement, overall drainage, incidence of biliary fistula and postoperative morbidity between those receiving fibrin glue application and controls.[54] Similar to the newer transection techniques, there is little evidence to justify the fibrin sealants, especially given the financial pressures on healthcare provision.

Laparoscopic liver surgery: less is more?

Laparoscopic surgery for hepatic neoplasms aims to provide curative resection while minimising complications. There are no randomised controlled trials assessing the use of laparoscopic hepatectomy and the evidence is based on retrospective series. A meta-analysis of series published between 1998 and 2005[55] included eight non-randomised studies, reporting on 409 resections of hepatic neoplasms, of which 165 (40.3%) were laparoscopic and 244 (59.7%) were open. Operative blood loss and duration of hospital stay were reduced significantly after laparoscopic surgery. These findings remained consistent when considering studies matched for the presence of malignancy and segment resection. There was no difference in postoperative adverse events and extent of oncological clearance. This paper concluded that laparoscopic liver resection has the potential to reduce operative blood loss and allow earlier recovery with oncological clearance comparable with open surgery.

The largest single-centre experience of laparoscopic resection of CRLMs included 83 resections within a series of 133 liver resections.[56] Resections comprised 42 wedge excisions, 10 segmentectomies, nine bisegmentectomies, three trisegmentectomies, 30 left lateral segmentectomies, four left hepatectomies, 31 right hepatectomies, three extended right hepatectomies and two caudate lobe resections. The authors reported a median operating time of

210 minutes (30–480 minutes), median blood loss of 300 mL (10–3000 mL) and a median postoperative stay of 4 days (1–15 days). Severe postoperative bleeding occurred in five patients (3.7%), requiring intensive care management or re-operation, and overall serious complications occurred in 16 patients (13%). Microscopically negative margins (R0/R1) were achieved in 96% of patients with CRLMs.

In 2008 a group of 45 experts in hepatobiliary surgery participated in a consensus conference and concluded that the laparoscopic approach to liver resection is a safe and effective technique for appropriately trained surgeons.[57]

The current evidence for laparoscopic liver resection is based on selective case series. Despite this, laparoscopic surgery has the potential to reduce operative blood loss and aid in earlier recovery, with oncological clearance comparable with open surgery. Randomised controlled trials would be useful to strengthen the evidence base and aid selection of appropriate cases.

Morbidity, mortality and survival after liver resection for CRLMs

The utility of surgical resection of CRLMs is clearly established. Prospective and retrospective studies consistently show 5-year survival rates following liver resection of 30–50%, depending on selection criteria. A major systematic review of surgical resection for CRLMs was undertaken to assess the published evidence for its efficacy and safety and to identify prognostic factors.[58] Thirty independent studies met all the eligibility criteria for the review and data on 30-day mortality and morbidity were included from a further nine studies. The best available evidence came from prospective case series, but only two studies reported outcomes for all patients undergoing surgery. The remainder reported outcomes for selected groups of patients: those undergoing hepatic resection or those undergoing curative resection.

Death within 30 days of hepatic resection was reported by 24 studies and ranged from 0% to 6.6% (median 2.8%). A further nine studies reported perioperative mortality within an undefined time period (1.3–4.6%, median 3.6%) and two studies reported 60-day mortality (3.4–5.5%). Mortality was not reported in four studies. Cause of death was reported in 15 studies for a total of 103 patients. The commonest specified causes of fatal complications were, in descending order of frequency: hepatic failure, postoperative haemorrhage, generalised sepsis, cardiac failure, multiorgan failure, pulmonary embolism, bile leak and anastomotic leak.[58]

Perioperative complications, including indicators of morbidity such as length of hospital stay, were reported in 29 studies. Commonest causes of morbidity, in descending order of frequency, were: wound infection (5.4%), generalised sepsis (4.6%), pleural effusion (4.3%), bile leak (4.0%), perihepatic abscess (3.0%), hepatic failure (2.8%), arrhythmia (2.8%), postoperative haemorrhage (2.7%), cardiac failure (2.4%) and pneumonia (1.9%).

Studies in which it was unclear whether resections were R0 or R1/2, or only presented data for both types of resection combined, had a median 5-year survival of 32% (9–63%). Sixteen studies presented 5-year survival for patients undergoing R0 resection, either for the whole study population or for subgroups of patients. Median 5-year survival for these studies was 30% (range 15–67%). Eleven studies reporting 5-year survival for non-radical resections had a median 5-year survival of 7.2% (range 0–30%) and six studies reporting patients who did not undergo resection had a median 5-year survival of 0% (range 0–6%). Disease-free survival was reported by fewer studies. Median disease-free survival was 14.3 months for radically resected patients and 17.2 months for patients with unspecified resections.

Twenty-two per cent of all patients experienced recurrence in the liver only, although this is likely to be underestimated as two studies did not specify the proportion of liver-only recurrences. Liver plus extrahepatic recurrences and extrahepatic-only recurrences were experienced by 16% and 24% of patients, respectively. In addition, one study reported recurrences in 235 (62.5%) radically resected patients, although sites of recurrence were not specified.

This systematic review was undertaken because ascertaining the benefits of surgical resection of CRLMs is difficult in the absence of randomised trials. However, it is clear that there is a biologically distinct group of patients with liver metastases who may become long-term disease-free survivors following hepatic resection. Such survival is rare in apparently comparable patients who do not have surgical treatment.

Classification of CRLMs

Staging systems and terminology

The present American Joint Committee on Cancer (AJCC) classifies all colorectal metastasis beyond the local lymphatic basin as stage IV colorectal cancer. This does not allow the distinction between patients who are currently incurable, with a prognosis of less than 6 months, from those who are potentially curable. This has led to the call for a new staging system for colorectal cancer that reflects these differing treatment pathways and prognostic outlook.[59] The 2003 French guidelines on the management of CRLMs recommended four categories that could be defined: (1) easily resectable liver metastases, (2) resectable liver metastases involving five to six liver segments and/or contralateral major vascular structures, (3) liver metastases that are initially unresectable but may become resectable after chemotherapy, and (4) definitely unresectable.[60] Based on the French classification system, the European Colorectal Metastases Treatment group has proposed a staging system:[26]

- IVa – easily resectable with curative intent at detection (French classification 1);
- IVb – technically difficult/borderline resectable at detection (French classification 2);
- IVc – potentially resectable after neotherapeutic chemotherapy (French classification 3);
- IVd – little or no hope of being rendered resectable with curative intent after conventional chemotherapy (French classification 4);
- Va – resectable extrahepatic disease;
- Vb – unresectable extrahepatic disease.

Other suggested systems include distinguishing between stage IV-R for patients with resectable disease and stage IV-U for patients with unresectable disease.[61] Furthermore, stage IV-R could be further divided into IV-Ra (resectable liver only), IV-Rb (resectable extrahepatic only) and IV-Rc (resectable hepatic and extrahepatic). Stage IV-U could be similarly subdivided, after assessment by an experienced site-specific surgical oncologist.

A number of scoring systems have been developed that take a different approach to the staging of CRLMs and attempt to classify patients based on clinical prognosis. The most popular of these were produced by Fong et al.,[20] Nordlinger et al.[62] and Rees et al.[63] The Fong classification (clinical risk score) was described earlier and is the most widely used owing to its ease of use. Nordlinger's classification ranges from 0 to 7, with 1 point being awarded for each of the following adverse risk factors:

1. Extension into serosa of primary tumour
2. Lymphatic spread of the primary tumour
3. Delay from primary tumour to resection <24 months
4. Number of liver metastases in preoperative imaging
5. Largest size of liver metastasis in preoperative imaging ≥5.0 cm
6. Preoperatively estimated clearance of normal parenchyma resected with liver metastasis <1 cm
7. Age ≥60.

These two scoring systems have been compared,[64,65] with the Fong classification proving to be more appropriate for use in clinical practice and better at differentiating between groups. Both scoring systems exclude patients with extrahepatic disease and fail to take into account many known adverse risk factors, meaning that their clinical utility may be limited.

Rees et al. proposed a scoring system that could be used in either the preoperative or postoperative setting.[63] In this risk prediction model, points were allocated up to a maximum of 30 (Table 6.1). Patients with a score of 0, 10, 20 and 30 on preoperative scoring had 5-year survival rates of 66%, 35%, 12% and 2%, respectively. This compared very well with the scores determined postoperatively. This scoring system is more complex than previously suggested models, which has limited its uptake as a clinical tool.

Table 6.1 • Basingstoke Predictive Index (BPI) of long-term cancer-specific survival after primary hepatic resection for colorectal liver metastasis

Risk factor	Preoperative	Postoperative
Primary tumour lymph node status		
Negative	0	0
Positive	2	2
Primary tumour differentiation		
Well	0	0
Moderate	3	2
Poor	5	4
CEA at hepatectomy		
<6 ng/mL	0	0
6–60 ng/mL	2	1
>60 ng/mL	3	3
Number of hepatic metastases		
1–3	0	n/a
>3	4	n/a
Largest tumour diameter		
<5 cm	0	0
5–10 cm	2	2
>10 cm	8	7
Hepatic resection margin		
Negative	n/a	0
Positive	n/a	11
Extrahepatic disease		
No	0	0
Yes	7	4

Whilst a consensus on a meaningful classification of metastatic colorectal disease is lacking, the proposed systems may be useful in guiding treatment decisions.

Chemotherapy for CRLMs

Agents

In the last 10 years, overall survival (OS) in patients with metastatic colorectal cancer has improved substantially,[66] reflecting improved chemotherapeutic manipulation of disease. Before 2000, 5-fluorouracil (5-FU) was the only available treatment. With the development of the cytotoxic agents oxaliplatin and irinotecan, doublet regimens are now considered standard therapy. In the last 5 years, major advances in the management of advanced colorectal cancer have been made by harnessing targeted monoclonal antibodies against extracellular receptors.

Extracellular growth factor receptor (EGFR) is a transmembrane glycoprotein that utilises tyrosine kinase activity for signal transduction with downstream signalling intrinsically involved in multiple biological processes essential for tumour survival. Cetuximab is a recombinant human/mouse chimeric antibody that binds specifically to the extracellular domain of human EGFR, inhibiting this pathway. It is now recognised that patients who have a mutation in the downstream *KRAS* proto-oncogene are resistant to cetuximab therapy, and so *KRAS* testing is routinely performed prior to commencing treatment.[67] Improved understanding of this signalling pathway has identified other common mutations in downstream effectors (including *BRAF*, *NRAS* and *PIK3CA*), which may also confer resistance to anti-EGFR treatments.[68]

Vascular endothelial growth factor (VEGF) is one of the most important regulators of the dynamic balance between pro- and anti-angiogenic factors that are crucial for tumour growth and metastasis, with signalling leading to angiogenic proliferation and increased microvascular permeability. Bevacizumab is a humanised monoclonal antibody directed against VEGF receptors. Proposed mechanisms of action includes inhibition of vessel development, regression of aberrant tumour vasculature and normalisation of tumour perfusion.[69]

Clarifying the intent of chemotherapy in CRLMs

Chemotherapeutic manipulation of advanced colorectal cancer has undergone a paradigm shift over the last 15 years. Previously, patients with unresectable disease were treated solely with the aim

of prolonging life. However, there is now growing recognition that a subgroup of patients who may not be resectable at presentation become resectable after chemotherapy. This approach is often referred to as 'induction' or 'conversion' chemotherapy.[61]

By contrast, chemotherapy may be given during the perioperative period with the aim of reducing occult disease burden. This approach is referred to as '(true) neoadjuvant' and 'adjuvant' therapy. The importance of correct nomenclature is vital when it comes to explaining the intent of any chemotherapeutic regimen.

Conversion/induction chemotherapy

Resectability rates after chemotherapy for initially unresectable disease vary widely, with modern regimes achieving conversion rates approaching 60%.[70] Attempting to bring unresectable disease to resection is worthwhile, with overall 5-year survival comparable between patients resectable at presentation and those converted to resectability after systemic chemotherapy[34] (**Fig. 6.8**). Response to chemotherapy is known to correlate with resection rate[70] and it seems sensible that patients with unresectable liver-only disease should be treated with the most aggressive regimen possible to provide the greatest chance of being bought to potentially curative resection (**Fig. 6.9**, Table 6.2).

The UK National Institute for Clinical Excellence (NICE) currently recommend the use of 5-FU, leucovorin- and oxaliplatin-based regimens (FOLFOX) as first-line therapy for all patients with non-resectable

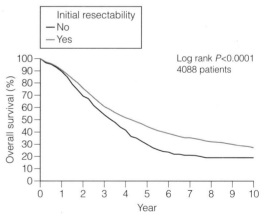

Figure 6.8 • LiverMetSurvey. Ten-year survival following hepatectomy for CRLMs comparing those who were initially resectable at presentation with those patients who were considered initially unresectable but were brought to resection using systemic chemotherapy. Reproduced with permission.

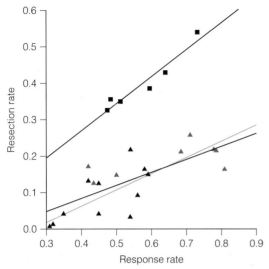

Figure 6.9 • Rate of liver resection following systemic chemotherapy for initially unresectable disease. The squares represent patients with non-resectable metastases confined to the liver ('selected patients', $r = 0.96$, $P = 0.002$). Studies with non-selected patients with colorectal cancer are shown as triangles. Due to the high heterogeneity of these studies, the observed correlation is less strong ($r = 0.74$, $P < 0.001$, solid line). A similar correlation was observed when the phase III trials (filled triangles) were separately analysed ($r = 0.67$, $P = 0.024$, dashed line). Reproduced from Folprecht G, Grothey A, Alberts S et al. Neoadjuvant treatment of unresectable colorectal liver metastases: correlation between tumour response and resection rates. Ann Oncol 2005; 16(8): 1311–9. With permission from Oxford University Press/European Society for Medical Oncology.

disease, with irinotecan-based regimens (FOLFIRI) for second-line therapy after failure of first-line treatment. Intensive triplet chemotherapy with FOLFOXIRI has been compared with FOLFIRI alone in a phase III randomised controlled trial. Response rates were higher after FOLFOXIRI, with a secondary resection rate of 36% in patients with liver-limited disease compared to 12% for those treated with standard FOLFIRI ($P = 0.017$).[71] However, toxicity was high and double-agent therapy therefore remains first-line treatment.

There is now growing evidence supporting the addition of targeted biological agents alongside a cytotoxic backbone. The randomised phase II OPUS trial compared FOLFOX with or without cetuximab in 337 patients with metastic colorectal cancer, with response rates of 46% and 36%, respectively ($P = 0.064$).[72] A subgroup analysis of 315 patients assessed *KRAS* status, demonstrating an overall response rate of 61% in wild-type patients, compared to 37% in *KRAS* mutants ($P = 0.01$).

The large CRYSTAL trial randomised 1198 patients to FOLFIRI with or without cetuximab as first-line treatment.[67] Retrospective analysis of *KRAS* status was performed on 1063 patients and found response rates of 59.3% and 43.2% for FOLFIRI and cetuximab compared to FOLFIRI alone in KRAS wild-type patients.[73] By contrast, cetuximab offered no survival advantage to the *KRAS* mutant group. Resectability rates for the entire group (irrespective of *KRAS* status) were 7% in the FOLFIRI plus cetuximab arm, compared to 3.7% in the FOLFIRI arm, with R0 rates of 4.8% and 1.7% ($P = 0.002$).

Table 6.2 • Response rate and resection rate for key trials of cytotoxic agents with the addition of targeted biological agents in patients with initially irresectable metastatic colorectal cancer

Study	Type	Regimen	No. of patients	Overall response rate	Patients undergoing resection	R0 resection
OPUS[72]	Randomised phase II	FOLFOX + cetuximab	169	61% (WT)*		9.8% (WT)
		FOLFOX	168	37% (WT)		4.1% (WT)
CRYSTAL[67]	Randomised phase III	FOLFIRI + cetuximab	599	59.3% (WT)	7%	4.8%
		FOFIRI	599	43.2% (WT)	3.7%	1.7%
CELIM[74]	Randomised phase II	FOLFOX + cetuximab	56	68%	40%	38%
		FOLFIRI + cetuximab	55	57%	43%	30%
POCHER[75]	Non-randomised phase II	FOLFOXIRI + cetuximab	43	79%	60.5%	36.3%
BEAT[76]	Phase IV	First-line cytotoxic + bevacizumab	704 liver only		15.2%	12.1%
GONO Group[77]	Non-randomised phase II	FOLFOXIRI + bevacizumab	57	76%	40% (liver only)	

*WT, *KRAS* wild type.

In 2010, the phase II CELIM study assessed FOLFOX/FOLFIRI and cetuximab for a more selected group of patients with unresectable metastatic liver-only disease and found response rates of 68% and 57%, respectively. Forty per cent of the FOLFOX and cetuximab arm underwent resection, compared to 43% of those who received FOLFIRI and cetuximab. In a combined analysis of both arms, 67 patients with *KRAS* wild-type tumours achieved a response rate of 79%.[74]

The 2010 phase II POCHER study assessed chronomodulated FOLFOXIRI alongside cetuximab in 43 patients with irresectable liver-only metastases.[75] Despite therapy not being allocated on the basis of *KRAS* status, the authors reported a 60% R0/R1 resection rate after a median of six cycles, with an objective response rate of 79.1%. Two-year survival was 80.6% in resected patients, compared to 47.1% in those who did not undergo resection ($P = 0.01$).

The largest experience of bevacizumab in unresectable patients remains the BEAT trial.[76] This large phase IV trial assessed the addition of bevacizumab to first-line chemotherapy for patients with unresectable metastatic colorectal cancer; 1914 patients were included, with a median progression-free survival (PFS) of 10.8 months (95% confidence interval (CI) 10.4–11.3) and median overall survival (OS) of 22.7 months (95% CI 21.7–23.8). In this unselected group, curative resection was performed in 7.6%. In 704 patients with metastatic disease limited to the liver, resection was achieved in 15.2%. Two-year survival was 89% in those undergoing resection, compared to 54% in those who did not.

The impressive response rates seen following systemic FOLFOXIRI led to the same group performing a single-arm phase II trial of FOLFOXIRI with the addition of bevacizumab.[77] Treatment was given as first line to 57 patients, with a 74% PFS at 10 months (95% CI 62–85). Curative resection was performed in 40% of those patients recruited with unresectable liver-only disease, and the same group has now developed a phase III randomised study comparing FOLFOXIRI plus bevacizumb with FOLFIRI plus bevacizumab. The results of this trial (the TRIBE trial) are eagerly awaited.

Perioperative chemotherapy

The precise role of adjuvant and neoadjuvant chemotherapy in the management of resectable disease remains a controversial topic.

In 2006, Portier et al. reported the results of the AURC 9002 trial assessing adjuvant 5-FU and leucovorin in patients that underwent liver resection for colorectal metastases, and demonstrated an improved 5-year disease-free survival following chemotherapy (33.5% vs. 26.7%, $P = 0.028$).[78]

The EORTC 40983 phase III trial (commonly referred to as EPOC) assessed perioperative chemotherapy by randomising patients to chemotherapy with perioperative FOLFOX and surgery (six cycles before surgery, six cycles after) or surgery alone. Although often criticised, this study clearly demonstrated a significantly improved 3-year progression-free survival in the chemotherapy arm and remains the best available evidence supporting perioperative chemotherapy[79] (**Fig. 6.10**).

Reddy et al. performed a retrospective analysis of 499 patients treated with perihepatectomy 5-FU and leucovorin, and demonstrated a survival advantage to adjuvant but not neoadjuvant therapy.[80] The role of neoadjuvant and adjuvant chemotherapy in CRLMs was further clouded by data from the LiverMetSurvey group. Adam et al. assessed 1471 patients with solitary liver metastases, and compared those who underwent resection without chemotherapy and those treated with perioperative chemotherapy followed by resection.[22] They found that preoperative chemotherapy had no impact on long-term outcome, but postoperative chemotherapy was associated with better overall and disease-free survival. A meta-analysis of trials assessing postoperative 5-FU based chemotherapy demonstrated a trend towards improved disease-free and overall survival, but did not achieve statistical significance.[81]

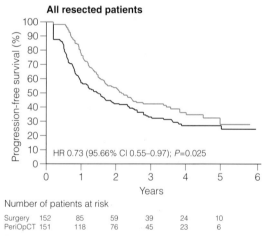

All resected patients

HR 0.73 (95.66% CI 0.55–0.97); *P*=0.025

Years

Number of patients at risk

Surgery	152	85	59	39	24	10
PeriOpCT	151	118	76	45	23	6

Figure 6.10 • The 7.3% improvement in 3-year disease-free survival demonstrated following perioperative chemotherapy (six cycles of FOLFOX before surgery, six cycles of FOLFOX after surgery) compared to surgery alone for CRLM in the EPOC trial (EORTC 40983).[79] Reproduced from Nordlinger B, Sorbye H, Glimelius B et al. Perioperative chemotherapy with FOLFOX4 and surgery versus surgery alone for resectable liver metastases from colorectal cancer (EORTC Intergroup trial 40983): a randomised controlled trial. Lancet 2008; 371(9617):1007–16. With permission from Elsevier.

Interestingly, there are no data to support the use of neoadjuvant, adjuvant or perioperative irinotecan-based regimens in this clinical setting.

Despite these controversies, expert consensus is that the majority of patients with colorectal liver disease should receive perioperative chemotherapy irrespective of their initial resectability,[82] with the rationale that this will result in the destruction of occult disease, allow a test of biology where progression despite chemotherapy signifies poor biology, as well as reduce lesion size, improving resectability.

Pathological response to chemotherapy as a predictor of long-term outcome

It now recognised that patients who exhibit good pathological response to chemotherapy have better overall survival.[83] Blazer et al. found complete pathological response to chemotherapy (absence of viable tumour cells on post-resection examination) only occurred in 9% of patients treated with systemic FOLFOX or FOLFIRI, but was associated with a 5-year survival of 75%.[84] This finding was supported by Adam et al., who found patients exhibiting complete pathological response had a 5-year survival of 76%, compared to 45% for those without.[85] The outstanding survival in this select group of complete pathological responders is similar to stage III and high-risk stage II colorectal disease, i.e. colorectal disease that has not metastasised.[86]

Complete pathological response is an impressive example of the effectiveness of modern chemotherapeutic regimens. Although oncologically desirable, it creates surgical difficulties. The correlation between complete radiological and pathological response is not clear, with around 80% of lesions showing complete radiological response containing residual disease.[87] Trying to locate a lesion that has disappeared is difficult, and results in patients undergoing blind resection on the basis of the last known location of that lesion. The difficulties associated with disappearing lesions highlight the importance of combined surgical and oncological planning to optimise the chemotherapeutic manipulation of disease, as well as the timing of any intervention. Improved preoperative assessment of pathological response by imaging will become increasingly important in deciding which patients can be managed with a 'watch and wait' policy.

Chemotherapy-associated hepatotoxicity

Increased use of neoadjuvant treatment has resulted in a rise in chemotherapy-associated hepatotoxicity. Oxaliplatin is associated with sinusoidal obstructive syndrome, characterised by a tender, congested and dilated liver, whilst patients treated with irinotecan develop fatty infiltration and scarring (steatohepatitis)[88,89] (**Fig. 6.11**). Vauthey et al. reported an incidence of 20.2% after a median of 16 weeks of FOLFIRI, compared to 4.4% for chemonaive patients.[88] Recognition of the growing number of patients coming to resection with chemotherapy-associated hepatotoxicity has led to growing interest in its impact on surgical outcome.

The EORTC 40983 trial[79] comparing upfront surgery and perioperative FOLFOX demonstrated a higher rate of minor complications in the chemotherapy and surgery arm (25% vs. 16%, $P = 0.04$).

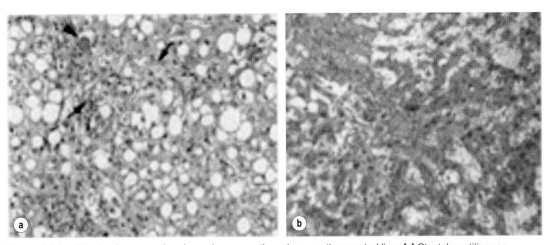

Figure 6.11 • Effects of preoperative chemotherapy on the subsequently operated liver. **(a)** Steatohepatitis seen following excessive pretreatment with irinotecan. The features of ballooned hepatocytes (arrowhead) and Mallory bodies (arrows) are shown. **(b)** Sinusoidal congestion and thrombosis seen after excessive pretreatment with oxaliplatin.

The MD Anderson group reported increased mean perioperative blood transfusion requirements in patients with oxaliplatin-induced sinusoidal injury (1.9 vs. 0.5 units, $P = 0.03$)[90] and also demonstrated an increased 90-day mortality in patients who had irinotecan-induced steatohepatitis compared to those who did not (14.7% vs. 1.6%, $P = 0.001$).[88] Other groups have reported similar outcomes[91] and marked steatohepatitis is now considered a contraindication to hepatic resection.[92]

Postoperative morbidity does appear to be related to the duration of neoadjuvant chemotherapy. Karoui et al. demonstrated a higher morbidity in those patients who received more than six cycles (54% vs. 19%, $P = 0.047$).[93] However, this increased risk does appear to be reversible. Welsh et al. showed complication rates of 2.6%, 5.5% and 11% for patients with intervals of 9–12, 5–8 and 4 weeks or less between cessation of chemotherapy and resection ($P = 0.009$), highlighting the need for close cooperation between medical and surgical oncologists to ensure the optimal timing for any interventions.[94]

Liver damage is often the result of potentially life-saving chemotherapy and research is therefore needed to elucidate the pathogenesis of this damage, as well as better methods of preoperative prediction that may enable tailoring of chemotherapeutic regimens. Currently, it is prudent to require a larger FLR of at least 30% after resection in patients who have received extensive preoperative systemic chemotherapy to compensate for impaired hepatic function.[5] The effects of modern biological therapies on operative morbidity and mortality also require further investigation, although preliminary work does suggest they are safe to use before surgery.[95,96]

> ✅✅ Appropriate chemotherapy can bring patients with irresectable disease to potentially curative surgery.[70] For patients with initially resectable disease, preoperative chemotherapy may improve long term outcome. Treatment can lead to disappearing lesions and chemotherapy induced liver damage. Decision making on the combined surgical and oncological management of these patients should be made by a multidisciplinary team including surgeons and oncologists.[116,117]

Liver-targeted therapies

Hepatic arterial infusion

The unique blood supply of the liver, with portal flow supplying healthy hepatic parenchyma and arterial flow supplying metastatic disease, has led to the concept of delivering liver-only chemotherapy in an effort to increase metastatic exposure to the agent whilst reducing systemic dose and off-target side-effects. Initial interest focused on hepatic arterial infusion (HAI) as a replacement for systemic chemotherapy. A catheter is inserted at laparotomy into the hepatic artery, through which a portable pump delivers an infusion of chemotherapeutic agent. A meta-analysis by Mocellin et al. found no evidence to support its use instead of systemic chemotherapy in the treatment of irresectable colorectal metastases.[97] Interest is now focused on the use of HAI alongside systemic therapies to maximise response in liver dominant disease.

Widescale adoption of HAI has been limited, possibly because of relatively high rates of technical complications. The Memorial Sloan Kettering group reported their experience of 544 consecutive insertions of HAI pump, and found a 16% failure rate within 2 years of insertion.[98]

Kemeny et al. published data from an early phase I trial of 49 patients treated with systemic oxaliplatin alongside HAI floxuridine in irresectable liver-only disease.[99] They reported an 8% complete response rate, an 84% partial response rate and a 47% conversion to resectability, which increased to 57% in chemonaive patients.[100,101] The same group recently reported their experience of adjuvant HAI alongside systemic FOLFOX/FOLFIRI in 125 resected patients, and reported improved overall and recurrence-free survival.[102] Further randomised studies are needed to accurately define the role for what would appear to be a biologically sensible approach.

Drug-eluting beads for TACE (DEB-TACE)

Drug-eluting beads are compressible microspheres produced from polyvinyl alcohol (PVA) hydrogel loaded with drug (usually irinotecan). DEB-TACE offers a theoretical advantage over HAI of simplified delivery (embolisation and chemotherapy are combined). Common side-effects include post-embolisation syndrome in around 10% of patients, characterised by abdominal pain, pyrexia and a transient rise in liver function tests.[103]

An international registry reported on 55 patients who had failed first- and second-line systemic therapy for metastatic colorectal cancer and were treated with DEB-TACE.[104] Response rates were 66% at 6 months and 75% at 12 months. Median overall survival from time of first treatment was 19 months, with a progression-free survival of 11 months. Six patients (10%) had their disease sufficiently downstaged to allow further treatment, with four undergoing resection and two undergoing radiofrequency ablation. These promising results have led to the development of further studies that aim to better define the precise role of DEBIRI-TACE within the chemotherapeutic armamentarium.

Selective internal radiation treatment (SIRT)

SIRT is the delivery of radiation treatment via intrahepatic arterial administration of yttrium-90 (Y-90) microspheres. Y-90 is a high-energy, beta-particle-emitting isotope bound to resin microspheres that is selectively delivered to a tumour via intra-arterial embolisation. Because of the half-life of Y-90 (2.67 days), 94% of the radiation dose is delivered during the 11 days following treatment.[105]

In selected patients, radioembolisation can downstage liver metastases so that further treatments, including ablation, are possible.[106] Encouraging results have also been reported in heavily pretreated patients with CRLMs.[107] Complications of SIRT include transient abdominal pain, fever, lethargy and nausea in up to one-third of patients. Gastroduodenal ulcers have been reported and are avoided by a meticulous administration technique that avoids reflux of Y-90 microspheres into the gastrointestinal vasculature.

The randomised phase III FOXFIRE trial comparing systemic FOLFOX chemotherapy with or without SIRT for unresectable liver-only or liver-predominant disease is currently recruiting, and will help clarify the role of SIRT in the management of CRLMs.

Ablative therapies for CRLMs

Ablative therapy takes numerous forms. Cryotherapy, laser hyperthermia and ethanol injection are decreasing in popularity due to high complication rates or lack of efficacy. Radiofrequency ablation (RFA) and microwave ablation (MWA) have significant advantages over older ablative techniques and are increasingly used. However, there remains a lack of clarity surrounding the precise role of ablation compared to surgery. Recent American Society of Clinical Oncology (ASCO) guidelines highlighted the wide variation in overall survival and local recurrence rates after ablation, and suggested that in the absence of adequate data, resection should remain the gold standard treatment for resectable disease.[108]

Despite these concerns, ablation still has a role as an adjunct to resection. Patients with small-volume resectable metastases who are not sufficiently fit to undergo liver resection should be considered for ablation, as should those with limited liver metastases who have insufficient liver volume to undergo resection.[109,110]

There is growing interest in the use of ablation alongside systemic chemotherapy for irresectable liver disease. Preliminary results of the EORTC 40004 (CLOCC) trial that compared systemic chemotherapy versus chemotherapy and RFA for unresectable metastatic colorectal liver disease suggested a survival advantage for the combined arm. The final results of this trial are eagerly awaited.[111]

Radiofrequency ablation

RFA is the most widely used ablative technique and relies on direct current transmission through tissue to generate heat and cause an ablation. Increasing lesion size leads to exponential increases in resistance to current, limiting the size of the effective ablation zone and explaining the increased risk of local recurrence and diminished survival with lesions greater than 3 cm.[108]

A recent meta-analysis of 95 published series reported a complication rate of 8.9%, with intra-abdominal bleeding, sepsis and biliary tree injury the most common complications.[112] Mortality rates range from 0 to 0.5%, with a reported local recurrence rate of 10–31%.[113] It is likely this high rate of recurrence is directly related to the type of lesions being treated by RFA. Ablations are often performed on metastases that are adjacent to major vascular structures where blood flow can operate as a heat sink, leading to incomplete ablation and local disease recurrence.

Microwave ablation

MWA has been designed to overcome some of the limitations of RFA. Electromagnetic waves agitate water molecules in tissue without the need for direct current conduction, producing friction and heat causing cell death. MWA offers higher intratumoral temperatures, larger tumour ablation volumes and faster ablation times,[114] as well as uniform ablation volumes irrespective of tissue type and moisture content,[115] allowing better prediction of ablation volume. Despite this, local recurrence after MWA has been reported between 5% and 13%, with a major complication rate ranging from 3% to 16%.[113]

> ✓✓ • Surgery remains standard of care for resectable disease.[108]
> • Ablative therapies offer an alternative treatment for patients who cannot be resected.[111]
> • RFA and microwave ablation are the modalities of choice.

Multidisciplinary team approach

The current management of advanced metastatic colorectal cancers is complex and is likely to become increasingly so in the future. Improved chemotherapeutic manipulation of disease and increasing understanding of who and what is technically and oncologically resectable will inevitably lead to more heterogeneous disease management. The rapidly changing and complex management of CRLMs means that these patients must have their treatment managed by highly specialised liver surgeons and oncologists. The UK system of local colorectal multidisciplinary teams (MDTs) organised into cancer networks, with recognised referral pathways to supraregional specialist liver MDTs, is designed to facilitate this process. However, even within this system there remains concern that not all patients with liver-only metastatic disease are being reviewed by appropriate specialists. A 2010 UK population-based study of 114 155 patients who underwent primary colorectal cancer resection between 1998 and 2004 identified 3116 (2.7%) who subsequently underwent resection for CRLMs, with the rate of hepatic resection varying widely between cancer networks (1.1–4.3%) and hospitals (0.7–6.8%).[116] The authors suggested that inconsistent use of first-line chemotherapy, or use of different thresholds to determine which patients should be considered for resection, may explain this variability and suggested that direct involvement of appropriate specialists was the only way to address these inequalities.

To help non-experts in decision making, a computer model (OncoSurge) has been created that recommends optimal treatment strategies on a case-specific basis.[117] An expert panel rated appropriateness of treatment (chemotherapy, resection or ablation) in 252 cases. A decision model was constructed, consensus measured, and results validated using 48 virtual cases and 34 real cases with known

outcomes. Consensus was achieved with overall agreement rates of 93.4–99.1%. This model combines the best available scientific evidence with the collective judgment of worldwide experts to yield a statement regarding the appropriateness of a particular treatment for each patient. The computer program can be accessed at www.evidis.com/oncosurge.

Multidisciplinary teams are becoming increasingly common but are not yet ubiquitous. It should be stressed that in order to exploit every opportunity to achieve cure, the management of CRLMs should be undertaken in a multidisciplinary setting, with specialist medical and surgical oncologists involved in the care of every patient.

Conclusions

The key recent advance in the management of CRLMs has been the availability of more effective and targeted cytotoxic and biological therapies. Better treatments are resulting in more initially unresectable patients being brought to potentially curative resection. Improved surgical technique has led to more patients being considered resectable, and the use of ablative and liver-targeted therapies alongside systemic chemotherapy and formal resection has further increased treatment options. It is clear that the optimal management of CRLMs requires close collaboration between specialist surgical and medical oncologists to identify the best biological and technical treatment for each individual patient.

Key points

- Surgery is the only treatment that offers the prospect of cure for CRLMs. The criteria now used for assessing resectability are based on whether a macroscopically and microscopically complete (R0) resection of the liver can be achieved, and whether the volume of the liver remaining after resection will be adequate.
- New surgical strategies to improve resectability include portal vein embolisation, two-stage hepatectomies, re-resection and serial liver resections, and resection of extrahepatic colorectal metastases with curative intent.
- Novel chemotherapeutic regimens combining 5-FU, folinic acid and oxaliplatin (FOLFOX) and/or irinotecan (FOLFIRI) can allow patients with initially unresectable disease to be successfully treated with liver surgery. Trials evaluating novel biological agents, such as bevacizumab and cetuximab, have shown that even more patients with initially unresectable CRLMs may respond to treatment with combinations of systemic treatments in the future.
- Increasing use of neoadjuvant treatment means that chemotherapy-associated liver injury has become more common and is associated with increased postoperative morbidity.
- The management of CRLM should be undertaken in a multidisciplinary setting, with a medical and surgical oncologist involved in the care of every patient.

References

1. Ferlay J, Shin H-R, Bray F, et al. Estimates of worldwide burden of cancer in 2008: GLOBOCAN 2008. Int J Cancer 2010;127(12):2893–917.

2. Weiss L, Grundmann E, Torhorst J, et al. Haematogenous metastatic patterns in colonic carcinoma: an analysis of 1541 necropsies. J Pathol 1986;150(3):195–203.

3. Stangl R, Altendorf-Hofmann A, Charnley RM, et al. Factors influencing the natural history of colorectal liver metastases. Lancet 1994;343(8910): 1405–10.

4. Poston GJ, Tait D, O'Connell S, et al., Guideline Development Group. Diagnosis and management of colorectal cancer: summary of NICE guidance. Br Med J 2011;343:d6751.

5. Abdalla EK, Adam R, Bilchik AJ, et al. Improving resectability of hepatic colorectal metastases: expert consensus statement. Ann Surg Oncol 2006;13(10):1271–80.

6. McLoughlin JM, Jensen EH, Malafa M. Resection of colorectal liver metastases: current perspectives. Cancer Control 2006;13(1):32–41.

7. Saini S. Imaging of the hepatobiliary tract. N Engl J Med 1997;336(26):1889–94.

8. Martínez L, Puig I, Valls C. Colorectal liver metastases: radiological diagnosis and staging. Eur J Surg Oncol 2007;33(Suppl. 2):S5–16.

9. Huppertz A, Balzer T, Blakeborough A, et al. Improved detection of focal liver lesions at MR imaging: multicenter comparison of gadoxetic acid-enhanced MR images with intraoperative findings. Radiology 2004;230(1):266–75.

10. Xu L-H, Cai S-J, Cai G-X, et al. Imaging diagnosis of colorectal liver metastases. World J Gastroenterol 2011;17(42):4654–9.

11. Israel O, Mor M, Gaitini D, et al. Combined functional and structural evaluation of cancer patients with a hybrid camera-based PET/CT system using ^{18}F-FDG. J Nucl Med 2002;43(9):1129–36.

12. Kochhar R, Liong S, Manoharan P. The role of FDG PET/CT in patients with colorectal cancer metastases. Cancer Biomark 2010;7(4):235–48.

13. Berger KL, Nicholson SA, Dehdashti F, et al. FDG PET evaluation of mucinous neoplasms: correlation of FDG uptake with histopathologic features. AJR Am J Roentgenol 2000;174(4):1005–8.

14. Mortensen FV, Zogovic S, Nabipour M, et al. Diagnostic laparoscopy and ultrasonography for colorectal liver metastases. Scand J Surg 2006;95(3):172–5.

15. Grobmyer SR, Fong Y, D'Angelica M, et al. Diagnostic laparoscopy prior to planned hepatic resection for colorectal metastases. Arch Surg 2004;139(12):1326–30.

16. Metcalfe MS, Close JS, Iswariah H, et al. The value of laparoscopic staging for patients with colorectal metastases. Arch Surg 2003;138(7):770–2.

17. de Castro SMM, Tilleman EHBM, Busch ORC, et al. Diagnostic laparoscopy for primary and secondary liver malignancies: impact of improved imaging and changed criteria for resection. Ann Surg Oncol 2004;11(5):522–9.

18. Koea J, Rodgers M, Thompson P, et al. Laparoscopy in the management of colorectal cancer metastatic to the liver. Aust N Z J Surg 2004;74(12): 1056–9.

19. Rahusen FD, Cuesta MA, Borgstein PJ, et al. Selection of patients for resection of colorectal metastases to the liver using diagnostic laparoscopy and laparoscopic ultrasonography. Ann Surg 1999;230(1):31–7.

20. Fong Y, Fortner J, Sun RL, et al. Clinical score for predicting recurrence after hepatic resection for metastatic colorectal cancer: analysis of 1001 consecutive cases. Ann Surg 1999;230(3):309–21.

21. Snowden CP, Prentis JM, Anderson HL, et al. Submaximal cardiopulmonary exercise testing predicts complications and hospital length of stay in patients undergoing major elective surgery. Ann Surg 2010;251(3):535–41.

22. Adam R, Frilling A, Elias D, et al. Liver resection of colorectal metastases in elderly patients. Br J Surg 2010;97(3):366–76.

23. de LiguoriCarino N, van Leeuwen BL, Ghaneh P, et al. Liver resection for colorectal liver metastases in older patients. Crit Rev Oncol Hematol 2008; 67(3):273–8.

24. Minagawa M, Makuuchi M, Torzilli G, et al. Extension of the frontiers of surgical indications in the treatment of liver metastases from colorectal cancer: long-term results. Ann Surg 2000;231(4): 487–99.

25. Elias D, Liberale G, Vernerey D, et al. Hepatic and extrahepatic colorectal metastases: when resectable, their localization does not matter, but their total number has a prognostic effect. Ann Surg Oncol 2005;12(11):900–9.

26. Van Cutsem E, Nordlinger B, Adam R, et al. Towards a pan-European consensus on the treatment of patients with colorectal liver metastases. Eur J Cancer 2006;42(14):2212–21.

27. Malde DJ, Khan A, Prasad KR, et al. Inferior vena cava resection with hepatecromy: challenging but justified. HPB (Oxford) 2011;13(11):802–10.

28. Carpizo DR, Are C, Jarnagin W, et al. Liver resection for metastatic colorectal cancer in patients with concurrent extrahepatic disease: results in 127 patients treated at a single center. Ann Surg Oncol 2009;16(8):2138–46.

29. Hemming AW, Reed AI, Langham MR, et al. Hepatic vein reconstruction for resection of hepatic tumors. Ann Surg 2002;235(6):850–8.

30. Abulkhir A, Limongelli P, Healey AJ, et al. Preoperative portal vein embolization for major liver resection: a meta-analysis. Ann Surg 2008;247(1):49–57.

31. Ribero D, Abdalla EK, Madoff DC, et al. Portal vein embolization before major hepatectomy and its effects on regeneration, resectability and outcome. Br J Surg 2007;94(11):1386–94.

32. Chun YS, Vauthey JN. Extending the frontiers of resectability in advanced colorectal cancer. Eur J Surg Oncol 2007;33(Suppl. 2):S52–8.

33. Covey AM, Brown KT, Jarnagin WR, et al. Combined portal vein embolization and neoadjuvant chemotherapy as a treatment strategy for resectable hepatic colorectal metastases. Ann Surg 2008;247(3):451–5.

34. Adam R, Delvart V, Pascal G, et al. Rescue surgery for unresectable colorectal liver metastases downstaged by chemotherapy: a model to predict long-term survival. Ann Surg 2004;240(4):644–58.

35. Jaeck D, Oussoultzoglou E, Rosso E, et al. A two-stage hepatectomy procedure combined with portal vein embolization to achieve curative resection for initially unresectable multiple and bilobar colorectal liver metastases. Ann Surg 2004;240(6):1037–51.

36. Antoniou A, Lovegrove RE, Tilney HS, et al. Meta-analysis of clinical outcome after first and second liver resection for colorectal metastases. Surgery 2007;141(1):9–18.

37. de Jong MC, Mayo SC, Pulitano C, et al. Repeat curative intent liver surgery is safe and effective for recurrent colorectal liver metastasis: results from an international multi-institutional analysis. J Gastrointest Surg 2009;13(12):2141–51.

38. Kondo S, Hirano S, Ambo Y, et al. Arterioportal shunting as an alternative to microvascular reconstruction after hepatic artery resection. Br J Surg 2004;91(2):248–51.

39. Azoulay D, Andreani P, Maggi U, et al. Combined liver resection and reconstruction of the suprarenal vena cava: the Paul Brousse experience. Ann Surg 2006;244(1):80–8.

40. Hemming AW, Reed AI, Langham MR, et al. Combined resection of the liver and inferior vena cava for hepatic malignancy. Ann Surg 2004;239(5):712–21.

41. Lodge JP, Ammori BJ, Prasad KR, et al. Ex vivo and in situ resection of inferior vena cava with hepatectomy for colorectal metastases. Ann Surg 2000;231(4):471–9.

42. Yedibela S, Klein P, Feuchter K, et al. Surgical management of pulmonary metastases from colorectal cancer in 153 patients. Ann Surg Oncol 2006;13(11):1538–44.

43. Shiono S, Ishii G, Nagai K, et al. Predictive factors for local recurrence of resected colorectal lung metastases. Ann Thorac Surg 2005;80(3):1040–5.

44. Pfannschmidt J, Muley T, Hoffmann H, et al. Prognostic factors and survival after complete resection of pulmonary metastases from colorectal carcinoma: experiences in 167 patients. J Thorac Cardiovasc Surg 2003;126(3):732–9.

45. Saito Y, Omiya H, Kohno K, et al. Pulmonary metastasectomy for 165 patients with colorectal carcinoma: a prognostic assessment. J Thorac Cardiovasc Surg 2002;124(5):1007–13.

46. Watanabe K, Nagai K, Kobayashi A, et al. Factors influencing survival after complete resection of pulmonary metastases from colorectal cancer. Br J Surg 2009;96(9):1058–65.

47. Kanzaki R, Higashiyama M, Oda K, et al. Outcome of surgical resection for recurrent pulmonary metastasis from colorectal carcinoma. Am J Surg 2011;202(4):419–26.

48. Adam R, de Haas RJ, Wicherts DA, et al. Concomitant extrahepatic disease in patients with colorectal liver metastases: when is there a place for surgery? Ann Surg 2011;253(2):349–59.

49. Pulitanò C, Bodingbauer M, Aldrighetti L, et al. Liver resection for colorectal metastases in presence of extrahepatic disease: results from an international multi-institutional analysis. Ann Surg Oncol 2011;18(5):1380–8.

50. Kooby DA, Stockman J, Ben-Porat L, et al. Influence of transfusions on perioperative and long-term outcome in patients following hepatic resection for colorectal metastases. Ann Surg 2003;237(6):860–70.

51. Lesurtel M, Selzner M, Petrowsky H, et al. How should transection of the liver be performed? A prospective randomized study in 100 consecutive patients: comparing four different transection strategies. Ann Surg 2005;242(6):814–23.

52. Gurusamy KS, Pamecha V, Sharma D, et al. Techniques for liver parenchymal transection in liver resection. Cochrane Database Syst Rev 2009;(1):CD006880.

53. Lupo L, Gallerani A, Panzera P, et al. Randomized clinical trial of radiofrequency-assisted versus clamp-crushing liver resection. Br J Surg 2007;94(3):287–91.

54. Figueras J, Llado L, Miro M, et al. Application of fibrin glue sealant after hepatectomy does not seem justified: results of a randomized study in 300 patients. Ann Surg 2007;245(4):536–42.

55. Simillis C, Constantinides VA, Tekkis PP, et al. Laparoscopic versus open hepatic resections for benign and malignant neoplasms – a meta-analysis. Surgery 2007;141(2):203–11.

56. Abu Hilal M, Di Fabio F, Abu Salameh M, et al. Oncological efficiency analysis of laparoscopic liver resection for primary and metastatic cancer: a single-center UK experience. Arch Surg 2012;147(1):42–8.

57. Buell JF, Cherqui D, Geller DA, et al. The international position on laparoscopic liver surgery:

the Louisville Statement, 2008. Ann Surg 2009;250(5):825–30.

58. Simmonds PC, Primrose JN, Colquitt JL, et al. Surgical resection of hepatic metastases from colorectal cancer: a systematic review of published studies. Br J Cancer 2006;94(7):982–99.

59. Poston GJ, Figueras J, Giuliante F, et al. Urgent need for a new staging system in advanced colorectal cancer. J Clin Oncol 2008;26(29):4828–33.

60. Lazorthes F, Navarro F, Ychou M, et al., ANAES. Therapeutic management of hepatic metastases from colorectal cancers. Gastroenterol Clin Biol 2003;27 Spec No 2B7.

61. Poston G, Adam R, Vauthey J-N. Downstaging or downsizing: time for a new staging system in advanced colorectal cancer? J Clin Oncol 2006;24(18):2702–6.

62. Nordlinger B, Guiguet M, Vaillant JC, et al. Surgical resection of colorectal carcinoma metastases to the liver. A prognostic scoring system to improve case selection, based on 1568 patients. Association Française de Chirurgie. Cancer 1996;77(7):1254–62.

63. Rees M, Tekkis PP, Welsh FKS, et al. Evaluation of long-term survival after hepatic resection for metastatic colorectal cancer: a multifactorial model of 929 patients. Ann Surg 2008;247(1):125–35.

64. Zakaria S, Donohue JH, Que FG, et al. Hepatic resection for colorectal metastases: value for risk scoring systems? Ann Surg 2007;246(2):183–91.

65. Merkel S, Bialecki D, Meyer T, et al. Comparison of clinical risk scores predicting prognosis after resection of colorectal liver metastases. J Surg Oncol 2009;100(5):349–57.

66. Kopetz S, Chang GJ, Overman MJ, et al. Improved survival in metastatic colorectal cancer is associated with adoption of hepatic resection and improved chemotherapy. J Clin Oncol 2009;27(22):3677–83.

67. Van Cutsem E, Köhne C-H, Hitre E, et al. Cetuximab and chemotherapy as initial treatment for metastatic colorectal cancer. N Engl J Med 2009;360(14):1408–17.

68. Roock WD, Claes B, Bernasconi D, et al. Effects of KRAS, BRAF, NRAS, and PIK3CA mutations on the efficacy of cetuximab plus chemotherapy in chemotherapy-refractory metastatic colorectal cancer: a retrospective consortium analysis. Lancet Oncol 2010;11(8):753–62.

69. Ellis LM. Mechanisms of action of bevacizumab as a component of therapy for metastatic colorectal cancer. Semin Oncol 2006;33(5, Suppl. 10):S1–7.

70. Folprecht G, Grothey A, Alberts S, et al. Neoadjuvant treatment of unresectable colorectal liver metastases: correlation between tumour response and resection rates. Ann Oncol 2005;16(8):1311–9.

71. Falcone A, Ricci S, Brunetti I, et al. Phase III trial of infusional fluorouracil, leucovorin, oxaliplatin, and irinotecan (FOLFOXIRI) compared with infusional fluorouracil, leucovorin, and irinotecan (FOLFIRI) as first-line treatment for metastatic colorectal cancer: the GruppoOncologico Nord Ovest. J Clin Oncol 2007;25(13):1670–6.

72. Bokemeyer C, Bondarenko I, Makhson A, et al. Fluorouracil, leucovorin, and oxaliplatin with and without cetuximab in the first-line treatment of metastatic colorectal cancer. J Clin Oncol 2009;27(5):663–71.

73. Van Cutsem E, Köhne C-H, Láng I, et al. Cetuximab plus irinotecan, fluorouracil, and leucovorin as first-line treatment for metastatic colorectal cancer: updated analysis of overall survival according to tumor KRAS and BRAF mutation status. J Clin Oncol 2011;29(15):2011–9.

74. Folprecht G, Gruenberger T, Bechstein WO, et al. Tumour response and secondary resectability of colorectal liver metastases following neoadjuvant chemotherapy with cetuximab: the CELIM randomised phase 2 trial. Lancet Oncol 2010;11(1):38–47.

75. Garufi C, Torsello A, Tumolo S, et al. Cetuximab plus chronomodulated irinotecan, 5-fluorouracil, leucovorin and oxaliplatin as neoadjuvant chemotherapy in colorectal liver metastases: POCHER trial. Br J Cancer 2010;103(10):1542–7.

76. Van Cutsem E, Rivera F, Berry S, et al. Safety and efficacy of first-line bevacizumab with FOLFOX, XELOX, FOLFIRI and fluoropyrimidines in metastatic colorectal cancer: the BEAT study. Ann Oncol 2009;20(11):1842–7.

77. Masi G, Loupakis F, Salvatore L, et al. Bevacizumab with FOLFOXIRI (irinotecan, oxaliplatin, fluorouracil, and folinate) as first-line treatment for metastatic colorectal cancer: a phase 2 trial. Lancet Oncol 2010;11(9):845–52.

78. Portier G, Elias D, Bouche O, et al. Multicenter randomized trial of adjuvant fluorouracil and folinic acid compared with surgery alone after resection of colorectal liver metastases: FFCD ACHBTH AURC 9002 trial. J Clin Oncol 2006;24(31):4976–82.

79. Nordlinger B, Sorbye H, Glimelius B, et al. Perioperative chemotherapy with FOLFOX4 and surgery versus surgery alone for resectable liver metastases from colorectal cancer (EORTC Intergroup trial 40983): a randomised controlled trial. Lancet 2008;371(9617):1007–16.

80. Reddy SK, Zorzi D, Lum YW, et al. Timing of multimodality therapy for resectable synchronous colorectal liver metastases: a retrospective multi-institutional analysis. Ann Surg Oncol 2009;16(7):1809–19.

81. Mitry E, Fields ALA, Bleiberg H, et al. Adjuvant chemotherapy after potentially curative resection of metastases from colorectal cancer: a pooled analysis of two randomized trials. J Clin Oncol 2008;26(30):4906–11.

82. Nordlinger B, Van Cutsem E, Gruenberger T, et al. Combination of surgery and chemotherapy and the role of targeted agents in the treatment of patients with colorectal liver metastases: recommendations from an expert panel. Ann Oncol 2009;20(6):985–92.

83. Rubbia-Brandt L, Giostra E, Brezault C, et al. Importance of histological tumor response assessment in predicting the outcome in patients with colorectal liver metastases treated with neo-adjuvant chemotherapy followed by liver surgery. Ann Oncol 2007;18(2):299–304.

84. Blazer DG, Kishi Y, Maru DM, et al. Pathologic response to preoperative chemotherapy: a new outcome end point after resection of hepatic colorectal metastases. J Clin Oncol 2008;26(33):5344–51.

85. Adam R, Wicherts DA, de Haas RJ, et al. Complete pathologic response after preoperative chemotherapy for colorectal liver metastases: myth or reality? J Clin Oncol 2008;26(10):1635–41.

86. O'Connell JB, Maggard MA, Ko CY. Colon cancer survival rates with the new American Joint Committee on Cancer sixth edition staging. J Natl Cancer Inst 2004;96(19):1420–5.

87. Benoist S, Brouquet A, Penna C, et al. Complete response of colorectal liver metastases after chemotherapy: does it mean cure? J Clin Oncol 2006;24(24):3939–45.

88. Vauthey J-N, Pawlik TM, Ribero D, et al. Chemotherapy regimen predicts steatohepatitis and an increase in 90-day mortality after surgery for hepatic colorectal metastases. J Clin Oncol 2006;24(13):2065–72.

89. Rubbia-Brandt L, Audard V, Sartoretti P, et al. Severe hepatic sinusoidal obstruction associated with oxaliplatin-based chemotherapy in patients with metastatic colorectal cancer. Ann Oncol 2004;15(3):460–6.

90. Aloia TA, Vauthey J-N, Loyer EM, et al. Solitary colorectal liver metastasis: resection determines outcome. Arch Surg 2006;141(5):460–7.

91. Fernandez FG, Ritter J, Goodwin JW, et al. Effect of steatohepatitis associated with irinotecan or oxaliplatin pretreatment on resectability of hepatic colorectal metastases. J Am Coll Surg 2005;200(6):845–53.

92. Chun YS, Vauthey J-N, Boonsirikamchai P, et al. Association of computed tomography morphologic criteria with pathologic response and survival in patients treated with bevacizumab for colorectal liver metastases. JAMA 2009;302(21):2338–44.

93. Karoui M, Penna C, Amin-Hashem M, et al. Influence of preoperative chemotherapy on the risk of major hepatectomy for colorectal liver metastases. Ann Surg 2006;243(1):1–7.

94. Welsh FKS, Tilney HS, Tekkis PP, et al. Safe liver resection following chemotherapy for colorectal metastases is a matter of timing. Br J Cancer 2007;96(7):1037–42.

95. Chaudhury P, Hassanain M, Bouganim N, et al. Perioperative chemotherapy with bevacizumab and liver resection for colorectal cancer liver metastasis. HPB (Oxford) 2010;12(1):37–42.

96. Kesmodel SB, Ellis LM, Lin E, et al. Preoperative bevacizumab does not significantly increase postoperative complication rates in patients undergoing hepatic surgery for colorectal cancer liver metastases. J Clin Oncol 2008;26(32):5254–60.

97. Mocellin S, Pilati P, Lise M, et al. Meta-analysis of hepatic arterial infusion for unresectable liver metastases from colorectal cancer: the end of an era? J Clin Oncol 2007;25(35):5649–54.

98. Allen PJ, Nissan A, Picon AI, et al. Technical complications and durability of hepatic artery infusion pumps for unresectable colorectal liver metastases: an institutional experience of 544 consecutive cases. J Am Coll Surg 2005;201(1):57–65.

99. Kemeny NE, Melendez FDH, Capanu M, et al. Conversion to resectability using hepatic artery infusion plus systemic chemotherapy for the treatment of unresectable liver metastases from colorectal carcinoma. J Clin Oncol 2009;27(21):3465–71.

100. Shitara K, Munakata M, Kudo T, et al. Combination chemotherapy with hepatic arterial infusion of 5-fluorouracil (5-FU) and systemic irinotecan (CPT-11) in patients with unresectable liver metastases from colorectal cancer. GanTo Kagaku Ryoho 2006;33(13):2033–7.

101. Gallagher DJ, Capanu M, Raggio G, et al. Hepatic arterial infusion plus systemic irinotecan in patients with unresectable hepatic metastases from colorectal cancer previously treated with systemic oxaliplatin: a retrospective analysis. Ann Oncol 2007;18(12):1995–9.

102. House MG, Kemeny NE, Gönen M, et al. Comparison of adjuvant systemic chemotherapy with or without hepatic arterial infusional chemotherapy after hepatic resection for metastatic colorectal cancer. Ann Surg 2011;254(6):851–6.

103. Martin RCG, Howard J, Tomalty D, et al. Toxicity of irinotecan-eluting beads in the treatment of hepatic malignancies: results of a multi-institutional registry. Cardiovasc Intervent Radiol 2010;33(5):960–6.

104. Martin RCG, Joshi J, Robbins K, et al. Hepatic intra-arterial injection of drug-eluting bead, irinotecan (DEBIRI) in unresectable colorectal liver metastases refractory to systemic chemotherapy: results of multi-institutional study. Ann Surg Oncol 2011;18(1):192–8.

105. Gulec SA, Fong Y. Yttrium 90 microsphere selective internal radiation treatment of hepatic colorectal metastases. Arch Surg 2007;142(7):675–82.

106. Hoffmann RT, Jakobs TF, Kubisch CH, et al. Radiofrequency ablation after selective internal radiation therapy with Yttrium90 microspheres in

metastatic liver disease – Is it feasible? Eur J Radiol 2010;74(1):199–205.

107. Cosimelli M, Golfieri R, Cagol PP, et al. Multi-centre phase II clinical trial of yttrium-90 resin microspheres alone in unresectable, chemotherapy refractory colorectal liver metastases. Br J Cancer 2010;103(3):324–31.

108. Wong SL, Mangu PB, Choti MA, et al. American Society of Clinical Oncology 2009 clinical evidence review on radiofrequency ablation of hepatic metastases from colorectal cancer. J Clin Oncol 2010;28(3):493–508.

109. Oshowo A, Gillams A, Harrison E, et al. Comparison of resection and radiofrequency ablation for treatment of solitary colorectal liver metastases. Br J Surg 2003;90(10):1240–3.

110. Jansen MC, van Duijnhoven FH, van Hillegersberg R, et al. Adverse effects of radiofrequency ablation of liver tumours in the Netherlands. Br J Surg 2005;92(10):1248–54.

111. Ruers T, van Coevorden F, Pierie J, et al. Radiofrequency ablation (RFA) combined with chemotherapy for unresectable colorectal liver metastases (CRC LM): interim results of a randomised phase II study of the EORTC-NCRI CCSG-ALM Intergroup 40004 (CLOCC). ASCO Meeting Abstr 2008;26(Suppl. 15):4012.

112. Mulier S, Ni Y, Jamart J, et al. Local recurrence after hepatic radiofrequency coagulation: multivariate meta-analysis and review of contributing factors. Ann Surg 2005;242(2):158–71.

113. Pathak S, Jones R, Tang JM, et al. Ablative therapies for colorectal liver metastases (CRLM): a systematic review. Colorectal Dis 2011;13(9):e252–65.

114. Simon CJ, Dupuy DE, Mayo-Smith WW. Microwave ablation: principles and applications. Radiographics 2005;25(Suppl. 1):S69–83.

115. Jones RP, Kitteringham NR, Terlizzo M, et al. Microwave ablation of ex vivo human liver and colorectal liver metastases with a novel 14.5 GHz generator. Int J Hyperthermia 2012;28(1):43–54.

116. Morris EJ, Forman D, Thomas JD, et al. Surgical management and outcomes of colorectal cancer liver metastases. Br J Surg 2010;97(7):1110–1118.

117. Poston GJ, Adam R, Alberts S, et al. OncoSurge; a strategy for improving resectability with curative intent in metastatic colorectal cancer. J Clin Oncol 2005;23:7125–34.

Non-colorectal hepatic metastases

Zaheer Kanji
Lynn Mikula
Carol-Anne Moulton
Steven Gallinger

Introduction

Colorectal cancer (CRC) is the most common source of secondary hepatic tumours, although almost any solid malignancy can metastasise to the liver. Tumour cells from gastrointestinal tract malignancies reach the liver directly via the portal circulation. Liver metastases may occur either in apparent isolation, as is sometimes seen in CRC, or in association with widespread systemic disease, as in pancreatic and gastric adenocarcinoma. In contrast, metastases from non-gastrointestinal tumours reach the liver via the systemic circulation and are generally indicative of disseminated disease.

The development of liver metastases was previously considered a preterminal event with treatment limited to palliation; however, the success of hepatectomy in improving outcomes in metastatic CRC has generated renewed enthusiasm in considering resection of liver metastases from non-colorectal primary cancers. Liver resection has become the standard of care for CRC liver metastases and many centres have adopted an increasingly aggressive approach, with reported 5-year survival rates exceeding 50%.[1,2] The complementary use of portal vein embolisation, radiofrequency ablation and staged resection strategies has increased the proportion of patients eligible for resection. At the same time, advances in surgical technique and knowledge of liver anatomy have reduced

significantly the morbidity and mortality associated with liver resection to less than 20% and 5%, respectively.[2,3]

Liver metastases of non-colorectal origin constitute a diverse group of tumours, most commonly arising from gastrointestinal sites. These tumours can be broadly divided into neuroendocrine and non-neuroendocrine malignancies, encompassing unique and markedly varied natural histories. Neuroendocrine tumours (NETs) have historically been described as indolent malignancies with hepatectomy for NET liver metastases associated with 5- and 10-year survival rates of 77.4% and 50.4%, respectively.[4] While hepatectomy is an increasingly accepted management strategy for NETs, it is performed less frequently for non-neuroendocrine tumours.

The evidence regarding hepatectomy for non-colorectal metastases originates largely from retrospective reviews spanning several decades of experience.[5-8] Many studies fail to distinguish between NET and non-NET metastases, and when that distinction is made, the non-NET metastases are usually considered a single entity despite comprising a heterogeneous set of pathologies. Reports focusing on a single tumour type are usually based on small case series. With advances in surgical techniques and promising results observed in CRC and NET hepatic metastases, the role of surgical treatments in non-NET liver tumours has once again become an area of active research.

✅ Due to the paucity of prospective, controlled data, the appropriate indications for hepatectomy for non-CRC metastases are unclear. Factors routinely associated with improved long-term outcomes include a long disease-free interval between treatment of the primary tumour and development of liver metastasis, little or no extrahepatic disease, the projected future liver remnant and well to moderately differentiated cancer.[9] The inability to resect all NET liver metastases does not appear to worsen overall survival.[4] Unfortunately, no single measure of tumour biology yet exists.

Pathophysiology and molecular basis of liver metastases

Achieving cure in cancer requires the complete eradication of all tumour cells. Thus, for most solid tumours, complete surgical excision is the cornerstone of treatment, often with adjuvant treatment to treat microscopic disease. In the presence of metastases there is an apparent contradiction in using a local therapy – surgery – to treat what is considered disseminated disease.

The rationale behind a surgical approach to metastatic disease is based on the concept of site-specific metastases. First proposed by Paget in 1889, this 'seed and soil' hypothesis argues that solid tumours have a distinct pattern of distant organ involvement created by the target organ microenvironment. Ewing proposed a 'mechanical' theory in which the metastatic pattern is determined by the venous drainage of the primary tumour.[10] Neither theory takes into account the complexity of the metastatic process, which requires that a cancer cell gains specific invasion and metastatic potential before it can disseminate. The clonal selection model of the metastatic process suggests that heterogeneity develops within a population of cancer cells through mutational events, allowing a subpopulation to randomly acquire the necessary traits to disseminate successfully.[11] Alternatively, it has been argued that within cancers of the same pathological type, i.e. breast cancer, some tumours are a priori more likely to develop metastases than others. This is supported by gene expression data where specific molecular signatures have been found to predict accurately prognosis in breast cancer,[12] ovarian cancer[13] and melanoma.[14] Similarly, in CRC the genotype of microsatellite instability correlates with a decreased likelihood of metastatic spread.[15]

A recent refinement to Paget's hypothesis, based on molecular genetic research, suggests that the primary tumour is itself capable of preparing the soil by creating a 'premetastatic niche'.[16] Every cancer has a type-specific pattern of cytokine expression that appears to direct both malignant and non-malignant cells to specific distant organs. The influx and clustering of bone-marrow-derived haematopoietic cells is one of the earliest events in the development of a metastatic deposit. This is closely followed by local inflammation and the release of matrix metalloproteinases. These local events appear to mediate remodelling of the extracellular matrix, creating a more permissive microenvironment for the eventual deposition and growth of malignant cells.[17] Thus, the primary tumour both chooses and alters the sites to which it metastasises. For reasons not yet understood, many solid tumours metastasise preferentially to the liver.

If the site-specific hypothesis of metastatic spread is correct, complete surgical excision of liver metastases can remove the only site of disease and offers a chance for cure. Nonetheless, residual micrometastatic disease may exist within the liver, and hepatic recurrences are a common cause of treatment failure following hepatectomy. Even in the presence of micrometastases, the removal of all macroscopic disease may have immunological benefits. The immune-suppressing effects of cancers are well accepted: malignant cells can induce both adaptive and innate immune suppression, facilitating tumour growth.[18] The degree of immune suppression correlates with the tumour burden[19] and if all gross metastatic disease can be removed, host defences may attack micrometastatic deposits more effectively. The use of neoadjuvant or adjuvant chemotherapy may improve cure rates by controlling micrometastases.[20,21]

The advent of next generation sequencing technologies and high-density oligonucleotide arrays has further deepened our understanding of the metastatic process. Whereas the ability of a cancerous cell to metastasise was once believed to occur following the accumulation of multiple somatic mutations in many cancer-causing genes, new findings, specifically in pancreatic cancer, have challenged this belief. Studies by Yachida et al.[22] and Campbell et al.[23] describe the existence of multiple subclones within a primary pancreas cancer tumour, each containing a unique genetic signature corresponding to an eventual site of metastatic spread. These subclones are present many years before an eventual metastasis is clinically detected, when disease is at an early stage. Furthermore, metastases seen in different organs share many common genetic mutations as well as site-specific changes that confer a selective growth advantage in the respective tissue. Future studies on the biology of metastases are likely to improve our understanding of this complex process, translating into more efficacious therapy.

Clinical approach to non-colorectal liver metastases

Routine clinical, radiological and serological assessments for liver metastases should be guided by the propensity for liver metastases of each specific tumour type and the ability of potential treatments to alter the outcome of the metastatic disease. In imaging the liver, the choice of transabdominal ultrasound, contrast-enhanced ultrasound, contrast-enhanced triphasic computed tomography (CT), magnetic resonance imaging (MRI) and positron emission tomography (PET) will be dictated by tumour type as well as local availability and expertise.

Some patients can be assessed for recurrence using more targeted techniques and biochemical markers (i.e. CA-125 for ovarian cancer, chromogranin A for NETs). Nuclear imaging can detect NETs expressing somatostatin receptors with 80–90% sensitivity. Whole-body PET scanning using a new somatostatin analogue, [68Ga]DOTA-TOC, has been found to be accurate for the detection of new metastases in NETs following radionuclide therapy.[24] Occasionally, the original presentation of an NET will be a liver metastasis from an unidentified primary, and the investigative focus is aimed at localisation of the primary tumour.

> ✅ When a patient is under consideration for hepatic metastasectomy, the most critical component of the clinical assessment is an accurate determination of the extent of metastatic spread, including a thorough assessment for extra-abdominal disease. The anatomical areas targeted for investigation (brain, lung, bone) will be determined by the known metastatic pattern of the primary tumour.

Certain tumours, such as gastric, breast and ovarian cancer, have a predilection for intraperitoneal spread. Although CT is the preferred modality for diagnosing peritoneal carcinomatosis, its accuracy is still limited by histological type, the anatomical site of spread and the size of tumour deposits.[25] For many of these equivocal cases, diagnostic laparoscopy has been recommended. Routine laparoscopy with laparoscopic ultrasound for patients with potentially resectable non-colorectal liver metastases has been found to result in a change in management in 20% of cases and may be used in preoperative staging.[26]

Treatment strategies

Several treatment modalities exist for metastatic disease, and the therapeutic approach must be tailored to the tumour type, the performance status of the patient and the extent of disease, determined in the setting of a multidisciplinary conference. Ablative strategies and systemic or locally delivered chemotherapy can be used as adjuncts to resection. Radiofrequency ablation (RFA) has been reported to be safe and successful at achieving local control in patients with liver metastases from breast cancer,[27] ovarian cancer[28] and NETs,[29] but its major limitation is the difficulty of achieving complete necrosis for tumours larger than 3 cm.

Transarterial embolisation (TAE) takes advantage of the differential blood supply of liver metastases, which depend mainly on the hepatic arteries, and the normal parenchyma, which relies more heavily on the portal vein. Transarterial chemoembolisation (TACE) involves the local delivery of a drug prior to occluding the artery and allows prolonged exposure of the tumour to the agent without increasing systemic toxicity. Both TAE and TACE have been well described for the treatment of unresectable hepatocellular carcinoma[30] and the symptomatic relief of NETs.[31]

Neuroendocrine tumours

Gastrointestinal NETs represent a diverse group of tumours originating throughout the gastrointestinal tract. They are classified into carcinoid and pancreatic histological subtypes. Carcinoid tumours arise most commonly in the midgut and may secrete serotonin and other bioactive amines. Pancreatic NETs (PNETs) can be non-functional or hormonally active (e.g. insulin, glucagon, gastrin, vasoactive intestinal peptide), manifesting varied clinical syndromes.

Most NETs of gastrointestinal origin demonstrate 'indolent' growth. Despite such a benign description, 46–93% of patients with NETs will have liver involvement at the time of diagnosis, with 5-year untreated survival of 0–20%.[32] Systemic chemotherapy with platinum-based regimens has shown a response rate of up to 67% in poorly differentiated NETs. Nevertheless, the survival benefit of chemotherapy is limited and associated with significant toxicity.[33] Somatostatin analogues such as octreotide can achieve symptomatic relief in 70–80% of patients, but an antiproliferative effect is seen in less than 10% of cases.[34] Furthermore, newer agents such as the receptor tyrosine kinase inhibitor sunitinib, the mammmalian target of rapamycin (mTOR) inhibitor everolimus, and the anti-vascular endothelial growth factor (anti-VEGF) bevacizumab have shown promise in PNETs.[33]

NETs metastasise preferentially to the liver, and in many patients the liver remains the only site of metastatic disease for a prolonged period of time. The majority of patients have multifocal, bilobar disease, of which less than 20% are candidates for surgery[32] (**Fig. 7.1a,b**). Liver resection may be

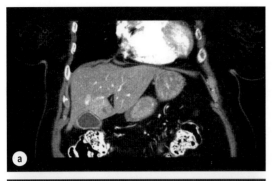

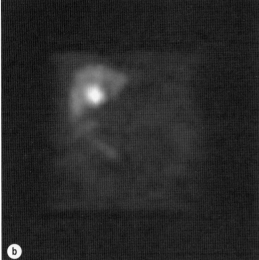

Figure 7.1 • (a) A 67-year-old female with a node-positive distal jejunal carcinoid tumour and synchronous solitary liver metastasis in segment 4B. **(b)** Octreotide scan of the same patient. Transaxial single-photon emission computed tomography (SPECT) demonstrates abnormal activity in segment 4B corresponding to known metastasis on CT.

performed with curative intent, symptom control or prolongation of survival in the palliative setting.

The choice of treatment for NET hepatic metastases is largely dependent on underlying tumour biology and pattern of metastatic spread.[35] According to the 2010 World Health Organization guidelines for the management of NETs, pathological grade (1-3) has been highlighted as an important marker for underlying tumour biology affecting survival.[36] Pathologic grade is determined microscopically by the number of cellular mitoses per high powered field (hpf) and through Ki-67 labelling of tumours. NETs with <2mitoses/10hpf and <3% Ki-67 index are classified as low grade (G1) well-differentiated tumours whereas NETs with >20/10hpf and >20% Ki-67 labelling are denoted as high grade (G3) and poorly differentiated. Recent studies have shown that G3 NETs exhibit a poor prognosis following

surgical management for hepatic metastases and are better treated non-operatively with chemotherapy.[36]

The metastatic pattern of spread in the liver for NETs also has prognostic implications and is categorized into three morphological subtypes:[35,36] (I) "restricted metastases" involving one lobe or two adjacent segments; (II) "dominant lesion with bilobar metastases" whereby a single major focus is accompanied by multiple contralateral satellite lesions; (III) diffuse, multifocal liver metastases affecting multiple segments within and between lobes. Patients with Type I or II (25% and 15% of cases respectively) disease, in the absence of metastases at distant extrahepatic sites are considered for curative surgical resection.[35,36]

The aim of liver resection with curative intent in NETs is to leave no residual disease (R0 resection) in both primary and secondary sites, and this may be associated with 5-year survival rates of up to 85%.[31,32] Surgical indications include the presence of a resectable well-differentiated NET without extra-abdominal metastases or peritoneal carcinomatosis, in a patient without right-sided cardiac dysfunction.[35] Optimal cytoreduction aims to reduce tumour volume by at least 90%.[32] Although there are no data from randomised trials, large series using historical controls or contemporary cases matched for stage have demonstrated that liver resection with optimal cytoreduction results in improved survival.[37-39]

> ✅ Hepatic resection for metastatic NETs results in improved overall survival compared to those receiving supportive care. Furthermore, R1 and R2 resections result in 5-year survival rates of 70% and 60%, respectively,[32] challenging the dogma that surgery should be reserved only for patients most likely to have an R0 resection. Cytoreduction similarly offers the most effective and durable palliation from symptoms.[38,40] As a result, surgical debulking has been advocated for both functional and non-functional tumours.[41] An aggressive approach, sometimes combining liver resection with other ablative strategies, is warranted (**Fig. 7.2a,b**).

Most series of hepatic resection for metastatic NETs include an occasional case with an unknown primary, despite thorough imaging and endoscopy. Although survival data are sparse, an aggressive resectional approach for these patients is reasonable (Fig. 7.2b).

Non-surgical treatment modalities include RFA, TAE and TACE. RFA in isolation can achieve symptomatic relief and local control of variable duration in up to 80% of NET patients with hepatic metastases. Although studies comparing RFA to other modalities are limited, RFA has been advocated in patients with bilobar disease with up to 14 hepatic lesions of less than 7cm in diameter, encompassing up to 20% of liver volume.[33,39] TAE

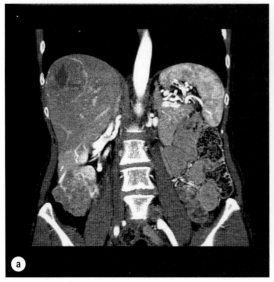
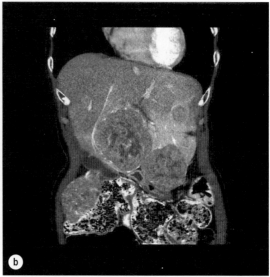

Figure 7.2 • **(a)** A 59-year-old female with an incidental finding of multiple NET metastases. There was no evidence of primary tumour on octreotide scan and endoscopy. Note multiple hypervascular, large metastases with central necrosis. **(b)** Same patient as in **(a)**. A debulking operation to remove 90% of tumour burden would be possible by performing an extended right hepatic lobectomy with wedge resections from segment 2.

and TACE appear to deliver comparable results and thus one modality is not favoured over the other. Embolisation is usually indicated for more extensive hepatic disease or for tumours in close proximity to biliary structures precluding RFA.[39] Duration of response is routinely short as the tumour rapidly develops collaterals and thus repeat treatments are often required.[41] Embolisation is contraindicated in patients with 50–75% liver involvement due to the risk of precipitating acute hepatic failure.

In general, aggressive multimodal therapy with embolic, ablative and systemic strategies is recommended to debulk or downstage metastatic NETs.[41] Despite complete resection, hepatic recurrence occurs in up to 84% of patients at 5 years post-surgery.[39] Recurrence is suspected by the elevation of tumour markers such as 5-hydroxyindoleacetic acid (5-HIAA) and chromogranin A. Chromogranin A is more sensitive than 5-HIAA in identifying disease progression and high levels have been shown to predict poorer outcomes. A reduction in chromogranin A levels of >80% predicts a good outcome following cytoreductive hepatectomy, even when complete resection has not been achieved.[42]

Liver transplantation has been advocated for patients with extensive, unresectable liver metastases with no extrahepatic disease. A recent retrospective study of 150 patients who underwent transplantation for metastatic NETs reported 5-year survival comparable to patients with hepatocellular carcinoma (HCC).[43] Of those transplanted, patients under the age of 55 without the need for concurrent major resection of the primary tumour had the best overall survival.[9]

Therefore, liver transplantation does appear to confer long-term survival in carefully selected patients and should be considered in the management of NETs.[44]

Gastrointestinal stromal tumours

Gastrointestinal stromal tumours (GISTs) are the most common gastrointestinal mesenchymal malignancies originating from the interstitial cells of Cajal. Approximately 70–80% of GISTs harbour a mutated c-Kit proto-oncogene, which results in the constitutive activation of the receptor tyrosine kinase and unregulated cell growth. Two thirds of c-Kit mutations are located on exon 11.[45] C-Kit exon 9 and PDGFRA mutations, encompassing a wild-type kinase domain that modulates receptor inhibitor sensitivity, account for another 5–10% of GISTs.[46]

Primary GISTs represent 1% of all gastrointestinal malignancies, and arise in the stomach (55%), small intestine (35%), colon/ rectum (10%) and oesophagus (5%), with the remainder found in various other sites (gallbladder, appendix or mesentery).[47] The primary tumour is usually classified into four prognostic categories, ranging from very low risk to high risk, according to site of the lesion, size of the lesion and the number of mitotic figures identified.[48] Surgery remains the gold standard for the treatment of primary GISTs.

Imatinib mesylate is a selective tyrosine kinase inhibitor that has revolutionised the treatment of unresectable GISTs.[44] Response to imatinib is greatest in tumours that harbour the c-Kit exon 11 mutation, with resistance rates higher in patients harbouring exon 9 or platelet-derived growth factor receptor α (PDGFRA) mutations.[44] Despite complete surgical resection with microscopic negative margins, recurrence (local or distant) occurs in 50% of patients.[48] The use of imatinib in the adjuvant setting was investigated in the phase III ACOSOG placebo controlled trial (Z9001) for patients with resected GISTs 3 cm or greater in size. A statistically significant 1-year recurrence-free survival (RFS) of 98% in the treatment group versus 83% in the placebo group was observed, prompting the inclusion of imatinib as an adjuvant treatment modality.[48] Currently, many nomograms have emerged to guide patient selection for those believed to be at highest risk of recurrence.

The treatment of metastatic GISTs has similarly been transformed by imatinib. Recurrence of GISTs most commonly occur with one of two metastatic patterns: local recurrence with peritoneal disease or intraparenchymal liver metastases.[49] Most patients with recurrent metastatic GISTs will receive imatinib as first-line treatment, with a clinical response demonstrated in 80%. This response is durable with a median survival of 48 months.[50] However, many patients develop imatinib resistance and disease progression caused by the development of secondary mutations.[51] Second- (e.g. sunitinib) and third-line agents (e.g. nilotinib and masitinib) have shown promise in patients resistant to imatinib.[52]

✅ The efficacy and low side-effect profile of imatinib prompted initial enthusiasm for the combined use of surgery and imatinib in the management of metastatic GISTs. Although evidence guiding surgical management in metastatic GISTs is limited, a recent study combining neoadjuvant imitanib with surgery and adjuvant imitanib in patients with previous R0 resection of the primary tumour has shown a favourable 3-year survival.[53] Nevertheless, future studies are warranted prior to recommending adjuvant imitanib in routine clinical practice for metastatic GISTs to the liver.

A subset of patients with GISTs develop a pattern of disease progression where isolated nodular foci progress within a pre-existing tumour mass in a patient already on imatinib. Such cases of partial progression have the same median survival as patients who meet standard criteria for disease progression.[54] There is currently no rationale for resection in this group. The benefit of surgical resection in the group of patients with disease that is stable or responding to imatinib is not clear.[55]

In general, GISTs metastatic to the liver are rarely amenable to resection. Therefore, imatinib is accepted as the first-line treatment for metastatic disease. Disease progression is managed by dose escalation followed by second-line agents such as sunitinib. In the event of tumour rupture or haemorrhage, surgery or hepatic artery embolisation may be performed in an emergency setting.

Breast cancer

The surgical management of breast cancer hepatic metastases is controversial. The widely held concept that liver metastases in breast cancer reflect diffuse systemic disease has led to a nihilistic view of the role of liver resection in this setting. However, an aggressive surgical approach has been adopted recently for patients presenting with the liver as the sole site of involvement. Unfortunately, the data are mostly retrospective and are based on heterogeneous indications, making it difficult to provide strong evidence-based guidelines.

Although breast cancer is common, isolated liver lesions in metastatic breast cancer are seen in only 7% of patients.[56] Sakamoto et al.[57] reported only 34 patients with resectable liver metastases among 11 000 breast cancer patients treated over an 18-year period. Selection criteria for such metastases are inconsistent in surgical series, with some centres considering resection only to disease confined to the liver while others advocate a more liberal approach. In short, there are no clear selection criteria for resection.

✅ Response to chemotherapy appears to be an important predictor of survival prior to liver resection for metastatic breast cancer. For those patients who progressed during prehepatectomy chemotherapy, 0% were alive at 5 years in comparison to 11% in responders. Therefore, surgery should only be considered in the setting of patients who have responded to preoperative chemotherapy or hormonal therapy, or both.[58]

Despite heterogeneous selection criteria, 5-year survival rates fall into two groups. Several reports describe 5-year overall survival of approximately 25%;[57,59] however, others report 5-year survival between 45% and 60%.[60,61] These disparate results cannot be explained by differences in study design or treatment factors. Outcomes following hepatic resection may therefore merely reflect differences in tumour biology, or publication bias. Furthermore, 5-year disease-free survival rates are much lower than overall survival rates, suggesting that liver resection may function as a cytoreductive rather than curative procedure in these highly selected patients.

Ovarian cancer

Epithelial ovarian cancer represents the most common malignancy of the ovary, of which surgery and platinum-based chemotherapy remain the mainstay of treatment. Unfortunately, most develop chemore-sistance after 24–36 months and median survival for advanced (stage III–IV) disease is 3.5 years.[62] Aggressive surgical debulking is advocated in advanced cases, with optimal cytoreduction targeted at <1 cm of residual disease.[63] Intraperitoneal (i.p.) chemotherapy has been demonstrated to further improve survival compared

---

✅ Although the liver is rarely the only site of metastatic disease in ovarian cancer, hepatectomy can be an important component of a primary cytoreduction strategy. Ovarian cancer can involve the liver through the development of peritoneal lesions on the surface of the liver (stage III – **Fig. 7.3**) or intraparenchymal metastases (stage IV – **Fig. 7.4**). Survival is improved for patients with stage IV disease who have undergone adequate debulking surgery including hepatectomy.[65,66]

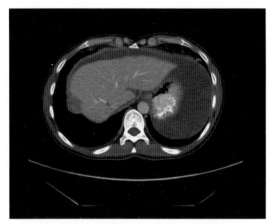

Figure 7.3 • Stage III ovarian cancer with hepatic involvement. Note direct invasion of liver capsule by peritoneal tumour plaque.

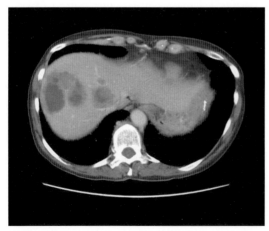

Figure 7.4 • Stage IV ovarian cancer with intraparenchymal liver metastases.

to intravenous therapy, and this is the current aim of treatment in many large centres. To be eligible for i.p. chemotherapy, patients must undergo maximal debulking.[64] Successful cytoreduction is thus a crucial step in the management of advanced ovarian cancer.

A recent phase II trial investigating combined i.p. carboplatin with i.v. paclitaxel in stage II–IV disease is under way, with preliminary results showing minimal toxicity and appropriate response in patients with suboptimal (>2 cm) surgical debulking.[67] Furthermore, various non-randomised observational studies have reported a benefit with varying degrees of cytoreductive surgery combined with hyperthermic intraperitoneal chemotherapy (HIPEC) in peritoneal carcinomatosis. The preliminary nature of these results precludes any definitive management recommendations.[25]

Survival following primary surgical debulking is inversely correlated with volume of residual disease, disease stage and tumour differentiation. Similarly, survival following hepatectomy for metastatic disease is dependent on optimal cytoreduction, negative margin status, greater pelvic than abdominal disease and a longer recurrence-free interval.[68] TACE offers a potential future therapeutic option in achieving local control in patients with unresectable hepatic disease.[69]

Renal cell carcinoma

Renal cell carcinoma (RCC), often termed the 'internist's tumour', represents the deadliest urological malignancy. Approximately 20–30% of patients with RCC present with synchronous metastatic disease and another 20–40% of patients with previous nephrectomy will develop more advanced disease.[70] Fewer than 5% of patients have metastases restricted to the liver.[71] Whereas interleukin-2 and interferon-α were previously used as first-line therapy for metastatic RCC, current regimens employ sunitinib, which has displayed a higher progression-free survival in phase III trials.[72]

The available data on hepatic resection for RCC metastases are limited to retrospective reports. A recent study from the Netherlands examined 33 patients who underwent resection or ablative therapy for RCC hepatic metastases. The study documented no operative mortality with 5-year disease-free and overall survival of 11% and 43%, respectively. The median overall survival was 33 months. Metachronous metastases and complete resection were highlighted as prognostic factors.[70]

Staehler et al. reported a 12-year retrospective comparative analysis of patients with metastatic RCC to the liver. In the study, 68 patients underwent surgery and were compared to a cohort of 20 patients who were eligible but refused an operation. Disease in these patients was mostly confined to the liver.

Overall 5-year survival in the treatment arm was 62% in comparison to 29% in the control group. Prognostic features included complete resection of liver lesions, negative margins, length of disease-free interval from resection of the primary and a left-sided primary lesion.[73] With ongoing improvements in surgical techniques coupled with an increasingly aggressive approach to metastatic disease in the liver, future prospective studies examining the role of hepatectomy in RCC should provide clearer treatment algorithms. Furthermore, an evidence-based approach to surgery combined with sunitinib or surafenib will hopefully be forthcoming.

Melanoma

The prognosis for patients with metastatic melanoma is poor and the median survival for patients with American Joint Committee on Cancer (AJCC) stage IV melanoma is 6–9 months.[74] Gastrointestinal and liver metastases occur in 2–4% of individuals with stage IV disease,[75] and palliative radiotherapy and systemic chemotherapy have largely been ineffective in conferring a survival advantage. Although biological agents such as interferon-α and interleukin-2 have yielded promising response rates, these are rarely durable and are associated with significant toxicity.[74] Favourable results in patients undergoing metastasectomy in the lung, soft tissues or abdomen have provided some enthusiasm for surgery in a selected patient population.

The available evidence for hepatectomy for metastatic melanoma is limited and consists largely of subset analyses from larger series of patients with non-colorectal liver metastases. A recent retrospective study evaluated all patients who presented with metastatic melanoma over the last decade at a single Australian institution. In this series, 13 of 23 patients underwent resection for liver metastases. Disease-free interval from resection of the primary was a median of 49 months. Overall 3-year survival was 40% with a median survival of 21 months, influenced largely by the number of metastases and the presence of multiple sites involved. The median disease-free interval observed prior to recurrence was 14 months.[75] Nevertheless, the authors have outlined the potential bias in their study, including only those patients who were most likely to achieve complete surgical resection in the operative cohort.

Recently, liver resection with postoperative tumour infiltrating lymphocyte (TIL) therapy has been explored. TIL involves the resection of metastatic lesions followed by extraction and culture of infiltrating lymphocytes ex vivo with interleukin-2. A direct comparison was performed between patients with complete surgical resection versus those with residual hepatic disease receiving postoperative TIL. The observed 3-year overall survival was 53% in the TIL cohort, with prognosis largely favoured by lack of extrahepatic disease and a single hepatic metastasis.[76]

The biological behaviour of metastatic melanoma depends in part on the site of origin of the primary tumour.[77] Cutaneous melanoma is more common than ocular melanoma.[78] While both metastasise to the liver, they appear to do so with distinct patterns and natural history. Ocular melanoma metastasises to the liver more frequently, but is more likely to be associated with isolated liver metastases than cutaneous melanoma.[77,78] Survival following hepatectomy appears to be more favourable in the highly selected but rare group of patients with melanoma of ocular origin. Pawlik et al. reported 5-year survival of 21% for liver resection for ocular primaries, with no 5-year survivors when the initial site of disease was cutaneous. However, 75% of resected patients in this study developed recurrent disease, and the rate of recurrence was similar between the ocular and cutaneous groups.[78]

✔ It is impossible from the available studies to estimate the impact that liver resection has on the survival of patients with metastatic melanoma. It seems reasonable to adopt a resectional approach in highly selected patients, i.e. patients with a long disease-free interval from primary to metastases, and patients that can be rendered disease free following surgery. This will occasionally lead to long-term survival, but patients with metastatic melanoma generally have a poor prognosis. Newer immune-based therapy combined with surgery may provide an added benefit in metastatic melanoma to the liver.

Non-colorectal gastrointestinal adenocarcinoma

Liver metastases from non-colorectal gastrointestinal (GI) adenocarcinomas can arise from the oesophagus, stomach, pancreas, gallbladder, ampulla of Vater, small bowel and distal bile duct. Hepatic resection is controversial for these tumours and the available literature is scant.

Metastatic oesophageal cancer is usually widely disseminated and is associated with a 5-year survival of 3–5% when multiple sites of disease are present and 7–8% when disease is limited to the liver.[79] Two case reports in the English-language literature describe hepatectomy for isolated, synchronous liver metastases.[80,81] In both cases hepatectomy was performed simultaneously with oesophagectomy and was followed by hepatic arterial chemotherapy. Both patients developed multiple liver metastases at 6[80] and 7[81] months postoperatively.

These recurrences responded partially to systemic chemotherapy, and patients were alive with disease at 14[80] and 18[81] months following hepatectomy. Thus, although rarely feasible, hepatectomy followed by hepatic arterial chemotherapy may provide a limited survival benefit in chemosensitive oesophageal cancer with isolated liver metastases.

Gastric adenocarcinoma is the second most common cause of cancer-related death worldwide, and the liver is a major site of spread in 9% of cases, generally in a bilobar distribution.[82] Overall 5-year survival in patients with liver metastases ranges from 0% to 10% and the role of surgery is unclear in this setting. A recent study of patients with isolated synchronous or metachronous liver metastases reported that surgery was performed if the tumour burden was deemed completely resectable, while lesions <5 cm were considered for RFA. Overall 5-year, survival in this cohort was 27% with a median survival of 48 months. In a comparison of patients who were not offered the above treatment modalities, no patients survived to 5 years, with a median survival of 9 months.[82] These results appear comparable to previously published studies.[83] Data regarding independent predictors of survival are limited and appear to correlate with absence of serosal invasion of the primary tumour and the presence of a solitary liver metastasis.

Primary small-bowel malignancies represent an exceedingly rare but histologically diverse subgroup accounting for 2% of all GI malignancies.[84] Small-bowel adenocarcinoma (SBA) represents the majority of these tumours and is seen in up to 5% of patients with familial adenomatous polyposis (FAP). By virtue of its non-specific clinical presentation and the limitations of radiological and endoscopic diagnostic modalities to examine the small bowel, approximately 80% of patients present with advanced disease. In addition, the low prevalence of SBAs limits our understanding of the natural history of tumour spread, restricting the development of clear treatment guidelines. A French multicentre retrospective study examining the efficacy of chemotherapy in 93 patients with advanced SBA compared various chemotherapeutic regimens for progression-free survival (PFS) and overall survival (OS). Median PFS and OS were 6.6 and 15.1 months, respectively, with best outcomes seen with FOLFOX therapy.[85] Negative prognostic factors include a poor baseline WHO performance status, elevated carbohydrate antigen (CA) 19-9/carcinoembryonic antigen (CEA) levels and the presence of a duodenal primary. The ability of surgery to prolong PFS in hepatic SBA metastases has only been described in a single case report of an FAP patient with a PFS of 3 years following neoadjuvant chemotherapy and surgery.[84] As such, future studies examining liver resections in metastatic SBA will provide further guidance as to its role in this disease.

Pancreatic ductal adenocarcinoma (PDAC) accounts for 90% of all histological subtypes of pancreatic cancer and confers the worst overall prognosis.[86] Over the last 50 years, PDAC has continued to rank as the tenth most common cancer in the western world and the fourth leading cause of cancer death. PDAC presents in a non-specific manner, often when disease is already at an advanced stage. Improvements in chemotherapy, surgical technique and knowledge of tumour biology have translated into marginal improvements in survival. Currently, only 15–20% of patients present with disease amenable to curative resection, of which 20% are alive at 5 years.[86] The overall average 5-year survival for unresectable PDAC is 5%, with a median survival of 6–9 months. Due to the dismal prognosis in patients with localised resectable disease, surgery in metastatic PDAC has been contraindicated. Yamada et al. examined the role of partial hepatectomy in non-neuroendocrine pancreatic cancer, including five patients with PDAC, one with adenosquamous carcinoma and one with cystadenocarcinoma.[87] Patients were chosen for surgery if complete excision of intrahepatic disease was deemed feasible, reliable control of the primary disease was possible and the liver was the only site of spread. Overall 5-year survival in this cohort was 16.7%; however, five patients experienced a recurrence and subsequently died of their disease within 4–52 months. Prognostic factors appear to correlate with disease-free interval from primary to metastasis and the presence of negative surgical margins at metastasectomy. Although the authors highlight the potential role of liver resection in metastatic PDAC, they acknowledge the need for future studies to clarify the true benefit of this approach.

✓ The available evidence for hepatectomy in the management of metastases from non-colorectal, non-neuroendocrine (NCRNNET) GI primaries is limited, and few meaningful statements can be made as to the utility of this treatment strategy. With improvements in safety of liver resections coupled with encouraging results from other malignancies metastasising to the liver, future prospective studies will shed light on the role of hepatic metastasecotomy in NCRNNETs.

Testicular cancer

Metastasectomy is well established in the management of disseminated non-seminomatous germ cell testicular carcinoma that does not completely respond to chemotherapy. Although it can be difficult to differentiate active residual tumour from post-treatment fibrosis or necrosis, the probability of achieving cure by surgical resection is high.

Residual teratoma has the potential for sarcomatous transformation and thus lymphadenectomy and visceral resection are performed whenever there is radiographic evidence of residual disease. The overall 10-year survival is 62% from diagnosis of hepatic metastasis.[88]

A single institution experience of 57 liver resections performed over the last two decades has demonstrated that surgery for hepatic metastases is safe and efficacious, depending on the histopathological characteristics of the resected specimen. Based on the presence and type of tumour in the liver, 40–70% of patients remain disease free at 20 months.[89] Negative prognostic indicators included viable tumour in the resected specimen, metastases greater than 3 cm in diameter and pure embryonal carcinoma in the primary lesion.

Urothelial cancer

Data for metastasectomy in the management of disseminated urothelial cancer are sparse, and no studies specifically address the role of hepatectomy. Of those patients treated for primary urothelial cancer 30% will recur, of which 75% will be with distant spread. Five-year survival of 28% has been reported following resection of lung, brain, adrenal, small-bowel or lymph node metastases with variation in the use of adjuvant chemotherapy.[90] Metastasectomy has also been employed for palliation.

Lung cancer

The management of metastatic lung cancer is largely restricted to radiation and chemotherapy. Although the surgical management of hepatic metastasis remains controversial, most cases have been reviewed within the broader context of NCRNNET. Hepatic metastases appear most commonly in right-sided non-small-cell lung tumours with concomitant bone metastases. A small case series of highly selected patients with one to two liver lesions has shown that surgery may confer a marginal survival benefit.[91] Nevertheless, the role of surgery as well as other treatment modalities (RFA, TAE/TACE) cannot be definitively made with current evidence.

Adrenocortical tumours

Adrenocortical tumours with liver metastases are rare, and literature on the management of this disease scenario is mostly anecdotal. Case reports have provided no clear guidance regarding the role of surgical or ablative strategies. It is possible that patients who develop metachronous liver metastases with a disease-free interval >1 year from primary to metastasis may derive benefit from surgery.[92]

Endometrial cancer

Metastatic endometrial cancer is usually multifocal and rarely managed operatively. A recent single-centre report described the results in five patients who developed metastatic disease to the liver ranging from 11 months to 10 years after primary resection. All patients underwent hepatic surgery, with disease-free survival between 8 and 66 months. Based on these results, the authors advocate referral to a hepatobiliary specialist with the intent of pursuing surgery.[93] Other isolated reports of long-term survivors exist within the context of larger studies focused on NCRNNET hepatic metastasis.

Conclusion

The recent success of an aggressive surgical approach in the management of CRC liver metastases has, in part, provided the impetus for liver resection in non-colorectal cancer hepatic metastatic disease. Extrapolating surgical strategies from one malignancy to another is reasonable in some cases; however, fundamental biological differences between various neoplasms require thoughtful consideration of differences in the natural history and non-surgical treatment modalities that are available for each tumour site. Unfortunately, strong evidence-based data are lacking and it is therefore necessary for the treating surgeon to have a good working knowledge of the biology and management of various malignancies. In many cases, this is augmented by the availability of multidisciplinary tumour boards and a critical mass of subspecialists to assist in decision-making.

It is worth emphasising that in most cases liver resection should be performed with curative intent. Exceptions include liver metastases from NETs, epithelial ovarian cancer and testicular malignancies, where 'debulking' is considered useful as a palliative manoeuvre to improve overall survival. The case for resection of breast cancer metastases is evolving, with some liver surgeons advocating resection in a selected patient population responsive to preoperative chemotherapy. There is no strong evidence that non-curative intent surgery is helpful for patients with liver metastases from gastrointestinal tract primaries, lung and other cancers.

The presence of extrahepatic disease is almost always a contraindication to liver resection, except within the context of a prospective trial or for specific malignancies such as ovarian cancer. The critical variables that usually predict cure after liver resection of secondary cancer of almost all types include prolonged disease-free interval from resection of the primary tumour, negative resection margins and performance status.

Future efforts should be directed toward the conduct of randomised trials designed to test the role of liver surgery for the common non-colorectal malignancies, and the discovery of genetic and proteomic signatures as better prognostic and predictive markers.

Key points

- The majority of patients with non-colorectal liver metastases have disseminated disease and are not candidates for hepatectomy.
- Treatment decisions must take into account clinical surrogates of tumour biology. Patients with synchronous liver metastases, a short disease-free interval and extrahepatic disease are believed to have more aggressive tumours and are less likely to gain significant survival benefit from liver resection.
- With few exceptions, liver resection for metastatic disease should be performed with curative intent. The ability to achieve negative resection margins is a significant prognostic factor.
- Debulking surgery including liver resection has been shown to significantly improve survival in metastatic neuroendocrine tumours. Aggressive cytoreduction, often using a multimodality approach, is indicated in most cases of metastatic NETs.
- Cytoreduction including hepatectomy, followed by intraperitoneal chemotherapy, appears to improve survival in stage III/IV ovarian adenocarconima. New studies are now focusing on combination adjuvant i.v./i.p. chemotherapy as well as combination surgery and HIPEC.
- Patients with breast cancer liver metastases that respond to preoperative chemotherapy appear to gain a survival benefit from hepatectomy.
- Level I and II evidence regarding hepatectomy for the treatment of non-colorectal liver metastases is lacking, and the indications for surgery are evolving.

References

1. Nguyen KT, Laurent A, Dagher, et al. Minimally invasive liver resection for metastatic colorectal cancer: a multi-institutional, international report of safety, feasibility and early outcomes. Ann Surg 2009;250:842–8.

2. Nanji S, Cleary SP, Ryan P, et al. Up front hepatic resection for metastatic colorectal cancer results in favorable long-term survival. Ann Surg Oncol 2013; 20(1): 295–304.

3. Abad A, Massuti B, Anton A, et al. Colorectal cancer metastasis resectability after treatment with the combination of oxaliplatin, irinotecan and 5-fluorouracil. Final results of a phase II study. Acta Oncol 2007;22:1–7.

4. Glazer ES, Tseng JF, Al-Refaie W, et al. Long-term survival after surgical management of neuroendocrine hepatic metastases. HPB (Oxford) 2010;12: 427–33.

5. Adam R, Chiche L, Aloia T, et al. Hepatic resection for noncolorectal nonendocrine liver metastases: analysis of 1,452 patients and development of a prognostic model. Ann Surg 2006;244:524–35.

6. O'Rourke TR, Tekkis P, Yeung S, et al. Long-term results of liver resection for non-colorectal, non-neuroendocrine metastases. Ann Surg Oncol 2008;15:207–18.

7. Lendoire J, Moro M, Andriani O, et al. Liver resection for non-colorectal, non-neuroendocrine metastases: analysis of a multicenter study from Argentina. HPB (Oxford) 2007;9:435–9.

8. Weitz J, Blumgart LH, Fong Y, et al. Partial hepatectomy for metastases from noncolorectal, non-neuroendocrine carcinoma. Ann Surg 2005;241: 269–76.

9. Lewis MA, Hubbard J. Multimodal liver-directed management of neuroendocrine hepatic metastases: review article. Int J Hepatol 2011;2011:452343.

10. Ribatti D, Mangialardi G, Vacca A. Stephen Paget and the 'seed and soil' theory of metastatic dissemination. Clin Exp Med 2006;6:145–9.

11. Fidler IJ. The pathogenesis of cancer metastasis: the 'seed and soil' hypothesis revisited. Nat Rev Cancer 2003;3:453–8.

12. van't Veer LJ, Dai H, van de Vijver MJ, et al. Gene expression profiling predicts clinical outcome of breast cancer. Nature 2002;415(31):530–6.

13. Spentzos D, Levine DA, Ramoni MF, et al. Gene expression signature with independent prognostic significance in epithelial ovarian cancer. J Clin Oncol 2004;22(1):4700–10.

14. Winnepenninckx V, Lazar V, Michiels S, et al. Gene expression profiling of primary cutaneous melanoma and clinical outcome. J Natl Cancer Inst 2006;98(5):472–82.

15. Gryfe R, Kim H, Hsieh ET, et al. Tumor microsatellite instability and clinical outcome in young patients with colorectal cancer. N Engl J Med 2000;342(13):69–77.

16. Kaplan RN, Rafii S, Lyden D. Preparing the "soil": the premetastatic niche. Cancer Res 2006;66(1):11089–93.

17. Kaplan RN, Riba RD, Zacharoulis S, et al. VEGFR 1-positive haematopoietic bone marrow progenitors initiate the pre-metastatic niche. Nature 2005;438(8):820–7.

18. Wojtowicz-Praga S. Reversal of tumor-induced immunosuppression by TGF-beta inhibitors. Invest New Drugs 2003;21(1):21–32.

19. Morton DL, Holmes EC, Golub SH. Immunologic aspects of lung cancer. Chest 1977;71:640–3.

20. Tabernero J, Van Cutsem E, Diaz-Rubio E, et al. Phase II trial of cetuximab in combination with fluorouracil, leucovorin, and oxaliplatin in the first-line treatment of metastatic colorectal cancer. J Clin Oncol 2007;25(20):5225–32.

21. Znajda TL, Hayashi S, Horton PJ, et al. Postchemotherapy characteristics of hepatic colorectal metastases: remnants of uncertain malignant potential. J Gastrointest Surg 2006;10:483–9.

22. Yachida S, Jones S, Bozic I, et al. Distant metastasis occurs late during the genetic evolution of pancreatic cancer. Nature 2010;467(7319):1114–7.

23. Campbell PJ, Yachida S, Mudie LJ, et al. The patterns and dynamics of genomic instability in metastatic pancreatic cancer. Nature 2010;467 (7319):1109–13.

24. Gabriel M, Oberauer A, Dobrozemsky G, et al. [68]Ga DOTA-Tyr3-octreotide PET for assessing response to somatostatin-receptor-mediated radionuclide therapy. J Nucl Med 2009;50(9):1427–34.

25. Sommariva A, Pilati P, Rossi CR. Cytoreductive surgery combined with hyperthermic intra-peritoneal chemotherapy for peritoneal surface malignancies: current treatment and results. Cancer Treat Rev 2012;38(4):258–68.

26. D'Angelica M, Jarnagin W, Dematteo R, et al. Staging laparoscopy for potentially resectable noncolorectal, nonneuroendocrine liver metastases. Ann Surg Oncol 2002;9:204–9.

27. Sofocleous CT, Nascimento RG, Gonen M, et al. Radiofrequency ablation in the management of liver metastases from breast cancer. Am J Roentgenol 2007;189:883–9.

28. Gervais DA, Arellano RS, Mueller PR. Percutaneous radiofrequency ablation of ovarian cancer metastasis to the liver: indications, outcomes, and role in patient management. Am J Roentgenol 2006;187:746–50.

29. Gillams A, Cassoni A, Conway G, et al. Radiofrequency ablation of neuroendocrine liver metastases: the Middlesex experience. Abdom Imaging 2005;30:435–41.

30. Ribero D, Curley SA, Imamura H, et al. Selection for resection of hepatocellular carcinoma and surgical strategy: indications for resection, evaluation of liver function, portal vein embolization, and resection. Ann Surg Oncol 2008;15:986–92.

31. Yao KA, Talamonti MS, Nemcek A, et al. Indications and results of liver resection and hepatic chemoembolization for metastatic gastrointestinal neuroendocrine tumors. Surgery 2001;130:677–85.

32. Harring TR, Nguyen NTN, Goss JA, et al. Treatment of liver metastases in patients with neuroendocrine tumors: a comprehensive review. Int J Hepatol 2011;2011:154541.

33. Strosberg JR, Cheema A, Kvols LK. A review of systemic and liver directed therapies for metastatic neuroendocrine tumors of the gastroenteropancreatic tract. Cancer Control 2011;18(2):127–37.

34. Faiss S, Pape UF, Bohmig M, et al. Prospective, randomized, multicenter trial on the antiproliferative effect of lanreotide, interferon alfa, and their combination for therapy of metastatic neuroendocrine gastroenteropancreatic tumors – the International Lanreotide and Interferon Alfa Study Group. J Clin Oncol 2003;21(15):2689–96.
Symptomatic relief but limited response to treatment.

35. Steinmuller T, Kianmanesh R, Falconi M, et al. Conscensus guidelines for the management of patients with liver metastases from the digestive (neuro)endocrine tumors: foregut, midgut, hindgut and unknown primary. Neuroendocrinology 2008;87:47–62.

36. Jagannath P, Chhabra D, Shrikhande S, et al. Surgical treatment of liver metastases in Neuroendocrine neoplasms. Int J Hepatol 2012;2012:782672.

37. Touzios JG, Kiely JM, Pitt SC, et al. Neuroendocrine hepatic metastases: does aggressive management improve survival? Ann Surg 2005;241(5):776–85.

38. Chamberlain RS, Canes D, Brown KT, et al. Hepatic neuroendocrine metastases: does intervention alter outcomes? J Am Coll Surg 2000;190:432–45.

39. Karabulut K, Akyildiz Y, Lance C, et al. Multimodality treatment of neuroendocrine liver metastases. J Surg 2011;150(2):316–25.

40. Osborne DA, Zervos EE, Strosberg J, et al. Improved outcome with cytoreduction versus embolization for symptomatic hepatic metastases of carcinoid and neuroendocrine tumors. Ann Surg Oncol 2006;13:572–581.

41. Hodul P, Malafa M, Choi J, et al. The role of cytoreductive hepatic surgery as an adjunct to the management of metastatic neuroendocrine carcinomas. Cancer Control 2006;13:61–71.

42. Jensen EH, Kvols L, McLoughlin JM, et al. Biomarkers predict outcomes following cytoreductive surgery for hepatic metastases from functional carcinoid tumors. Ann Surg Oncol 2007;14:780–5.

43. Gedaly R, Daily MF, Davenport D, et al. Liver transplantation for the treatment of liver metastases from neuroendocrine tumors: an analysis of the UNOS database. Arch Surg 2011;146(8):953–8.

44. van Vilsteren FG, Baskin-Bey ES, Nagorney DM, et al. Liver transplantation for gastroenteropancreatic neuroendocrine cancers: defining selection criteria to improve survival. Liver Transpl 2006;12:448–56.

45. Florman S, Toure B, Kim L, et al. Liver transplantation for neuroendocrine tumors. J Gastrointest Surg 2004;8:208–12.

46. Corless CL, Barnett CM, Heinrich MC. Gastrointestinal stromal tumors: origin and molecular oncology. Nat Rev Cancer 2011;11(12):865–78.

47. Stamatakos M, Douzinas E, Stefanaki C, et al. Review: gastrointestinal stromal tumors. World J Surg Oncol 2009;7:61.

48. Pisters PWT, Colombo C. Adjuvant imatinib therapy for gastrointestinal stromal tumors. J Surg Oncol 2011;104:896–900.

49. DeMatteo RP, Lewis JJ, Leung D, et al. Two hundred gastrointestinal stromal tumors: recurrence patterns and prognostic factors for survival. Ann Surg 2000;231:51–8.

50. Zhu J, Yang Y, Zhou L, et al. A long-term follow-up of the imatinib mesylate treatment for the patients with recurrent gastrointestinal stromal tumor (GIST): the liver metastasis and the outcome. BMC Cancer 2010;10:199.

51. Gorre ME, Mohammed M, Ellwood K, et al. Clinical resistance to STI-571 cancer therapy caused by BCR-ABL gene mutation or amplification. Science (New York) 2001;293:876–80.

52. Kim EJ, Zalupski MM. Systemic therapy for advanced gastrointestinal stromal tumors: beyond imatinib. J Surg Oncol 2011;104:901–6.

53. Xia L, Zhang MM, Ji L, et al. Resection combined with imatinib therapy for liver metastases of gastrointestinal stromal tumors. Surg Today 2010;40:936–42.

54. Desai J, Shankar S, Heinrich MC, et al. Clonal evolution of resistance to imatinib in patients with metastatic gastrointestinal stromal tumors. Clin Cancer Res 2007;13(15):5398–405.

55. Gronchi A, Fiore M, Miselli F, et al. Surgery of residual disease following molecular-targeted therapy with imatinib mesylate in advanced/metastatic GIST. Ann Surg 2007;245:341–6.

56. Rubino A, Doci R, Foteuh JC, et al. Hepatic metastases from breast cancer. Updates Surg 2010;62:143–8.

57. Sakamoto Y, Yamamoto J, Yoshimoto M, et al. Hepatic resection for metastatic breast cancer: prognostic analysis of 34 patients. World J Surg 2005;29:524–7.

58. Lermit E, Marzano E, Chereau E, et al. Surgical resection of liver metastases from breast cancer. J Surg Oncol 2010;19:79–84.

59. Selzner M, Morse MA, Vredenburgh JJ, et al. Liver metastases from breast cancer: long-term survival after curative resection. Surgery 2000;127:383–9.

60. Vlastos G, Smith DL, Singletary SE, et al. Long-term survival after an aggressive surgical approach in patients with breast cancer hepatic metastases. Ann Surg Oncol 2004;11:869–74.

61. Carlini M, Lonardo MT, Carboni F, et al. Liver metastases from breast cancer. Results of surgical resection. Hepatogastroenterology 2002;49:1597–601.

62. Chi DS, McCaughty K, Diaz JP, et al. Guidelines and selection criteria for secondary cytoreductive surgery in patients with recurrent, platinum-sensitive epithelial ovarian carcinoma. Cancer 2006;106(1):1933–9.

63. Ellatar A, Bryant A, Winter-Roach BA, et al. Optimal primary surgical treatment for advanced epithelial ovarian cancer. Cochrane Database Syst Rev 2011;(8):CD007565.

64. Armstrong DK, Bundy B, Wenzel L, et al. Intraperitoneal cisplatin and paclitaxel in ovarian cancer. N Engl J Med 2006;354(5):34–43.

65. Bristow RE, Montz FJ, Lagasse LD, et al. Survival impact of surgical cytoreduction in stage IV epithelial ovarian cancer. Gynecol Oncol 1999;72:278–87.

66. Naik R, Nordin A, Cross PA, et al. Optimal cytoreductive surgery is an independent prognostic indicator in stage IV epithelial ovarian cancer with hepatic metastases. Gynecol Oncol 2000;78:171–5.

67. Fujiwara K, Nagao S, Kigawa J, et al. Phase II study of intraperitoneal carboplatin with intravenous paclitaxel in patients with suboptimal residual epithelial ovarian or primary peritoneal cancer: a Sankai gynecology cancer study group study. Int J Gynecol Cancer 2009;19:834–7.

68. Roh HJ, Kim DY, Joo WD, et al. Hepatic resection as part of secondary cytoreductive surgery for recurrent ovarian cancer involving the liver. Arch Gynecol Obstet 2011;284:1223–9.

69. Vogl TJ, Naguib NN, Lehnert T, et al. Initial experience with repetitive transarterial chemoembolization (TACE) as a third line treatment of ovarian cancer metastasis to the liver: Indications, outcomes and role in patient's management. Gynecol Oncol 2012;124(2):225–9.

70. Ruys AT, Tanis PJ, Iris ND, et al. Surgical treatment of renal cell carcinoma liver metastases: a population based study. Ann Surg Oncol 2011;18:1932–8.

71. Dekernion JB, Ramming KP, Smith RB. The natural history of metastatic renal cell carcinoma: a computer analysis. J Urol 1978;120:148–52.

72. Motzer RJ, Hutson TE, Tomczak P, et al. Sunitinib versus interferon alfa in metastatic renal cell carcinoma. N Engl J Med 2007;356:115–24.

73. Staehler MD, Kruse J, Haseke N, et al. Liver resection for metastatic disease prolongs survival in renal cell carcinoma: a 12-year result from a retrospective comparative analysis. World J Urol 2010;28:543–7.

74. McGettigan S. A review of treatments for patients with metastatic melanoma. Continuing Education Modules: The Abramson Cancer Center of the University of Pennsylvania 2009, http://www.oncolink.org/resources/article.cfm?c=16&s=59&ss=224&id=972 [accessed 04.10.12].

75. Chua TC, Saxena A, Morris DL. Surgical metastasectomy in AJCC stage IV M1c melanoma patients with gastrointestinal and liver metastases. Ann Acad Med Singapore 2010;39:634–9.

76. Ripley RT, Davis JL, Klapper JA, et al. Liver resection for metastatic melanoma with postoperative tumor-infiltrating lymphocyte therapy. Ann Surg Oncol 2010;17:163–70.

77. Albert DM, Ryan LM, Borden EC. Metastatic ocular and cutaneous melanoma: a comparison of patient characteristics and prognosis. Arch Ophthalmol 1996;114:107–8.

78. Pawlik TM, Zorzi D, Abdalla EK, et al. Hepatic resection for metastatic melanoma: distinct patterns of recurrence and prognosis for ocular versus cutaneous disease. Ann Surg Oncol 2006;13:712–20.

79. Daly JM, Karnell LH, Menck HR. National Cancer Data Base report on esophageal carcinoma. Cancer 1996;78(15):1820–8.

80. Yamamoto T, Tachibana M, Kinugasa S, et al. Esophagectomy and hepatic arterial chemotherapy following hepatic resection for esophageal cancer with liver metastasis. J Gastroenterol 2001;36:560–3.

81. Hanazaki K, Kuroda T, Wakabayashi M, et al. Hepatic metastasis from esophageal cancer treated by surgical resection and hepatic arterial infusion chemotherapy. Hepatogastroenterology 1998;45:201–5.

82. Dittmar Y, Altendorf-Hofmann A, Rauchfuss F, et al. Resection of liver metastases is beneficial in patients with gastric cancer: a report on 15 cases and review of the literature. Gastric Cancer 2012;15(2):131–6.

83. Koga R, Yamamoto J, Ohyama S, et al. Liver resection for metastatic gastric cancer: experience with 42 patients including eight long term survivors. Jpn J Clin Oncol 2007;37:836–42.

84. Eigenbrod T, Kullman F, Klebl F. Resection of small bowel adenocarcinoma liver metastasis combined with neoadjuvant and adjuvant chemotherapy results in extended disease free period – a case report. Int J Gastrointest Cancer 2006;37:94–7.

85. Zaanan A, Costes L, Gauthier M, et al. Chemotherapy of advanced small-bowel adenocarcinoma: a multicenter AGEO Study. Ann Oncol 2010;21(9):1786–93.

86. Samuel N, Hudson TJ. The molecular and cellular heterogeneity of pancreatic ductal adenocarcinoma. Nat Rev Gastroenterol Hepatol 2011;9(2):77–87.

87. Yamada H, Hirano S, Tanaka E, et al. Surgical treatment of liver metastases from pancreatic cancer. HPB (Oxford) 2006;8:85–8.

88. You YN, Leibovitch BC. Hepatic metastasectomy for testicular germ cell tumors: is it worth it? J Gastrointest Surg 2009;13:595–601.

89. Mallucio M, Einhorn LH, Goulet RJ. Surgical therapy for testicular cancer metastatic to the liver. HPB (Oxford) 2007;9:199–200.

90. Lehmann J, Suttmann H, Albers P, et al. Surgery for metastatic urothelial cancer with curative intent: the German experience. Eur Urol 2009;55(6):1293–9.

91. Ercolani G, Ravaioli M, Grazi GL, et al. The role of liver resections for metastases from lung carcinoma. HPB (Oxford) 2006;8:114–5.

92. Di Carlo I, Toro A, Sparatore F, et al. Liver resection for hepatic metastases from adrenocortical carcinoma. HPB (Oxford) 2006;8:106–9.

93. Knowles B, Bellamy COC, Oniscu A, Wigmore, SJ. Hepatic resection for metastatic endometrioid carcinoma. HPB (Oxford) 2010;12:412–7.

8

Portal hypertension

Geoffrey H. Haydon
John Isaac
John A.C. Buckels
Simon P. Olliff

Introduction

The management of portal hypertension has evolved from a surgical discipline into one with the majority of patients successfully treated by medical and radiological therapies. Surgery still has a distinct role for a limited number of patients, chiefly those with extrahepatic portal hypertension and those suitable for liver transplantation (which can cure both the complications and the underlying liver disease). As patients with gastrointestinal (GI) bleeding will often be referred for a surgical opinion, it is important that the surgeon has a good understanding of the pathophysiology of variceal bleeding as well as the treatment options.

Portal hypertension itself does not require treatment, but intervention is indicated when the risk of bleeding from varices is present or when complications such as actual variceal haemorrhage or the formation of ascites occur. The management of many patients commences with a herald variceal bleed, which requires effective therapy before a plan can be made for longer-term treatment. A significant choice of options is now available, many of which are evidence based. These include: pharmacotherapy to both prevent and treat variceal bleeding; endoscopic options of injection therapy or variceal ligation; radiologically placed transjugular intrahepatic portosystemic shunts (TIPS); and surgical options (surgical shunts and liver replacement). The selection of these options needs to be tailored

to the individual patient, taking into account their general fitness, including severity of any underlying liver disease and the local medical facilities and expertise available.

This chapter will briefly outline the causes, pathophysiology and natural history of portal hypertension, but will concentrate on the evaluation and management of both asymptomatic patients and patients who present with an acute bleed, together with longer-term strategies. In addition, specific recommendations will be made for the management of ascites and for patients with hepatic venous outflow obstruction due to Budd–Chiari syndrome.

Aetiology and pathophysiology of portal hypertension

Traditionally, portal hypertension has been classified as prehepatic, intrahepatic or posthepatic, with the intrahepatic causes subdivided into presinusoidal, sinusoidal and postsinusoidal (Table 8.1). Prehepatic causes are usually due to portal vein thrombosis, which is discussed later in this chapter. The main cause of portal hypertension in the West is cirrhosis. This is a sinusoidal obstruction to portal flow with varying causes. Viral hepatitis and alcoholic liver disease are the most common causes, but others include primary biliary cirrhosis, primary sclerosing

Table 8.1 • Causes of portal hypertension

Presinusoidal	Sinusoidal	Postsinusoidal
Extrahepatic	Cirrhotic	Budd–Chiari syndrome
Portal vein thrombosis	Postviral (B, C)	Veno-occlusive disease
Splenic vein thrombosis	Alcoholic	Caval web
Increased splenic flow (tropical splenomegaly, myelofibrosis)	Cryptogenic Primary biliary cirrhosis	Constrictive pericarditis
	Primary sclerosing cholangitis	
Intrahepatic	Chronic active hepatitis	
Schistosomiasis	Haemochromotosis	
Congenital hepatic fibrosis	Wilson's disease	
Sarcoidosis	Non-cirrhotic	
	Acute alcoholic hepatitis	
	Cytotoxic drugs	

cholangitis and haemochromatosis. Presinusoidal obstruction due to hepatic fibrosis occurs in schistosomiasis. Worldwide, this is one of the commonest causes of portal hypertension and, as it is usually associated with normal liver function, has a better prognosis. The main causes of postsinusoidal portal hypertension are hepatic venous thrombosis (Budd–Chiari syndrome) and veno-occlusive disease.

Experimental studies have demonstrated that the initial factor in the pathophysiology of portal hypertension is the increase in vascular resistance to portal blood flow. In cirrhosis, this increase in resistance occurs in the hepatic microcirculation (sinusoidal portal hypertension), and is a consequence of both a 'passive' and an 'active' component. The 'passive' component is the mechanical consequence of the hepatic architectural disorder resulting from histological cirrhosis, and the 'active' component is the active contraction of portal/septal myofibroblasts, activated stellate cells and portal venules. The increase in intrahepatic tone is probably a consequence of an imbalance between an increase in the endogenous vasoconstrictor substances, such as endothelin, noradrenaline, leukotrienes and angiotensin II, and a relative decrease in the endogenous vasodilator nitric oxide.[1] Vasodilatory drugs (for example, calcium channel blockers) may restore the equilibrium in intrahepatic tone, although they are not used for this indication in clinical practice.

The other major pathophysiological factor contributing to portal hypertension is an increase in portal venous blood flow through the portal circulation resulting from splanchnic arteriolar vasodilatation caused by an excessive release of endogenous arteriolar vasodilators (endothelial, neural and humoral). This can be corrected by means of splanchnic vasoconstrictors such as terlipressin and non-selective beta-blockers. Many drugs that lower portal pressure both reduce intrahepatic vascular resistance and decrease portal venous inflow.

An important but rare form, segmental or left upper quadrant portal hypertension, occurs in patients with splenic vein thrombosis. This should be suspected in patients with bleeding gastric varices but normal liver function, particularly if there is a history of either acute or chronic pancreatitis.

The natural history of portal hypertension

The prevalence of oesophageal varices in patients with cirrhosis and portal hypertension is high. When cirrhosis is diagnosed, varices are present in 40% of compensated and 60% of decompensated cirrhotics.[2] After the initial diagnosis of cirrhosis, varices develop with an incidence of 5% per year; subsequently, they may progress from small to large at an incidence of 10–15% per year.[3] Rapid progression of hepatic decompensation is associated with a rapid increase in size, whilst improvement in liver function, particularly when associated with removal of the injurious agent (e.g. abstinence from alcohol), may result in a decrease in size or disappearance of the varices.[4,5]

The overall incidence of variceal bleeding following diagnosis is of the order of 25% in unselected patients. The most important predictive factors of variceal bleeding are severity of liver dysfunction, size of varices and intravariceal wall pressure (which although difficult to measure may correlate at endoscopy with the presence of red spots or red weals).[6] Traditionally, liver dysfunction has been classified using the Child–Pugh score[7] (Table 8.2), but a more recent scoring system, the MELD (Model for End-stage Liver Disease), may be a better prognostic indicator (Box 8.1).[8] Variceal size may be the best single predictor of variceal bleeding and generally it is used to decide whether a patient should be given prophylactic therapy or not. Whether a patient dies from a variceal bleed depends on the severity of the accompanying liver failure; those with a high Child–Pugh or MELD score have been reported to have as high a risk of mortality

Table 8.2 • Child–Pugh classification

	Number of points		
	1	2	3
Bilirubin (µmol/L)*	<34	34–51	>51
Albumin (g/L)	>35	28–35	<28
Prothrombin time prolonged by (s)	<3	3–10	>10
Ascites	None	Slight to moderate	Moderate to severe
Encephalopathy	None	Slight to moderate	Moderate to severe

Grade A 5–6 points; Grade B 7–9 points; Grade C 10–15 points.
* In primary biliary cirrhosis, the point scoring for bilirubin level is adjusted as follows: 1, <68; 2, 68–170; 3, >170.

Box 8.1 • Model for End-stage Liver Disease (MELD)

MELD is calculated for patients over the age of 12 based on the following variables:

- Serum creatinine (mg/dL)
- Total bilirubin (mg/dL)
- INR (international normalised ratio).

The formula incorporates these variables as:

$$MELD = 3.78 \left[Ln\,serum\,bilirubin\,(mg/dL) \right]$$
$$+ 11.2 (Ln\,INR) + 9.57$$
$$\left[Ln\,serum\,creatinine\,(mg/dL) \right] + 6.43$$

The following rules must be observed when using this formula:

- 1 is the minimum acceptable value for any of the three variables.
- The maximum acceptable value for serum creatinine is 4.
- The maximum value for the MELD score is 40. All values higher than 40 are given a score of 40.
- If the patient has been dialysed twice within the last 7 days, then the value for serum creatinine used should be 4.0.

In being considered for liver transplantation, patients with a diagnosis of liver cancer are assigned a MELD score based on how advanced the cancer is, using the TNM staging system.

as 30–50% within 6 weeks of the index bleed.[9] However, a more realistic figure would be 20% at 6 weeks with an immediate mortality from uncontrolled bleeding as low as 5–8%. Indeed, in 40–50% of patients who bleed and develop hypotension, variceal bleeding stops spontaneously, probably as a result of reflex splanchnic vasoconstriction with associated reduction in

portal pressure and blood flow; this beneficial response is nullified by over-transfusing the patient.

The incidence of re-bleeding ranges between 30% and 40% within the first 6 weeks; this risk peaks in the first 5 days following the index bleed. Bleeding gastric varices, active bleeding at emergency endoscopy, low serum albumin levels, renal failure and a hepatic venous pressure gradient >20 mmHg have all been reported as significant indicators of an early risk of re-bleeding.[10–12] Patients surviving a first episode of variceal bleeding have a very high risk of re-bleeding (63%) and death (33%), and this is the basis for treating all patients to prevent further bleeding.[9]

Presentation

Portal hypertension may present acutely with variceal bleeding or be discovered during the investigation of a patient with liver disease. Varices are usually easily diagnosed at endoscopy and patients will then be investigated systematically. A classification of the grading of varices is given in Table 8.3. Presentation of patients with liver disease is variable and ranges from nonspecific tiredness to advanced encephalopthy with decompensation. External features of advanced liver disease such as spider naevi, palmar erythema and ascites are easy to detect, although these signs will be lacking in many patients. Splenomegaly is probably the most useful physical sign, although some patients will have the classic sign of dilated umbilical vein collaterals (caput medusae).

Imaging

Doppler ultrasonography is a useful and easily obtained initial imaging modality for patients with suspected portal hypertension. Spleen size and the state of the liver parenchyma can be assessed together with portal and hepatic vein patency and flow velocity, and the presence or absence of varices can often be inferred. Computed tomography (CT) and magnetic resonance imaging (MRI) now give detailed roadmaps of vascular anatomy prior to any surgical intervention with no need for invasive angiography in most cases.

Management of varices

The management of oesophageal varices will be considered in three sections: the prevention of bleeding in patients with varices who have never bled (primary prophylaxis); the longer-term management of patients who have bled to prevent

Table 8.3 • Classification of oesophageal and gastric varices

Classification of varices		
Oesophageal varices	Grade 0 (or absent)	
	Grade 1 (or small)	Varices that collapse on insufflation of oesophagus with air
	Grade 2 (or medium)	Varices that do not collapse on air insufflation
	Grade 3 (or large)	Varices that are large enough to occlude the lumen
Gastric varices	GOV1	Gastro-oesophageal varices extending <5 cm from the oesophagus across gastro-oesophageal junction
	GOV2	Gastro-oesophageal varices extending into the fundus across gastro-oesophageal junction
	IGV1	Isolated gastric varices in the fundus
	IGV2	Isolated non-fundic varices

future bleeding episodes (secondary prophylaxis); and the emergency resuscitation and initial control of the acute bleeding episode. Though the emergency management of many patients will be in a district general hospital, patients may require referral to specialised centres with expertise in liver diseases and where recourse to specialised radiological intervention is available. As pharmacological therapy is employed in the majority of cases, the treatment aims of this will be discussed first.

Therapeutic aims for pharmacological therapy in portal hypertension

The hepatic venous pressure gradient (HVPG) reflects accurately portal pressure in sinusoidal portal hypertension and is readily measured by hepatic vein catheterisation.

✔✔ Varices do not develop until the HVPG increases to 10–12 mmHg and the HVPG must be greater than 12 mmHg for the appearance of complications such as variceal bleeding and ascites.[13] Longitudinal studies of patients with complications of portal hypertension have demonstrated that when an HVPG decreases to less than 12 mmHg with pharmacological therapy, TIPS or an improvement in liver function, variceal bleeding is prevented and varices may decrease in size or disappear altogether.[14] When this target is not reached, a substantial reduction in portal pressure by more than 20% still offers protection against variceal bleeding[15] and thus these two parameters are regarded as the end-points to therapeutic strategies to lower portal pressure.

Recent evidence suggests that these therapeutic end-points may also reduce the risk of other complications of portal hypertension, including ascites, spontaneous bacterial peritonitis and hepatorenal syndrome.[16,17]

Oesophageal varices

Primary prophylaxis for the prevention of variceal haemorrhage

All patients with cirrhosis should be screened for varices at the time of first diagnosis of their cirrhosis. In patients with grade I varices at index endoscopy, a follow-up endoscopy should be performed after 12 months to detect the progression from grade II to III varices. Patients without varices should be re-evaluated 2–3 years after their index endoscopy.

The mainstay of primary prophylactic therapy in the prevention of variceal haemorrhage is the non-selective β-adrenergic receptor blocker (beta-blocker). Twelve trials using beta-blockers in this context have been reported.

✔✔ A meta-analysis has indicated that indefinite treatment with propanolol or nadolol significantly reduces the bleeding risk from 25% with non-active treatment or placebo to 15% with beta-blockers over a median follow-up period of 24 months; there was no significant reduction in mortality.[3] The benefit of therapy was only proven in those patients with grade II (or larger) varices; there was no evidence to support the use of primary prophylactic therapy in patients with grade I varices.

> ✅ Withdrawal of therapy was associated with a return to the same bleeding risk (25%) as the untreated subpopulation; indeed, there may also be an increased risk of mortality over untreated patients in those individuals who stop therapy.[18,19]

Assessment of the success of primary prophylactic therapy is ideally undertaken by measurement of the HVPG before and after initiating therapy, with the aim being to reduce the HVPG to <12 mmHg or to reduce it by >20% from its baseline value.[14] In practice, however, measurement of HVPG does require specific training and is probably not cost-effective for assessing primary prophylactic therapy. Thus, the clinician faces the question of how to adjust the dose of beta-blocker to maximise its beneficial effects. Traditional practice has recommended a stepwise increase in dose until the heart rate decreases by 25%, is <55 beats per minute, or there is arterial hypotension or clinical intolerance. This means that the dose of the beta-blocker is titrated against its β_1 effects (cardiac) and clinical tolerance; however, a fall in portal pressure results from blockade of both β_1 and β_2 receptors, and the fall in portal pressure does not readily correlate with the fall in heart rate or blood pressure. Therefore, titration solely against clinical tolerance may be the most useful surrogate marker of the maximal dose of beta-blocker in the absence of HVPG measurement.

There appears to be no advantage of one non-selective beta-blocker over another. However, the newest approach to increase response to beta-blockers has been the use of carvedilol, a drug that combines a non-selective beta-blocker action with an α_1-adrenoceptor blocker action. This causes a marked decrease in portal pressure, but has the side-effect of systemic hypotension.

When compared with propanolol, carvedilol significantly increased the number of patients achieving a target reduction of HVPG (<12 mmHg or >20% reduction from baseline HVPG).[19] There is considerable controversy about how to give the carvedilol because of its hypotensive side-effects; however, the above study demonstrated that lower doses (12.5 mg/day) result in good tolerance. In practice, the usual starting dose is 6.25 mg/day and the usual maintenance dose 12.5 mg/day.

In patients who are unable to tolerate beta-blockers (15–20%) because of side-effects or relative/absolute contraindications (for example, asthma), treatment with nitrates is ineffective, despite its portal pressure-lowering properties.[20] Therefore, variceal band ligation (VBL) therapy is the only option for patients with high-risk varices (grade II or above) and contraindications to beta-blockers. More controversially, a meta-analysis has suggested that VBL is a more effective mode of treatment than beta-blockers for primary prophylaxis.[21] However, this analysis included four trials, only two of which have been published in full; therefore, it seems reasonable to recommend that, for the time being, beta-blockers remain the primary prophylactic therapy of choice in terms of cost and convenience. Of course, VBL does not reduce portal pressure (and therefore measurement of HVPG following endoscopic monotherapy is of no value) and this may leave the patient at risk of developing other complications of portal hypertension. An algorithm for the primary prevention of variceal bleeding is given in **Fig. 8.1**.

Prevention of re-bleeding from oesophageal varices (secondary prophylaxis)

Following a variceal bleed, patients with cirrhosis should be managed in two ways: firstly, they should receive urgent and active treatment for the prevention of re-bleeding; secondly, they should be examined for signs of physiological stress following their bleed, which might indicate a need for an elective liver transplant assessment (**Fig. 8.2**). Management of non-cirrhotic patients is discussed later in this chapter.

Endoscopic variceal band ligation therapy or beta-blocker therapy are the treatments of choice for the prevention of re-bleeding from oesophageal varices.

> ✅✅ Meta-analyses of studies using beta-blocker therapy to prevent re-bleeding have demonstrated both a significantly decreased mortality (27% in controls to 20% in beta-blocker-treated individuals) and a decreased incidence of re-bleeding (63% to 42%).[3]

VBL also both improves survival and significantly decreases re-bleeding rates; it is superior to endoscopic sclerotherapy since it is associated with significantly fewer complications.[22,23] Currently, it is unclear whether pharmacological therapy is better than VBL or vice versa; studies have demonstrated a variety of outcomes with reference to re-bleeding rates, but none have indicated any clear difference in survival.[15,24,25] A combination of pharmacological therapy and endoscopic therapy is commonly used, but evidence suggesting a better outcome with this combination compared with monotherapy is hard to find. Likewise, combination therapy of nitrates and beta-blockers has not been consistently shown to be more effective than beta-blockers alone or VBL.[15,26]

Re-bleeding is still common with pharmacological or endoscopic therapy (30–50% at 2 years) and in these cases second-line therapies should be offered.

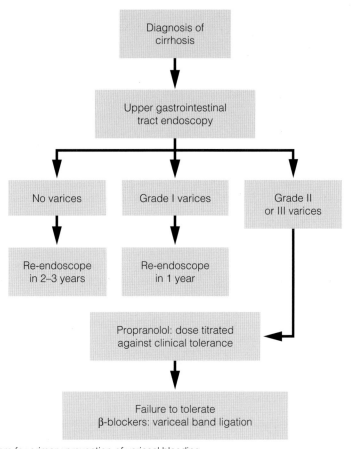

Figure 8.1 • Algorithm for primary prevention of variceal bleeding.

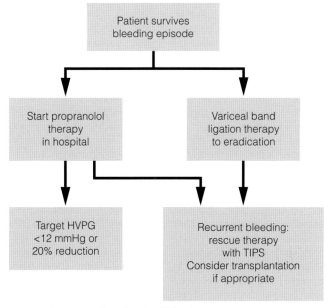

Figure 8.2 • Algorithm for secondary prevention of variceal bleeding.

This will depend on the underlying aetiology and fitness and age of the patient, and may be TIPS, shunt surgery or liver transplantation; these are considered later in this chapter.

Treatment for bleeding oesophageal varices

Variceal bleeding is a medical emergency and the first priority is to achieve adequate resuscitation of the patient in a safe environment, preferably a high-dependency or intensive care unit. On presentation, airway protection is essential, especially for intoxicated patients or those withdrawing from alcohol. Subsequent therapy is aimed at correcting hypovolaemic shock. Over-transfusion should be avoided because of the risk of a rebound increase in portal pressure with continued bleeding or re-bleeding.

✓✓ Antibiotics should be instituted from admission, since these increase the survival of bleeding patients; norfloxacin 400 mg/12 hours or ciprofloxacin 250 mg/12 hours are the antibiotics of choice.[27,28]

Finally, early therapy should also involve starting a vasoactive drug from admission (usually terlipressin or octreotide); a number of randomised controlled trials demonstrate that early administration of vasoactive drugs facilitates endoscopy, improves control of bleeding and reduces the 5 day re-bleeding rate.[29,30] Initiation of these measures in association with endoscopic therapy at the time of diagnostic endoscopy will control bleeding in approximately 75% of patients. However, as in most trials, in acute variceal bleeding this combined approach failed to improve overall mortality compared with drug or endoscopic therapy alone. The optimal duration of vasoactive drug therapy is not well established and requires evaluation; current recommendations are to continue the drug for 5 days, since this covers the period of maximum risk of re-bleeding.

Endoscopic therapy should be performed at the time of diagnostic endoscopy, within 12 hours of admission in a resuscitated patient. However, if the patient is stable, endoscopic therapy can probably be postponed until within normal working hours. There are multiple randomised controlled trials examining modes of endoscopic therapy in acute variceal bleeding. These have compared: endoscopic therapy with no therapy; endoscopic therapy with vasoactive drug therapy; endoscopic sclerotherapy with variceal band ligation therapy; combined endoscopic therapy with variceal band ligation therapy; and endoscopic therapy with TIPS. Endoscopic therapy is certainly superior to no therapy;[31] of the two endoscopic therapies, variceal band ligation therapy should be considered the treatment of choice since it is associated with significantly fewer complications (oesophageal stricturing or oesophageal ulcer formation) and significantly fewer sessions of therapy to eradicate the varices. However, there is probably no difference in re-bleeding or mortality rates between the two therapies. Likewise, there is little evidence to support combined endoscopic therapy for the treatment of bleeding varices.[32] In practice, however, it is sometimes beneficial for the endoscopist to use a small volume of sclerosant initially to improve vision in order to place some variceal bands to achieve eventual haemostasis. If endoscopic therapy fails to control bleeding, balloon tamponade should be used as a 'bridge' until definitive therapy can be offered. In practice, this usually means a further attempt at endoscopic band ligation therapy followed by second-line therapies. An algorithm for the management of variceal bleeding in cirrhotics is given in **Fig. 8.3**.

Gastric varices

Gastric varices are most commonly caused by cirrhosis complicated by portal hypertension and are the source of 5–10% of all upper GI bleeding episodes. Patients with pancreatic disease, especially inflammatory pancreatic disease, can also develop splenic vein thromboses with subsequent formation of isolated gastric varices. There have been sporadic reports of gastric varices developing after endoscopic therapy for bleeding oesophageal varices, particularly after endoscopic sclerotherapy. The risk of bleeding from gastric varices is no greater than from oesophageal varices and it is probable that pharmacological therapy is equally as effective as primary prophylactic therapy in oesophageal varices, so patients with gastric varices should also receive non-selective beta-blockers as first-line therapy. There are no reports of primary attempts at prophylactic therapy using endoscopic-based therapy.

Treatment of acute gastric variceal bleeding is very challenging. Medical management is similar to the treatment of oesophageal varices. Terlipressin and octreotide are useful for control of acute bleeding, while beta-blockers may also be as effective as secondary prophylactic therapy. The Sengstaken–Blakemore tube may have some utility for controlling bleeding from junctional (GOV1 or GOV2) varices but has little effect on controlling bleeding varices in the fundus or further down the stomach. Some endoscopic therapies are promising, but quality data are scarce; sclerotherapy, glue injection, thrombin and variceal band ligation therapy have all been reported. Control of bleeding using sclerotherapy with cyanoacrylate has been

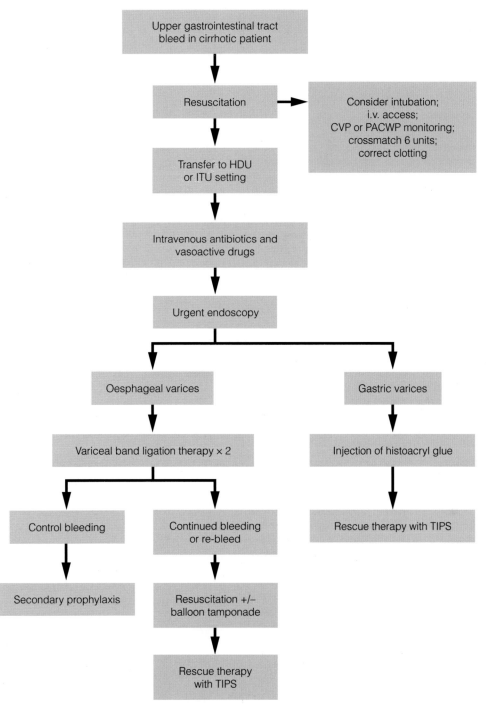

Figure 8.3 • Algorithm for the management of variceal bleeding.

reported as efficacious in 62–100% of cases, with successful obliteration of varices in 0–94%.[33,34]

> ✔✔ A randomised controlled trial from Taiwan has confirmed that endoscopic sclerotherapy with cyanoacrylate was more effective and also safer than band ligation in the management of bleeding gastric varices.[35]

The major rescue therapy (indeed, some may consider it the primary therapy) for bleeding gastric varices used in the UK is TIPS, which has a success rate for initial haemostasis of greater than 90% and re-bleeding rates of 20–30%.

> ✔✔ Recently, the first prospective, randomised controlled trial comparing TIPS with cyanoacrylate injection in the prevention of gastric re-bleeding was published. This concluded that TIPS was more effective than glue injection in preventing re-bleeding from gastric varices, although the two modalities shared a similar mortality rate and frequency of complications.[36]

It is imperative that all patients treated with any of the above-mentioned interventions (for bleeding oesophageal and gastric varices), except medical management, also receive treatment with a proton-pump inhibitor (PPI) to suppress acid secretion and to prevent complications related to acid interaction with bands, injection sites and treatment-related ulcers.

Portal hypertensive gastropathy

The presence of portal hypertensive gastropathy (PHG) is strongly correlated with the severity of cirrhosis, its overall prevalence in cirrhosis being about 80%.[37] However, the incidence of acute bleeding is low, occurring in about 2.5% of patients over an 18-month follow-up period, with an associated mortality of 12.5%; the incidence of chronic bleeding is significantly higher at 12%. Propanolol, octreotide and terlipressin have all been proposed for the treatment of acute bleeding from PHG based on their ability to decrease portal blood flow. In a randomised controlled trial, propanolol was found to reduce recurrent bleeding from PHG.[38] Once again, TIPS is considered as the rescue therapy of choice in patients who have repeated bleeding from PHG despite propanolol therapy.

Second-line therapies

Second-line therapies include the less invasive radiological techniques of TIPS or open surgery, which can range from direct oversewing of bleeding veins to surgical shunts and ultimately liver replacement.

TIPS (transjugular intrahepatic portosystemic shunt)

TIPS is a non-surgical method of creating a portocaval shunt. Its principal use is in treating active variceal bleeding not controlled by medical and endoscopic means or preventing re-bleeding. It therefore has a role in both elective and emergency situations. TIPS is appropriate in selected cases of refractory ascites, hepatic hydrothorax, portal hypertensive gastropathy, Budd–Chiari syndrome and hepatorenal syndrome. TIPS may facilitate surgery in patients with portal hypertension requiring hepatic or other abdominal surgery, although it is not generally used prior to liver transplant without other specific indications.

TIPS is created by needle puncture from a hepatic vein to a major intrahepatic portal vein branch. The track is maintained by a stent.

> ✔ The degree of shunting can be tailored to some extent by adjusting the diameter of the balloon-dilated shunt against the resulting pressure gradient, directly measured through the catheter.[39]

Occasionally there are severe and life-threatening complications but in the majority of cases few and only minor complications occur. Simpler radiological interventions can restore and maintain most narrowed or occluded TIPS, providing satisfactory secondary patency. Patients require regular follow-up by Doppler ultrasound, and elective venography may be performed to treat stenoses before significant bleeding recurs. As with any shunt there is a risk of encephalopathy. This is greater in older patients, wider diameter shunts and in those with prior encephalopathy or more advanced liver disease. Patients with precarious liver function may deteriorate into liver failure as a result of reduced portal perfusion.

> ✔✔ An early disadvantage of TIPS was the poor primary patency rate, but this can be significantly improved by the use of covered stents, as demonstrated in a recent randomised trial.[40]

TIPS has been compared unfavourably with surgery (see later section on surgical shunts) because of the high rate of reintervention, yet overall survival has been similar in randomised trials of both H-graft portocaval shunts and distal splenorenal shunts versus TIPS.[41,42] However, TIPS is usually preferred in patients with more advanced liver disease and in those likely to need future transplantation. Patients with more severe liver disease may be candidates for liver transplantation, but TIPS can stabilise some to enable survival long enough to receive a successful transplant. Moreover, the MELD score can be used to predict likely survival following TIPS.[43]

TIPS for variceal bleeding

Uncontrolled bleeding from oesophagogastric or ectopic varices in the presence of a patent portal vein can usually be controlled by TIPS. The procedure can be performed on patients considered too sick for surgery. The mortality of these patients is due more to their general condition rather than the TIPS procedure. The 30-day mortality after TIPS in the UK National Confidential Enquiry into Perioperative Death study was 17%.[44] In this study, 80% of patients dying after TIPS had the procedure performed urgently or as an emergency for bleeding varices.

TIPS can be combined with embolisation of varices as there is direct access to the portal system. This is done particularly in acute bleeding to further reduce the risk of haemorrhage. Reduction of extrahepatic portosystemic shunting may also improve portal venous flow towards the liver and the TIPS. In some cases this may counter encephalopathy as well as helping to maintain flow in the TIPS.

Meta-analyses of several trials compare TIPS with endoscopic sclerotherapy and/or banding for prevention of recurrent variceal bleeding.[45,46] Additional medical therapy was included in some. TIPS was more successful at preventing re-bleeding but with no overall improvement in mortality. Encephalopathy was overall more frequent in the TIPS patients, but not in every trial. In some studies patients in the endoscopic groups were rescued by TIPS because of significant recurrent bleeding. General consensus is that endoscopic and medical therapy should be the primary treatment and TIPS reserved for those cases where control is not achieved. TIPS may be combined effectively with medical treatment or endoscopic variceal eradication after bleeding has been controlled. Long-term TIPS surveillance and reintervention may then be less necessary.[47,48]

Other procedures have been used to control bleeding from varices when venous anatomy permits catheter access. Retrograde balloon occlusion of gastric varices has been mainly used in Asia as an alternative to TIPS when there is a patent gastrorenal venous connection.[49,50]

Surgical options

Until endoscopic sclerotherapy was introduced in the early 1970s, the only practical options were surgical. These ranged from oesophageal transection and devascularisation procedures, to portosystemic shunt procedures and, more recently, liver transplantation, which is the treatment of choice for patients with variceal bleeding who meet the acceptance criteria.

Devascularisation procedures have been popular in Japan but were rarely used in the West and have been largely superseded by TIPS.

Portal systemic shunts

The variety of surgical shunts described for portal hypertension is perhaps a testament to the ingenuity of surgeons (**Fig. 8.4**). With the passing of the 'shunt era' most surgical trainees will not have seen a shunt, which now has a limited application for a selected group of patients. These are mainly those with non-cirrhotic portal hypertension and patients living in areas where newer therapies are not available. However, in some units where an active interest in shunt surgery has been maintained, a combination of very experienced surgeons and an excellent organisation has allowed for good results with emergency shunt surgery.[51]

✔✔ A controlled crossover trial comparing distal splenorenal (Warren) shunt (DSRS) with endoscopic sclerotherapy showed that shunting produced better control of bleeding but did not produce any survival advantage.[52]

Shunt operations can be classified into selective or non-selective shunts. The former carry lower rates of hepatic encephalopathy but are less successful in controlling acute bleeding. The two main procedures that have achieved popularity are the DSRS and the interposition portocaval or mesocaval shunt utilising a small-diameter prosthetic H-graft (see Fig. 8.4e,f). Direct primary portocaval anastomosis produces the most effective lowering of portal pressure but with the highest encephalopathy rates, and the advantage of the small-diameter portocaval H-graft is that it is selective and maintains some portal flow. This shunt has been compared to TIPS in a single-centre randomised trial in which the entry criterion was variceal bleeding in patients who had failed or 'were not amenable to' sclerotherapy or banding; recruitment was rapid, which suggests a low threshold to proceed with second-line therapies.[53] There was a higher 30-day mortality in shunt patients but a better long-term control of bleeding than that seen in the TIPS patients. It should be recognised that the expertise needed for TIPS insertion and the protocols for subsequent surveillance will vary between centres, such that results should be interpreted with caution as they may reflect local interest and expertise. It had previously been established that shunt surgery for cirrhotics carries significant postoperative mortality rates, being as high as 26.1% for Child C patients even in specialised centres.[54] Furthermore 5-year survival

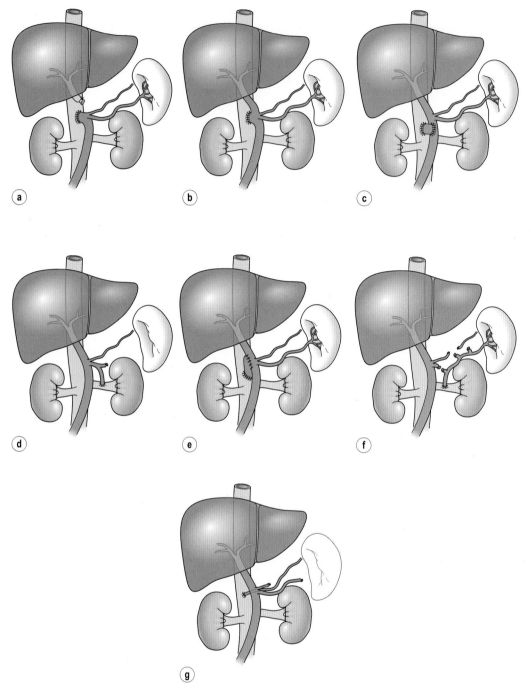

Figure 8.4 • Non-selective **(a–d)** and selective **(e–g)** portosystemic shunts. **(a)** End-to-side portocaval. **(b)** Side-to-side portocaval. **(c)** Mesocaval (jugular vein graft or prosthesis). **(d)** Proximal splenorenal. **(e)** Small-diameter PTFE H-graft portocaval. **(f)** Distal splenorenal (Warren). **(g)** Left gastric-to-IVC (Inokuchi).

rates in patients with advanced liver disease are poor and shunt surgery carries an additional burden due to the risks of hepatic encephalopathy.

> ✓✓ A recently reported multicentre randomised trial of TIPS versus DSRS showed no overall difference in survival and a tendency for TIPS to be more cost-effective in terms of lives saved.[42,55]

On current evidence there is no role for routine shunting in cirrhotic patients. Shunts should be avoided in patients in whom transplantation is an option as they significantly increase the risk of surgery. If endoscopic and radiological approaches fail, surgery away from the liver hilum is recommended either as a splenorenal or interposition mesocaval shunt.[56]

Liver transplantation

With the improved results and wider application of liver transplantation, this has become the definitive treatment for many patients with variceal bleeding. However, results are inferior for patients transplanted around the time of an acute bleed. Furthermore, there are reports of oesophageal complications, including perforation in grafted patients who have undergone recent endoscopic therapy. Thus, the indications for liver replacement are more to do with the stage of the underlying liver disease, although the priority for grafting will be influenced by a history of recent bleeding or a high risk for re-bleeding.

In 1997, minimal selection criteria, based on studies of the natural history of compensated chronic liver diseases, were developed to aid such a process.[57] The minimal listing criteria were: an estimated 1-year survival ≤90%; Child–Pugh score ≥7 (Class B or C); or portal hypertensive bleeding; or an episode of spontaneous bacterial peritonitis regardless of the Child–Pugh score. The basis of these criteria is that the expected outcome of the untreated patient would be significantly worse than that of the outcomes from liver transplantation. This recognises the significantly worse prognosis of decompensated cirrhosis, which in those with hepatitis C, for example, dramatically reduces from a 91% 5-year survival to 50%.[58] Spontaneous bacterial peritonitis carries an adverse outcome in these patients, with 1-year survival falling from 66% to 38% in one report,[59] and despite the many therapeutic modalities available for treatment, the only definitive therapy for recurrent variceal bleeding is liver transplantation.[60]

Broadly, liver transplantation should be considered in any patient who is able to cooperate with the treatment and in whom an anticipated survival rate of at least 50% at 5 years postgrafting is likely to be achieved. The decisions to proceed to liver replacement should be made by a multidisciplinary team including an experienced hepatologist. Today, MELD scoring is widely used to list patients for liver transplant. Transplanting a patient with a MELD of <15 is associated with a poorer outcome than would be expected on the waiting list and transplanting these patients may not be the best use of the limited organ pool (see Box 8.1).

Selection of second-line therapy

Non-cirrhotic

The easiest groups to consider are those without cirrhosis. If such patients fail with pharmacological or endoscopic therapy then a surgical shunt is the treatment of choice. For those with portal vein thrombosis, a distal splenorenal shunt is recommended and has the advantage of preserving the spleen. For non-cirrhotics with a patent portal vein, the choice rests between a portocaval or distal splenorenal depending on local expertise.

Cirrhotic

It is clear that if the patient is a potential transplant candidate they should be assessed for this once the initial bleeding has been controlled. If the bleeding cannot be controlled they should be considered for urgent TIPS insertion and then for liver replacement. Patients who are unsuitable for transplantation may be candidates for TIPS provided they do not have significant encephalopathy as this may worsen following the procedure. Once the transplant candidates, patients who are high risk because of comorbidity, and uncooperative patients who are actively drinking are identified as unsuitable for shunting, there are relatively few potential candidates for a TIPS procedure. Clearly, in areas where transplantation is not available as an option, patients should be considered for shunting provided they are Child A or B.

Management of ascites

Ascites is a common feature of portal hypertension, although the exact mechanisms remain under debate.[61] Ascites in chronic liver disease can be effectively treated by a number of medical, surgical or radiological techniques. The new development of ascites should be investigated for bacterial peritonitis, portal vein thrombosis or hepatic malignancy. Initial treatment involves dietary sodium restriction and diuretic therapy. Unresponsive patients may benefit from regular large-volume paracentesis with concurrent intravenous administration of

20% human albumin.[62] Though peritoneovenous shunting is effective in controlling ascites, potential risks include disseminated intravascular coagulation, sepsis and cardiac failure. It has few advantages over large-volume paracentesis and is not recommended for patients who are transplant candidates.[63] Refractory ascites is an indication for transplant assessment.

TIPS can also be very effective in controlling ascites refractory to medical treatment, but many such patients have very advanced liver disease with poor prognosis. The immediate risk is worsening liver failure and hepatic encephalopathy, and advice from an experienced hepatologist should be sought before TIPS. Older patients and those with renal dysfunction fare worse, and if patients with severe ascites are liver transplant candidates this may be a better option than TIPS. Patients with better liver function and disproportionate ascites, especially those with liver disease that can improve, e.g. by withdrawal from alcohol, respond well to TIPS. Some trials have shown TIPS to be more effective than medical treatment plus paracentesis, but patient selection is most important. Some studies have shown an improved survival and quality of life in patients having TIPS for ascites, whereas others have not.[64–66] Surgical shunts are no longer recommended for resistant ascites due to high perioperative mortality and encephalopathy rates.

Budd–Chiari syndrome

Budd–Chiari syndrome is a rare condition resulting from occlusion of the hepatic veins. Presenting features include acute abdominal pain, ascites, acute fulminant liver failure or chronic liver failure, and can mimic many other conditions. Ultrasonography (US) will show absent or abnormal hepatic venous drainage. CT will often reveal abnormal liver perfusion that can be difficult to interpret and cases may be initially misdiagnosed as advanced hepatic malignancy. One common feature is the compensatory hypertrophy of the caudate lobe of the liver. This occurs as it has venous drainage separate from the three main hepatic veins. This regenerated liver is clearly life preserving, although pressure from the caudate may compound a tendency to caval thrombosis, which is seen in a proportion of patients. The majority of patients will have or will develop evidence of a thrombophilic state and should all be assessed by an expert haematologist. Given the lifetime risks of further thromboses, all patients require long-term anticoagulation. Referral to a specialised centre with suitable hepatology, radiology and surgical expertise is advised.

Acute Budd–Chiari syndrome

In the acute presentation there will usually be abdominal pain and swelling. If there is a short stenosis or occlusion of the hepatic vein(s) and/or inferior vena cava (IVC), balloon dilatation or stenting is very effective. Transjugular, transfemoral or transhepatic access may be required. Occlusion or stenosis of the IVC (sometimes a web) may similarly respond to balloon dilatation. If the dilated or recanalised segment of hepatic vein is not satisfactorily maintained after balloon inflation, a metal stent can be inserted to maintain the patent lumen.[67] These approaches have the benefit of restoring physiological hepatic vein outflow in at least one of the main hepatic veins. Adjunctive pharmacological or mechanical thrombolysis may assist these procedures in selected cases, especially when acute thrombosis complicates an otherwise successful vein recanalisation. There are individual case reports of systemic thrombolysis producing improvement but these are rare.[68]

✅ TIPS can be used in both acute and chronic Budd–Chiari, and would now be regarded as the treatment of choice for those not responding to medical therapy and/or hepatic vein recanalisation.[69,70]

A recent study has shown that TIPS was the most frequent treatment modality applied in a 2-year multicentre European study of new Budd–Chiari presentations.[71] The advantage of TIPS is decompression of the portal vein above the compressed part of the IVC within the caudate lobe and avoidance of laparotomy. With their tendency to thrombosis, Budd–Chiari patients have a greater need for reintervention than other TIPS patients but covered stents have shown improved patency.[72]

Extended TIPS can be a successful treatment for patients with Budd–Chiari syndrome complicated by portal and mesenteric vein thrombosis. A few cases have been described in which TIPS was a stabilising factor before liver transplantation, but most patients improve sufficiently after TIPS to avoid the need for transplantation. If TIPS cannot be achieved then surgical shunt can be performed or liver transplant when there is significant liver failure. In summary, there is a progressive hierarchy of radiological procedures that can manage the majority of Budd–Chiari patients according to their individual venous anatomy. These procedures are effective in combination with appropriate medical therapy.[73]

If the radiological approach fails, the type of surgical shunt will depend on the patency of the vena cava. If the cava is patent a mesocaval shunt using a length of autologous internal jugular vein between the superior mesenteric vein and the infrarenal vena cava is recommended. For cases with caval occlusion, a meso-atrial shunt using a graft of reinforced polytetrafluoroethylene (PTFE) between the superior mesenteric vein and the right atrium can be performed. Selection of patients for shunting is not easy and our experience suggests that patients with jaundice as an early symptom are at risk of decompensation and should be considered for liver grafting. If the patient develops fulminant hepatic failure, then emergency liver transplantation is the only potential option. High success rates are reported but recurrence can occur and all patients will require long-term anticoagulation.

Chronic Budd–Chiari syndrome

Many patients present with significant ascites and marked changes on liver biopsy, which include significant fibrosis or even cirrhosis. It is likely that for some patients the hepatic venous obstruction is sequential and that the condition is asymptomatic until a second or final (third) hepatic vein is occluded. Either hepatic vein dilatation or TIPS should be performed based on the presence of identifiable hepatic veins within the liver.[70,73] Shunt procedures should be reserved for radiological approach failures. Our local experience is that significant jaundice is an adverse prognostic sign and in these cases liver transplantation may be required.

Non-cirrhotic portal hypertension

Portal hypertension is uncommon in the absence of cirrhosis. The causes are mainly portal vein thrombosis, periportal fibrosis and segmental, usually left upper quadrant, portal hypertension associated with splenic vein thrombosis.

Portal vein thrombosis

Portal vein thrombosis is rare in the West but is seen more frequently in Third World countries and is thought to be the result of umbilical sepsis in the neonatal period. Presentation can be in early childhood but is usually delayed to the early teenage years. The symptoms are usually that of a sudden variceal bleed, although some patients may be picked up by the presence of significant splenomegaly with or without haematological features of hypersplenism. The management of the acute bleed is similar to patients with cirrhosis. Re-bleeding or the presence of large gastric varices should be considered as a clear indication for a surgical shunt. Given the risks of splenectomy

in the young, a spleen-preserving procedure is recommended. In a small child, splenorenal shunts are less practical because of the small size of the vessels and interposition mesocaval shunts using autologous jugular vein have high success rates with good long-term patency.[74] In larger children, the distal splenorenal (Warren) shunt is usually favoured, although side-to-side splenorenal shunts have been reported in significant numbers from centres with a high prevalence of portal vein thrombosis.[75] The natural history of these patients is interesting in that as they grow the varices become less symptomatic, and certainly shunting is not indicated unless bleeding episodes occur.

Extensive mesenteric venous thrombosis is a potentially lethal complication seen in a few patients with portal vein thrombosis. Many patients will present with gut infarction but those presenting late pose major management problems. Careful angiography may reveal particularly dilated mesenteric collaterals, which might allow ad hoc shunts to the cava, but currently only medical therapies to lower portal pressure can be recommended.

Segmental portal hypertension

Segmental portal hypertension should always be considered as the potential cause of bleeding in patients with pancreatic pathology as they may have splenic vein thrombosis. Those with advanced pancreatic malignancy can usually be controlled with medical therapy or sclerotherapy. Patients with chronic pancreatitis who develop variceal bleeding secondary to splenic vein thrombosis should be considered for splenectomy, which will usually be curative.

TIPS and portal vein thrombosis

Interventions have extended into the portal venous system by percutaneous transhepatic, transjugular and even the trans-splenic routes in selected cases.[76] Limited acute portal vein thrombus is relatively easily treated by TIPS combined with thrombolysis, including clot disruption by balloon or other devices.[77] Patients with normal liver may only require transhepatic portal vein procedures for success, but those with hepatic portal hypertension benefit from TIPS improved outflow as well. Chronic portal vein thrombosis is often associated with extensive portal collaterals forming a portal vein cavernoma. If there is an appropriate clinical indication, then these can be traversed and the main portal vein flow can be restored by balloon dilatation and/or stent insertion.[78] More extensive occlusion involving the splenic and superior mesenteric veins may respond but with more difficulty, and those with underlying liver disease fare worse.

Key points

- Patients with grade II varices or worse who have not bled should be treated with beta-blockers unless there are medical contraindications.
- Endoscopic band ligation is the initial treatment of choice for acute variceal bleeding.
- After bleeding, patients should enter a programme of variceal ligation or beta-blockade to prevent recurrent bleeding.
- TIPS should be considered in patients in whom endoscopic therapy is unsuccessful.
- Liver transplantation should be considered in appropriate cases once variceal bleeding is problematic.
- Shunt surgery should be considered for non-cirrhotic patients with recurrent variceal bleeding and for Child–Pugh stage A and B patients who live in areas where TIPS or transplantation is unavailable.

References

1. Rodríguez-Vilarrupla A, Fernández M, Bosch J, et al. Current concepts on the pathophysiology of portal hypertension. Ann Hepatol 2007;6:28–36.

2. Schepis F, Camma C, Nicefero D, et al. Which patients should undergo endoscopic screening for esophageal varices detection? Hepatology 2001;33:333–8.

3. D'Amico G, Pagliaro L, Bosch J. Pharmacological treatment of portal hypertension: an evidence based approach. Semin Liver Dis 1999;19:475–505.
   Meta-analysis illustrating the benefits of treating patients with beta-blockers after an episode of bleeding oesophageal varices both in terms of decreasing risk of re-bleeding and decreasing mortality.

4. Zoli M, Merkel C, Magalotti D, et al. Natural history of cirrhotic patients with small esophageal varices: a prospective study. Am J Gastroenterol 2000;95:503–8.

5. Vorobioff J, Grozmann RJ, Picabea E, et al. Prognostic value of hepatic venous pressure gradient measurements in alcoholic cirrhosis: a 10 year prospective study. Gastroenterology 1996;111:701–9.

6. The North Italian Endoscopic Club for the Study and Treatment of Esophageal Varices. Prediction of the first variceal haemorrhage in patients with cirrhosis of the liver and esophageal varices: a prospective multicenter study. N Engl J Med 1988;319:983–9.

7. Albers I, Hartmann H, Bircher J, et al. Superiority of the Child–Pugh classification to quantitative liver function tests for assessing prognosis of liver cirrhosis. Scand J Gastroenterol 1989;24:269–76.

8. Kamath PS, Wiesner RH, Malinchoc M, et al. A model to predict survival in patients with end-stage liver disease. Hepatology 2001;33:464–70.

9. D'Amico G, Luca A. Natural history. Clinical–haemodynamic correlations. Prediction of the risk of bleeding. Baillière's Best Pract Res Clin Gastroenterol 1997;11:243–56.

10. Ben Ari Z, Cardin F, McCormik AP, et al. A predictive model for failure to control bleeding during acute variceal haemorrhage. J Hepatol 1999;31:443–50.

11. Goulis J, Armonis A, Patch D, et al. Bacterial infection is independently associated with failure to control bleeding in cirrhotic patients with gastrointestinal haemorrhage. Hepatology 1998;27:1207–12.

12. Moitinho E, Escorsell A, Bandi JC, et al. Prognostic value of early measurements of portal pressure in acute variceal bleeding. Gastroenterology 1999;117:626–31.

13. Garcia-Tsao G, Grozsmann RJ, Fisher RL, et al. Portal pressure, presence of gastroesophageal varices and variceal bleeding. Hepatology 1985;5:419–24.

14. Feu F, Garcia-Pagan JC, Bosch J, et al. Relation between portal pressure response to pharmacotherapy and risk of recurrent variceal bleeding in patients with cirrhosis. Lancet 1995;346:1056–9.

15. Villaneuva C, Minana J, Ortiz J, et al. Endoscopic ligation compared with combined treatment with nadolol and isosorbide mononitrate to prevent variceal bleeding. N Engl J Med 2001;345:647–55.
    References 13–15 provide the rationale for the therapeutic aim of pharmacological therapy to decrease the HVPG to <12 mmHg or reduce it to 20% of its baseline value.

16. Tarantino I, Abraldes JG, Turnes J, et al. The HVPG response to pharmacological treatment of portal hypertension predicts prognosis and the risk of developing complications of cirrhosis. J Hepatol 2002;36(Suppl. 1):15A.

17. Bosch J, Abraldes JG, Groszmann R. Current management of portal hypertension. J Hepatol 2003;38:S54–68.

18. Abraczinskas DR, Ookubo R, Grace ND, et al. Propanolol for the prevention of first esophageal haemorrhage: a lifetime commitment? Hepatology 2001;34:1096–102.

19. Banares R, Moitinho E, Matilla A, et al. Randomised comparison of long-term carvedilol and propanolol administration in the treatment of portal hypertension in cirrhosis. Hepatology 2002;36:1367–73.
    References 18 and 19 provide the rationale for the use of long-term beta-blockade to reduce the risk of bleeding in grade II or III varices.

20. Borroni G, Salerno F, Cazzaniga M, et al. Nadolol is superior to isosorbide mononitrate for the prevention of the first variceal bleeding in cirrhotic patients with ascites. J Hepatol 2002;37:315–21.

21. Imperiale TF, Chalasani N. A meta-analysis of endoscopic variceal ligation for primary prophylaxis of esophageal variceal bleeding. Hepatology 2001;33:908–14.

22. De Franchis R, Primignami M. Endoscopic treatments for portal hypertension. Semin Liver Dis 1999;19:439–55.

23. Laine L, El Newihi HM, Migikovsky B, et al. Endoscopic ligation compared with sclerotherapy for the treatment of bleeding esophageal varices. Ann Intern Med 1993;119:1–7.

24. Patch D, Sabin CA, Goulis J, et al. A randomised, controlled trial of medical therapy versus endoscopic ligation for the prevention of variceal rebleeding in patients with cirrhosis. Gastroenterology 2002;123:1013–9.

25. Lo GH, Chen WC, Chen MH, et al. Banding ligation versus nadolol and isosorbide mononitrate for the prevention of esophageal rebleeding. Gastroenterology 2002;123:728–34.

26. Gournay J, Masliah C, Martin T, et al. Isosorbide mononitrate and propanolol compared with propanolol alone for the prevention of variceal re-bleeding. Hepatology 2000;31:1239–45.

27. Bernard B, Grange JD, Khac EN, et al. Antibiotic prophylaxis for the prevention of bacterial infections in cirrhotic patients with gastrointestinal bleeding: a meta-analysis. Hepatology 1999;29:1655–61.

28. Rimola A, Garcia-Tsao G, Navasa M, et al. Diagnosis, treatment and prophylaxis of spontaneous bacterial peritonitis: a consensus document. International Ascites Club. J Hepatol 2000;32:142–53.
    References 27 and 28 illustrate the benefit to cirrhotic patients of prophylactic antibiotics following a variceal bleed by decreasing mortality.

29. Avgerinos A, Nevens F, Raptis S, et al. Early administration of somatostatin and efficacy of sclerotherapy in acute variceal bleeds: the European acute bleeding oesophageal variceal episodes (ABOVE) randomised trial. Lancet 1997;350:1495–9.

30. Cales P, Masliah C, Bernard B, et al. Early administration of vapreotide for variceal bleeding in patients with cirrhosis. French Club for the Study of Portal Hypertension. N Engl J Med 2001;344:23–8.

31. Infante-Rivard C, Esnaola S, Villeneuve JP. Role of endoscopic variceal sclerotherapy in the long-term management of variceal bleeding: a meta-analysis. Gastroenterology 1989;96:1087–92.

32. Singh P, Pooran N, Indaram A, et al. Combined ligation and sclerotherapy versus ligation alone for secondary prophylaxis of esophageal variceal bleeding: a meta-analysis. Am J Gastroenterol 2002;97:623–9.

33. Huang YH, Yeh HZ, Chen GH, et al. Endoscopic treatment of bleeding gastric varices by N-butyl-2-cyanoacrylate (Histoacryl) injection: long-term efficacy and safety. Gastrointest Endosc 2000;52:512–9.

34. Kind R, Guglielmi A, Rodella L, et al. Bucrylate treatment of bleeding gastric varices: 12 years' experience. Endoscopy 2000;32:512–9.

35. Lo GH, Lai KH, Cheng JS, et al. A prospective randomised trial of butyl cyanoacrylate injection versus band ligation in the management of bleeding gastric varices. Hepatology 2001;33:1060–4.
    This was the first study to compare banding with the injection of 'glue' in the treatment of gastric varices as a prospective randomised trial.

36. Lo GH, Liang HL, Chen WC, et al. A prospective, randomised controlled trial of transjugular intrahepatic portosystemic shunt versus cyanoacrylate injection in the prevention of gastric variceal rebleeding. Endoscopy 2007;39:679–85.
    A further rare, randomised controlled trial in gastric variceal bleeding from the same institution. This study compared the efficacy and complications of TIPS with glue injections in preventing re-bleeding from gastric varices. TIPS was more effective than glue injection in preventing re-bleeding, but was associated with a similar risk of mortality and frequency of complications.

37. Primignani M, Carpinelli L, Preatoni P, et al. Natural history of portal hypertensive gastropathy in patients with liver cirrhosis. The New Italian Endoscopic Club for the study and treatment of esophageal varices (NIEC). Gastroenterology 2000;119:181–7.

38. Perez-Ayuso RM, Pique JM, Bosch J, et al. Propanolol in the prevention of recurrent bleeding from severe portal hypertensive gastropathy in cirrhosis. Lancet 1991;337:1431–4.

39. Rossle M, Siegerstetter V, Olchewski M, et al. How much reduction in portal pressure is necessary to prevent variceal rebleeding? A longitudinal study in 225 patients with transjugular intrahepatic portosystemic shunts. Am J Gastroenterol 2001;96:3379–83.
    Observations on 225 patients having TIPS follow-up. Reduction of pressure gradient by 25–50% of original may be sufficient to prevent re-bleeding rather than the target of 12 mmHg.

40. Bureau C, Pagan JC, Layrargues GP, et al. Patency of stents covered with polytetrafluoroethylene in patients treated by transjugular intrahepatic portosystemic shunts: long-term results of a randomized multicentre study. Liver Int 2007;27:742–7.
    PTFE-covered stents require less reintervention with no disadvantage at 2 years.

41. Rosemurgy AS, Zervos EE, Blooston M, et al. Post shunt resource consumption favors small-diameter prosthetic H-graft portocaval shunt over TIPS for patients with poor hepatic reserve. Ann Surg 2003;237:820–5.

42. Henderson JM, Boyer TD, Kutner MH, et al. Distal splenorenal shunt versus transjugular intrahepatic portal systematic shunt for variceal bleeding: a randomized trial. Gastroenterology 2006;130:1643–51.

43. Ferral H, Gamboa P, Postoak DW, et al. Survival after elective transjugular intrahepatic portosystemic shunt creation: prediction with model for end-stage liver disease score. Radiology 2004;231:231–6.

44. NCEPOD report on Vascular Interventional Radiology, www.ncepod.org.uk; 2000.

45. Burroughs AK, Vangeli M. Transjugular intrahepatic portosystemic shunt versus endoscopic therapy: randomized trials for secondary prophylaxis of variceal bleeding: an updated meta-analysis. Scand J Gastroenterol 2002;37:249–52.

46. Khan S, Tudur Smith C, Williamson P, et al. Portosystemic shunts versus endoscopic therapy for variceal rebleeding in patients with cirrhosis. Cochrane Database Syst Rev 2006;18:CD000553.

47. Brensing KA, Horsch M, Textor J, et al. Hemodynamic effects of propranolol and nitrates in cirrhotic patients with transjugular intrahepatic portosystemic stent-shunt. Scand J Gastorenterol 2002;37:1070–6.

48. Tripathi D, Lui HF, Helmy A, et al. Randomised controlled trial of long term portographic follow up versus variceal band ligation following transjugular intrahepatic portosystemic stent shunt for preventing oesophageal variceal rebleeding. Gut 2004;53:431–7.

49. Hiraga N, Aikata H, Takaki S, et al. The long-term outcome of patients with bleeding gastric varices after balloon-occluded retrograde transvenous obliteration. J Gastroenterol 2007;42:663–72.

50. Cho SK, Shin SW, Lee IH, et al. Balloon-occluded retrograde transvenous obliteration of gastric varices: outcomes and complications in 49 patients. AJR Am J Roentgenol 2007;189:W365–72.

51. Orloff MJ, Isenberg JI, Wheeler HO, et al. A randomised trial of liver transplantation in a randomized controlled trial of emergency treatment of acutely bleeding esophageal varices in cirrhosis. Transplant Proc 2010;42(10):4101–8.

52. Henderson JM, Kutner MH, Millikan Jr WJ, et al. Endoscopic variceal sclerosis compared with distal splenorenal shunt to prevent recurrent variceal bleeding in cirrhosis. A prospective, randomized trial. Ann Intern Med 1990;112:262–9.
Shunting produced better control of bleeding but did not produce any survival advantage.

53. Rosemurgy A, Serafini F, Zweibel B, et al. Transjugular intrahepatic portosystemic shunt vs. small-diameter prosthetic H-graft portacaval shunt: extended follow-up of an expanded randomized prospective trial. J Gastrointest Surg 2000;4:589–97.

54. Rikkers LF. The changing spectrum of treatment for variceal bleeding. Ann Surg 1998;228:536–46.

55. Boyer TD, Henderson JM, Heerey AM, et al. Cost of preventing variceal rebleeding with transjugular intrahepatic portal systemic shunt and distal splenorenal shunt. J Hepatol 2008;48:407–14.

56. Dell'Era A, Grande L, Barros-Schelotto P, et al. Impact of prior portosystemic shunt procedures on outcome of liver transplantation. Surgery 2005;137:620–5.

57. Lucey MR, Brown KA, Everson GT, et al. Minimal criteria for placement of adults on liver transplant waiting list: a report of a national conference organized by the American Association for the Study of Liver Diseases. Liver Transpl Surg 1997;3:628–37.

58. Fattovich G, Giustina G, Degos F, et al. Morbidity and mortality in compensated cirrhosis type C: a retrospective follow up study of 384 patients. Gastroenterology 1997;112:463–72.

59. Andreu M, Sola R, Sitges-Serra A, et al. Risks for spontaneous bacterial peritonitis in cirrhotic patients with ascites. Gastroenterology 1993;104:1133–8.

60. D'Amico G, Pagliaro L, Bosch J. The treatment of portal hypertension: a meta-analytic review. Hepatology 1995;22:332–54.

61. Jalan R, Hayes PC. Hepatic encephalopathy and ascites. Lancet 1997;350:1309–15.

62. Gines A, Fernandez-Esparrach G, Monescillo A, et al. Randomized trial comparing albumin, dextran 70, and polygeline in cirrhotic patients with ascites treated by paracentesis. Gastroenterology 1996;111:1002–10.

63. Gines P, Arroyo V, Vargas V, et al. Paracentesis with intravenous infusion of albumin as compared with peritoneovenous shunting in cirrhosis with refractory ascites. N Engl J Med 1991;325:829–35.

64. Salerno F, Camma C, Enea M, et al. Transjugular intrahepatic portosystemic shunt for refractory ascites: a meta-analysis of individual patient data. Gastroenterology 2007;133:825–34.

65. Deltenre P, Mathurin P, Dharancy S, et al. Transjugular intrahepatic portosystemic shunt in refractory ascites: a meta-analysis. Liver Int 2005;25:349–56.

66. Saab S, Nieto JM, Lewis SK, Runyon BA. TIPS versus paracentesis for cirrhotic patients with refractory ascites. Cochrane Database Syst Rev 2006;18:CD004889

67. Beckett D, Olliff S. Interventional radiology in the management of Budd Chiari syndrome. Cardiovasc Intervent Radiol 2008;31:839–47.

68. Sharma S, Texeira A, Texeira P, et al. Pharmacological thrombolysis in Budd Chiari syndrome: a single

centre experience and review of the literature. J Hepatol 2004;40:172–80.

69. Perello A, Garcia Pagan JC, et al. TIPS is a useful long-term derivative therapy for patients with Budd Chiari syndrome uncontrolled by medical therapy. Hepatology 2002;35:132–9.

70. Eapen CE, Velissaris D, Heydtmann M, et al. Favourable medium term outcome following hepatic vein recanalisation and/or transjugular intrahepatic portosystemic shunt for Budd Chiari syndrome. Gut 2006;55:878–84.

71. Heydtmann M, Raffa S, Olliff S, et al. One year survival in Budd–Chiari syndrome treated with TIPS: an international study. Gut 2007;56(Suppl. II):A2.

72. Hernández-Guerra M, Turnes J, Rubinstein P, et al. PTFE-covered stents improve TIPS patency in Budd–Chiari syndrome. Hepatology 2004;40:1197–202.

73. Olliff SP. Transjugular intrahepatic portosystemic shunt in the management of Budd Chiari syndrome. Eur J Gastroenterol Hepatol 2006;18:1151–4.

74. Gauthier F, De Dreuzy O, Valayer J, et al. H-type shunt with an autologous venous graft for treatment of portal hypertension in children. J Pediatr Surg 1989;24:1041–3.

75. Mitra SK, Rao KL, Narasimhan KL, et al. Side-to-side lienorenal shunt without splenectomy in non-cirrhotic portal hypertension in children. J Pediatr Surg 1993;28:398–401.

76. Tuite DJ, Rehman J, Davies MH, et al. Percutaneous transsplenic access in the management of bleeding varices from chronic portal vein thrombosis. J Vasc Interv Radiol 2007;18:1571–5.

77. Uflacker R. Applications of percutaneous mechanical thrombectomy in transjugular intrahepatic portosystemic shunt and portal vein thrombosis. Tech Vasc Interv Radiol 2003;6:59–69.

78. Bilbao JI, Elorz M, Vivas I, et al. Transjugular intrahepatic portosystemic shunt (TIPS) in the treatment of venous symptomatic chronic portal thrombosis in non-cirrhotic patients. Cardiovasc Intervent Radiol 2004;27:474–80.

9

The spleen

Chee-Chee H. Stucky
Richard T. Schlinkert

Introduction

The history of the spleen, including surgery, anatomy and physiology, has been nicely detailed by McClusky et al. and will not be reviewed here.[1,2] The spleen lies in the posterior left upper quadrant superior to the level of the costal margin. It is attached to adjacent structures via a series of ligaments including the splenophrenic, splenorenal, splenocolic and gastrosplenic ligaments.

The splenic artery arises from the coeliac trunk. Aberrant anatomy may include direct origination from the aorta, the superior mesenteric, middle colic or left gastric arteries. The splenic artery gives off pancreatic branches (the largest of which is the pancreatic magna) as well as the left gastroepiploic artery before branching and entering the spleen. The hilum may consist of a single, long splenic artery that branches late into the spleen, or an artery branching much earlier after its origin. Each artery ends in the sinusoids of a segment of the spleen. The spleen also receives blood flow from the short gastric vessels.

The splenic vein leaves the hilum and runs along the posterior aspect of the pancreas, providing venous drainage of the pancreas as well. It is joined by the inferior mesenteric vein before merging with the superior mesenteric vein to form the portal vein.

The spleen is composed of two or three lobes and two to ten segments with unique arterial supplies. Accessory spleens occur in approximately 10–15% of patients and are most commonly located near the splenic hilum, but may also be located at distant sites.

The spleen plays a significant role in fighting infections, particularly of encapsulated organisms. It also serves to filter aged blood cellular elements and removes intracellular inclusions, a process known as pitting. There are extensive T-cell and dendritic cell populations located primarily in the periarterial lymphatic sheaths. B cells are located in the lymphoid nodules while macrophages are distributed widely.

While the spleen provides important immune and housekeeping functions, it may also be a source of massive blood loss from trauma, excessive cellular destruction or sequestration, certain lymphomatous or myeloid diseases, symptomatic splenomegaly, or tumours. Splenic preservation is always preferred due to its many functions, but splenectomy may be necessary in these instances.

Postsplenectomy sepsis

Asplenic patients are at increased risk of developing overwhelming sepsis throughout their lives. This lifetime risk of postsplenectomy sepsis is approximately 0.02% for adults.[3] In a recent large population-based study from Scotland, Kyaw et al.[4] showed severe infection, defined as need for hospitalisation, occurred with an incidence of 7 per 100 person-years. The risk of overwhelming infection, defined as septicaemia or meningitis, was 0.89 per 100 person-years.

✔️✔️ A high mortality is associated with overwhelming postsplenectomy infection and therefore prevention is of utmost importance. Davies et al.[5] in 2002 revised the guidelines of the British Committee for Standards in Haematology published in 1996.[6] Ideally, vaccinations should be administered a minimum of 2 weeks prior to splenectomy. Vaccinations should include polyvalent pneumococcal, haemophilus influenza type B and meningococcal C vaccines (Box 9.1). Pneumococcal vaccines should be repeated after 3–5 years.[7] Shatz et al.[8] prospectively studied 59 patients in a randomised fashion to determine the ideal timing of postoperative immunisation in patients who did not receive preoperative vaccines. Improved functional antibody responses to certain serotypes and serogroups were identified if immunisations were delayed for 14 days. Surgeons globally must be fastidious regarding compliance with vaccination guidelines.[7,9]

Trauma

The most common cause of splenic injury is blunt trauma.[10] Rupture may also occur from penetrating trauma, iatrogenic injury or, rarely, diseases such as mononucleosis or typhoid. Management of splenic trauma has evolved significantly over the last several years. Non-operative management is used in 60–80% of blunt injury cases, with success rates of 95%.[11] Initial management of all traumas should begin with primary and secondary surveys completed according to the Advanced Trauma Life Support guidelines.[12] Diagnostic evaluation for splenic injury follows and is based on the haemodynamic status of the patient. Haemodynamically unstable patients should undergo rapid focused assessment by sonography for trauma (FAST).[11,13] If FAST is not available or inconclusive, diagnostic

Box 9.1 • Immunisation recommendations

Vaccine recommendations:
- Polyvalent pneumococcus
- Haemophilus influenza B
- Meningococcus

Timing:
- Ideal: >2 weeks preoperative
- If postoperative:
  - delay 2 weeks if possible
  - better to give sooner than 2 weeks **if** follow-up is unlikely

Repeat pneumococcus vaccine once at 5 years

peritoneal lavage may be used. Scant fluid on the FAST exam should prompt a search for other causes of shock. A large amount of intraperitoneal blood on FAST is an indication for emergent laparotomy. Currently, exploration for traumatic splenic injury is performed in an open fashion.

Haemodynamically stable patients with physical findings of abdominal trauma should undergo abdominal computed tomography (CT) to assess all potential injuries. A grading system for splenic injury based on CT findings has been developed by the American Association for the Surgery of Trauma (AAST)[14] and is presented in Table 9.1. The decision to proceed to operative exploration, however, is not based solely upon these grades. All grades of injury have undergone successful non-operative management. Patients with higher grade injuries or age >55 years, however, are at increased risk for failure of non-operative management and warrant a low threshold to proceed with operative intervention.[15–17]

Indications for operative intervention in splenic trauma from the Society for Surgery of the Alimentary Tract (SSAT) Patient Care Guidelines[18] are shown in Box 9.2. The group also suggests an

Table 9.1 • American Association for the Study of Trauma (AAST) splenic injury scale based on CT criteria

Grade		Injury description
I	Haematoma	Subcapsular, <10% surface area
	Laceration	Capsular tear, <1 cm parenchymal depth
II	Haematoma	Subcapsular, 10–50% surface area. Intraparenchymal, <5 cm in diameter
	Laceration	1–3 cm parenchymal depth, which does not involve a trabecular vessel
III	Haematoma	Subcapsular, >50% surface area or expanding; ruptured subcapsular or parenchymal haematoma; intraparenchymal haematoma ≥5 cm or expanding
	Laceration	>3 cm parenchymal depth, or involving trabecular vessels
IV	Laceration	Laceration involving segmental or hilar vessels producing major devascularisation (>25% of spleen)
V	Laceration	Completely shattered spleen
	Vascular	Hilar vascular injury that devascularises spleen

Advance one grade for multiple injuries, up to grade III.

Box 9.2 • Accepted indications for operative intervention in trauma of the spleen based on Society for Surgery of the Alimentary Tract (SSAT) Patient Care Guidelines

- Haemodynamic instability
- Bleeding >1000 mL
- Transfusion of more than 2 units of blood
- Other evidence of ongoing blood loss

More aggressive non-operative approach in children <14 years of age

aggressive non-operative approach for children <14 years of age.

The use of selective arterial embolisation in the management of splenic trauma was initially described by Sclafani et al.[19] but remains somewhat controversial. Protocol-driven strategies utilising both conservative and aggressive indications for implementing embolisation have yielded excellent results.[20,21] Other groups, however, have highlighted difficulties in using CT grading systems and selective arterial embolisation, hence the conflict preventing widespread use.[22,23]

✅ The decisions implicit in non-operative management are difficult and protocols will be useful to aid this process.[14] Ultimately, decisions will be determined by clinical acumen and resources available at the centre treating the patient. The risk of postsplenectomy-related sepsis of 0.02% in adults[3] will need to be weighed against the risks of transfusions, ongoing haemorrhage and late re-bleeding.

As many as 40% of splenectomies are performed as a result of iatrogenic splenic injury.[24,25] Such injuries usually result from excess traction against either the splenic ligaments or adhesions to the spleen. The standard use of laparoscopic procedures may lower the risk of splenic injury by providing better visualisation, application of less traction, improved instrumentation for perisplenic dissection, and better control of capsular haemorrhage by the pressure of the pneumoperitoneum.[26] Haemostatic control of splenic injuries begins with direct pressure. Haemostatic agents such as microfibrillar collagen, microporous polysaccharide hemispheres or injectable haemostatic matrices may be applied to aid haemostasis.[27] Haemostatic instruments such as argon-beam coagulators may also be helpful. Ligation of selected arteries in the hilum may help control bleeding but potentially lead to a need for partial splenectomy. Splenorrhaphy and partial splenectomy have been described for splenic trauma; however, Holubar et al.[28] showed the most

important factor in preventing adverse outcome after iatrogenic splenic injury is prompt cessation of bleeding by whatever means. Splenectomy, while not desirable, is preferable to significant blood loss and should be performed when bleeding is excessive, if the patient cannot tolerate prolonged procedures, or if there are other factors that would make re-bleeding a greater risk than splenectomy.

Elective indications for splenectomy

Most recommendations for elective splenic surgery are based on level III or IV evidence. This is likely due to the relative rarity of diseases requiring splenectomy and the length of follow-up required to assess results. Recent literature reviews are referenced in this chapter when the supporting literature is composed largely of smaller non-prospective studies regarding a particular disease.

Immune thrombocytopenic purpura

The most common non-traumatic indication for splenectomy is immune thrombocytopenic purpura (ITP). This disease is characterised by low platelet count, normal bone marrow (increased megakaryocytes) and absence of other causes of thrombocytopenia. The destruction of platelets in this condition is mediated by platelet antibodies and the spleen is typically the site of destruction of the platelets. ITP remains a diagnosis of exclusion as tests for antiplatelet antibodies are not reliable indicators of the disease. The spleen is usually normal in size. Platelet function is also normal and while spontaneous bruising is common, severe haemorrhage is less likely unless platelet levels drop below 10 000.

✅✅ Corticosteroid therapy is frequently instituted with platelet counts of 20 000–30 000.[29–31] Most patients will respond to medical therapy, at least initially. If counts respond and are sustained, the treatment is stopped and patients are observed. Intravenous immunoglobulin may be used to increase platelet counts temporarily, but the response lasts days to weeks only. Patients who require prolonged treatment or do not respond to medical therapy should be considered for splenectomy.

Approximately 80% of patients respond to splenectomy and 65–85% of patients sustain response long term.[31] There is no widely accepted factor to predict response to splenectomy. If platelet counts drop after splenectomy, peripheral blood smears may show absence of nuclear inclusions (e.g. Howell–Jolley bodies) indicating residual splenic tissue. Nuclear medicine scans, magnetic resonance imaging or CT may help localise such remnants for re-exploration or embolisation. Mild to moderate degrees of thrombocytopenia without symptoms of purpura or bleeding postsplenectomy may be observed without resuming medical therapy.[31]

Evans syndrome

Evans syndrome is characterised by autoimmune haemolytic anaemia and autoimmune thrombocytopenia. Splenectomy may be curative in up to 40% of patients and improve the situation in up to 60%; however, failures are common.[32]

Hereditary spherocytosis

Hereditary spherocytosis results from abnormalities of membrane proteins, particularly spectrin. The degree of spectrin deficiency varies, as does the pattern of inheritance. Approximately 75% of cases demonstrate an autosomal dominant pattern. Autosomal recessive patients have a greater degree of spectrin deficiency and unlike the autosomal dominant patients do not respond to splenectomy. The disease is characterised by extravascular destruction of red cells, particularly in the spleen.[33]

✔✔ Guidelines from the General Haematology Task Force of the British Committee for Standards in Haematology state that patients with severe disease presenting in childhood require splenectomy.[34] If possible, surgery should be delayed until after 6 years of age to allow maturation of the immune system. Patients with mild disease may be safely observed. Otherwise, patients should be selected for splenectomy based on clinical symptoms and associated complications such as gallstones. Cholecystectomy should be performed if gallstones are present at the time of splenectomy.[34]

Several groups have reported the use of subtotal splenectomy for the treatment of hereditary spherocytosis and demonstrated amelioration of anaemia and maintenance of immune function. Mild to moderate haemolysis, however, may persist and gallstone formation and aplastic crises still developed in some patients.[35–37]

Elliptocytosis

The protein spectrin is also abnormal in elliptocytosis. Many mild cases require no therapy; however, if greater than 90% of cells are affected anaemia, is substantive, and splenectomy should be considered.

Thallassaemias

Genetic abnormalities resulting in abnormal haemoglobin structure, such as thalassaemias, may require splenectomy. Defective alpha chains and beta chains in the haemoglobin tetramer lead to alpha thalassaemia and beta thalassaemia, respectively. The alpha chains precipitate in the absence of the beta chains and create the more severe beta thalassaemia. Blood transfusions and chelation therapy are the mainstays of treatment; however, stem cell transplantation is playing a greater role in the management of this disease.[38] Splenectomy is rarely required. Thalassaemia patients are at increased risk of infective complications postoperatively.

Sickle cell anaemia

Sickle cell anaemia is characterised by high HgF levels. Major indications for splenectomy are recurrent acute splenic sequestration crisis, hypersplenism, splenic abscess and massive splenic infarction.[39] Cholecystectomy is recommended if gallstones are present, also simplifying the diagnosis if abdominal crisis occurs in the future.

Autoimmune haemolytic anaemia

Autoimmune haemolytic anaemia caused by IgG may respond to splenectomy in perhaps 50% of cases. Failure of medical therapy or need for high-dose steroids should prompt consideration of splenectomy. IgM haemolytic anaemias are not splenic driven and will not respond to splenectomy.

Lymphoma

Laparotomy was formerly necessary for the diagnosis and/or staging of Hodgkin's lymphoma; however, it is now rarely indicated due to advancement of treatment algorithms and diagnostic imaging. Surgery plays essentially no role in the treatment of non-Hodgkin's lymphoma. Splenectomy may be required for symptomatic splenomegaly, hypersplenism, diagnosis (in cases of isolated splenic disease) or 'debulking' of splenic predominant disease.

Myeloid disease

Splenectomy plays little or no role in the treatment of chronic myelogenous leukaemias. Similarly, systemic therapy has replaced splenectomy as the primary treatment of hairy cell leukaemia, reserving splenectomy for refractory disease.

The spleen may reach truly massive proportions in primary myelofibrosis. This may lead to symptomatic splenomegaly, thrombocytopenia, hypercatabolic state with resultant high output heart failure, and forward flow portal hypertension. Medical therapy has delayed splenectomy until the last stages of the disease. Splenectomy may improve quality of life; however, it does not alter the course of the underlying disease. Mortality rates are high due to severe bleeding complications, heart failure and advanced stage of underlying disease at the time of splenectomy.

Volvulus

Some spleens have elongated or absent ligamentous attachments, leading to a 'wandering' spleen. These spleens may undergo torsion on their vascular pedicle. Patients present with severe abdominal pain and a right lower quadrant mass, occasionally occurring intermittently. A viable spleen should be returned to the left upper quadrant and fixed in place using a mesh sac tacked to the diaphragm.[40] A necrotic spleen requires splenectomy.

Haemangiomas

Haemangiomas are the most common benign neoplasm in the spleen. Small lesions (less than 4 cm) may be safely watched.[41] Risks presented by larger haemangiomas are unclear. Therefore, splenectomy versus observation must be individually determined.

Cysts

Cystic lesions of the spleen are often classified as parasitic or non-parasitic. Cyst size and symptoms determine surgical intervention. Asymptomatic cysts with reassuring radiographic features may be observed. Cysts greater than 5 cm in diameter are at potentially higher risk of rupture, so intervention may be indicated either by laparoscopic deroofing or resection. Percutaneous drainage and alcohol ablation have also been used with unreliable results. Bacterial abscesses may be drained either by percutaneous or surgical means. Occasionally, splenectomy is required.[42]

Parasitic cysts are usually echinococcal in origin and the diagnosis is often confirmed by serological studies. Splenic conserving techniques may be appropriate for early disease or disease located at the perimeter of the spleen.[43] Spillage of hydatid cyst contents must be meticulously avoided as anaphylactic shock may occur.

Portal hypertension

Sinistral (left-sided) portal hypertension secondary to splenic vein thrombosis may lead to bleeding gastric varices. Splenectomy is curative. This is a situation where preoperative splenic artery embolisation should be considered to decrease venous pressure in the splenic collaterals, thereby increasing the safety of surgery. Embolisation can be performed under the same anaesthesia as the splenectomy, since splenic embolisation is extremely painful to the patient.

Preparation for splenectomy

Preoperative preparation for splenectomy, as for other procedures, is designed to prevent or minimise complications. Splenectomy carries the usual risk of other abdominal operations and, depending on the disease, increased risks such as bleeding, coagulopathies including disseminated intravascular coagulation, infection (both immediate and delayed) and altered cardiovascular performance.

Efforts should be made to correct all coagulopathies and optimise blood counts preoperatively if possible. In patients with ITP, laparoscopic splenectomy can be performed safely with very low platelet counts. If platelets are to be given in destructive or consumptive states, transfusion should be withheld if possible until the splenic artery is ligated to prevent the rapid breakdown of the transfused platelets.

Patients with massive splenomegaly secondary to primary myelofibrosis may have hypertrophied cardiac dysfunction, pulmonary hypertension, ascites and pleural effusions. The patient's cardiac and pulmonary conditions should be optimised preoperatively. Appropriate preoperative antibiotics should be given to reduce the risk of infection, particularly in immunocompromised states.

Technique

Open splenectomy

Open splenectomy remains the standard for trauma surgery and should be considered in patients with massive splenomegaly or portal hypertension.

The patient is placed in the supine position and prepped from nipples to pubis. An upper midline or left subcostal incision may be used. Our preference is for an upper midline approach, which may be extended in the case of massive splenomegaly. Four-quadrant packing can control traumatic bleeding temporarily. Once packs are removed sequentially and bleeding controlled, the spleen is mobilised from its lateral attachments. The hilum may be compressed by the surgeon's hands to secure haemostasis while the remaining vessels are controlled. The remaining vascular attachments are divided and the spleen removed. Haemostasis is ensured, in particular by inspecting the ligated short gastric vessels.

Alternatively, early entrance to the lesser sac and ligation of the splenic hilum facilitates platelet transfusions as necessary, as well as control of bleeding as the spleen is further mobilised. Hilar vessels are divided between clamps and ligated or divided with a linear stapler when appropropriate. Accessory spleens should be sought and removed if surgery is designed to correct a destructive or sequestration state.

Laparoscopic splenectomy

✓ Laparoscopic splenectomy has been shown to be safe and provides comparative haematological results, with a lower risk of postoperative complications and reduced length of hospital stay when compared to open splenectomy. Laparoscopic splenectomy is the preferred procedure for non-traumatic splenectomy in patients with normal to moderately enlarged spleens. Hand-assisted laparoscopic splenectomy should be considered in cases of significant splenomegaly.[44,45] Open splenectomy is preferred when spleens are so large that an adequate laparoscopic working space is not feasible.

The operative goal of laparoscopic splenectomy is circumferential mobilisation of the splenic hilum for transection. Reported techniques vary in the sequence in which the ligaments are divided, but all procedures involve the same steps.[46,47] The patient is placed in the right lateral semidecubitus position and is rolled back slightly from full lateral decubitus so that the midline is exposed should urgent conversion to open surgery be required. The surgeon and camera operator stand in front of the patient and one assistant stands behind the patient. We prefer a five-port technique but others report a four-port technique.[47] The omentum and transverse mesocolon are examined for accessory spleens. A wary eye is kept to identify accessory spleens throughout the procedure. Steps of dissection are illustrated

in **Figs 9.1–9.6**.[46] Dissection begins by dividing the splenocolic ligament and then proceeds anteriorly. The lesser sac is opened and the gastrosplenic ligament, including the short gastric vessels, is divided. The main splenic artery is isolated and ligated, if feasible, to facilitate later hilar transaction and decrease bleeding at the staple line. The lateral

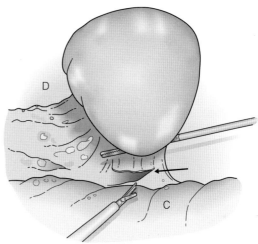

Figure 9.1 • After exploration, dissection of the splenic attachments is begun with the splenocolic ligament (arrow). Traction is always placed toward the spleen with countertraction, if necessary. C, colon; D, diaphragm. Reprinted with permission from Schlinkert RT, Teotia SS. Laparoscopic splenectomy. Arch Surg 1999; 134:100–1. Copyright © 1999, American Medical Association. All rights reserved.

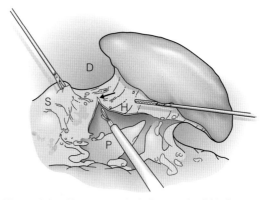

Figure 9.2 • The gastrosplenic ligament is divided (arrow). Dissection is begun at the inferior aspect and continued until all short gastric vessels are divided. The superior medial aspect of the splenophrenic ligament is also divided. D, diaphragm; H, hilum; P, pancreas; S, stomach. Reprinted with permission from Schlinkert RT, Teotia SS. Laparoscopic splenectomy. Arch Surg 1999; 134:100–1. Copyright © 1999, American Medical Association. All rights reserved.

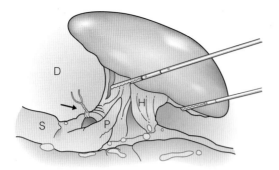

Figure 9.3 • If the splenic artery can be identified superior to the tail of the pancreas, it is ligated (arrow). D, diaphragm; H, hilum; P, pancreas; S, stomach. Reprinted with permission from Schlinkert RT, Teotia SS. Laparoscopic splenectomy. Arch Surg 1999; 134:100–1. Copyright © 1999, American Medical Association. All rights reserved.

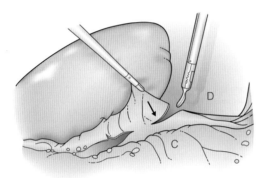

Figure 9.4 • The splenorenal ligament (arrow) is divided, retracting the spleen anteriorly. Areolar connective tissue between this ligament and the splenic hilum is gently divided. C, colon; D, diaphragm. Reprinted with permission from Schlinkert RT, Teotia SS. Laparoscopic splenectomy. Arch Surg 1999; 134:100–1. Copyright © 1999, American Medical Association. All rights reserved.

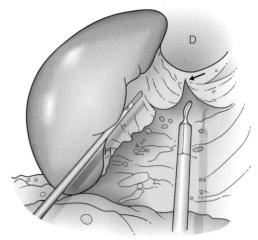

Figure 9.5 • The gastrophrenic ligament is divided (arrow) and areolar connective tissue again is dissected. At the completion of this step, the splenic hilum has been mobilised circumferentially. D, diaphragm; H, hilum. Reprinted with permission from Schlinkert RT, Teotia SS. Laparoscopic splenectomy. Arch Surg 1999; 134:100–1. Copyright © 1999, American Medical Association. All rights reserved.

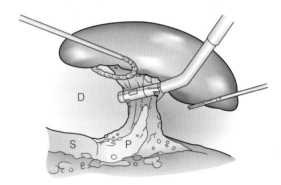

Figure 9.6 • The splenic hilum is now divided with the spleen retracted far into the left upper quadrant. After transection, the spleen is placed in a bag, morcellated and removed. D, diaphragm; P, pancreas; S, stomach. Reprinted with permission from Schlinkert RT, Teotia SS. Laparoscopic splenectomy. Arch Surg 1999; 134:100–1. Copyright © 1999, American Medical Association. All rights reserved.

attachments are divided. Some surgeons will leave the highest end of the splenophrenic ligament attached until after hilar transection to prevent rotation; this is known as the 'hanged spleen' technique.[48]

The hilar vessels are freed from the pancreas and staple ligation is performed. The hilum may also be controlled using clips or energy devices. The spleen is placed into a bag and morcellated after the open end of the bag is brought through a trocar site.

Resection of large spleens is facilitated by rotating the patient more towards a supine position to enhance exposure of the splenic artery. The length of the spleen is often a misleading indicator of the success of the laparoscopic approach. More often the bulk of the spleen, as assessed by its anterior–posterior and lateral–medial dimensions, has a greater effect on exposure. Hand-assisted techniques are valuable aids for removing larger spleens, allowing safer dissection of the hilum and easier vascular control should trouble arise. The spleen may be removed intact through the lower abdominal hand incision or morcellated as needed. Spleens that are so large as to prevent creation of a laparoscopic working space should be removed using an open approach.

Most patients that undergo laparoscopic splenectomy for ITP leave the hospital on the day following surgery. Recovery varies with greater degrees of splenomegaly or hypersplenism.

Postoperative management and complications

Major postoperative complications include haemorrhage, subphrenic abscess, pancreatitis, pancreatic fistula or overwhelming sepsis. Venous thrombosis is also a serious complication of splenectomy, particularly when involving the portal vein or mesenteric veins. All complications should be treated immediately upon diagnosis.

Asplenic patients should be treated with a high index of suspicion for overwhelming sepsis and broad-spectrum antibiotic therapy should be initiated with early signs of infection. Those patients not receiving immunisations preoperatively should be vaccinated 2 weeks after splenectomy. This should be performed prior to discharge from hospital if there is concern for poor compliance or follow-up.

Summary

Laparoscopic splenectomy is the preferred method of splenic removal for most haematological conditions. Hand-assisted laparoscopic splenectomy may be useful in cases of significant splenomegaly. Open splenectomy is reserved for trauma, extreme splenomegaly and at the discretion of the surgeon. Attention to preoperative preparation, meticulous technique and careful postoperative care allow excellent results for these procedures.

Key points

- Most splenic injuries can be safely managed non-operatively. Management protocols may improve success.
- Vaccinations are mandatory for patients undergoing splenectomy and are ideally administered more than 2 weeks preoperatively.
- ITP is the most common haematological indication for splenectomy, with response rates of approximately 80%.
- Laparoscopic splenectomy is the procedure of choice for haematological diseases when the spleen is normal to moderately enlarged. Hand-assisted techniques may improve success rates for significantly enlarged spleens.
- Open splenectomy is preferred for trauma, extreme splenomegaly or at the surgeon's discretion.

References

1. McClusky 3rd DA, Skandalakis LJ, Colborn GL, et al. Tribute to a triad: history of splenic anatomy, physiology, and surgery – part 1. World J Surg 1999;23:311–25.

2. McClusky 3rd DA, Skandalakis LJ, Colborn GL, et al. Tribute to a triad: history of splenic anatomy, physiology, and surgery – part 2. World J Surg 1999;23:514–26.

3. Galvan DA, Peitzman AB. Failure of nonoperative management of abdominal solid organ injuries. Curr Opin Crit Care 2006;12:590–4.

4. Kyaw MH, Holmes EM, Toolis F, et al. Evaluation of severe infection and survival after splenectomy. Am J Med 2006;276(119):271–7.

5. Davies JM, Barnes R, Milligan D. Update of guidelines for the prevention and treatment of infection in patients with an absent or dysfunctional spleen. Clin Med 2002;2:440–3.

6. Working Party of the British Committee for Standards in Haematology Clinical Haematology Task Force. Guidelines for the prevention and treatment of infection in patients with an absent or dysfunctional spleen. Br Med J 1996;312:430–4.
   Evidence-based guidelines outlining prevention of sepsis in splenectomised patients.

7. Mourtzoukou EG, Pappas G, Peppas G, et al. Vaccination of asplenic or hyposplenic adults. Br J Surg 2008;95:273–80.
   Evidence-based guidelines outlining prevention of sepsis in splenectomised patients.

8. Shatz DV, Schinsky MF, Pais LB, et al. Immune responses of splenectomized trauma patients to the 23-valent pneumococcal polysaccharide vaccine at 1 versus 7 versus 14 days after splenectomy. J Trauma 1998;44:760–6.

9. Kyaw MH, Holmes EM, Chalmers J, et al. A survey of vaccine coverage and antibiotic prophylaxis in splenectomised patients in Scotland. J Clin Pathol 2002;55:472–4.

10. Savage SA, Zarzaur BL, Magnotti LJ, et al. The evolution of blunt splenic injury: resolution and progression. J Trauma 2008;64:1085–91.

11. Schroeppel TJ, Croce MA. Diagnosis and management of blunt abdominal solid organ injury. Curr Opin Crit Care 2007;13:399–404.

12. American College of Surgeons. Advanced trauma life support for doctors. 8th ed Chicago: American College of Surgeons; 2008.

13. Rozycki GS. Surgeon-performed ultrasound: its use in clinical practice. Ann Surg 1998;228:16–28.

14. Tinkoff G, Esposito TJ, Reed J, et al. American Association for the Surgery of Trauma Organ Injury Scale I: spleen, liver, and kidney, validation based on National Trauma Data Bank. J Am Coll Surg 2008;207:646–55.

15. Harbrecht BG, Peitzman AB, Rivera L, et al. Contribution of age and gender to outcome of blunt splenic injury in adults: multicenter study of the Eastern Association for the Surgery of Trauma. J Trauma 2001;51:887–95.

16. McIntyre LK, Schiff M, Jurkovich GJ. Failure of nonoperative management of splenic injuries: causes and consequences. Arch Surg 2005;140:563–9.

17. Smith Jr JS, Wengrovitz MA, DeLong BS. Prospective validation of criteria, including age, for safe, nonsurgical management of the ruptured spleen. J Trauma 1992;33:363–9.

18. Patient Care Committee of the Society for Surgery of the Alimentary Tract (SSAT). Surgical treatment of injuries and diseases of the spleen. J Gastrointest Surg 2005;9:453–4.

19. Sclafani SJ, Shaftan GW, Scalea TM, et al. Nonoperative salvage of computed tomography-diagnosed splenic injuries: utilization of angiography for triage and embolization for hemostasis. J Trauma 1995;39:818–27.

20. Cooney R, Ku J, Cherry R, et al. Limitations of splenic angioembolization in treating blunt splenic injury. J Trauma 2005;59:926–32.

21. Haan J, Ilahi ON, Kramer M, et al. Protocol-driven nonoperative management in patients with blunt splenic trauma and minimal associated injury decreases length of stay. J Trauma 2003;55:317–22.

22. Barquist ES, Pizano LR, Feuer W, et al. Inter- and intrarater reliability in computed axial tomographic grading of splenic injury: why so many grading scales? J Trauma 2004;56:334–8.

23. Harbrecht BG, Ko SH, Watson GA, et al. Angiography for blunt splenic trauma does not improve the success rate of nonoperative management. J Trauma 2007;63:44–9.

24. Cassar K, Munro A. Iatrogenic splenic injury. J R Coll Edinb 2002;47:731–41.

25. Merchea A, Dozois EJ, Wang JK, et al. Anatomic mechanisms for splenic injury during colorectal surgery. Clin Anat 2012;25(2):212–7.

26. Malek MM, Greenstein AJ, Chin EH, et al. Comparison of iatrogenic splenectomy during open and laparoscopic colon resection. Surg Laparosc Endosc Percutan Tech 2007;17:385–7.

27. Chung BI, Desai MM, Gill IS. Management of intraoperative splenic injury during laparoscopic urological surgery. BJU Int 2011;108:572–6.

28. Holubar SD, Wang JK, Wolff BG, et al. Splenic salvage after intraoperative splenic injury during colectomy. Arch Surg 2009;144:1040–5.

29. Ruggeri M, Rodeghiero F, Tosetto A. Steroids and intravenous immune globulines for the treatment of acute idiopathic thrombocytopenic purpura in adults. Cochrane Database Syst Rev 2007;4.
Evidence base for medical therapy of ITP.

30. Portielje JE, Westendorp RG, Kluin-Nelemans HC, et al. Morbidity and mortality in adults with idiopathic thrombocytopenic purpura. Blood 2001;97:2549–54.

31. Provan D, Stasi R, Newland AC, et al. International consensus report on the investigation and management of primary immune thrombocytopenia. Blood 2010;115:168–86.
Evidence base for medical therapy of ITP.

32. Duperier T, Felsher J, Brody F. Laparoscopic splenectomy for Evans syndrome. Surg Laparosc Endosc Percutan Tech 2003;13:45–7.

33. Smedley JC, Bellingham AJ. Current problems in haematology. 2: Hereditary spherocytosis. J Clin Pathol 1991;44:441–4.

34. Bolton-Maggs PH, Langer JC, Iolascon A, et al. Guidelines for the diagnosis and management of hereditary spherocytosis – 2011 update. Br J Haematol 2011;156:37–49.
Evidence base for medical therapy of hereditary spherocytosis.

35. Stoehr GA, Stauffer UG, Eber SW. Near-total splenectomy: a new technique for the management of hereditary spherocytosis. Ann Surg 2005;241:40–7.

36. Bader-Meunier B, Gauthier F, Archambaud F, et al. Long-term evaluation of the beneficial effect of subtotal splenectomy for management of hereditary spherocytosis. Blood 2001;97:399–403.

37. Buesing KL, Tracy ET, Kiernan C, et al. Partial splenectomy for hereditary spherocytosis: a multi-institutional review. J Pediatr Surg 2011;46:178–83.

38. Locatelli F, De Stefano P. Innovative approaches to hematopoietic stem cell transplantation for patients with thalassaemia. Haematologica 2005;90:1592–4.

39. Al-Salem AH. Indications and complications of splenectomy for children with sickle cell disease. J Pediatr Surg 2006;41:1909–15.

40. Rescorla FJ, West KW, Engum SA, et al. Laparoscopic splenic procedures in children: experience in 231 children. Ann Surg 2007;246:683–8.

41. Willcox TM, Speer RW, Schlinkert RT, et al. Hemangioma of the spleen: presentation, diagnosis, and management. J Gastrointest Surg 2000;4:611–3.

42. Hansen MB, Moller AC. Splenic cysts. Surg Laparosc Endosc Percutan Tech 2004;14:316–22.

43. Kalinova K, Stefanova P, Bosheva M. Surgery in children with hydatid disease of the spleen. J Pediatr Surg 2006;41:1264–6.

44. Habermalz B, Sauerland S, Decker G, et al. Laparoscopic splenectomy: the clinical practice guidelines of the European Association for Endoscopic Surgery (EAES). Surg Endosc 2008;22:821–48.

45. Park AE, Birgisson G, Mastrangelo MJ, et al. Laparoscopic splenectomy: outcomes and lessons learned from over 200 cases. Surgery 2000;128:660–7.

46. Schlinkert RT, Teotia SS. Laparoscopic splenectomy. Arch Surg 1999;134:99–103.

47. Katkhouda N, Hurwitz MB, Rivera RT, et al. Laparoscopic splenectomy: outcome and efficacy in 103 consecutive patients. Ann Surg 1998;228:568–78.

48. Delaitre B. Laparoscopic splenectomy. The "hanged spleen" technique. Surg Endosc 1995;9:528–9.

10

Gallstones

Leslie K. Nathanson

Introduction

In the UK it has been estimated from autopsy studies that approximately 12% of men and 24% of women of all ages have gallstones present.[1] The prevalence in North America is comparable to that in the UK, and it is believed that 10–30% of gallstones become symptomatic. There is a high prevalence in native Americans, who have an incidence of 50% in men and 75% in women in the age group 25–44 years, and this points to the importance of genetic factors in the aetiology of gallstones. In the UK more than 40 000 cholecystectomies are performed each year,[2] whereas in the USA approximately 500 000 operations are performed annually.[3] The incidence of common bile duct stones found before or during cholecystectomy is approximately 12%,[4] indicating that in the UK alone more than 4000 common bile ducts require stone clearance annually.

Composition, formation and risk factors

Gallstones are usually designated as cholesterol stones, mixed stones or pigment stones.[5] Pure cholesterol and pure pigment stones account for only 20% of gallstones, and mixed stones are considered as variants of cholesterol stones as they usually contain over 50% cholesterol and account for about 80% of gallstones in Western countries. Chemical analysis shows a continuous spectrum of stone composition rather than three mutually exclusive stone types, and 10–20% contain enough calcium to be rendered radio-opaque.

The two most important determinants of gallstone frequency in any population are age and gender; gallstones become more common with increasing age and are at least twice as common in women.[6] The increased frequency in women becomes manifest at puberty, and an increased risk of gallstones is conferred by parity and by the ingestion of oral contraceptives.[7] Other factors related to the development of cholesterol gallstones include obesity, ileal disease or resection, cirrhosis, cystic fibrosis, diabetes mellitus, long-term parenteral nutrition, impaired gallbladder emptying, ingestion of clofibrate,[8] heart transplant,[9] and periods of dieting on a very low fat diet.[10] A positive family history of previous cholecystectomy also increases the risk of developing symptomatic gallstone disease.[11] Increasing evidence is emerging that impaired colonic motility contributes to stone formation, and speculation arises for this as a means of prevention.[12]

Pigmented gallstones are composed mainly of calcium hydrogen bilirubinate, in a polymerised and oxidised form in 'black' stones and in unpolymerised form in 'brown' stones. Black stones form in sterile gallbladder bile, but brown stones form secondary to stasis and anaerobic infection in any part of the biliary tree (**Fig. 10.1**).

Black stones form only in the gallbladder due to hyperbilirubinbilia caused by haemolysis of any cause, ineffective erythropoiesis due to vitamin B_{12} and folate deficiency, and induced enterohepatic cycling of uncojugated bilirubinate.

Brown stones form in any part of the biliary tree from any cause of chronic stasis and anaerobic infection. Anaerobes secrete enzymes that hydrolyse

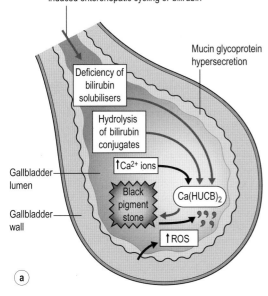

Increased bilirubin conjugate secretion (hyperbilirubinbilia):
Causes:
  bilirubin overproduction
  (haemolysis, ineffective erythropoesis)
  induced enterohepatic cycling of bilirubin

Mucin glycoprotein hypersecretion

Deficiency of bilirubin solubilisers

Hydrolysis of bilirubin conjugates

↑Ca^{2+} ions

Gallbladder lumen

Gallbladder wall

Black pigment stone

Ca(HUCB)$_2$

↑ROS

(a)

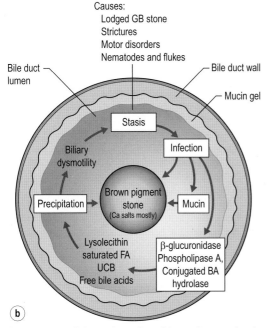

Causes:
  Lodged GB stone
  Strictures
  Motor disorders
  Nematodes and flukes

Bile duct lumen

Bile duct wall

Mucin gel

Stasis

Biliary dysmotility

Infection

Precipitation

Brown pigment stone (Ca salts mostly)

Mucin

Lysolecithin saturated FA UCB Free bile acids

β-glucuronidase Phospholipase A, Conjugated BA hydrolase

(b)

Figure 10.1 • Schematic outline of the pathogenesis of 'black' pigmented stones in sterile gallbladder bile **(a)** and 'brown' pigmented stones in an obstructed biliary tree (gallbladder infrequently) infected with a mixed anaerobic microflora derived from the colon **(b)**. Adapted from Vitek L, Carey MC. New pathophysiologic concepts underlying pathogenesis of pigment gallstones. Clin Res Hepatol Gastroenterol 2012; 36(2):122–9.

ester and amide linkages in biliary lipids into calcium-sensitive anions that phase separately as insoluble anions or calcium salts. These precipitates deposit on obstructing elements such as small cholesterol crystals, black stones from the gallbladder, parasite eggs and dead worms or flukes. Oriental hepatolithiasis syndrome is the most serious manifestation of brown pigment stone disease.[13]

Presentation

Gallstones present with symptoms related to the site of the gallstones and are therefore considered according to site.

Cholecystolithiasis

Gallstones confined to the gallbladder may present with an acute episode of pain from acute cholecystitis, biliary colic, chronic recurrent abdominal discomfort from repeated episodes of mild biliary colic, or from a vague collection of symptoms usually referred to as flatulent dyspepsia.

Pathophysiology

Impaction of a stone in the neck of the gallbladder is thought to result in gallbladder spasm, which produces biliary colic. As the stone falls back, the gallbladder empties and the pain stops, whereas continuing impaction of the stone in the gallbladder neck produces continuing pain. The trapped bile alters in composition, producing local inflammation, which creates a more constant pain that may take several days to resolve. The gallbladder contents may become infected, adding to the patient's toxaemia, and may lead to the development of empyema or possible gangrene and perforation. An empyema will produce pain, right upper quadrant tenderness and a swinging pyrexia. Urgent intervention at this point is required since conservative measures rarely succeed in resolution. Increasing oedema and intramural vascular compromise may result in infarction of the gallbladder wall, with consequent perforation of the organ.

The pathophysiology behind 'flatulent dyspepsia' is not understood. The gallbladder may be shrunken and contracted from episodes of subclinical inflammation, but it is not unusual to find a normal-looking gallbladder at cholecystectomy in patients with gallstones causing 'flatulent dyspepsia'. Contraction of the gallbladder against stones is the traditional explanation for postprandial discomfort, but there is a poor correlation between such symptoms and the presence of gallstones in a general population. A mucocoele may develop when a gallstone impacts in Hartmann's pouch in an empty gallbladder. The gallbladder secretes mucus behind the obstructing stone, producing a steady increase in the size of the gallbladder, which may be easily palpable.

Clinical features

There is a poor correlation between pathological findings in the gallbladder wall and the presenting clinical features. Typically, acute cholecystitis presents with sharp, constant, right upper quadrant pain, which frequently is of sudden onset but may have been preceded by years of postprandial epigastric discomfort. It will be worse on inspiration or movement and frequently radiates to the back or to the tip of the right shoulder blade. It may be associated with nausea, vomiting or loss of appetite, and may persist for several days. Examination may reveal signs of toxaemia; the abdomen is tender in the right upper quadrant and classically a positive Murphy's sign is elicited. In more advanced cases, there may be a palpable inflammatory mass, which is usually due to an enlarged oedematous gallbladder surrounded by adherent omentum. Clinical signs of swinging pyrexia, tachycardia and impaired cardiorespiratory function should raise clinical suspicion of an empyema. The development of diffuse upper abdominal peritonism is a sign of perforation of the gallbladder. The presence of jaundice suggests choledocholithiasis, although the possibility of common bile duct compression from an inflamed and oedematous gallbladder may need to be considered (Mirizzi's syndrome type 1).

Biliary colic presents in a similar fashion to acute cholecystitis but is usually not affected by movement and lasts only for several hours. It is often precipitated by ingestion of fatty foods but resolution is spontaneous. Chronic pain due to gallstones is attributed to the occurrence of 'flatulent dyspepsia' characterised by bouts of postprandial fullness, belching, nausea and a sensation of regurgitation of food. A family history of gallstone disease is not unusual, and factors predisposing to the development of gallstones may be present. Patients presenting with flatulent dyspepsia or recurrent episodes of biliary colic have little to find on examination.

Choledocholithiasis

Pathophysiology

It is uncertain whether all common bile duct (CBD) stones produce symptoms. It is traditionally held that the CBD cannot produce colicky pain as it does not contain smooth muscle, but pain in the right upper quadrant following cholecystectomy may be a sign of retained bile duct stones. A stone impacted in the lower end of the CBD may also be associated with nausea and vomiting, and undoubtedly the muscular spasms of the sphincter of Oddi or duodenum could account for the pain that is often felt radiating through to the back. Obstructive jaundice results when a stone becomes impacted within the CBD, in the tapered portion within the pancreas or ampulla. A stone may pass spontaneously or fall back into the CBD ('ball-valving') with spontaneous regression of the jaundice, or it may remain impacted until it is removed. A stone at the lower end of the CBD may also cause pancreatitis by temporary obstruction of the pancreatic duct, and this may be associated with transient jaundice (see Chapter 13). Ascending cholangitis results from infection within an obstructed or poorly draining biliary system. In patients with CBD stones, coliforms are identified within the bile in around 80% of cases.[14] The classic Charcot's triad of symptoms produced by bile duct stones with cholangitis consists of pain, obstructive jaundice and fever (with or without rigors). Acute cholangitis may progress to acute obstructive suppurative cholangitis with pain, obstructive jaundice, fever, hypotension and mental obtundation (Reynolds' pentad) requiring early recognition and prompt endoscopic retrograde cholangiopancreatography (ERCP) drainage to save life.[15]

Clinical features

Presentation of a patient with right upper quadrant pain some time after cholecystectomy may indicate choledocholithiasis. However, CBD stones are more likely to be either silent and found at the time of cholecystectomy or present due to one of the complications of obstructive jaundice, pancreatitis or ascending cholangitis. Pain is associated more frequently with obstructive jaundice due to gallstones as opposed to an underlying malignancy. In addition to the presence of bilirubin in the urine and pale stool, obstructive jaundice may be associated with pruritus and steatorrhoea. Examination will not normally reveal a palpable gallbladder, and features of pancreatitis should be sought. Ascending cholangitis should be suspected in the presence of rigors and swinging pyrexia associated with jaundice. The patient may demonstrate signs of bacteraemia or septicaemia with a flushed appearance, tachycardia and hypotension.

Investigation

The diagnosis of gallstone disease is suspected on clinical grounds but relies on the relevant laboratory or radiological investigations for confirmation. The differentiation between gallstone causes for pain and other acute intra-abdominal disease should include an erect chest radiograph and plain radiograph of the abdomen. Less than 10% of gall-stones are radio-opaque and therefore the yield from abdominal radiographs is low. Occasionally, in cases of intestinal obstruction, air is seen in the biliary tree, suggesting a cholecyst–enteric fistula and gallstone ileus.

Blood tests

Liver function tests (LFTs) should be performed routinely in patients with suspected gallstones. Although these may not be affected by the presence of cholecystolithiasis, they may be abnormal in the presence of choledocholithiasis. An isolated increase of unconjugated bilirubin is present in prehepatic jaundice such as is seen with excessive haemolysis. The biochemical picture of hepatic jaundice, as seen with hepatitis, is one of raised conjugated and unconjugated bilirubin, high aspartate (AST) and alanine (ALT) transaminase levels, but associated with a relatively normal or slightly raised alkaline phosphatase (ALP). Posthepatic (obstructive) jaundice is associated with a raised conjugated bilirubin only, high ALP, and normal AST and ALT. In late cases of obstructive jaundice or in acute cholangitis, the transaminase levels will rise as hepatocellular damage proceeds. Minor abnormalities in the LFTs occur with non-obstructing stones in the CBD. These minor abnormalities may prompt the undertaking of an operative cholangiogram at the time of surgery if a selective operative cholangiogram policy is being pursued.[16,17]

Approximately 60% of patients with CBD stones (including asymptomatic stones) will have one or more abnormal LFTs, although a substantial number of patients with an abnormal LFT will not have CBD stones. Bilirubin, ALP and γ-glutamyl transpeptidase (GGT) are the most sensitive tests routinely used.[18] In the acute situation, a serum amylase or lipase level should also be ascertained to exclude a diagnosis of pancreatitis, and a raised white blood cell count may support a clinical diagnosis of acute cholecystitis.

Ultrasonography

Ultrasound is the investigation used most widely to confirm the diagnosis of cholelithiasis. It is easy to perform, causes little discomfort to the patient, avoids irradiation and potentially toxic contrast media, and may be useful in demonstrating and assessing other structures in the upper abdomen. The gallbladder wall, as well as its contents, can be assessed and this may give additional information useful for planning management. CBD stones may be harder to identify, although the presence of a dilated CBD and small stones within the gallbladder give clues as to their presence. If the gallbladder cannot be identified, the presence of an echogenic focus in the gallbladder area is nearly as specific a finding as that of calculi in a distended gallbladder. With high-quality ultrasound scanning, gallstones should be detected in at least 95% of patients with stones. Its reliability in detecting CBD stones varies between 23% and 80% depending on body habitus and experience of the ultrasonographer.[19]

Endoscopic ultrasound (EUS)

Prat et al. have reported EUS with a sensitivity of 93% and specificity of 97% in detecting CBD stones, showing some promise of approaching values achieved by ERCP (89% and 100%).[20] EUS has also been reported as more sensitive than the transabdominal approach. Norton and Alderson reported confirmation of gallstone disease in 15 of 44 patients with 'idiopathic' pancreatitis who underwent EUS.[21]

Computed tomography (CT)

CT may be more accurate than ultrasound in identifying CBD stones, with a sensitivity of 75% for CBD stones causing obstructive jaundice.[22] However, the relatively low rate of gallbladder stone detection may be due, in part, to cholesterol stones being isodense with bile on CT. The newer generation spiral CT and magnetic resonance imaging (MRI) may be better but their potential advantage over abdominal ultrasound scanning is not readily apparent. Spiral CT following intravenous infusion cholangiography has been shown to allow accurate reconstruction of cystic duct/CBD anatomy and providing severe jaundice is not present rivals magnetic resonance cholangiopancreatography (MRCP) in its capacity to outline CBD stones.[23]

Radioisotope scanning

Technetium-labelled hydroxy-imino-diacetic acid (HIDA) is excreted in the bile after intravenous injection. It may be useful for demonstrating the patency of the biliary tree or of biliary–enteric anastomoses, but its use with gallstones is limited. Failure to demonstrate a gallbladder due to a blocked cystic duct may assist in the diagnosis of acute cholecystitis but images are too poor to reveal CBD stones. HIDA scanning may be helpful in patients with right upper quarter pain, fever, gallstones and right lower lobe pneumonia. Referred pain and tenderness can give confusing clinical signs, and the presence of a functional gallbladder makes the diagnosis of cholecystitis much less likely. HIDA scanning is of no value in cases of severe jaundice, since the isotope is not excreted into an obstructed system.

Magnetic resonance cholangiopancreatography (MRCP)

Fast image acquisition in a few seconds and improved software have allowed imaging of the biliary and pancreatic tree in enough detail to approach the resolution of ERCP.[24] The technique relies on the principle of imaging fluid columns that are static and so give detail of bile and static fluid in the duodenum and stomach. Better images are obtained with dilated ducts, and bile flow can be a source of error in false-positive stone detection. The presence of CBD calculi can be detected with a sensitivity of 95%, specificity of 89% and accuracy of 92%. The ability to detect anatomical variation of the extrahepatic bile ducts is less established.[25] Following standard non-invasive tests, Liu et al. stratified suspicion of CBD stones into four categories. Patients at extremely high risk of CBD stone underwent ERCP. Patients at high risk underwent MRCP followed by ERCP if stones were seen. With diagnostic accuracies greater than 90% many patients were spared unnecessary ERCP.[26]

Percutaneous transhepatic cholangiography (PTC)

PTC is best performed in patients who have a dilated biliary tree, but is not employed routinely in patients with suspected gallstone biliary obstruction. Despite the use of a fine-gauge needle, there is a risk of bile leakage and haemorrhage in patients with abnormal clotting.

Endoscopic retrograde cholangiopancreatography (ERCP)

ERCP is considered the gold standard in preoperative CBD imaging. With direct visualisation of the papilla using a side-viewing duodenoscope, the papilla can be cannulated selectively to provide images of both the pancreatic and common bile ducts. Water-soluble contrast medium is injected to outline the biliary tree, and offers the advantage over other biliary tree imaging techniques of therapeutic intervention with sphincterotomy and stone extraction at the time of examination (**Fig. 10.2**). The role of ERCP in the management of CBD stones is discussed later in this chapter.

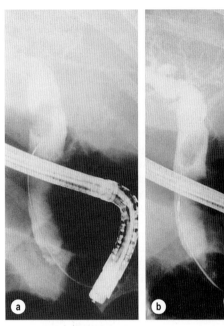

Figure 10.2 • (a) A large stone has been demonstrated by endoscopic retrograde cholangiography within the common bile duct. **(b)** The common bile duct stone has been snared by a Dormia basket ready for extraction.

Management of gallbladder stones

Asymptomatic stones

There has been much debate regarding the need for surgical intervention in patients with asymptomatic gallstones. In one American study, which assessed the natural history of subjects with asymptomatic stones, individuals with gallstones were diagnosed by ultrasound scan on entry to a large university healthcare plan.[27] Only 2% of patients with incidentally diagnosed gallstones became symptomatic each year and presented with biliary colic or cholecystitis rather than the more serious complications of jaundice, empyema or cholangitis.[27] Only 10% of the asymptomatic patients, followed for a mean of almost 5 years by McSherry and Glenn, developed symptoms, and only 7% required operation.[28] Although stones are undoubtedly associated with an increased risk of gallbladder cancer, only one of the 691 gallstone patients followed in this study was found eventually to have an incidental carcinoma at operation, and further data are required to clarify this issue.

Recent Swedish population postcholecystectomy follow-up data after a mean of 15 years revealed a weak increased risk of oesophageal adenocarcinoma with a standardised incidence ratio of 1.29. This is hypothesised to be due to increased oesophageal bile acid exposure.[29]

Further randomised data have revealed that surgery remains the best treatment for symptomatic gallstones, but conservative management may in selected circumstances be used in the elderly.[30]

> ✓✓ There is no evidence to support interventional treatment of patients with asymptomatic gallstones since natural history studies have shown that symptoms develop at a rate of less than 2% per year.

Non-operative treatments for gallstones

Dissolution

In the early 1970s there was great interest in the use of dissolution agents, principally chenodeoxycholic acid (CDCA), in the treatment of gallstones.[31] Prerequisites for attempting dissolution therapy were a functioning gallbladder, multiple small stones (which have a greater total surface area for contact with the dissolution agent rather than a smaller number of larger stones) and radiolucency (indicative of pure cholesterol stones without a calcium or pigment matrix to impede dissolution). Success was slow to be achieved in most subjects, usually taking 6–12 months as judged by the disappearance of stones on ultrasound. Side-effects of treatment included abdominal cramps, diarrhoea and occasional LFT abnormalities. Ursodeoxycholate (UDCA) has been shown to be equally effective as CDCA in dissolving gallstones. In patients administered dissolution agents, O'Donnell and Heaton[32] found that recurrence rates increased rapidly in the first few years, with rates of 13% at 1 year, 31% at 3 years, 43% at 4 years and 49% at 11 years. Although recurrent stones were readily redissolved, they generally recurred when therapy ceased.

Lithotripsy

Success with lithotripsy for renal stones led to the use of the same techniques for gallbladder stones. Early lithotripters, with immersion in large water baths, were soon succeeded by smaller devices with a limited area of contact via a water-filled cushion. Biliary anatomy, however, did not lend itself to a repeat of the success observed with renal stones. The tidal flow of bile into and out of the gallbladder, along with the presence of multiple gallstones, were factors that contributed to the failure of the technique. Ahmed et al.[33] reported that 45% of patients undergoing lithotripsy required subsequent

cholecystectomy. Lithotripsy has therefore been retained only for the management of ductal stones resistant to endoscopic removal.[34]

> ✓ The potential role of oral dissolution therapy and lithotripsy has been superseded by the advent of laparoscopic cholecystectomy.

Operative treatment of gallbladder stones

Open cholecystectomy

The operative mortality of open cholecystectomy for cholelithiasis had fallen in the years before the introduction of laparoscopic surgery, with many series reporting operative mortality rates of less than 1%.[35] Common duct exploration was regarded as increasing the risk of open cholecystectomy by four- to eight-fold.[36] In a comparative study between a North American and a European centre, 12–14% of patients developed complications, and the bile duct was explored in 8.6% of the patients in Toronto as opposed to 17.9% in Geneva, the incidences of positive exploration being 61% and 73%, respectively. Factors increasing the risk of postoperative mortality were advancing age, acute admission, admission to hospital within 3 months of the index admission, and the number of discharge diagnoses.[36] Only 18% of postoperative deaths in this study were related to the gallstone disease or the surgery, with underlying cardiovascular or respiratory disease contributing to 48% of deaths.

There has been considerable uncertainty regarding the true incidence of bile duct injury at open cholecystectomy, and the surveys available cite figures of one injury per 300–1000 operations.[37] At cholecystectomy, injury results from imprecise dissection and inadequate demonstration of the anatomical structures.[38] Although some patients do have anatomical anomalies or pathological changes that increase the risk of duct injury, it is noteworthy that in the extensive Swedish review, the patients most at risk appeared to be young, slim females who had not undergone previous surgery.[37]

In a detailed analysis of a consecutive group of patients undergoing cholecystectomy for presumed biliary pain in a District General Hospital between 1980 and 1985, Bates et al.[39] compared the outcome of an age- and sex-matched control group of surgical patients without gallstone disease. Flatulent dyspepsia was more frequent in gallstone patients but operation markedly reduced these symptoms to an incidence almost identical to that of the control group. However, within 1 year of cholecystectomy, no less than 34% of patients still suffered some abdominal pain and none of the 35 patients referred back to hospital for investigation had evidence of retained ductal stones. Multivariate analysis showed that preoperative flatulence and long durations of attacks of pain were risk factors for postoperative dissatisfaction.

> ☑☑ Given that the basis for symptoms before cholecystectomy often remains uncertain, it is evident that a substantial number of patients continue to experience problems after operation.

Mini-laparotomy cholecystectomy

In the few years before the advent of laparoscopic cholecystectomy, there had been a resurgence of interest in open cholecystectomy through a small incision, the so-called mini-laparotomy cholecystectomy, in an effort to reduce the trauma of open surgery.

There have been few controlled trials; of those that have been performed, one showed laparoscopic cholecystectomy to be superior and the other showed mini-laparotomy cholecystectomy as superior.[40,41] The most recent randomised trial has again confirmed a smoother convalescence for laparoscopic cholecystectomy, although operating times remained longer.[42]

The technique relies on retractors to provide exposure for a fundus-first cholecystectomy carried out without the surgeon's hands entering the abdominal cavity. Cholangiography is possible but is not performed in most reports of the technique. The author's limited first-hand experience of the technique has not persuaded him that the view of the cystic duct/CBD junction is comparable to that achieved by laparoscopic cholecystectomy. The true incidence of bile duct injury with this technique is unknown and cannot be equated to the open era of large incisions.

> ☑ There is no evidence to support the routine use of mini-cholecystectomy in the treatment of symptomatic gallstone disease.

Laparoscopic cholecystectomy

Despite the paucity of randomised controlled trials, enthusiasm for the technique of laparoscopic cholecystectomy continues unabated, driven predominantly by patient satisfaction, with less pain and an earlier return to normal activities. Surgeons are attracted by the excellent view of the gallbladder and biliary tree afforded by the laparoscope, and health providers and purchasers are attracted by the short hospital stay, which offers significant cost savings.

Symptomatic gallstones

The laparoscopic procedure can be offered to all patients with symptomatic gallstones, providing their cardiorespiratory status does not preclude laparoscopy. Of all patients presenting for operation, 95% can be completed successfully by laparoscopic means. Obesity, acute inflammation, adhesions and previous abdominal surgery do not usually prevent a laparoscopic cholecystectomy, but may require some adaptations of technique to complete the procedure.[43–51] Techniques of laparoscopic cholecystectomy have been well described previously,[43,44] including cases performed under regional anaesthesia in patients with chronic pulmonary disease.[45] Laparoscopic cholecystectomy has been widely reported in pregnancy[46] and in patients with cirrhosis.[47] In a substantial audit of seven European centres,[43,44] 96% of procedures were completed successfully in the 1236 patients and only four bile duct injuries were reported. There were no postoperative deaths, median hospital stay was 3 days and the median return to normal activities was only 11 days.

Acute cholecystitis

Fears that laparoscopic cholecystectomy in the management of acute cholecystitis could carry an unacceptable risk of disseminating infection or of perpetuating an injury to the bile duct appear unfounded.[51] Several large series report success and safety with this procedure, although the incidence of bile duct injury and conversion to open operation remain slightly higher.[52] In difficult cases, improvement in the exposure of Calot's triangle may require additional or different positioning of the laparoscopic cannulae, the use of oblique viewing telescopes and placement of endoscopic retractors. Decompression of a distended or inflamed gallbladder may also improve access.

Complications

The mortality rate in a good-risk patient undergoing elective operation is less than 1% and operative risks usually arise from comorbid conditions. The laparoscopic technique is associated with lower wound infection rates than open surgery.[53] Furthermore, a recent meta-analysis has shown that antibiotic prophylaxis is not warranted in low-risk patients undergoing laparoscopic cholecystectomy.[54]

Day-case laparoscopic cholecystectomy

Worldwide, laparoscopic cholecystectomy is being performed in the day-case setting with good preoperative patient selection, improved techniques, and improved postoperative control of pain, nausea and vomiting.[55]

Needlescopic cholecystectomy

This technique has been described using 2- and 3-mm instruments and a 3-mm laparoscope. A randomised trial has shown less pain and smaller scars when this technique was used in patients with chronic cholecystitis.[56]

Evolution of technical aspects of multiport exposure, decreasing port sizes and instrumentation continues. There is currently no evidence of a benefit for single-incision laparoscopic port techniques,[57] with impaired ergonomic performance and probable increased incisional hernia rate.

Bile duct injury

Anxieties regarding an increased incidence of bile duct injury with the introduction of laparoscopic cholecystectomy have not been substantiated by multicentre studies from Europe[48] and the USA,[49] with a reported incidence of injury to the CBD of 1 in 200–300 cases. In a study in the West of Scotland, a prospective audit of laparoscopic cholecystectomy was undertaken.[58] A total of 5913 laparoscopic cholecystectomies were undertaken by 48 surgeons, and 37 laparoscopic bile duct injuries were reported. Major bile duct injuries were defined as those where laceration to more than 25% of the bile duct diameter occurred, where the common hepatic duct or CBD was transected, or in those instances when a bile duct stricture developed in the postoperative period. Of the 37 injuries, 20 were classified in this way, giving an incidence of 0.3%. Delayed identification of bile duct injury occurred in 19 patients and, although it was noted by the author that cholangiography did not play a part in the identification of bile duct injuries, it was noteworthy that imaging was used in only 8.8% of all laparoscopic procedures. During the course of this 5-year study, the annual incidence of bile duct injury peaked at 0.8% in the third year but had fallen to 0.4% in the final year of the audit. A meta-analysis of more than 100 000 cases reported an injury rate of 0.5%.[59] Archer et al. emphasised the importance of supervised surgical training to allow attenuation of the trainee surgeon's learning curve by the experience of his/her proctoring surgeon. The importance of cholangiography in the early detection of bile duct injury was also emphasised.[60] Way et al. analysed bile duct injuries from a cognitive psychological perspective and concluded that errors that led to bile duct injury stemmed from anatomical misperceptions as opposed to errors of skill or judgment (**Fig. 10.3**). This analysis concluded with a list of rules to help prevent injuries.[61]

Cholecystostomy

For patients whose symptoms of acute cholecystitis did not settle in the past, cholecystostomy was often undertaken in those cases where open cholecystectomy was thought to carry an unacceptable risk of injury to the biliary tree. The procedure could be undertaken under local anaesthesia and, following decompression of the gallbladder and stone removal, a drain could be left in situ. With the demonstration that acute cholecystectomy could be undertaken safely,[52] cholecystostomy has become an infrequent surgical procedure. The technique now is most often undertaken percutaneously under ultrasound or CT guidance and is most used in the frail patient with cardiorespiratory instability requiring time to control or when anticoagulation precludes surgery. It may rarely be of value during a difficult laparoscopic cholecystectomy when the risk of conversion to an open procedure may be considered unacceptable. In such instances, a drain can be inserted through one of the 5-mm cannulae, which can be introduced directly into the gallbladder by reinsertion of a trocar.

Subtotal cholecystectomy

This is another strategy to consider if dense fibrosis or large vessels are present in the area of Calot's triangle and the cystic duct is clearly identified and confirmed by cholecystogram. The cystic duct is ligated and excision of the gallbladder is undertaken, leaving its posterior wall intact on the liver. This situation probably arises most in those patients with cirrhosis and portal hypertension.

> ✔✔ Laparoscopic cholecystectomy is associated with less pain, shorter hospital stay, faster return to normal activity and less abdominal scarring than open surgery, and is therefore preferred to open surgery in the management of symptomatic gallstone disease.[62]

Intraoperative cholangiography (IOC)

The debate over the potential benefit of operative cholangiography has spanned the open and laparoscopic eras.

Routine IOC

Many surgeons who had previously performed the technique routinely at open cholecystectomy abandoned cholangiography during laparoscopic cholecystectomy, since it was thought to be too difficult to undertake. In a large population-based study in Western Australia, Fletcher et al.[63] concluded that operative cholangiography had a protective effect for complications of cholecystectomy. In a large study of over 1.5 million Medicare patients undergoing cholecystectomy, Flum et al.[64] demonstrated that surgeons performing operative cholangiography routinely had a lower rate of bile duct

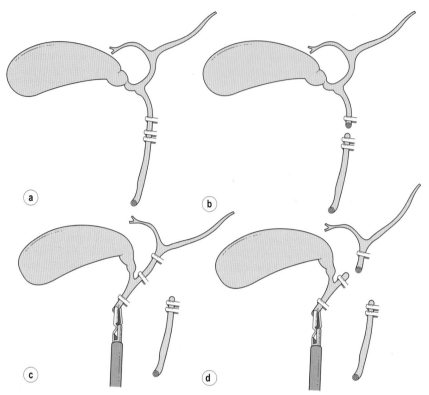

Figure 10.3 • The 'classical' laparoscopic bile duct injury. **(a)** The common duct is misidentified as the cystic duct and is doubly clipped. **(b)** The common duct is then divided. **(c)** The gallbladder is retracted to the right, stretching the common hepatic duct and placing it in contact with the gallbladder. This is identified as an accessory duct and double clipped. **(d)** A high transection of the common hepatic duct results in the excision of most of the extrahepatic biliary tree.

injuries than those who did not, and this difference disappeared when IOC was not used. The author believes that operative cholangiography has an important role in laparoscopic cholecystectomy, not only to detect CBD stones but also to confirm, beyond doubt, the anatomy of the biliary tree, since the severity of bile duct injury appears far greater in laparoscopic surgery. The addition of cholangiography to the total dissection time of laparoscopic cholecystectomy is relatively short. On the basis that the time to learn operative cholangiography is not during the management of a difficult case, it is recommended that it should be performed as a routine but should not be seen as a substitute for careful dissection of the infundibulum of the gallbladder and the cystic duct close to the gallbladder. By dissecting these structures both anteriorly and posteriorly, the gallbladder is displaced (sometimes called the 'flag' technique, or 'critical view') to enable the surgeon to see behind the gallbladder and thus minimise the risk of injury to the portal structures. Routine IOC also improves the surgeon's skills to enable successful transcystic exploration of the CBD.

Selective IOC

There are data supporting a selective approach to IOC at open[17] and laparoscopic cholecystectomy.[65] Unsuspected stones on routine cholangiography at laparoscopic cholecystectomy occurred in only 2.9%, and residual CBD stones causing symptoms in patients not undergoing routine cholangiography were found in only 0.30%. The strength of any selective policy for IOC will depend on the predictive values of preoperative investigations. Numerous studies have examined risk factors for choledocholithiasis but, from multivariate analysis, it would appear that an increased diameter of the CBD and the presence of multiple (>10) gallstones are the only significant independent indicators.[17]

Bile duct injury

The principal cause of damage is due to misidentification of the CBD as the cystic duct. As dissection proceeds an 'accessory duct' (in reality the common hepatic duct) is visualised, clipped and divided, resulting in resection of most of the extrahepatic biliary tree (Fig. 10.3). Operative cholangiography adds to the certainty that the cannula is in the cystic duct.

If only the distal biliary tree is filled, the surgeon is alerted to the error before any duct is completely divided. Although critics of operative cholangiography will argue that the CBD has been injured by the incision through which the cholangiogram catheter is introduced, the injury at this point is recoverable, either by direct suture or insertion of a T-tube (**Fig. 10.4**). In the rarer situation when the cystic duct arises from the right hepatic duct, and dissection has not progressed correctly, cholangiography identifies such anomalies and helps to avert more major injury (**Fig. 10.5**).

Laparoscopic ultrasound (LUS)

The emergence of ultrasound probes that can be passed down the laparoscopic ports has further improved the accurate measurement of CBD diameter, as well as the stone load within the gallbladder. Both mechanical sectoral and linear array laparoscopic ultrasound probes have been shown to be as useful as cholangiography in the detection of CBD stones.[66,67] LUS is less invasive, less time-consuming, allows less radiation exposure and has similar failure rates to IOC when performed in well-trained hands. In a large series, the common hepatic duct and the CBD were identified in 93% and 99% of cases, respectively. Sensitivity and specificity for identifying bile duct stones were 92% and 100%, respectively. A normal CBD diameter at LUS was also an excellent negative predictor of CBD stones.[68] The same authors later concluded that LUS could

replace IOC.[69] Others feel IOC and LUS should be seen as complementary tests rather than competitive.[70] LUS may facilitate a policy of selective cholangiography. Despite reports of accurate identification of anatomy it remains to be seen whether this will translate to prevention of bile duct injury. A cost benefit also remains to be demonstrated, given the capital outlay for the equipment.

✔✔ The use of intraoperative cholangiography allows detection of CBD stones during cholecystectomy and when interpreted appropriately is associated with a lower risk of CBD injury.

Management of common bile duct stones

The natural history of a given CBD stone remains difficult to predict. In a prospective study of 1000 cases of symptomatic gallstones it was found that 73% of cases that presented with features suggestive of CBD stones had no CBD stone at the time of operation and were therefore considered to have passed the stone spontaneously. Cases of cholangitis or jaundice were less likely to pass stones spontaneously.[71]

Primary bile duct stones form within the CBD, usually due to ampullary stenosis, diverticula or impaired bile duct motility. Management of these

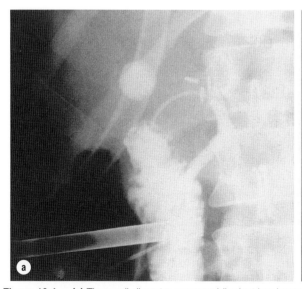 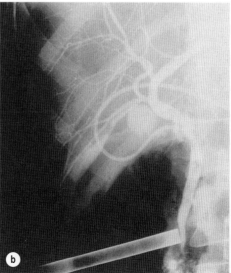

Figure 10.4 • (a) The small-diameter common bile duct has been mistaken for the cystic duct. Only the distal common bile duct and duodenum are shown, with no proximal filling of the ducts. Recognition of the error at this stage averts a major injury to the common duct. **(b)** After further dissection, the cystic duct was identified and a T-tube placed in the incision in the common duct. A subsequent T-tube cholangiogram confirms the normal anatomy, and laparoscopic cholecystectomy was completed successfully.

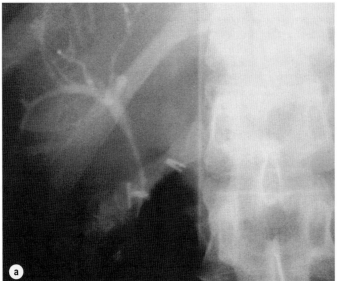

Figure 10.5 • (a) During what appeared to be a very straightforward laparoscopic cholecystectomy, the routine operative cholangiogram showed only the right hepatic duct and right hepatic biliary tree. **(b)** Repositioning of the catheter and the LigaClip showed the remainder of the biliary tree and made clear that the structure initially thought to be the cystic duct was the distal right hepatic duct below an anomalous origin of the cystic duct.

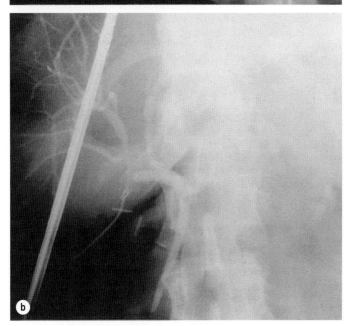

stones will often require choledochojejunostomy, depending on the circumstances and patient age.[72,73] Treatment of primary duct stones with choledochotomy and T-tube drainage alone is associated with recurrence rates up to 41%.[74] Laparoscopic choledochoduodenostomy remains an option for the advanced laparoscopic surgeon,[75,76] although there may be concerns regarding the longer-term consequences of bilioenteric reflux.

Secondary bile duct stones are stones that originate within the gallbladder and are found in the CBD prior to, at the time of, or within 2 years of cholecystectomy. Approximately 12% of patients undergoing surgery for symptomatic gallbladder stones will also have stones in the CBD. More than 90% of these patients will have preoperative indications such as a history of jaundice or pancreatitis or abnormal LFTs, but 5–10% have no indication of stones in the bile duct other than a positive finding (filling defect, absence of filling of the terminal segment of the common duct, delay or absence of flow into the duodenum) on the perioperative cholangiogram.

The best management of CBD stones is still a matter of debate.[77] Discussion of different practices is presented here in the order the author considers most practical, and a suggested algorithm is presented.

Laparoscopic transcystic common bile duct exploration

Laparoscopic CBD exploration has been described through the cystic duct or common duct using either fibreoptic instruments or radiologically guided wire baskets or balloons.[78–81] The increased emphasis on improving techniques via the transcystic route is because of the ease of closure without the added need for intracorporeal suture technique, combined with postoperative recovery similar to cholecystectomy alone. Careful evaluation of the CBD diameter and stone load from the cholangiogram is required to determine the best approach.

The author's preferred initial method of laparoscopic exploration is by fluoroscopic means using a C-arm image intensifier, which is mobile and provides dynamic images with angulation. We employ a 5.5-Fr 70-cm radio-opaque nylon catheter with soft tip and end hole along with a side arm that connects to a catheter for injection of contrast (**Fig. 10.6**). Once the cystic duct is opened for insertion of the cholangiogram catheter, absence of bile backflow is a signal to milk the cystic duct backwards to extrude stones caught in transit to the CBD, rather than push them onwards into the CBD. A cholangiogram is performed (**Fig. 10.7a**), note being taken of the cystic duct and bile duct diameter, number of stones, stone size and their distribution in the biliary tree. CBD stones that appear to be of a size suitable for removal via the cystic duct and are not too numerous indicate that transcystic clearance has a high chance of success. Transcystic clearance proceeds by passing a 75-cm-long stone extractor (Cook®, Wilson-Cook Medical GI Endoscopy Inc., North Carolina). The basket tip should be positioned well back from the cannula tip to avoid perforation of the duct. Once the cannula tip is progressed, under image intensification, the basket is advanced within the cannula to allow engagement of the stone, which is withdrawn into the basket and extracted via the cystic duct (**Fig. 10.7b**). It is useful to remove the proximal stones first, and vital to avoid opening the basket within the duodenum or withdrawing through the ampulla with the basket wires open. Any impacted stones can be dislodged by passing a 4-Fr Fogarty catheter beyond the stone and withdrawing the catheter with the balloon inflated. Failed disimpaction may require choledochoscopy and lithotripsy (**Fig. 10.7c–f**, Box 10.1).

Traditionally at open surgery, the common duct was decompressed postoperatively with a T-tube until it was known that the bile was draining satisfactorily through the ampulla and there was no bile leak. Most series of laparoscopic transcystic common duct explorations do not report the routine use of drainage of the common duct. A subhepatic drain is routine.

There is accumulating evidence, including three randomised trials, that 60–70% of patients are able to have their calculi cleared via the cystic duct.[82–88]

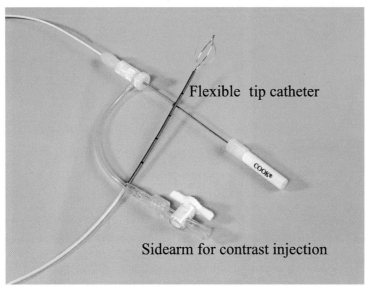

Flexible tip catheter

Sidearm for contrast injection

Figure 10.6 • Composite cholangiogram catheter and stone extraction basket used for laparoscopic transcystic exploration of the common bile duct. Reproduced with permission of Cook Australia.

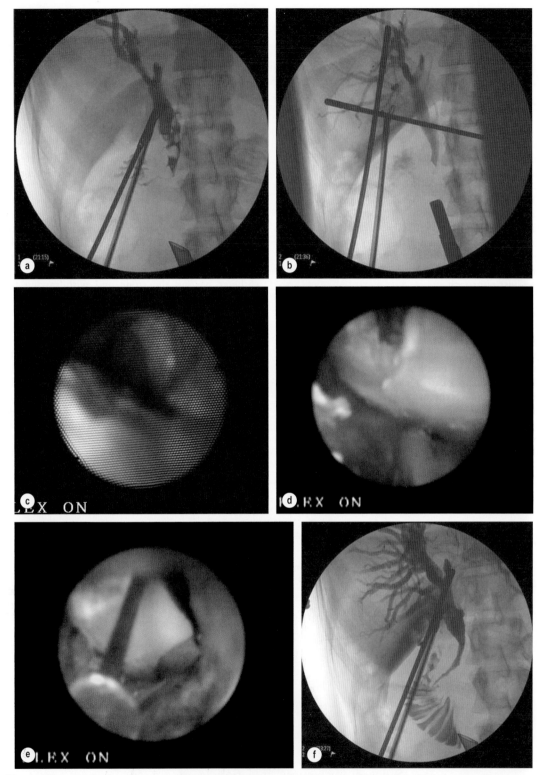

Figure 10.7 • **(a)** Cholangiogram of a 21-year-old jaundiced patient demonstrating multiple CBD stones with one impacted 3 cm proximal to ampulla. **(b)** Fluoroscopic view of bile duct showing after rapid transcystic four-wire basket retrieval of all except the impacted stone. **(c)** Transcystic choledochoscopic view of impacted stone, unable to be dislodged with a balloon catheter. **(d)** Transcystic ureteroscopic lithoclast stone fragmentation. **(e)** Wire basket stone retrieval under vision. **(f)** Fluoroscopic view of cleared bile duct.

- Careful dissection of cystic duct/CBD junction
- Avoidance of the spiral valves when incising cystic duct
- Careful examination of cholangiogram ('did that stone pass through the cystic duct?')
- Approach cystic duct from different or extra ports
- Choledochoscopy via cystic duct, with lithotripsy if required
- Vary retraction on fundus

Laparoscopic choledochotomy

In up to 35% of patients, laparoscopic transcystic exploration of the CBD will fail to clear the CBD.[82–88] Choledochotomy then needs to be considered. The only absolute contraindication to choledochotomy is a CBD diameter of less than 8 mm (Box 10.2). It should also be borne in mind that approximately one-third of stones detected at cholangiography may be passed spontaneously, and that exploration of a small duct may result in increased morbidity for the patient.[89] Therefore, laparoscopic choledochotomy is only an option for appropriately trained surgeons (Box 10.3).

Once clearance of the duct has been confirmed by choledochoscopy (see below), a T-tube is inserted or primary closure can be considered with the insertion of an antegrade stent across the ampulla.[82] Antegrade stenting, placement of a T-tube or cystic

Box 10.2 • Indications for choledochotomy

- Unsuccessful transcystic exploration
- Cystic duct diameter smaller than size of stones
- CBD diameter >8 mm
- Multiple large stones
- Ampullary diverticulum on IOC
- Previous Billroth II gastrectomy
- Previous failed ERCP
- Contraindication to postoperative ERCP
- ERCP unavailable

Box 10.3 • Useful tips in performing laparoscopic choledochotomy

- Deflate duodenum with nasogastric tube (NGT)
- Extra port to retract duodenum
- Leave cholangiocatheter in to prevent deflation
- Sharp scissors choledochotomy
- Intraoperative lithotripsy preferably by lithoclast

duct tube decompression of the CBD is wise where doubt exists about free postoperative bile drainage through the ampulla. This is most likely where a stone was impacted, ampullary manipulation has been extensive or in patients with established cholangitis. Placement of a subhepatic drain is essential.

Open choledochotomy

Successful exploration of the CBD can only be achieved through an adequately sized choledochotomy to facilitate both removal of any obvious stones and choledochoscopy. The gradual adoption of operative choledochoscopy during the 1970s and 1980s saw a decline in the incidence of retained CBD stones following surgery, from about 10% to 1.2%, with a number of surgeons reporting large series of patients with no retained stones.[90] On initial examination of the proximal ducts, it is normally possible to visualise several generations of ducts when these are dilated. Once it has been ascertained that the upper ducts are clear, the distal biliary tree can be examined. It is mandatory to clearly visualise the rather ragged appearance of the ampulla of Vater and then withdraw the choledochoscope. If a stone is visualised it can be retrieved with a stone basket and the procedure repeated until the duct is clear. The common duct is closed with or without a T-tube.[91] The latter is probably unnecessary for an experienced choledochoscopist but, for the less experienced surgeon, it allows access to the biliary tree for postoperative cholangiography to confirm ductal clearance and to allow re-exploration of the duct without the need for re-operation.

Following the evolution of laparoscopic exploration of the bile duct, the most important area for laparotomy is for Mirizzi type 2–4 erosion of the bile duct by large stones and chronic inflammation. Reconstruction of the bile duct with the remaining gallbladder wall, or bilioenteric bypass in these circumstances, is best approached by laparotomy.

Endoscopic retrograde cholangiopancreatography (ERCP)

With the advent of laparoscopic cholecystectomy, ERCP and endoscopic sphincterotomy (ES) have become the usual procedure for treating common duct stones, since laparoscopic common duct exploration is not yet a widely practised technique (Box 10.4). Moreover, cholecystectomy without cholangiography is commonly performed in the expectation that ERCP and ES will be effective in dealing with unrecognised retained common duct stones at a later date. Such a policy, however, does expose the patient to an additional and often unnecessary procedure. Laparoscopic common duct exploration by whatever route has the advantage for the patient of being able to deal with both gallbladder and CBD stones at the same time.[92]

There is general agreement that endoscopic removal of bile duct stones is preferable to surgery in postcholecystectomy patients, and in high-risk surgical patients when the gallbladder is still present – that is, patients with severe acute cholangitis and selected patients with acute biliary pancreatitis.[93–95] The author believes ERCP becomes an option when transcystic CBD exploration has failed, but should not be considered the first-line management of all CBD stones.

Duct clearance can be expected in 90–95% of patients undergoing successful sphincterotomy, and this results in an overall success rate for endoscopic stone clearance of 80–95%, the highest success rates being recorded as experience increases.[93,95,96] Major complications occur in up to 10% of patients, and include haemorrhage, acute pancreatitis, cholangitis and retroduodenal perforation, but the overall procedure-related mortality is less than 1%.[93] However, the 30-day mortality can reach 15%, reflecting the severity of the underlying disease. In selected patients with calculi less than 15 mm in diameter, morbidity may be reduced by papillary dilatation rather than sphincterotomy.[94] Difficulties in removing CBD stones endoscopically may be due to unfavourable or abnormal anatomy, such as a periampullary diverticulum or previous surgery. Stones larger than 15 mm and those situated intrahepatically or proximal to a biliary stricture may be difficult to remove (Box 10.5). Adjuvant techniques include mechanical lithotripsy, extracorporeal shockwave lithotripsy and chemical dissolution.[95,97,98] Although successful stone fragmentation has been reported in up to 80% of patients, the major drawback is the need for multiple treatment sessions and at least one subsequent ERCP to extract stone fragments.

The establishment of ERCP in the prelaparoscopic era was based on the avoidance of an open exploration of the CBD, a procedure that was believed to have significant morbidity.[99] ERCP was therefore generally reserved for the high-risk surgical patients but open cholecystectomy and exploration of the CBD was reserved for the younger patient. In the laparoscopic era, management strategies vary considerably and are based on local endoscopic and laparoscopic resources and expertise.

ERCP stent insertion

In the 5% or less of situations where extraction of CBD stones is incomplete or impossible, a nasobiliary tube or stent should be inserted to provide biliary decompression and prevent stone impaction of the distal CBD (**Fig. 10.8**).[100] Such manoeuvres may allow improvement of the patient's clinical condition until complete stone clearance can be achieved by further endoscopic manoeuvres or subsequent surgery. Temporary biliary endoprosthesis placement avoids accidental or intentional dislodgement

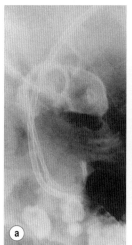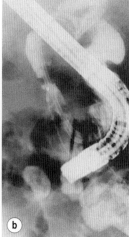

Figure 10.8 • Multiple common bile duct stones lying above a mid-common bile duct stricture and not amenable to endoscopic extraction. Biliary drainage is maintained with two endoscopically placed stents.

of the nasobiliary catheter by a confused or unco-operative patient. The stent may become blocked after a few months, but bile drainage often continues around the stent, and the presence of the stent alone may be sufficient to prevent stones from becoming impacted at the lower end of the CBD. In the surgically unfit patient, a change of stent may be required if jaundice recurs. Recurrent episodes of cholangitis may result in secondary biliary cirrhosis in the long term, and careful consideration of the patient's level of fitness must be made before surgery is totally discounted.

Preoperative ERCP

For some, ERCP is the chosen method of preoperative CBD stone clearance, after imaging documentation of CBD stones with MRI or CT cholangiogram. The advantage of this strategy is that duct clearance preoperatively removes the dilemma as to how to manage CBD stones found at operation. ERCP as a tool to detect suspected stones without imaging exposes a substantial number of patients to an unnecessary endoscopic intervention.

A randomised study has shown no significant advantage for patients treated by preoperative sphincterotomy as opposed to open cholecystectomy and exploration of CBD alone.[101] Despite this, ERCP and ES have become popular practice in the management of CBD stones, with an increased reliance on ERCP and a reluctance among surgeons to perform surgical exploration of the CBD.[102]

Cholecystectomy should routinely follow clearance of the CBD except in those considered too frail or unfit for general anaesthetic. It can be expected that if the gallbladder is left intact following ERCP and ES, up to 47% of patients will develop at least one recurrent biliary event, with many requiring cholecystectomy.[86]

Intraoperative ERCP

There have been several reports over the years describing this technique with success but few centres consider this the most appropriate use of resources.[103]

Postoperative ERCP

If ductal stones are not suspected preoperatively, their presence can be determined at laparoscopic cholecystectomy by IOC. CBD stones identified in this way could be referred for postoperative endoscopic clearance if the surgeon was unable to explore the duct. Such a policy would reduce dramatically the number of ERCPs undertaken by a policy of routine or selective preoperative ERCP. This would leave only a small proportion of patients in whom stones could not be cleared by ERCP, requiring a second operation.[104] If the surgeon is trained in laparoscopic exploration of the CBD, ERCP should be

reserved for the few patients in whom laparoscopic ductal clearance fails. A recent randomised trial lends some evidence that this approach is safe and represents an effective management plan.[88]

At the present time, the precise role of ERCP remains to be defined but is likely to be dictated by local expertise and practice (see 'Laparoscopic choledochotomy' above). A number of acceptable algorithms have been proposed to manage laparoscopic cholecystectomy patients suspected of harbouring CBD stones.

There is also an argument for leaving small stones (<5 mm) found intraoperatively. On follow-up for up to 33 months in a small group of patients, 29% in this category developed symptoms, but were safely managed with ERCP.[105]

Laparoscopic exploration of the CBD versus preoperative or postoperative ERCP

At present, the array of management strategies for common duct stones requires data to guide us, with the techniques employed depending on local circumstances. In hospitals with ready access to ERCP, a surgeon may see little need for ascending the learning curve of laparoscopic CBD exploration, whereas those units with less ready access to ERCP see many attractions in dealing with common duct stones by laparoscopic means.

Preoperative ERCP and laparoscopic clearance of the CBD have been shown to be equivalent in overall outcomes.[83] However, those patients whose ductal stones were cleared transcystically experienced a far shorter hospital stay.

Postoperative ERCP clearance in a small single-surgeon study showed equivalent overall outcome to laparoscopic CBD clearance.[84] However, the number of choledochotomies was small and the retained stone rate high. Placement of biliary stents at the time of operation may improve the success of postoperative ERCP and stone clearance.

With experience, the majority of CBD stones can be treated at the time of surgery provided a flexible approach is employed.[85] No single technique will be applicable to the management of all stones. In general, if the stones are few in number, small (<1 cm) in size, situated in the common duct or distal to cystic duct entry, then transcystic exploration has a high chance of success. If the stone or stones are large and numerous, or if the stones are situated in the common hepatic duct or intrahepatic biliary tree, a choledochotomy and exploration with the larger 5-mm choledochoscope is the preferred option.

Intraoperative stone fragmentation remains an option for stones found at operation that are unable to be dislodged at laparoscopic or open surgery, especially at the ampulla. This requires skills using the lithoclast for certain circumstances and laser or electrohydrolic fragmentation for others. Expertise in this area renders the transduodenal sphinctero-plasty approach obsolete.

For those embarking on laparoscopic exploration, careful consideration of the strategies to be employed, equipment required and adequacy of assistance will go a long way to simplifying a potentially complex procedure. When laparoscopic transcystic exploration fails, the surgeon has three options:

- to ligate the cystic duct, complete the cholecystectomy and rely on postoperative ERCP;
- to perform a laparoscopic choledochotomy;
- to perform a laparotomy and open exploration of the CBD.

If laparoscopic choledochotomy fails, the options include: insertion of a T-tube and subsequent extraction of the retained stones via the T-tube track after 6 weeks; postoperative ERCP and sphincterotomy; or conversion to open exploration CBD. Individual circumstances will dictate which option is the most suitable, although this should be discussed carefully with the patient before a management strategy is implemented.

It has been suggested that preoperative ERCP is the most cost-effective management of patients at high risk for CBD stones.[106] There is evidence accumulating, however, that where transcystic clearance is successful this leads to less morbidity and more rapid recovery.[83,88] The author believes the most cost-effective approach is laparoscopic cholecystectomy, IOC and transcystic clearance of CBD stones, reserving ERCP for retained stones. Learning the techniques to achieve this seems worthwhile.

In a recent extensive review of the literature, it was concluded that laparoscopic CBD exploration is safe and effective for all patients presenting with gallstones and may be a better way of removing CBD stones than ERCP.[107,108]

Recurrent or retained CBD stones

Recurrent CBD stones occur in up to 10% of cases. In a retrospective series of 169 patients followed for up to 19 years, recurrences were more common in patients with primary duct stones, large CBD diameter (around 16 mm) and periampullary diverticula. Lowest recurrence rates were found in those patients undergoing choledochoduodenostomy.[73]

Retained CBD stones found at postoperative T-tube cholangiography are best dealt with by ERCP. If ERCP is unsuccessful or not available,

exploration of the CBD via the T-tube tract is indicated. It usually takes approximately 6 weeks for the T-tube track to mature, at which time percutaneous choledochoscopy or radiologically guided extraction can be performed. A cholangiogram is obtained immediately prior to the procedure as a proportion of stones will have passed spontaneously.

The T-tube is removed, a guidewire is left in situ, and either a steerable catheter or choledochoscope is advanced down the track and into the CBD. With choledochoscopy, the remainder of the technique is identical to that carried out at open operation.[109] With the steerable catheter technique, fluoroscopy and further cholangiograms are taken as the stones are retrieved with a stone basket.[110]

If there is uncertainty as to the completeness of clearance, a straight tube may be inserted to keep the track open for a further attempt a few days later. Both techniques are successful in more than 95% of cases and carry less risk of complications such as pancreatitis or haemorrhage than ERCP. Providing there are no time constraints and the patient is happy to be managed as an outpatient with a T-tube, the technique is effective.

✔✔ Transcystic exploration of the common bile duct at the time of cholecystectomy is an effective means of managing choledocholithiasis with low morbidity and cost.

✔✔ ERCP is effective in managing the remaining patients in whom this is not achievable and is the accepted means of managing the patient presenting with acute cholangitis.

Transhepatic stone retrieval

In a few patients, particularly those who have previously undergone a Pólya gastrectomy, the ampulla will not be readily accessible for ERCP. Access to the common duct can be achieved using a percutaneous transhepatic technique. Over a percutaneously inserted guidewire, a series of dilators are advanced into the biliary tree, so as to develop a transhepatic tract. Following insertion of a sheath, a choledochoscope or steerable catheter can be inserted and stones retrieved.[111]

Acalculous biliary pain

Given the poor understanding of the mechanisms of pain production in patients with acalculous biliary disease, the outcome for patients following cholecystectomy is uncertain. There is gathering evidence that some patients have abnormal motility of the sphincter of Oddi, in addition to the gallbladder. Some authors have reported improvement in symptoms in as many as 85–95% of patients with acalculous biliary pain after cholecystectomy,[112] but it is conceivable that surgery confers a placebo effect. Controversy exists over the use of cholecystokinin (CCK) provocation tests as a means of reproducing symptoms and predicting which patients might benefit from cholecystectomy. In one study, all 26 patients with positive CCK tests showed improvement after removal of the gallbladder,[113] whereas 10 of the 16 patients with negative tests

were found to have other pathology accounting for their pain. Despite these encouraging results, other investigators have failed to demonstrate differences in outcome in patients with positive CCK tests when compared to those with negative tests.[114] Objective criteria on which to base the decision to recommend cholecystectomy in such patients are difficult to define. It is clear, however, that despite the minimally invasive nature of laparoscopic cholecystectomy, there should be no relaxation in the indications for cholecystectomy in patients with acalculous biliary pain.

Key points

- Asymptomatic gallstones do not require surgical intervention.
- The standard treatment for symptomatic gallstones is now laparoscopic, and there are few exceptions to a trial of a laparoscopic approach in all comers.
- All surgeons undertaking cholecystectomy, by whatever technique, should be capable of performing operative cholangiography.
- The use of operative cholangiography appears to be associated with a lower incidence of bile duct injury.
- Experience is accumulating that transcystic clearance of the CBD at the time of cholecystectomy is effective, with low morbidity and cost. In the one-third of patients where this is not achievable, ERCP is probably the best means of clearance.
- An algorithm for the management of common bile duct stones is shown in **Fig. 10.9**. The management strategy chosen will depend on personal experience, equipment availability, time and the availability of other departmental expertise. There is no consensus as to the ideal approach.

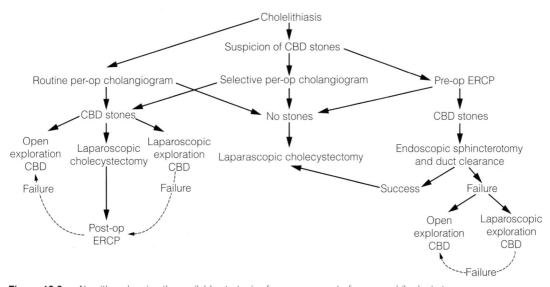

Figure 10.9 • Algorithm showing the available strategies for management of common bile duct stones.

References

1. Godfrey PJ, Bates T, Harrison M, et al. Gallstones and mortality: a study of all gallstone related deaths in a single health district. Gut 1984;25:1029–33.

2. Hospital In-patient Inquiry Main tables Department of Health and Social Security/Office of Population Census and Surveys. London: HMSO; 19801989.

3. American College of Surgeons. Socio-economic fact book for surgery. Chicago: Socioeconomic Affairs Department, American College of Surgeons; 1988.

4. Motson RW. Operative cholangiography. In: Motson RW, editor. Retained common duct stones. Prevention and treatment. London: Grune & Stratton; 1985. p. 8–9.

5. Neoptolemos JP, Hofmann AF, Moossa AR. Chemical treatment of stones in the biliary tree. Br J Surg 1986;73:515–24.

6. Bennion LJ, Grundy SM. Risk factors for the development of cholelithiasis in man. N Engl J Med 1978;299:1161–221.

7. Scragg RK, McMichael AJ, Seamark RF. Oral contraceptives, pregnancy and endogenous oestrogen in gallstone disease – a case controlled study. Br Med J (Clin Res Ed) 1984;288:1795–9.

8. Scragg RK, McMichael AJ, Paghurst PA. Diet, alcohol and relative weight in gallstone disease: a case controlled study. Br Med J (Clin Res Ed) 1984;288:1113–8.

9. Richardson WS, Surowiec WJ, Carter KM, et al. Gallstone disease in heart transplant recipients. Ann Surg 2003;237:273–6.

10. Festi D, Colecchia A, Orsini M, et al. Gallbladder motility and gallstone formation in obese patients following very low calorie diets. Int J Obes Relat Metab Disord 1998;22(6):592–600.

11. Nakeeb A, Comuzzie AG, Martin L, et al. Gallstones: genetics versus environment. Ann Surg 2002;235(6):842–9.

12. Dowling RH, Veysey MJ, Pereira SP, et al. Role of intestinal transit in the pathogenesis of gallbladder stones. Can J Gastroenterol 1997;11(1):57–64.

13. Vitek L, Carey MC. New pathophysiologic concepts underlying pathogenesis of pigment gallstones. Clin Res Hepatol Gastroenterol 2012;36(2):122–9.

14. Keighley MRB. Micro-organisms in the bile. A preventable cause of sepsis after biliary surgery. Ann R Coll Surg Engl 1977;59:328–34.

15. Glenn F, Moody FG. Acute obstructive suppurative cholangitis. Surg Gynecol Obstet 1961;113:265–73.

16. Taylor TV, Torrance B, Rimmer S, et al. Operative cholangiography: is there a statistical alternative? Am J Surg 1983;145:640–3.

17. Wilson TG, Hall JC, Watts JM. Is operative cholangiography always necessary? Br J Surg 1986;73:637–40.

18. Prat F, Meduri B, Ducot B, et al. Prediction of common bile duct stones by noninvasive tests. Ann Surg 1999;229(3):362–8.

19. Lindsel DRM. Ultrasound imaging of pancreas and biliary tract. Lancet 1990;335:390–3.

20. Prat F, Amouyal G, Amouyal P, et al. Prospective controlled study of endoscopic ultrasonography and endoscopic retrograde cholangiography in patients with suspected common bile duct lithiasis. Lancet 1996;347(8994):75–9.
A study making the case for endoscopic ultrasonography as an alternative to ERCP for the detection of common bile duct stones.

21. Norton SA, Alderson D. Endoscopic ultrasonography in the evaluation of idiopathic acute pancreatitis. Br J Surg 2000;87:1650–5.

22. Baroll RL. Common bile duct stones. Reassessment of criteria for CT diagnosis. Radiology 1987;162:419–24.

23. Ichii H, Takada M, Kashiwagi R, et al. Three-dimensional reconstruction of biliary tract using spiral computed tomography for laparoscopic cholecystectomy. World J Surg 2002;26:608–11.

24. Hochwalk SN, Dobransky M, Rofsky NM, et al. Magnetic resonance cholangiopancreatography accurately predicts the presence or absence of choledocholithiasis. J Gastrointest Surg 1998;2(6):573–9.

25. Masui T, Takehara Y, Fujiwara T, et al. MR and CT cholangiography in evaluation of the biliary tract. Acta Radiol 1998;39(5):557–63.

26. Liu TH, Consorti ET, Kawashima A, et al. Patient evaluation and management with selective use of magnetic resonance cholangiography and endoscopic retrograde cholangiopancreatography before laparoscopic cholecystectomy. Ann Surg 2001;234(1):33–40.

27. Gracie WA, Ransahoff DF. The natural history of silent gallstones: the innocent gallstone is not a myth. N Engl J Med 1982;307:798–800.

28. McSherry CK, Glenn F. The incidence and causes of death following surgery for non-malignant biliary tract disease. Ann Surg 1980;191:271–5.

29. Lagergren J, Mattsson F. Cholecystectomy as a risk factor for oesophageal adenocarcinoma. Br J Surg 2011;98:1133–7.

30. Schmidt M, Søndenaa K, Vetrhus M, et al. A randomized controlled study of uncomplicated gallstone disease with 14-year follow-up showed that operation was the preferred treatment. Dig Surg 2011;28:270–6.

31. Iser JH, Dowling RH, Mok HYI, et al. Chenodeoxycholic acid treatment of gallstones. N Engl J Med 1975;293:333–78.

32. O'Donnell LDJ, Heaton KW. Recurrence and re-recurrence of gallstones after medical dissolution: a long-term follow-up. Gut 1988;29:655–8.

33. Ahmed R, Freeman JV, Ross B, et al. Long term response to gallstone treatment – problems and surprises. Eur J Surg 2000;166:447–54.

34. Sauerbruch T, Stern M. Fragmentation of bile duct stones by extracorporeal shockwaves. A new approach to biliary calculi after failure of routine endoscopic measures. Gastroenterology 1989;96:146–52.

35. Clavien PA, Sanabria JR, Mentha G, et al. Recent results of elective open cholecystectomy in a North American and a European centre – comparison of complications and risk factors. Ann Surg 1992;216:618–26.

36. Bredesen J, Jorgensen T, Andersen TF, et al. Early postoperative mortality following cholecystectomy in the entire female population of Denmark – 1977–1991. World J Surg 1992;16:530–5.
    Both these papers document the results of open cholecystectomy prior to the advent of laparoscopic cholecystectomy.

37. Andren-Sandberg A, Alinder A, Bengmark S. Accidental lesions of the common bile duct at cholecystectomy: pre- and peroperative factors of importance. Ann Surg 1985;201:328–33.
    Frequently cited study that documents risk factors implicated in injury to the common bile duct during open cholecystectomy.

38. Connor S, Garden OJ. Bile duct injury in the era of laparoscopic cholecystectomy. Br J Surg 2006;93:158–68.

39. Bates T, Ebbs SR, Harrison M, et al. Influence of cholecystectomy on symptoms. Br J Surg 1991;78:964–7.

40. MacMahon AJ, Russell IT, Baxter JN, et al. Laparoscopic versus minilaparotomy cholecystectomy: a randomised trial. Lancet 1994;343:135–8.

41. Majeed AW, Troy G, Nicholl JP, et al. Randomised, prospective, single-blind comparison of laparoscopic versus small-incision cholecystectomy. Lancet 1996;347:989–94.

42. Ros A, Gustafsson L, Krook H, et al. Laparoscopic cholecystectomy versus mini-laparotomy cholecystectomy: a prospective, randomised, single-blind study. Ann Surg 2001;234(6):741–9.
    No evidence to support routine mini-cholecystectomy.

43. Dubois F, Icard P, Berthelot G, et al. Coelioscopic cholecystectomy. Ann Surg 1990;211:60–2.

44. Nathanson LK, Shimi S, Cuschieri A. Laparoscopic cholecystectomy: the Dundee technique. Br J Surg 1991;78:155–9.

45. Gramatica L, Brasesco OE, Mercado LA, et al. Laparoscopic cholecystectomy performed under regional anaesthesia in patients with chronic obstructive pulmonary disease. Surg Endosc 2002;16:472–5.

46. Ghumman E, Barry M, Grace PA. Management of gallstones in pregnancy. Br J Surg 1997;84:1646–50.

47. Yeh CN, Chen MF, Jan YY. Laparoscopic cholecystectomy in 226 cirrhotic patients. Experience of a single centre in Taiwan. Surg Endosc 2002;16:1583–7.

48. Cuschieri A, Dubois F, Mouiel J, et al. The European experience of laparoscopic cholecystectomy. Am J Surg 1991;161:385–7.

49. The Southern Surgeons Club. A prospective analysis of 1518 laparoscopic cholecystectomies. N Engl J Med 1991;324:1073–8.

50. Wilson P, Leese T, Morgan WP, et al. Elective laparoscopic cholecystectomy for 'all comers'. Lancet 1991;338:795–7.

51. Unger SW, Rosenbaum G, Unger HM, et al. A comparison of laparoscopic and open treatment of acute cholecystitis. Surg Endosc 1993;7:408–11.

52. Navez B, Mutter D, Russier Y, et al. Safety of laparoscopic approach for acute cholecystitis: retrospective study of 609 cases. World J Surg 2001;25(10):1352–6.

53. Richards C, Edwards J, Culver D, et al. Does using a laparoscopic approach to cholecystectomy decrease the risk of surgical site infection? Ann Surg 2003;3:358–62.

54. Al-Ghnaniem R, Benjamin IS, Patel AG. Meta-analysis suggests antibiotic prophylaxis is not warranted in low-risk patients undergoing laparoscopic cholecystectomy. Br J Surg 2003;90:365–6.

55. Lau H, Brooks DC. Contemporary outcomes of ambulatory laparoscopic cholecystectomy in a major teaching hospital. World J Surg 2002;26:1117–21.

56. Cheah WK, Lenzi JE, So BY, et al. Randomised trial of needlescopic versus laparoscopic cholecystectomy. Br J Surg 2001;88:45–7.

57. Lai ECH, Yang GPC, Tang CN, et al. Prospective randomized comparative study of single incision laparoscopic cholecystectomy versus conventional four-port laparoscopic cholestectomy. Am J Surg 2011;202:254–8.

58. Richardson MC, Bell G, Fullarton GM, The West of Scotland Laparoscopic Cholecystectomy Audit Group. Incidence and nature of bile duct injuries following laparoscopic cholecystectomy: an audit of 5913 cases. Br J Surg 1996;83:1356–60.

59. MacFadyen BV, Vecchio R, Ricardo AE, et al. Bile duct injury after laparoscopic cholecystectomy. Surg Endosc 1998;12:315–21.

60. Archer SB, Brown DW, Hunter JG, et al. Bile duct injury during laparoscopic cholecystectomy: results of a national survey. Ann Surg 2001;234(4):549–59.

61. Way LW, Stewart L, Hunter JG, et al. Causes and prevention of laparoscopic bile duct injuries. Analysis of 252 cases from a human factors and cognitive psychology perspective. Ann Surg 2003;4:460–9.

62. Keus F, de Jong JAF, Gooszen HG, et al. Laparoscopic versus open cholecystectomy for patients with symptomatic cholecystolithiasis. Cochrane Database Syst Rev 2006;(4):CD006231.

63. Fletcher DR, Hobbs M, Tan P, et al. Complications of cholecystectomy. Risks of the laparoscopic approach and protective effects of operative cholangiography: a population-based study. Ann Surg 1999;229(4):449–57.

64. Flum DR, Dellinger EP, Cheadle A, et al. Intraoperative cholangiography and risk of common bile duct injury during cholecystectomy. JAMA 2003;289:1639–44.
    Large study on 1.5 million patients demonstrating an increased risk of common bile duct injury when intraoperative cholangiography was not used during laparoscopic cholecystectomy.

65. Snow LL. Evaluation of operative cholangiography in 2043 patients undergoing laparoscopic cholecystectomy. A case for the selective operative cholangiogram. Surg Endosc 2001;15:14–20.

66. John TG, Banting SW, Pye S, et al. Preliminary experience with intracorporeal laparoscopic ultrasonography using a sector scanning probe. A prospective comparison with intraoperative cholangiography in the detection of choledocholithiasis. Surg Endosc 1994;8:1176–81.

67. Greig JD, John TG, Mahadaven M, et al. Laparoscopic ultrasonography in the evaluation of the biliary tree during laparoscopic cholecystectomy. Br J Surg 1994;84:1202–6.

68. Tranter SE, Thompson MH. Potential of laparoscopic ultrasonography as an alternative to operative cholangiography in the detection of bile duct stones. Br J Surg 2001;88:65–9.

69. Tranter SE, Thompson MH. A prospective single-blinded controlled study comparing laparoscopic ultrasound of the common bile duct with operative cholangiography. Surg Endosc 2003;17:216–9.

70. Catheline JM, Turner R, Paries J. Laparoscopic ultrasonography is a complement to cholangiography for the detection of choledocholithiasis at laparoscopic cholecystectomy. Br J Surg 2002;89:1235–9.

71. Tranter SE, Thompson MH. Spontaneous passage of bile duct stones: frequency of occurrence and relation to clinical presentation. Ann R Coll Surg Engl 2003;85:174–7.

72. Lygidakis NJ. A prospective randomised study of recurrent choledocholithiasis. Surg Gynecol Obstet 1982;155(5):679–84.

73. Panis Y, Fagniez PL, Brisset D, et al. Long-term results of choledochoduodenostomy versus choledochojejunostomy for choledocholithiasis. Surg Gynecol Obstet 1993;177(1):33–7.
    Two studies stressing the need to consider a surgical drainage procedure if ductal stones are thought to represent primary calculi.

74. Uchiyama K, Onishi H, Tani M, et al. Long-term prognosis after treatment of patients with choledocholithiasis. Ann Surg 2003;238(1):97–102.

75. Jeyapalan M, Almeida JA, Michaelson RL, et al. Laparoscopic choledochoduodenostomy: review of a 4-year experience with an uncommon problem. Surg Laparosc Endosc 2002;12(3):148–53.

76. Rhodes M, Nathanson L. Laparoscopic choledochoduodenostomy. Surg Laparosc Endosc 1996;6(4):318–21.

77. Strömberg C, Nilsson M. Nationwide study of the treatment of common bile duct stones in Sweden between 1965 and 2009. Br J Surg 2011;98:1766–74.

78. Petelin JB. Clinical results of common bile duct exploration. Endosc Surg Allied Technol 1993;1(3):125–9.

79. Berci G, Morgenstern L. Laparoscopic management of common bile duct stones. A multiinstitutional SAGES study. Society of American Gastrointestinal Endoscopic Surgeons. Surg Endosc 1994;8:1168–74.

80. Rhodes M, Nathanson L, O'Rourke N, et al. Laparoscopic exploration of the common bile duct: lessons learned from 129 consecutive cases. Br J Surg 1995;82:666–8.

81. Khoo D, Walsh CJ, Murphy C, et al. Laparoscopic common bile duct exploration: evolution of a new technique. Br J Surg 1996;83:341–6.

82. Martin IJ, Bailey IS, Rhodes M, et al. Towards T-tube free laparoscopic bile duct exploration: a methodologic evolution during 300 consecutive procedures. Ann Surg 1998;228(1):29–34.

83. Cuschieri A, Lezoche E, Morino M, et al. E.A.E.S. multicentre prospective randomised trial comparing two-stage vs. single-stage management of patients with gallstone disease and ductal calculi. Surg Endosc 1999;13(10):952–7.

84. Rhodes M, Sussman L, Cohen L, et al. Randomised trial of laparoscopic exploration of common bile duct versus postoperative endoscopic retrograde cholangiography for common bile duct stones. Lancet 1998;351:159–61.
    Two important randomised studies indicating success of laparoscopic bile duct exploration.

85. Buddingh KT, Weersma RK, Savenije RAJ, et al. Lower rate of major bile duct injury and increased intraoperative management of common bile duct stones after implementation of routine intraoperative cholangiography. J Am Coll Surg 2011;213:267–74.

86. Boerma D, Rauws EAJ, Keulemans YCA, et al. Wait-and-see policy of laparoscopic cholecystectomy after endoscopic sphincterotomy for bile-duct stones: a randomised trial. Lancet 2002;360:761–5.

87. Riciardi R, Islam S, Canete JJ, et al. Effectiveness and long-term results of laparoscopic common bile duct exploration. Surg Endosc 2003;17:19–22.

88. Nathanson LK, O'Rourke NA, Martin IJ, et al. Postoperative ERCP versus laparoscopic choledochotomy for clearance of selected bile duct calculi: a randomized trial. Ann Surg 2005;242(2):188–92.

89. Collins C, Maguire D, Ireland A, et al. A prospective study of common bile duct calculi in patients undergoing laparoscopic cholecystectomy: natural history of choledocholithiasis revisited. Ann Surg 2004;239(1):28–33.

90. Finnis D, Rowntree T. Choledochoscopy in exploration of the common bile duct. Br J Surg 1977;64:661–4.

91. Williams JA, Treacy PJ, Sidey P, et al. Primary duct closure versus T-tube drainage following exploration of the common bile duct. Aust N Z J Surg 1994;64(12):823–6.

92. Tanaka M. Bile duct clearance, endoscopic or laparoscopic? J Hepatobiliary Pancreat Surg 2002;9:729–32.

93. Leese T, Neoptolemos JP, Carr-Locke DL. Successes, failures, early complications and their management: results of 394 consecutive patients from a single centre. Br J Surg 1985;72:215–9.

94. Ochi Y, Mukawa K, Kiyosawa K, et al. Comparing the treatment outcomes of endoscopic papillary dilation and endoscopic sphincterotomy for removal of bile duct stones. J Gastroenterol Hepatol 1999;14(1):90–6.

95. Vaira D, Ainley C, Williams S, et al. Endoscopic sphincterotomy in 1000 consecutive patients. Lancet 1989;ii:431–4.
Three reports supporting use of endoscopic removal of common bile duct stones in high-risk surgical patients.

96. Lambert ME, Betts CD, Hill J, et al. Endoscopic sphincterotomy – the whole truth. Br J Surg 1991;78:473–6.

97. Webber J, Ademak HE, Riemann JF. Extracorporeal piezo-electric lithotripsy for retained bile duct stones. Endoscopy 1992;24:239–43.

98. Shaw MJ, Mackie RD, Moore JP, et al. Results of a multi-centre trial using a mechanical lithotriptor for the treatment of large bile duct stones. Am J Gastroenterol 1993;88:730–3.

99. Leese T, Neoptolemos JP, Baker AR, et al. Management of acute cholangitis and the impact of endoscopic sphincterotomy. Br J Surg 1986;73:988–92.

100. Leung JWC, Cotton PB. Endoscopic nasobiliary catheter drainage in biliary and pancreatic disease. Am J Gastroenterol 1991;86:389–94.

101. Neoptolemos JP, Carr-Locke DL, Fossard NP. A prospective randomised study of pre-operative endoscopic sphincterotomy versus surgery alone for common bile duct stones. Br Med J 1987;294:470–4.

102. Barwood NT, Valinsky LJ, Hobbs M, et al. Changing methods of imaging the common bile duct in the laparoscopic cholecystectomy era in Western Australia Implications for surgical practice. Ann Surg 2002;235(1):41–50.

103. Tatulli F, Cuttitta A. Laparoendoscopic approach to treatment of common bile duct stones. J Laparoendosc Adv Surg Tech 2000;10(6):315–7.

104. Ng T, Amaral J. Timing of endoscopic retrograde cholangiopancreatography and laparoscopic cholecystectomy in the treatment of choledocholithiasis. J Laparoendosc Adv Surg Tech Part A 1999;9(1):31–7.

105. Ammori BJ, Birbas K, Davides D, et al. Routine vs 'on demand' postoperative ERCP for small bile duct calculi detected at intraoperative cholangiography. Surg Endosc 2000;14:1123–6.

106. Urbach DR, Khanjanchee YS, Jobe BA, et al. Cost-effective management of common bile duct stones. Surg Endosc 2001;15:4–13.

107. Tranter SE, Thompson MH. Comparison of endoscopic sphincterotomy and laparoscopic exploration of the common bile duct. Br J Surg 2002;89:1495–504.

108. Martin DJ, Vernon DR, Toouli J. Surgical versus endoscopic treatment of bile duct stones. Cochrane Database Syst Rev 2006;(2): CD003327.
Similar clearance rates and more procedures with ERCP.

109. Menzies D, Motson RW. Percutaneous flexible choledochoscopy: a simple method for retained common bile duct stone removal. Br J Surg 1991;78(8):959–60.

110. Mason R. Percutaneous extraction of retained gallstones via the T-tube track – British experience of 131 cases. Clin Radiol 1980;31:587–97.

111. Nussinson E, Cairns SR, Vaira D, et al. A 10-year single centre experience of percutaneous and endoscopic extraction of bile duct stones with T-tube in situ. Gut 1991;32:1040–3.

112. Nathan MH, Newman MA, Murray DJ, et al. Cholecystokinin cholecystography. Four years evaluation. AJR Am J Roentgenol 1970;110:240–51.

113. Lennard TWJ, Farndon JR, Taylor RMR. Acalculous biliary pain: diagnosis and selection for cholecystectomy using the cholecystokinin test for pain reproduction. Br J Surg 1984;71:368–70.

114. Sunderland GT, Carter DC. Clinical application of the cholecystokinin provocation test. Br J Surg 1988;75:444–9.

11

Benign biliary tract diseases

Benjamin N.J. Thomson
O.James Garden

Introduction

Apart from those disorders related to choledocho-lithiasis, benign diseases of the biliary tree are relatively uncommon (Box 11.1). The most challenging issues are in patients who present with symptoms associated with biliary strictures, which arise more commonly following iatrogenic injury during cholecystectomy. Congenital abnormalities such as choledochal cysts and biliary atresia are usually in the domain of the paediatric surgeon, although later presentation of cysts may occur after missed diagnosis or when revisional surgery is required. Most of the published literature regarding benign non-gallstone biliary disease is retrospective or at best prospectively gathered, non-randomised data, but clear guidelines can be followed based upon observation.

Congenital anomalies

Biliary atresia

Biliary atresia occurs in approximately 1 per 10 000 live births but its aetiology remains unclear. There is experimental evidence for a primary perinatal infection as well as cellular and humoral autoimmunity. An inflammatory process before birth may result in failure of the biliary lumen to develop in all or part of the extrahepatic biliary tree.

Presentation is usually in the early neonatal period with prolongation of neonatal jaundice. Most patients are treated in specialist neonatal surgical units; however, occasionally patients may be referred to adult units for assessment for liver transplantation following previous unsuccessful treatment. Management in the neonate is by porto-enterostomy (Kasai's operation), which involves anastomosis of a Roux limb of jejunum to the tissue of the hilum. Restoration of bile flow has been reported in 86% of infants treated before 8 weeks of age, but only 36% in older children.[1] Four-year survival is dependent on the timing of surgery. Of 349 North American children with biliary atresia, 210 (60%) required later liver transplantation, with a 4-year transplantation survival of 82%.[2] Recent evidence has suggested better outcomes following maternal liver-related liver transplantation, potentially due to tolerance to non-inherited maternal antigens.[3]

Choledochal cysts

The earliest description of a choledochal cyst was by Douglas in 1952,[4] who described a 17-year-old girl with jaundice, fever and a painful mass in the right hypochondrium. However, presentation is usually in childhood and around 25% are diagnosed in the first year, although prenatal diagnosis is now possible with improvements in antenatal ultrasonography. Adult centres treat a small proportion of those presenting with delayed diagnosis as well as those with complications from previous cyst surgery.

The incidence of choledochal cysts in Western countries is around 1 in 200 000 live births but it is much higher in Asia. There is frequent association with other hepatobiliary disease such as hepatic fibrosis, as well as an aberrant pancreatico-biliary duct junction.[5]

Strictures of the extrahepatic biliary tree
Iatrogenic biliary injury
Postcholecystectomy
Trauma
Other
Gallstone related
Mirizzi's syndrome
Inflammatory
Recurrent pyogenic cholangitis
Parasitic infestation
  Clonorchis sinensis
  Opisthorchis viverrini
  Echinococcus
  Ascaris
Primary sclerosing cholangitis
Benign strictures imitating malignancy
  Pancreatitis
    Lymphoplasmacytic pancreatitis
  Inflammatory pseudotumour
  Idiopathic strictures
HIV cholangiopathy

Magnetic resonance cholangiopancreatography (MRCP) now allows images that are superior to traditional cholangiography (**Fig. 11.1**), and it should be recommended due to its non-invasive nature.[6]

Classification

The modified Todani classification is employed to describe the various forms of choledochal cyst[7] (**Fig. 11.2**). Type I, the most common, represents a solitary cyst characterised by fusiform dilatation of the common bile duct. Type II comprises a diverticulum of the common bile duct, whilst type III cysts are choledochocoeles. Type IV is the second most common, with extension of cysts into the intrahepatic ducts. Lastly, type V involves intrahepatic cystic disease with no choledochal cyst, which merges into the syndrome of Caroli's disease.

Risk of malignancy

In the Western literature, the incidence of cholangiocarcinoma is reported to be approximately 12% (Fig. 11.1),[8] compared to Todani et al.'s Japanese experience of 16% in 1353 patients.[9] The incidence of malignancy is reported to be 2% at 20 years, increasing to 43% for those in their sixties.[10] Cyst drainage without cyst excision does not prevent later malignant change, and there is continuing debate regarding the precise ongoing risk following cyst resection. Takeshita et al. reported 180 patients who underwent primary surgery for a choledochal cyst. Synchronous malignancy was found in 36 patients (20%), with only one of the remaining 144 patients developing malignancy during follow-up.[11]

Management

Surgical resection is required to prevent recurrent episodes of sepsis and pain, to prevent the risk of pancreatitis from passage of debris and calculi, and because of the association with cholangiocarcinoma. Complete cyst excision with preservation of the pancreatic duct is required, with hepaticojejunostomy for reconstruction. Some authors advocate liver resection for type IV cysts with intrahepatic extension for complete removal of the cyst, although the advantage is debatable. For those patients with Caroli's disease, resection may be feasible if the biliary involvement is localised to one part of the liver. For other patients, endoscopic or radiological techniques may be required to address biliary sepsis by improving biliary drainage, while others may need to be considered for hepatic replacement if liver failure develops.

For extrahepatic cysts, cyst-enterostomy, or drainage of the cyst into the duodenum, should no longer be performed as the cyst epithelium remains unstable and malignant potential exists. If previous drainage has been performed, symptoms of cholangitis generally persist and conversion to a Roux-en-Y hepaticojejunostomy is advisable.

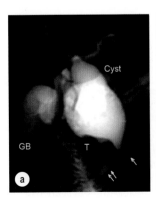 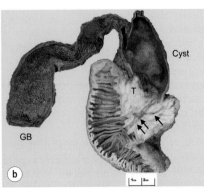

Figure 11.1 • MRCP **(a)** and macroscopic photograph **(b)** demonstrating a type I choledochal cyst with a distal cholangiocarcinoma in a 42-year-old Caucasian woman requiring a pancreaticoduodenectomy. Gallbladder (GB), tumour (T), pancreatic duct (single arrow) and aberrant common channel (double arrow) are shown. Courtesy of Professor Prithi S. Bhathal, Pathology Department, University of Melbourne, Australia.

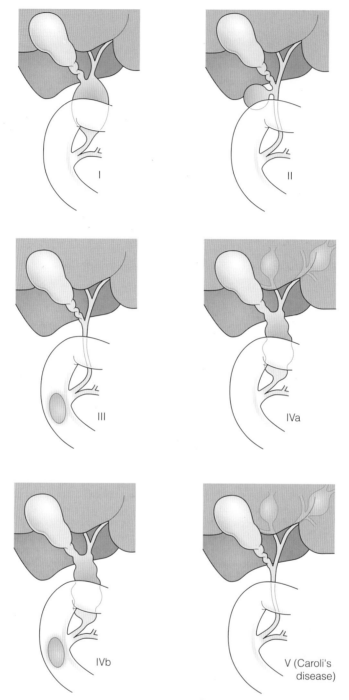

Figure 11.2 • Modified Todani classification for choledochal cysts.[7] Reproduced from Todani T, Watanabe Y, Narusue M et al. Congenital bile duct cysts: classification, operative procedures, and review of thirty-seven cases including cancer arising from choledochal cyst. Am J Surg 1977; 134:263–9. With permission from Elsevier.

Special operative techniques

During operative exposure, intraoperative ultrasound is very useful to identify the biliary confluence, the intrahepatic extension of the cyst, and the relationship to the right hepatic artery above and to the pancreatic duct below (**Fig. 11.3**). Small aberrant hepatic ducts may enter the cyst below the biliary confluence and these are missed frequently on preoperative imaging.[12] Such aberrant ducts are usually identified once the cyst has been opened. The cyst is

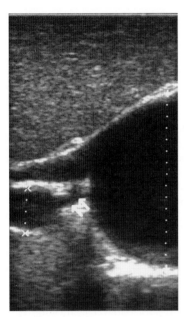

Figure 11.3 • Operative ultrasound scan of a type I choledochal cyst. The junction of the undilated proximal biliary tree with the cyst (long dotted line) is demonstrated. The right hepatic artery is posterior (two arrows), as is the right branch of the portal vein (short dotted line).

normally best excised in its entirety and this is facilitated by opening it along its anterior length. This aids identification of the vessels from which the cyst is freed. Early identification of the biliary confluence aids the surgeon in planning the incorporation of any segmental duct into the eventual hepaticojejunal Roux-en-Y anastomosis. Dissection into the head of the pancreas is made easier by use of bipolar scissors and the CUSA™ (ultrasonic surgical aspiration system, ValleyLab, Boulder, CO) if the plane of dissection is obscured by fibrosis or inflammation. It may be necessary to leave a small oversewn lower common bile duct stump to avoid compromise to the pancreatic duct lumen; however, recurrent pancreatitis and possible malignant transformation remain possible complications.

✓✓ There is an accepted association between choledochal cyst and cholangiocarcinoma. The cyst should be excised and the biliary tree reconstructed by means of a hepatico-jejunostomy Roux-en-Y.

Iatrogenic biliary injury

The commonest cause of an injury to the extrahepatic biliary tree is as a result of an iatrogenic injury at the time of cholecystectomy. Although it is recognised that injury may also occur during other gastric or pancreatic procedures, this is much less common with the reduction in ulcer surgery and increasing specialisation in pancreatico-biliary surgery. Rarely, the injury may be related to abdominal trauma, injection of scolicidal agents in the management of hydatid cyst, ablation of hepatic tumours or radiotherapy.

The true incidence of biliary injury following laparoscopic cholecystectomy remains obscure. It has been suggested that there was a slight increase in the incidence of injuries following initial introduction of the laparoscopic technique,[13] with a reported incidence of 0.3–0.7%.[14–16] Open cholecystectomy is said to have a lower incidence of biliary injury, with a rate of 0.13%.[17] Recent variations in technique such as single-incision laparoscopic surgery (SILS) cholecystectomy are not immune to biliary injury. Han et al. recently reported two (1.5%) bile duct injuries in 150 patients having single-port laparoscopic surgery.[18]

Aetiology

Previous reports of injury during laparoscopic cholecystectomy suggested that injury was more likely to occur when performed for pancreatitis, cholangitis or acute cholecystitis.[19] However, in a prospective analysis of patients referred following biliary injury, 71% occurred in patients in whom the indication for cholecystectomy was biliary colic alone,[20] and thus surgeons should always be vigilant regardless of the indication.

In the majority of patients the problem is misinterpretation of the biliary anatomy, with the common bile duct being confused with the cystic duct. Associated injury to the right hepatic artery often occurs as it is mistaken for the cystic artery. Partial injury may occur to the common bile duct after a diathermy burn or due to rigorous traction on the cystic duct, leading to its avulsion from the bile duct.

Techniques to avoid injury

Many techniques have been described to decrease the risk of injury to the common bile duct during cholecystectomy. The main risk factors are thought to be inexperience, aberrant anatomy and inflammation.[19,21] However, in an analysis of 252 laparoscopic bile duct injuries, the authors suggested that the primary cause of error was a visual perceptual illusion in 97% of cases, whilst faults in technical skill were thought to have been present in only 3% of injuries.[22]

Correct identification of the biliary anatomy is essential in avoiding injury to the extrahepatic bile duct. Dissection of Hartmann's pouch should start at the junction of the gallbladder and cystic duct and continue lateral to the cystic lymph node, thus staying as close as possible to the gallbladder. The biliary tree and hepatic arterial anatomy is highly variable and therefore great care must be taken in identifying all structures within Calot's triangle before ligation. In Couinaud's published study of biliary anatomy, 25% had drainage of a right sectoral duct directly into the common hepatic duct.[23] Sometimes this structure may follow a prolonged extrahepatic course, where it can be at greater risk from cholecystectomy. The right hepatic artery may also course through this area. All structures should be traced into the gallbladder to minimise the risk of injury (**Fig. 11.4** and **11.5**).

Calot's original description of gallbladder anatomy described a triangle formed by the cystic duct, common hepatic duct and superior border of the cystic artery.[24] For satisfactory visualisation of the structures, dissection should also extend above the cystic artery to the liver. Extensive dissection should be avoided in Calot's triangle as diathermy injury may occur to the lateral wall of the common hepatic duct. Furthermore, arterial bleeding in this area should not be cauterised or clipped blindly. Most bleeding can be controlled with several minutes of direct pressure with a laparoscopic forceps compressing Hartmann's pouch on to the bleed point. During the era of open cholecystectomy many advocated complete excision of the cystic duct to its insertion into the common bile duct to avoid a cystic duct stump syndrome. However, extensive dissection around the common bile duct with or without diathermy may cause an ischaemic stricture due to damage to the intricate blood supply of the common hepatic duct.

Many authors argue that operative cholangiography is essential to avoid biliary injury.[16,19] Fletcher et al. reported an overall twofold reduction in biliary injuries with the use of operative cholangiography, with an eightfold decrease in complex cases.[19] Flum and colleagues analysed retrospectively the Medicare database in the USA and identified 7911 common bile duct injuries following cholecystectomy. After adjusting for patient-level factors and surgeon-level factors the relative risk

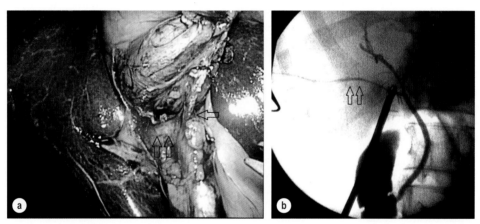

Figure 11.4 • Aberrant biliary anatomy. The normal biliary anatomy is a trifurcation of the right sectoral and left hepatic ducts forming the common hepatic duct which receives the cystic duct after a variable distance. Operative photograph **(a)** and a cholangiogram **(b)** of a short cystic duct (single arrow) draining into the right posterior sectoral duct (double arrow), which has a long extrahepatic course.

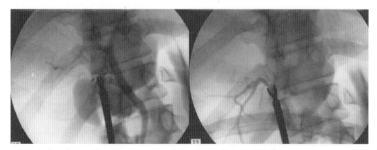

Figure 11.5 • Operative cholangiography of an aberrant right sectoral duct. The injury was recognised after division of the duct following cholangiography. The cholangiogram catheter was used to obtain a cholangiogram of the aberrant duct. The surgeon obtained advice by telephone and a decision was made to ligate the duct. The patient remains asymptomatic.

was 1.49 when intraoperative cholangiography was not used.[16] When the use of intraoperative cholangiography has undergone cost analysis, routine cholangiography has been found to be the most cost-effective during high-risk operations when employed by less experienced surgeons.[25]

Unfortunately, many operative cholangiograms are interpreted incorrectly and injuries are missed. Although this event should be less frequent with the use of modern C-arm imaging, in reported series of biliary injuries only 6–33% of operative cholangiograms are interpreted correctly.[20,26] For correct anatomical interpretation of the proximal biliary tree, both right sectoral/sectional ducts and the left hepatic duct should be visualised. In the presence of an endoscopic sphincterotomy, contrast will preferentially flow into the duodenum and the patient may need to be placed in a head-down position to fill the intrahepatic ducts. If the anatomy is unclear no proximal clip should be placed on what is presumed to be the cystic duct, to avoid a crush injury to what may be the common hepatic duct.

Retrograde cholecystectomy has been described previously as a safe technique when inflammation around Calot's triangle makes identification of the anatomy difficult. Nonetheless, care still needs to be exercised during dissection to avoid injury to the right hepatic artery and common hepatic duct, which may be adherent to an inflamed gallbladder. Eight such patients have recently been described by Strasberg and Gouma.[27] If identification remains impossible then the gallbladder can be opened to facilitate identification of the cystic duct. A subtotal cholecystectomy should be considered if a safe plane of dissection cannot be established, thus avoiding injury to the common hepatic or left hepatic ducts. Originally described for open cholecystectomy, these techniques have now also been performed laparoscopically.[28]

✔✔ Bile duct injury can be avoided by careful identification of the biliary anatomy, dissection close to the gallbladder and avoidance of diathermy in Calot's triangle. The use of operative cholangiography and its correct interpretation is associated with a reduced incidence of bile duct injury.

Classification

Injury to the distal biliary tree is less technically demanding to repair than involvement of the biliary confluence. The success of reconstruction depends on the type of injury and the anatomical location.[29] Bismuth first described a classification system for biliary strictures reflecting the relationship of the injury to the biliary confluence (Table 11.1).[30] Strasberg et al. further proposed a broader classification to include a number of biliary complications,

Table 11.1 • Bismuth classification of biliary strictures

Bismuth classification	Definition
Bismuth 1	Low common hepatic duct stricture – hepatic duct stump >2 cm
Bismuth 2	Proximal common hepatic duct stricture – hepatic duct stump <2 cm
Bismuth 3	Hilar stricture with no residual common hepatic duct – hepatic duct confluence intact
Bismuth 4	Destruction of hepatic duct confluence – right and left hepatic ducts separated
Bismuth 5	Involvement of aberrant right sectoral hepatic duct alone or with concomitant stricture of the common hepatic duct

including cystic stump leaks, biliary leaks and partial injuries to the biliary tree (**Fig. 11.6**).[17]

Presentation

It is preferable that injuries are recognised at the time of surgery to allow the best chance of repair, but this occurs in less than a third of patients. An unrecognised injury may present early with a postoperative biliary fistula, symptoms of biliary peritonitis or jaundice. Early symptoms or signs may be lacking but ductal injury should be suspected in the patient whose recovery is not immediate or is complicated by symptoms of peritoneal or diaphragmatic irritation and/or associated with deranged liver function tests in the first 24–48 hours of surgery. Signs may range from localised abdominal tenderness through to generalised peritonitis with overwhelming sepsis. Ligation of the bile duct will present early with jaundice; however, later presentation may occur as a result of stricture formation from a partial injury, localised inflammation or ischaemic insult.

Ligation of sectoral ducts may cause subsequent or late atrophy of the drained liver segments, which may become infected secondarily. Occasionally liver resection or transplantation may be required for fulminant hepatic failure secondary to combined biliary and vascular injuries.[31,32] More commonly, injuries may present late with secondary biliary cirrhosis, which may require liver transplantation when liver failure results.[31,32]

In many patients there is a delay until referral, despite evidence of a biliary injury. In a report by Mirza et al., the median interval until referral was 26 days.[33] This delay is not inconsequential as the

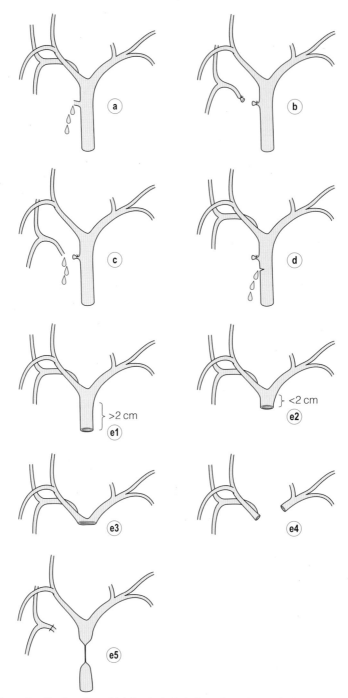

Figure 11.6 • Strasberg classification. Type A injuries include leakage from the cystic duct or subvesical ducts. Type B involves occlusion of part of the biliary tree, most usually an aberrant right hepatic duct. If the former injury involves transection without ligation this is termed a type C injury. A lateral injury to the biliary tree is a type D injury. Type E injuries are those described by Bismuth and subdivided into his classification (Table 11.1). Adapted from Strasberg SM, Hertl M, Soper NJ et al. An analysis of the problem of biliary injury during laparoscopic chole cystectomy. J Am Coll Surg 1995; 180:102–25. With permission from the American College of Surgeons.

opportunity for an early repair is lost and results in the liver sustaining further damage.

Management

Intraoperative recognition

In a review by Carroll et al., only 27% of patients underwent a successful repair by the primary surgeon responsible for the injury, whilst 79% of repairs performed following referral had a successful outcome.[34] If experienced help is not at hand, no attempt should be made to remedy the situation since this may compromise subsequent successful management. A T-tube or similar drain should be placed to the biliary injury and drains left in the subhepatic space, followed by referral to a specialist centre. No attempt should be made to repair a transection or excision of the bile duct.

A partial injury to the bile duct may sometimes be managed by direct closure with placement of a T-tube through a separate choledochotomy. Primary repair with or without a T-tube for complete transection of the common bile duct is nearly always unsuccessful. This may result from unappreciated loss of common duct or an associated arterial injury, or result from local diathermy injury or devascularisation of the duct from overzealous dissection of the common bile duct[35] (**Fig. 11.7a,b**). Succesful endoscopic treatment is possible for failed primary repair; however, as many as 32% will require subsequent hepatico-jejunostomy.[36]

✅✅ If an injury to the biliary tree is suspected during cholecystectomy, help must be sought from an experienced hepatobiliary surgeon. A successful repair by the surgeon who has caused the injury is far less likely than one performed by a surgeon experienced in performing a hepatico-jejunostomy.

Postoperative recognition: biliary fistula

Any patient who is not fit for discharge at 24 hours due to ongoing abdominal pain, vomiting, fever or bile in an abdominal drain should be considered to have a biliary leak. The lack of bile in an abdominal drain does not exclude the possibility of a biliary leak, particularly if there is liver function test derangement. Symptoms and signs vary widely, and widespread soiling of the abdominal cavity may be present with few signs.

Initial investigation should include full blood examination and determination of serum levels of urea, electrolytes, creatinine and liver function tests. Ultrasound is usually the initial investigation but it cannot readily differentiate bile and blood from a residual fluid collection following uneventful cholecystectomy. It may provide important information about the presence of intra-abdominal or pelvic fluid, biliary dilatation or retained stones within the bile duct.

If there is evidence of significant peritoneal irritation from widespread biliary peritonitis, laparoscopy allows confirmation of this and provides an opportunity for abdominal lavage. The porta hepatis can be inspected to determine the cause of the bile leak. Whilst dislodged clips from the cystic duct can be managed by application of further clips or suture, any other form of bile leak should lead to specialist referral. Drains can be placed to the subhepatic space as well as the subdiaphragmatic space and pelvis if required. No attempt should be made to repair an injury laparoscopically. If laparotomy is required, this should be considered in conjunction with specialist assistance if bile duct injury is suspected.

Further assessment depends on the clinical situation. The majority of biliary fistulas are due to leaks from the cystic duct stump or subvesicle ducts, and endoscopic retrograde cholangiopancreatography (ERCP) allows anatomical definition, endoscopic sphincterotomy or stent placement. As complete transection of the bile duct precludes ERCP, computed tomography intravenous cholangiography (CT-IVC) or MRCP can determine continuity of the biliary tree prior to endoscopy. Occasionally, persistent bile drainage is associated with choledocholithiasis requiring sphincterotomy and stone extraction. Most simple cystic duct stump leaks can be resolved by endoscopic stenting if cannulation is possible at ERCP[37] and occasionally side injury to the biliary tree can be controlled with endoscopic stent placement.[38]

If ERCP is unsuccessful or the bile duct is ligated or occluded by clips, percutaneous transhepatic cholangiography may facilitate biliary decompression but it is less frequently employed for diagnosis or delineation of the biliary anatomy. Occasionally, both sides of the liver may need to be externally drained to gain control of a biliary fistula, especially with E4 injuries to the biliary confluence. However, injury to the biliary tree detected in this way may allow surgical repair to be considered within the first week of injury in the stable non-septic patient, and again such further investigation or management decisions should only be considered following specialist referral.

Where the diagnosis of bile duct injury has been delayed, the aim should be to control the biliary fistula with external drainage using surgical or radiologically placed drains. Further control may be required with endoscopic stenting or external biliary drainage. Delayed repair can be considered subsequently once sepsis and intra-abdominal soiling have resolved, as a planned elective procedure in a specialist unit usually 2–3 months following injury. Such an initial conservative approach renders a potentially difficult operation into a repair that will be considerably easier.

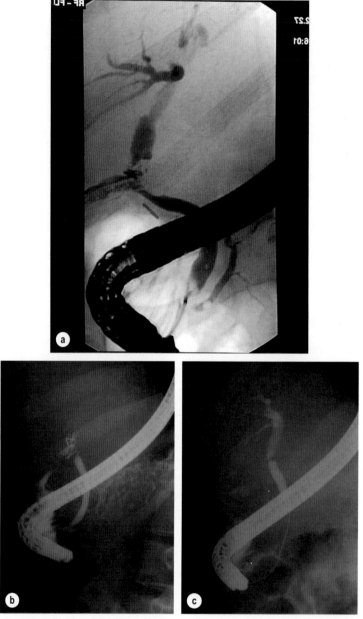

Figure 11.7 • (a) Failure of primary repair with T-tube. Primary repair was performed for an injury to the common bile duct presenting with biliary peritonitis. A T-tube was inserted through the anastomosis and this was removed at 4 weeks. An anastomotic stricture developed and the patient required a hepatico-jejunostomy 2 months later. **(b)** Failure of primary repair for ligation of the common bile duct. A complete transection of the common bile duct identified at postoperative endoscopic retrograde cholangiopancreatography (ERCP). Immediate repair was performed with a direct duct-to-duct repair. **(c)** A tight anastomotic stricture is demonstrated at a later ERCP.

✓✓ Diagnosis of a bile duct injury in the postoperative period should lead to immediate referral to a specialist centre since inappropriate attempts to manage this outwith a specialist centre will compromise the outcome.

Postoperative recognition: biliary obstruction

Ligation or inadvertent clipping of the biliary tree presents early in the postoperative period with jaundice. Later, stricture formation may occur as a result of direct trauma during dissection, clips placed inadvertently on the cystic duct but compromising the bile duct, or from damage to the intricate vascular supply of the bile duct by extensive mobilisation or diathermy. Initial investigation should include haematology, assessment of coagulation by estimation of prothrombin time, and liver function tests. Ultrasound may indicate the level of obstruction or exclude the presence of a correctable cause of obstructive jaundice, such as a retained stone in the common bile duct.

ERCP will identify a stricture or complete transection of the bile duct; however, identification of complete transection with MRCP will avoid the risks of an unnecessary ERCP. Overzealous instillation of contrast should be avoided, and placement of an endoscopic stent should only be considered after consultation with a specialist unit since this may introduce sepsis into the biliary tree and compromise further management. Furthermore, an undrained biliary tree may allow proximal biliary dilatation, thereby facilitating later reconstruction. Although some have reported satisfactory resolution of biliary strictures with endoscopic stenting alone, the follow-up has usually been short and almost all patients require later surgery in our experience. Partial occlusion of the duct by a clip may be remedied by balloon dilatation with or without placement of a stent; however, delay in diagnosis may result in subsequent recurrent stricture formation. Nonetheless, de Reuver et al. reported 110 patients with bile duct strictures following cholecystectomy that were treated with endoscopic stenting, 48 (44%) of which had already undergone attempted surgical repair. At a mean follow-up of 7.6 years, 74% of patients had a successful outcome.[37] The development of removable endoscopic expandable metal stents has recently been described, although long-term results and large series are not yet available. Furthermore stent migration can complicate treatment.

> ✔ If the diagnosis of ductal obstruction is made early within the first week postsurgery, the bilirubin level is only moderately elevated and there is no coexisting coagulopathy or sepsis, immediate repair offers the best chance of a successful outcome.

> ✔ If repair needs to be delayed, stent placement may still be avoidable and a decision will generally be made based on the individual patient circumstances. Suspicion or evidence of arterial injury may influence the management decision.

> ✔ For strictures that declare late, appropriate indications for stent placement are the presence of sepsis, severe itch resistant to medical therapy, or significant hepatic dysfunction.

The timing of repair

Early repair

When an injury is recognised in the early postoperative period and there is minimal peritoneal contamination or sepsis, a definitive repair by an experienced surgeon can be successful (**Fig. 11.8**). In our series of 123 patients referred with injury to the biliary tree, 22 patients underwent primary biliary repair in the first 2 weeks following injury and three had revision of a failed biliary repair. Between 2 weeks and 6 months, a further 22 injuries were repaired selectively. Successful repair was possible in 22 of 25 early repairs compared with 20 of 22 delayed repairs.[39]

Delayed repair

Many injuries continue to be unrecognised or referral delayed. In a prospective audit of major bile duct injuries from Australia, the median delay before referral was 9 days (2–28 days), and this included five patients with generalised peritonitis.[20]

Controlling the biliary injury and associated sepsis is the first treatment aim, which may require endoscopic or percutaneous biliary decompression, allowing jaundice to settle or biliary sepsis to be drained. Intra-abdominal collections may be drained percutaneously, or in the early postoperative period this may be better achieved by laparoscopic means. It is accepted, however, that bile collections are frequently loculated and difficult to

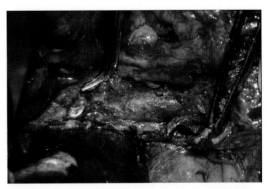

Figure 11.8 • Operative picture of an early repair of an E4 injury. A right-angle forceps is placed in the opening of the left hepatic duct whilst the open right hepatic duct is visible below. The portal vein is skeletonised with ligation and excision of both the extrahepatic biliary tree and right hepatic artery (held by forceps).

eradicate in patients with intra-abdominal sepsis or widespread biliary contamination or peritonitis. The most effective treatment may be laparotomy with extensive lavage and the placement of large intra-abdominal drains. Definitive repair should not be contemplated if there is severe peritoneal soiling since injudicious attempts to repair the injury may aggravate the injury and result in a poor outcome.

Once these objectives have been met, the patient should be allowed to recover from the combined insult of surgery and sepsis. A period of rehabilitation at home is generally required before repair is contemplated in these compromised patients. Abdominal and biliary drainage can be managed on an outpatient basis with community nursing support. Nutritional supplementation may be required, particularly in those who have required a prolonged admission to the intensive care unit and hospital. Attention should be paid to the consequences of prolonged external biliary drainage and consideration given to recycling of bile.

Associated vascular injury

Abdominal CT is required to ensure resolution of intra-abdominal collections and before repair to exclude the presence of liver atrophy. Atrophy can occur from prolonged obstruction to the segmental, sectional or hepatic ducts, but is generally associated with the presence of a vascular injury, most usually of the right hepatic artery. Liver resection may occasionally be needed at the time of definitive repair to remove a source of ongoing sepsis, or if satisfactory reconstruction to the left or right duct is not possible.

Buell et al. identified associated vascular injury as an independent predictor of mortality, with 38% of patients dying compared to 3% (P<0.001) where no arterial injury was present.[40] Some authors advocate arteriography before repair to identify such associated vascular injury as a repair is less likely to be successful,[41] or for consideration of hepatic arterial reconstruction at the time of hepatico-jejunostomy.[41,42] However, a recent paper described 55 patients with postcholecystectomy strictures who underwent surgical reconstruction with a left duct approach and preoperative coeliac axis and superior mesenteric artery angiography.[43] Twenty-six patients (47%) had an associated vascular injury, of which 20 (36%) were of the right hepatic artery. In this series only one patient in each group (vascular injury vs. no injury) developed a recurrent stricture after repair.[43] A proximal anastomosis may offer a better blood supply, minimising the risk of anastomotic stricturing (**Fig. 11.9**). In support of this theory, Mercado et al. demonstrated that an anastomosis fashioned below the biliary confluence was more likely to

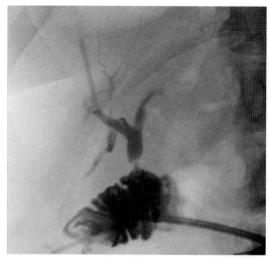

Figure 11.9 • Anastomotic stricture following repair of biliary injury. Percutaneous transjejunal cholangiogram (PTJC) of a Bismuth 1 injury repaired by hepatico-jejunostomy at the level of the transection of the common bile duct (not to the left hepatic duct). Three months later the patient required reconstruction of the anastomotic stricture.

require revisional surgery (16%) compared to an anastomosis performed at the biliary confluence (0%; P<0.05).[44] Recent improvements in magnetic resonance imaging (MRI) and spiral CT are producing impressive arterial and venous anatomical reconstructions, which may negate the need for invasive arteriography.

Injury to the hepatic arterial supply (usually the right hepatic artery) may present with haemobilia or intra-abdominal haemorrhage from a false aneurysm, usually associated with ongoing subhepatic sepsis. If suspected, urgent angiography is required (**Fig. 11.10**). Haemorrhage may be controlled by embolisation of the feeding vessel, although rebleeding can occur and necessitate further embolisation. However, in our experience, further bleeding in the presence of ongoing sepsis usually requires laparotomy for control of bleeding and drainage of any subhepatic collection.

Rarely, combined injury to the hepatic artery and portal vein can occur with resultant infarction of the affected hepatic parenchyma, usually the right liver. Such injuries may require urgent hepatic resection or transplantation.[31,32,45]

Further imaging

For patients with injury to the biliary confluence (E3 and E4), preoperative imaging will help in the planning of future repair. In the presence of a biliary stricture, invasive cholangiography by

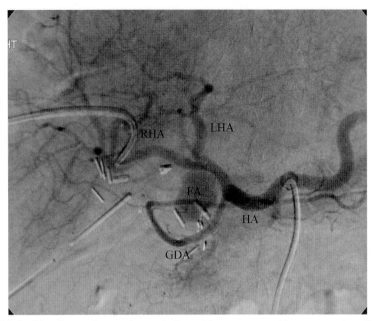

Figure 11.10 • Digital subtraction angiogram demonstrating a false aneurysm of the common hepatic artery. Embolisation was required for control. The patient has undergone a primary repair for a complete transection of the common bile duct. FA, false aneurysm; GDA, gastroduodenal artery; HA, common hepatic artery; LHA, left hepatic artery; RHA, right hepatic artery.

ERCP or percutaneous transhepatic cholangiogram (PTC) risks introducing sepsis. However, if PTC is required for external biliary drainage, an adequate cholangiogram may be obtained at this time. The quality of MRCP continues to improve, and detailed biliary anatomical reconstructions can be produced, thereby negating the need for more invasive imaging.

Operative techniques

Biliary reconstruction should be performed under optimal circumstances at the time of injury or soon thereafter. Once this opportunity has been lost, repair should only be considered when the patient has been optimised, in the absence of intra-abdominal sepsis, and when sufficient time has elapsed to allow for maturation of adhesions and the tissues at the porta hepatis.

A right subcostal incision is used for access, which can be extended across the midline if required. Retraction is provided with Doyen's blades and the Omni-tract® (Omni-tract surgical, St Paul, MN) mechanical retractor. Laparotomy is undertaken to assess the liver and to allow adhesiolysis, thereby freeing the small bowel for reconstruction. Frequently the omentum, hepatic flexure, duodenum and hepatoduodenal ligament are involved in a dense inflammatory mass, and occasionally an unsuspected fistula between bile duct and duodenum or colon is identified. Dissection is often easier if

commenced laterally and then directed towards the biliary structures. The common bile duct can be difficult to identify, particularly in the presence of extensive fibrosis, and intraoperative ultrasound is a useful tool in allowing its location and relationship to vessels to be determined.

For injuries that involve the biliary confluence, lowering of the hilar plate allows easier identification of the left and right hepatic ducts. This may be aided by the use of an ultrasonic dissector (CUSA), which is also employed to break down the contracted fibrotic tissue in the gallbladder bed and facilitate the division of any bridge of liver tissue between segments 3 and 4. Opening these two planes on the right and left sides facilitates identification of and access to the biliary confluence.

Since the blood supply to the bile duct is often damaged at the time of injury, the common hepatic duct should be opened as proximally as possible, although frequently there has been retraction of the fibrotic remnant superiorly. Extension of the incision into the left hepatic duct allows a wide anastomosis to be fashioned with adequate views of the left- and right-sided ducts. Care should be taken since there may be a small superficial arterial branch crossing the left duct anteriorly and running above to segment 4. For injuries with separation of the confluence, the right and left hepatic ducts can be anastomosed together before formation of a hepatico-jejunostomy, allowing a single biliary anastomosis. If possible, injuries to an isolated right sectoral duct are best repaired or drained into a Roux limb of bowel (Fig. 11.5). Simple ligation will lead to atrophy of the drained segments, which may become a nidus for sepsis. However, enteric drainage of a small sectoral duct may also lead to sepsis if an anastomotic stricture occurs.

Repair should be effected by a hepatico-jejunostomy with a 70-cm Roux limb of jejunum, thereby minimising the risk of enteric reflux and chronic damage to the biliary tree. Moraca et al. advocate hepatico-duodenostomy for biliary injury on the basis that it is more physiological, quicker to perform, and allows later ERCP for imaging and intervention.[46] They found no difference in outcome following hepatico-duodenostomy when compared with hepatico-jejunostomy, although median follow-up was only 54 months. Hepatico-duodenostomy has largely been abandoned in the treatment of other benign biliary disease due to ongoing enteric reflux. There have been anecdotal reports of the late development of cholangiocarcinoma,[47] as well as the need to undertake liver transplantation in patients so managed when secondary biliary cirrhosis due to enteric reflux has resulted. Our own view is that hepatico-duodenostomy has no role in the management of bile duct injury.

Fine absorbable interrupted sutures of 4/0 or 5/0 polydioxanone sulphate (PDS II) should be used to fashion an end-to-side hepatico-jejunostomy, with care being taken to produce good mucosal apposition. Some authors advocate the use of an access limb, particularly for E3 and E4 injuries, to allow subsequent radiological intervention for dilatation of recurrent strictures.[48] However, others believe that advances in percutaneous transhepatic techniques have made this unnecessary and have achieved satisfactory results without using this surgical approach.

Rarely, there may be no recognisable bile ducts visible in the porta hepatis. In such cases a variation of porto-enterostomy (Kasai procedure) can be considered with the Roux limb sutured to the fibrous structure of the hilar plate (S.W. Banting, personal communication).[49]

Partial injury to the biliary tree can be repaired with fine interrupted sutures, although when resulting from diathermy dissection, formal hepatico-jejunostomy may be necessary as conduction of the thermal injury may cause later stricture formation. If a T-tube is placed to protect a primary duct repair, this should be placed through a separate choledochotomy.

Management of complications related to repair

Revisional surgery

Many patients with biliary injury continue to suffer from complications despite reconstruction. Factors such as the experience of the initial surgeon, the level of injury, the associated sepsis and liver atrophy all increase the chance of an unsuccessful repair. Following primary repair of a ductal tear or laceration, further stricture formation may result if there has been extensive dissection around the common hepatic duct. In such instances, surgical revision with the formation of a Roux-en-Y hepatico-jejunostomy is indicated.

The majority of patients requiring revisional surgery will have undergone a previous biliary enteric drainage procedure. Anastomotic stricturing will require revision of the anastomosis, with extension of the choledochotomy into the left hepatic duct (Fig. 11.9).

Liver resection and transplantation

In the acute setting of bile duct injury, long-term damage to the hepatic parenchyma is difficult to predict. Major vascular injury or unrecognised segmental biliary obstruction may lead to atrophy of the liver, chronic intrahepatic infection, abscess formation or secondary biliary cirrhosis. In such patients, careful operative assessment is required; CT should be performed to identify areas of associated liver atrophy and to exclude portal vein thrombosis.

In our experience, the majority of patients requiring liver resection are those with ongoing sepsis in an obstructed segment or those where drainage of the extrahepatic biliary tree is not possible due to sectoral duct damage or fibrosis.[31] A recent review identified 99 patients (5.6%) requiring hepatectomy among 1756 postcholecystectomy bile duct injury patients,[50] with combined arterial and Strasberg E4 and E5 injuries more likely to require hepatic resection.[50] Occasionally, early hepatic resection is required for combined arterial, portal venous and biliary injury, although results are poor.[45] Very rarely, resection may be needed to gain access to the biliary tree, especially when the injury involves the biliary confluence (E4), although some authors routinely advocate resection of segments IVb and V for access to the right hepatic ducts.[51] The right lobe is most commonly affected by sepsis and atrophy as the right-sided sectoral ducts and arterial supply are more likely to be damaged during cholecystectomy, although both left- and right-sided hepatic resections have been reported in patients with severe biliary injury. Resection of the right liver can be performed, for example at the time of delayed reconstruction if there is any doubt regarding the integrity of the anastomosis to the right sectoral or hepatic duct and when a satisfactory anastomosis can be achieved to the long extrahepatic left duct.

Failed reconstruction and persistent cholangitis may lead to end-stage liver failure within a few years and this may require liver transplantation[31] (**Fig. 11.11**). A long interval between injury and

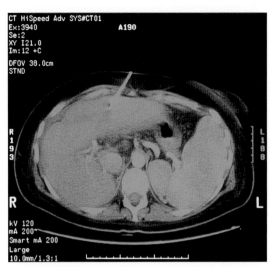

Figure 11.11 • Contrast-enhanced CT image of the liver after unsuccessful revisional hepatico-jejunostomy. The surgeon who performed the laparoscopic cholecystectomy performed the hepatico-jejunostomy for an E4 injury. A revisional hepatico-jejunostomy was performed before referral, which was complicated by an anastomotic stricture and portal vein thrombosis. The CT scan shows evidence of right lobe atrophy and splenomegaly as well as a percutaneous biliary drain.

referral is known to be associated with end-stage liver disease.[52] Rarely, liver transplantation may be needed when the combined biliary and vascular injury is so severe as to preclude attempted reconstruction, although the results are universally poor.[31]

Prognosis

Success of repair

Successful repair has been well described and can be achieved in 90% of patients in a specialised unit.[20,26] As for laparoscopic cholecystectomy, a learning curve for biliary repair has also been described for tertiary centres managing bile duct injury. Over a 20-year period, Mercado et al. reported an improvement with experience and a reduction of post-repair strictures from 13% to 5%.[53] As well as anastomotic strictures, liver atrophy and cirrhosis may also occur many years following repair. Predictors of a poor outcome include involvement of the biliary confluence,[29,52] repair by the injuring surgeon,[34,54,55] three or more previous attempted repairs[29] and recent active inflammation.[55]

Survival

Mortality following injury to the biliary tree is significant. Death may follow the acute injury itself, following the biliary repair, or occur later as a result of biliary sepsis or cirrhosis. In a recent report of a nationwide analysis of survival following biliary injury after cholecystectomy, Flum et al. identified 7911 (0.5%) injuries from 1 570 361 cholecystectomies.[54] Within the first year after cholecystectomy the mortality rate was 6.6% in the uninjured group and 26.1% in those with injury to the common bile duct. The adjusted hazard ratio for death during follow-up was higher for those with an injury (2.79; 95% confidence interval 2.71–2.88). The risk of death increased significantly with advancing age and comorbidities. If the initial repair was performed by the injuring surgeon then the adjusted hazard of death increased by 11%.

Quality of life

Boerma et al. first undertook an assessment of quality of life in patients who had sustained biliary injury or leak that required additional intervention.[56] Five years after injury, quality of life in the physical and mental domains was significantly worse than controls, despite a successful outcome in 84% of treated patients and regardless of the type of treatment or severity of injury. However, the length of treatment was an independent predictor of a poor mental quality of life. Melton et al. report that quality of life in 89 patients who had undergone biliary repair following laparoscopic cholecystectomy showed no difference in the physical or social domains when compared to controls.[57] However, in the psychological domain, patients were significantly worse, particularly in the 31% of patients who sought legal recourse for their injury.

Associated malignancy

A small number of reports exist about the development of cholangiocarcinoma at the site of anastomosis 20–30 years following repair.[47] It is possible that enteric reflux into the biliary tree with sepsis and the production of mutagenic secondary bile salts may be responsible. Furthermore, hepatocellular carcinoma may develop due to secondary biliary cirrhosis (**Fig. 11.12**).

Benign biliary strictures

Mirizzi's syndrome

Mirizzi first described the syndrome of extrahepatic biliary stricture in association with cholelithiasis in 1948,[58] a condition that occurs in fewer than 0.5% of cholecystectomies.[59] Obstruction of the common hepatic duct may occur for two reasons: (i) a stone impacted in the cystic duct may cause direct pressure or oedema (Mirizzi type I; **Fig. 11.13**), or (ii) occasionally the stone may erode through the wall of the gallbladder or cystic duct and into the common hepatic duct (Mirizzi type II).

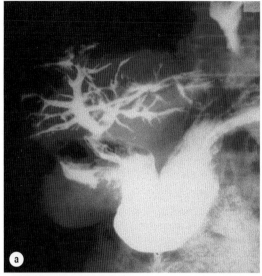

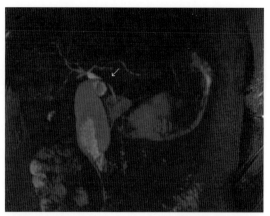

Figure 11.13 • Mirizzi syndrome (type I). Magnetic resonance cholangiopancreatography (MRCP) demonstrating compression of the common bile duct (single arrow) secondary to acute cholecystitis from a stone impacted in Hartmann's pouch.

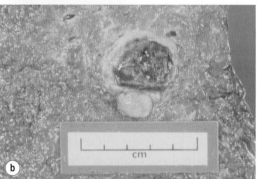

Figure 11.12 • Hepatocellular carcinoma as a consequence of biliary injury. This patient required a liver transplant for secondary biliary cirrhosis, which developed following hepato-duodenostomy for a biliary injury **(a)**. At pathological examination a hepatocellular carcinoma was detected in the explanted liver **(b)**.

Presentation

Diagnosis can be difficult as symptoms may be the same as for acute cholecystitis, but all patients with the disease process will have abnormal liver function tests and some may present with jaundice. Occasionally the diagnosis is made at the time of laparoscopic cholecystectomy.

Management

The investigations may be aimed at excluding a diagnosis of bile duct or gallbladder cancer. Ultrasound assessment will identify dilatation of the biliary tree proximal to the stricture and may even have features suggestive of a Mirizzi syndrome. An ultrasound finding of a decompressed gallbladder with stones involving the common hepatic duct

would be more suggestive of a Mirizzi syndrome. An associated mass or lymphadenopathy would be more in keeping with biliary malignancy, but associated sepsis or an empyema of the gallbladder may lead the operator to diagnose Mirizzi's syndrome as cancer. Both conditions may coexist. ERCP allows endoscopic stent placement to relieve jaundice and may demonstrate a fistula between the gallbladder and common hepatic duct (type II). A smooth, tapered stricture is more typical of a benign rather than malignant cause of jaundice. Endoscopic stenting provides resolution of jaundice, an anatomical roadmap and also may help with identification of the common hepatic duct at operation. Occasionally a stone impacted in the cystic duct may produce a distal biliary stricture. This occurs when there is a low insertion of the cystic duct with stone impaction at the cystic duct/common bile duct junction. It can be difficult to visualise or extract the stone at ERCP and therefore MRCP will be required to confirm the diagnosis.

When Mirizzi's syndrome is difficult to distinguish from a malignant stricture, CT may aid in the diagnosis. Contrast-enhanced ultrasound may allow better delineation of a benign or malignant cause; however, availability of contrast is limited at present. Occasionally laparoscopic ultrasound may be necessary to further delineate the stricture and exclude tumour dissemination. Although the two conditions may appear similar, vascular invasion may be seen and targeted biopsy may confirm a malignant diagnosis.[60]

Successful completion of cholecystectomy by laparoscopic means has been reported for apparent type I Mirizzi's syndrome,[61] although this would be inappropriate where there was a clear fistulous communication between gallbladder and common hepatic duct. One of these reported patients has subsequently developed a biliary stricture (O.J. Garden, personal communication). The conventional approach for type I strictures is to perform an open cholecystectomy or to convert from a laparoscopic procedure to allow adequate assessment of the associated biliary stricture. Operative cholangiography should be performed, and in those with persistent strictures a hepatico-jejunostomy should be performed. For type II, where a defect results from the removal of the gallbladder and stent, the common bile duct should be explored. The majority of patients will require a hepatico-jejunostomy, although apparently successful reconstructions using grafts of Hartmann's pouch have been described.[62] Long-term results of this innovative approach are awaited.

In a recent report, Schafer et al. identified Mirizzi's syndrome in 39 of 13 023 patients (0.3%) undergoing a laparoscopic cholecystectomy.[63] Thirty-four (87%) patients had a type I Mirizzi syndrome. Of these, 23 patients underwent cholecystectomy alone, 10 patients required bile duct exploration and T-tube insertion, and one patient had a Roux-en-Y reconstruction. Twenty-four of the 34 patients (74%) required open conversion. Of the remaining five patients with a type II Mirizzi syndrome, three underwent a hepatico-jejunostomy and two had simple closure with T-tube drainage. All had required open conversion and, interestingly, four patients (10%) were found to have a gallbladder carcinoma on histopathology.

✔ Mirizzi's syndrome is an uncommon cause of obstructive jaundice secondary to gallstone disease. This condition will normally necessitate conversion to open surgery if a laparoscopic cholecystectomy is attempted, and a hepatico-jejunostomy will normally be required for a type II lesion.

Hepatolithiasis

Intrahepatic gallstone disease (hepatolithiasis) is also known as oriental cholangiohepatitis or recurrent pyogenic cholangitis. It is most common in Taiwan, south-east Asia and Hong Kong. Symptoms include abdominal pain and jaundice as well as cholangitis.

Recently there has been a decline in incidence, possibly related to improved economic conditions and changes in diet.[64] The cause is unknown, although *Clonorchis sinensis*, ascariasis and nutritional insufficiency have been suggested as associated factors in its causation.

Pathologically there is gross irregular dilatation and intrahepatic stricture formation of the biliary tree, which frequently contains stones, debris and pus. Bile duct proliferation, portal and periportal inflammation and fibrosis are seen, and occasionally there is liver abscess formation. Stone formation is frequently associated with bacterial superinfection and the bile is infected in 96% of patients with hepatolithiasis, most usually with *Escherichia coli*.[65] There is a strong association between hepatolithiasis and cholangiocarcinoma, particularly in the presence of liver atrophy.[66] Diagnosis is based on history and demographic features, and investigation includes liver biochemistry and abdominal ultrasonography. Ultrasound is usually diagnostic, although abdominal CT may add further information regarding associated liver atrophy or abscess formation. ERCP will provide important anatomical detail and will allow endoscopic stenting if required. If stricture formation or stones prevent filling of the intrahepatic ducts, MRCP should provide further information, avoiding the risk of PTC.

Management

In an acute attack, treatment of cholangitis is initiated with broad-spectrum antibiotics. A third-generation cephalosporin and metronidazole with the addition of ampicillin for resistant enterococci will provide broad cover for most biliary pathogens. Intravenous fluid resuscitation and analgesia are required. Conservative treatment fails in around 30% of cases, which is more likely in those with obstruction of the extrahepatic biliary tree rather than an isolated segment. When conservative treatment fails, biliary decompression is required by either an endoscopic, radiological or surgical approach.

Following resolution of an acute attack definitive surgery is required. A multidisciplinary approach is required involving radiologists, surgeons and gastroenterologists. A full spectrum of interventions from simple exploration and stone removal, hepatico-jejunostomy or liver resection through to liver transplantation may be required. Of 97 Japanese patients treated for hepatolithiasis, 49% undergoing hepatico-jejunostomy, 25% drained with T-tube and 10% treated with percutaneous transhepatic cholangioscopic lithotripsy were found to have residual stones. No patients treated with hepatic resection had residual stone disease. Furthermore, recurrent stones were found in 14% of hepatectomy patients compared to 25% or more for the other treatment options.[67]

Parasitic infestation causing jaundice

Liver flukes (trematodes)

Infestation with liver flukes is caused through consuming inadequately cooked, pickled or salted infected fish. The immature fluke passes into the biliary tree, where it grows to maturity. Ova are passed into the gastrointestinal tract and subsequently to water supplies, infecting molluscs and fish. Infection with *Clonorchis sinensis* occurs in China, Japan and south-east Asia, whilst *Opisthorchis viverrini* is found in parts of eastern Europe and Siberia. Infection may be asymptomatic or the patient may present with an acute febrile illness or chronic symptoms. Chronic infestation results in hepatolithiasis and should be managed as detailed above.

Diagnosis is possible by the detection of ova within the stool or in duodenal aspirates, and an eosinophilia may also be present on blood film. ERCP may demonstrate slender filling defects within the bile duct as well as associated changes of fibrosis and calculus formation.

Echinococcus

Hydatid cysts involving the liver remain endemic in parts of the Mediterranean and Far East, as well as sheep farming areas of Australia, New Zealand, South America and South Africa. Infection is from *Echinococcus granulosus*, and less commonly *Echinococcus multilocularis* in central Europe.

Biliary obstruction can occur due to local compression of the common hepatic duct by the expanding cyst, or when daughter cysts pass down the common hepatic duct following rupture of the cyst into intrahepatic radicles. Secondary sclerosing cholangitis has been described following inappropriate injection of scolicidal agents into the hepatic cyst when there is communication with the biliary tree.[68]

Treatment

Preoperative endoscopic cholangiography may identify debris within the biliary tree, and endoscopic sphincterotomy may prevent further episodes of biliary obstruction. Endoscopic stenting may also allow resolution of obstruction secondary to a large intrahepatic cyst.

The secondary sclerosing cholangitis produced by inappropriate instillation of a scolicidal agent into the biliary tree will often only be amenable to hepatic replacement. Surgical bypass may be possible for localised strictures.

Ascaris lumbricoides

The roundworm *Ascaris lumbricoides* is the commonest worm to infect humans. Rarely, an infected patient can present with obstructive jaundice due to migration of the worm into the biliary tree and this is difficult to distinguish from stone disease. The more frequent presentation is from cholangitis due to the worm traversing the ampulla. *Ascaris* has also been associated with recurrent pyogenic cholangitis.

Ultrasound sometimes identifies a long, linear filling defect within the biliary tree. Identification may occur at the time of ERCP where endoscopic extraction may be possible. Medical treatment exists with the anthelmintics mebendazole or albendazole, which are often curative. The late complication of papillary stenosis can be treated with endoscopic sphincterotomy.

Primary sclerosing cholangitis

Aetiology

Primary sclerosing cholangitis is a rare condition, and although the precise cause has yet to be determined there is increasing evidence of an immunological basis as well as an overall increase in the incidence.[69] Around 70% of patients will have ulcerative colitis, or more rarely Crohn's disease. There are other reports of association with Riedel's thyroiditis, retroperitoneal fibrosis, lymphoplasmacytic sclerosing pancreatitis[70] as well as a strong association with a number of human leucocyte antigens.[71]

Presentation

Primary sclerosing cholangitis is a progressive obliterative fibrosis of the intrahepatic and extrahepatic biliary tree with a wide clinical spectrum and frequent remissions and relapses. In the early stages of disease most patients are asymptomatic but later in the disease process patients may have pruritus, ill-defined pain, fever, jaundice and weight loss. Many asymptomatic patients are diagnosed by detection of abnormal liver function tests during the investigation of inflammatory bowel disease. Although some patients may present at an advanced stage, signs of liver failure develop over a period of time. Sudden deterioration may suggest the development of cholangiocarcinoma, with which there is a strong association.

Investigation

Liver biochemistry demonstrates a cholestatic picture. Although antineutrophil cytoplasmic antibodies are present in the majority of patients, testing for autoantibodies is usually performed to exclude primary biliary cirrhosis, a condition from which it can be difficult to differentiate.

The mainstay of investigation is cholangiography, which usually demonstrates a diffuse picture of stricturing and attenuated intrahepatic bile ducts. As well as providing anatomical details of the biliary tree, ERCP enables endoscopic therapy and the opportunity for brush cytology if malignancy is suspected. MRCP is highly sensitive, with a diagnostic accuracy comparable to ERCP, and is now preferred as a means of both diagnosing and assessing the extent of disease to avoid the introduction of bacteria, possibly causing severe biliary sepsis. CT intravenous cholangiography also provides a good alternative when MRCP is contraindicated.

Management

The prognosis of primary sclerosing cholangitis is poor, with a median survival of only 9.6 years from diagnosis to death or liver transplantation.[72] Survival may improve with earlier diagnosis and liver transplantation; however, subsequent development of cholangiocarcinoma and colorectal cancer has now become the leading cause of death.[73] The use of ursodeoxycholic acid in the treatment of pruritus has been associated with improvements in biochemical function and histological appearance.[74] Episodes of cholangitis can be treated with antibiotics covering biliary pathogens. There is no evidence that colectomy for inflammatory bowel disease alters disease progression.

Endoscopic or transhepatic dilatation of short dominant strictures with or without endoscopic stenting has been described as effective, safe and well tolerated, although no randomised trials have been performed. Dilatation achieves palliation at 1 and 3 years in 80% and 60% of patients, respectively.[75] In those patients without cirrhosis but with jaundice secondary to a dominant stricture, surgical drainage with an access limb has been described.

Liver transplantation is necessary to treat end-stage liver disease. However, it is now more usual for patients to be considered if there is persistent jaundice, intractable pruritus, recurrent cholangitis, malnutrition or fatigue. Many patients are now transplanted before liver failure, with survival rates of greater than 80% at 5 years.[76]

Exclusion of associated malignant stricture

Cholangiocarcinoma and gallbladder cancer complicate 10–36% of patients with primary sclerosing cholangitis,[72] and need to be excluded before liver transplantation.

In the majority of patients, concern regarding occult cholangiocarcinoma is small, and liver transplantation is undertaken in the absence of a dominant stricture. Serum carbohydrate antigen (CA) 19-9 has been used in an attempt to identify cases with an occult biliary malignancy. Patients with a sudden rapid deterioration in their clinical state or with a dominant stricture must be considered to have a cholangiocarcinoma and be investigated extensively. Brush cytology at ERCP may provide the diagnosis if a malignant smear is obtained. CT or MRI may demonstrate a mass lesion in association with the biliary tree, although the usual appearance is of a stricture indistinguishable

from a benign disease. Positron emission tomography (PET) scanning is superior to conventional radiological investigations to differentiate primary sclerosing cholangitis and cholangiocarcinoma.[77]

Laparoscopy identifies the majority of patients with unresectable biliary tract cancer,[78] and may be of use in assessing those considered for transplantation in whom a cholangiocarcinoma is suspected since tumour dissemination often occurs early. Laparoscopic ultrasound may further aid assessment, and occasionally laparotomy may be required if there is diagnostic doubt regarding cholangiocarcinoma.

Biliary strictures imitating malignancy

It is not unusual for benign biliary pathology to be found in resected specimens of the pancreatic head that had been thought to be malignant. Around 10% of Whipple resections for malignancy will be found to have benign pathology. Most commonly the pathology is chronic pancreatitis related to alcohol or gallstone disease. However, other confounding pathologies include lymphoplasmacytic sclerosing pancreatitis, primary sclerosing cholangitis, choledocholithiasis and inflammatory pseudotumours.

Up to 14% of patients undergoing surgery for presumed malignant hilar obstruction are found to have a benign fibrotic stricture of the bile duct.[79] It is usually impossible to differentiate them from malignancy preoperatively and thus resection is often attempted and nearly always feasible. Successful treatment has been described with the use of steroids.

Lymphoplasmacytic sclerosing pancreatitis

Lymphoplasmacytic sclerosing pancreatitis is also known as autoimmune pancreatitis, sclerosing pancreatitis or primary inflammatory pancreatitis. The disease is associated with other autoimmune diseases such as Sjögren's syndrome, Riedel's thyroiditis, retroperitoneal fibrosis, ulcerative colitis and primary sclerosing cholangitis.[80] Although only accounting for about 2.4% of pancreatic resections, the condition is important since a proportion of patients will develop either biliary anastomotic strictures or intrahepatic strictures following resection. In a series of 31 patients, eight (28%) went on to develop recurrent jaundice after resection.[80]

Increased levels of IgG4 have been described in association with the disease, and successful treatment with steroids has been described, although disease recurrence is reported.[81] As yet the value of steroid treatment in the prevention and treatment of recurrent strictures is not well described.

Functional biliary disorders

Most patients who present for investigation of sphincter of Oddi dysfunction have already undergone cholecystectomy for presumed gallbladder pain. However, up to 39–90% of patients with idiopathic recurrent pancreatitis may also have sphincter of Oddi dysfunction.[82] In those patients with postcholecystectomy pain, the presentation and investigation identifies three types:[83]

- Type 1 – Abdominal pain, obstructive liver function tests, biliary dilatation and delayed emptying of contrast at ERCP.
- Type 2 – Pain with only one or two of the above-mentioned criteria.
- Type 3 – Recurrent biliary pain only.

Between 65% and 95% of group 1 patients will be found on biliary manometry to have sphincter of Oddi dysfunction compared to only 12–28% of type 3.[82] Diagnosis is usually by exclusion of other causes of abdominal pain such as peptic ulcer disease and irritable bowel syndrome. Liver function tests, abdominal ultrasonography, CT, endoscopy and MRCP have often been already performed. Morphine–neostigmine and secretin provocation MRCP studies may also be of diagnostic value.

At ERCP, biliary manometry is not required if there is delayed drainage of contrast in type 1 or 2 patients. This investigation should be reserved for those patients in whom the diagnosis remains unclear.

Medical therapy with calcium channel blockers, nitrates and botulinum toxin is available but long-term results are unknown. Avoidance of opiate analgesia, particularly over-the-counter preparations containing codeine, may prevent the onset of pain in the majority. Endoscopic sphincterotomy is a potential treatment; however, 5–16% of patients will develop postprocedural pancreatitis[84] and good or excellent responses are only reported in 69% of patients at long-term follow-up.[85] Surgical sphincterotomy is now indicated rarely due to the lower cost and lower morbidity of endoscopic sphincterotomy but it may be required if the endoscopic approach has been unsuccessful.

Key points

- Choledochal cysts should be treated with complete cyst excision and hepatico-jejunostomy due to the risk of malignancy in the remaining biliary epithelium.
- Identification of the biliary anatomy and minimisation of diathermy near the common bile duct are essential during laparoscopic cholecystectomy to avoid biliary injury.
- Operative cholangiography is useful for delineating the biliary anatomy during cholecystectomy; however, many cholangiograms are not interpreted correctly at the time of biliary injury.
- Following laparoscopic cholecystectomy, any patient who is not fit for discharge at 24 hours due to ongoing abdominal pain, vomiting, fever or bile in an abdominal drain should be considered to have a biliary leak.
- Diagnosis of a bile duct injury in the postoperative period should lead to immediate referral to a specialist centre since inappropriate attempts to manage this outwith a specialist centre will compromise the outcome.
- In the absence of sepsis, repair of injuries to the biliary tree can be performed successfully within the first week.

References

1. Mieli-Vergani G, Howard ER, Portmann B, et al. Late referral for biliary atresia: missed opportunities for effective surgery. Lancet 1989;i:421–3.

2. Schreiber RA, Barker CC, Roberts EA, et al. Canadian Pediatric Hepatology Research Group. Biliary atresia: the Canadian experience. J Pediatr 2007;151:659–65.

3. Nijagal A, Fleck S, Hills NK, et al. Decreased risk of graft failure with maternal liver transplantation in patients with biliary atresia. Am J Transplant 2012;12(2):409–19.

4. Douglas AH. Case of dilatation of the common bile duct. Monthly J M Sci 1952;14:97–101.

5. Suda K, Miyano T, Suzuki F, et al. Clinicopathologic and experimental studies on cases of abnormal pancreatico-choledocho-ductal junction. Acta Pathol Jpn 1987;37:1549–62.

6. Kim SH, Lim JH, Yoon HK, et al. Choledochal cyst: comparison of MR and conventional cholangiography. Clin Radiol 2000;55:378–83.

7. Todani T, Watanabe Y, Narusue M, et al. Congenital bile duct cysts: classification, operative procedures, and review of thirty-seven cases including cancer arising from choledochal cyst. Am J Surg 1977;134:263–9.

8. Lenriot JP, Gigot JF, Segol P, et al. Bile duct cysts in adults: a multi-institutional retrospective study. French Associations for Surgical Research. Ann Surg 1998;228:159–66.

9. Todani T, Watanabe Y, Toki A, et al. Carcinoma related choledochal cysts with internal drainage operations. Surg Gynecol Obstet 1987;164:61–4.

10. Voyles CR, Smadja C, Shands WC, et al. Carcinoma in choledochal cysts. Age-related incidence. Arch Surg 1983;118:986–8.

11. Takeshita N, Ota T, Yamamoto M. Forty-year experience with flow-diversion surgery for patients with congenital choledochal cysts with pancreaticobiliary maljunction at a single institution. Ann Surg 2011;254(6):1050–3.

12. Narasimhan KL, Chowdhary SK, Rao KL. Management of accessory hepatic ducts in choledochal cysts. J Pediatr Surg 2001;36:1092–3.

13. Morgenstern L, McGrath MF, Carroll BJ, et al. Continuing hazards of the learning curve in laparoscopic cholecystectomy. Am Surg 1995;61:914–8.

14. Waage A, Nilsson M. Iatrogenic bile duct injury: a population-based study of 152 776 cholecystectomies in the Swedish Inpatient Registry. Arch Surg 2006;141:1207–13.
Population-based study in Sweden of 152 776 cholecystectomies with 613 (0.40%) requiring biliary reconstruction.

15. Richardson MC, Bell G, Fullarton GM, The West of Scotland Laparoscopic Cholecystectomy Audit Group. Incidence and nature of bile duct injuries following laparoscopic cholecystectomy: an audit of 5913 cases. Br J Surg 1996;83:1356–60.
A prospective audit of biliary injury following cholecystectomy in Scotland. One of the first studies to record the rate of biliary injury and the more severe nature of the injuries at laparoscopic surgery.

16. Flum DR, Dellinger EP, Cheadle A, et al. Intraoperative cholangiography and risk of common bile duct injury during cholecystectomy. JAMA 2003;289:1691–2.
A retrospective analysis of more than 1.5 million cholecystectomies detailing the risk of injury and the decreased risk if operative cholangiography is used.

17. Strasberg SM, Hertl M, Soper NJ. An analysis of the problem of biliary injury during laparoscopic cholecystectomy. J Am Coll Surg 1995;180:102–25.
This paper describes a very useful classification system for biliary injury that includes the Bismuth classification as well as other less major injuries.

18. Han HJ, Choi SB, Park MS, et al. Learning curve of single port laparoscopic cholecystectomy determined using the non-linear ordinary least squares method based on a non-linear regression model: an analysis of 150 consecutive patients. J Hepatobiliary Pancreat Sci 2011;18(4):510–5.

19. Fletcher DR, Hobbs MS, Tan P, et al. Complications of cholecystectomy: risks of the laparoscopic approach and protective effects of operative cholangiography: a population-based study. Ann Surg 1999;229:449–57.
A retrospective audit of biliary injury in Western Australia that identified the increased risk of biliary injury after laparoscopic cholecystectomy compared to open cholecystectomy. This study also identified a significantly reduced risk of injury if operative cholangiography was performed.

20. Thomson BNJ, Cullinan MJ, Banting SW, et al. Recognition and management of biliary complications after laparoscopic cholecystectomy. Aust N Z J Surg 2003;73:183–8.

21. Strasberg SM. Avoidance of biliary injury during laparoscopic cholecystectomy. J Hepatobiliary Pancreat Surg 2002;9:543–7.

22. Way LW, Stewart L, Gantert W, et al. Causes and prevention of laparoscopic bile duct injuries: analysis of 252 cases from a human factors and cognitive psychology perspective. Ann Surg 2003;237:460–9.
Analysis of 252 bile duct injuries according to the principles of the cognitive science of visual perception judgment and human error showing that the majority of errors result from misperception, not errors of skill, knowledge or judgment.

23. Couinaud C. Le foi. Etudes anatomiques et chirurgicales. Paris: Masson; 1957.

24. Calot F. De la cholecystectomie. 1891. Doctoral thesis, Paris.

25. Flum DR, Flowers C, Veenstra DL. A cost-effectiveness analysis of intra-operative cholangiography in the prevention of bile duct injury during laparoscopic cholecystectomy. J Am Coll Surg 2003;196:385–93.

26. Slater K, Strong RW, Wall DR, et al. Iatrogenic bile duct injury: the scourge of laparoscopic cholecystectomy. Aust N Z J Surg 2002;72:83–8.

27. Strasberg SM, Gouma DJ. 'Extreme' vasculobiliary injuries: association with fundus-down cholecystectomy in severely inflamed gallbladders. HPB (Oxford) 2012;14(1):1–8.

28. Philips JA, Lawes DA, Cook AJ, et al. The use of laparoscopic subtotal cholecystectomy for complicated cholelithiasis. Surg Endosc 2008;22(7):1697–700.

29. Chapman WC, Halevy A, Blumgart LH, et al. Postcholecystectomy bile duct strictures. Arch Surg 1995;130:597–604.

30. Bismuth H. Postoperative strictures of the bile duct. In: Blumgart LH, editor. The biliary tract. Clinical surgery international. Edinburgh: Churchill Livingstone; 1982. p. 209–18.

31. Thomson BN, Parks RW, Madhavan KK, et al. Liver resection and transplantation in the management of iatrogenic biliary injury. World J Surg 2007;31:2363–9.

32. Ardiles V, McCormack L, Quiñonez E, et al. Experience using liver transplantation for the treatment of severe bile duct injuries over 20 years in Argentina: results from a National Survey. HPB (Oxford) 2011;13(8):544–50.

33. Mirza DF, Narsimhan KL, Ferras Neto BH, et al. Bile duct injury following laparoscopic cholecystectomy: referral pattern and management. Br J Surg 1997;84:786–90.

34. Carroll BJ, Birth M, Phillips EH. Common bile duct injuries during laparoscopic cholecystectomy that result in litigation. Surg Endosc 1998;12:310–3.

35. Stewart L, Way LW. Bile duct injuries during laparoscopic cholecystectomy: factors that influence the results of treatment. Arch Surg 1995;130:1123–9.

36. de Reuver PR, Busch OR, Rauws EA, et al. Long-term results of a primary end-to-end anastomosis in peroperative detected bile duct injury. J Gastrointest Surg 2007;11:296–302.

37. de Reuver PR, Rauws EA, Vermeulen M, et al. Endoscopic treatment of post-surgical bile duct injuries: long term outcome and predictors of success. Gut 2007;56:1599–605.

38. Sandha GS, Bourke MJ, Haber GB, et al. Endoscopic therapy for bile leak based on a new classification: results in 207 patients. Gastrointest Endosc 2004;60:567–74.

39. Thomson BN, Parks RW, Madhavan KK, et al. Early specialist repair of biliary injury. Br J Surg 2006;93:216–20.

40. Buell JF, Cronin DC, Funakii B. Devastating and fatal complications associated with combined vascular and bile duct injuries during cholecystectomy. Arch Surg 2002;137:703–8.

41. Schmidt SC, Settmacher U, Langrehr JM, et al. Management and outcome of patients with combined bile duct and hepatic arterial injuries after laparoscopic cholecystectomy. Surgery 2004; 135:613–8.

42. Li J, Frilling A, Nadalin S, et al. Management of concomitant hepatic artery injury in patients with iatrogenic major bile duct injury after laparoscopic cholecystectomy. Br J Surg 2008;95:460–5.

43. Alves A, Farges O, Nicolet J, et al. Incidence and consequence of an hepatic artery injury in patients with postcholecystectomy bile duct strictures. Ann Surg 2003;238:93–6.

44. Mercado MA, Chan C, Orozco H, et al. Acute bile duct injury. The need for a high repair. Surg Endosc 2003;17:1351–5.

45. Strasberg SM, Helton WS. An analytical review of vasculobiliary injury in laparoscopic and open cholecystectomy. HPB (Oxford) 2011;13(1):1–14.

46. Moraca RJ, Lee FT, Ryan JA, et al. Long-term biliary function after reconstruction of major bile duct injuries with hepaticoduodenostomy or hepaticojejunostomy. Arch Surg 2002;137:889–93.

47. Bettschart V, Clayton RA, Parks RW, et al. Cholangiocarcinoma arising after biliary–enteric drainage procedures for benign disease. Gut 2002; 51:128–9.

48. Al-Ghnaniem R, Benjamin IS. Long-term outcome of hepaticojejunostomy with routine access loop formation following iatrogenic bile duct injury. Br J Surg 2002;89:1118–24.

49. Gao JB, Bai LS, Hu ZJ, et al. Role of Kasai procedure in surgery of hilar bile duct strictures. World J Gastroenterol 2011;17(37):4231–4.

50. Truant S, Boleslawski E, Lebuffe G, et al. Hepatic resection for post-cholecystectomy bile duct injuries: a literature review. HPB (Oxford) 2010; 12(5):334–41.

51. Mercado MA, Chan C, Orozco H, et al. Long-term evaluation of biliary reconstruction after partial resection of segments IV and V in iatrogenic injuries. J Gastrointest Surg 2006;10(1):77–82.

52. Nordin A, Halme L, Makisalo H, et al. Management and outcome of major bile duct injuries after laparoscopic cholecystectomy: from therapeutic endoscopy to liver transplantation. Liver Transpl 2002;8:1036–43.

53. Mercado MA, Franssen B, Dominguez I, et al. Transition from a low- to a high-volume centre for bile duct repair: changes in technique and improved outcome. HPB (Oxford) 2011;13(11):767–73.

54. Flum DR, Cheadle A, Prela C, et al. Bile duct injury during cholecystectomy and survival in medicare beneficiaries. JAMA 2003;290:2168–74.
A retrospective analysis of survival following bile duct injury among Medicare beneficiaries in the USA. This study demonstrates the increased hazard ratio of death following injury in comparison to a control group of routine cholecystectomy patients.

55. Huang CS, Lien HH, Tai FC, et al. Long-term results of major bile duct injury associated with laparoscopic cholecystectomy. Surg Endosc 2003;17:1362–7.

56. Boerma D, Rauws EA, Keulemans YC, et al. Impaired quality of life 5 years after bile duct injury during laparoscopic cholecystectomy: a propsective analysis. Ann Surg 2001;234:750–7.
A prospective analysis of quality of life that demonstrated a poor outcome at 5 years, despite successful repair.

57. Melton GB, Lillemoe KD, Cameron JL, et al. Major bile duct injuries associated with laparoscopic cholecystectomy: effect of surgical repair on quality of life. Ann Surg 2002;235:888–95.
A study of the impact of biliary injury on quality of life that demonstrated a significantly worse psychological domain, especially in those pursuing legal action.

58. Mirizzi PL. Sindrome del conducto hepatico. J Int Chir 1948;8:731–77.

59. Johnson LW, Sehon JK, Lee WC, et al. Mirizzi's syndrome: experience from a multi-institutional review. Am Surg 2001;67:11–4.

60. Garden OJ, Paterson-Brown S. The gallbladder and bile ducts. In: Garden OJ, editor. Intraoperative and laparoscopic ultrasonography. Oxford: Blackwell Science; 1995. p. 17–43.

61. Binnie NR, Nixon SJ, Palmer KR. Mirizzi syndrome managed by endoscopic stenting and laparoscopic cholecystectomy. Br J Surg 1992;79:647.

62. Shah OJ, Dar MA, Wani MA, et al. Management of Mirizzi syndrome: a new surgical approach. Aust N Z J Surg 2001;71:423–7.

63. Schafer M, Schneiter R, Krahenbuhl L. Incidence and management of Mirizzi syndrome during laparoscopic cholecystectomy. Surg Endosc 2003;17:1186–90.

64. Lo CM, Fan ST, Wong J. The changing epidemiology of recurrent pyogenic cholangitis. Hong Kong Med J 1997;3:302–4.

65. Tabata M, Nakayama F. Bacteriology of hepatolithiasis. Prog Clin Biol Res 1984;152:163–74.

66. Suzuki Y, Mori T, Abe N, et al. Predictive factors for cholangiocarcinoma associated with hepatolithiasis determined on the basis of Japanese Multicenter study. Hepatol Res 2012;42(2):166–70.

67. Uchiyama K, Kawai M, Ueno M, et al. Reducing residual and recurrent stones by hepatectomy for hepatolithiasis. J Gastrointest Surg 2007;11:626–30.

68. Belghiti J, Benhamou JP, Houry S, et al. Caustic sclerosing cholangitis. A complication of the surgical treatment of hydatid disease of the liver. Arch Surg 1986;121:1162–5.

69. Molodecky NA, Kareemi H, Parab R, et al. Incidence of primary sclerosing cholangitis: a systematic review and meta-analysis. Hepatology 2011;53(5):1590–9.

70. Montefusco PP, Geiss AC, Bronzo RL, et al. Sclerosing cholangitis, chronic pancreatitis, and Sjögren's syndrome: a syndrome complex. Am J Surg 1984;147:822–6.

71. Chapman RW, Kelly PM, Heryet A, et al. Expression of HLA-DR antigens on bile duct epithelium in primary sclerosing cholangitis. Gut 1988;29:422–7.

72. Tischendorf JJ, Hecker H, Krüger M, et al. Characterization, outcome, and prognosis in 273 patients with primary sclerosing cholangitis: a single center study. Am J Gastroenterol 2007;102:107–14.

73. Fevery J, Henckaerts L, Van Oirbeek R, et al. Malignancies and mortality in 200 patients with primary sclerosering cholangitis: a long-term single-centre study. Liver Int 2012;32(2):214–22.

74. Beuers U, Spengler U, Kruis W, et al. Ursodeoxycholic acid for treatment of primary sclerosing cholangitis: a placebo-controlled trial. Hepatology 1992;16:707–14.
A prospective randomised double-blind trial that demonstrated the efficacy of ursodeoxycholic acid in the treatment of primary sclerosing cholangitis.

75. Aljiffry M, Renfrew PD, Walsh MJ, et al. Analytical review of diagnosis and treatment strategies for dominant bile duct strictures in patients with primary sclerosing cholangitis. HPB (Oxford) 2011;13(2):79–90.

76. Roberts MS, Angus DC, Bryce CL, et al. Survival after liver transplantation in the United States: a disease-specific analysis of the UNOS database. Liver Transpl 2004;10:886–97.

77. Prytz H, Keiding S, Björnsson E, et al. Dynamic FDG-PET is useful for detection of cholangiocarcinoma in patients with PSC listed for liver transplantation. Hepatology 2006;44:1572–80.

78. Weber SM, DeMatteo RP, Fong Y, et al. Staging laparoscopy in patients with extrahepatic biliary carcinoma. Analysis of 100 patients. Ann Surg 2002;235:392–9.

79. Uhlmann D, Wiedmann M, Schmidt F, et al. Management and outcome in patients with Klatskin-mimicking lesions of the biliary tree. J Gastrointest Surg 2006;10:1144–50.

80. Weber SM, Cubukcu-Dimopulo O, Palesty JA, et al. Lymphoplasmacytic sclerosing pancreatitis: inflammatory mimic of pancreatic carcinoma. J Gastrointest Surg 2003;7:129–37.

81. Church NI, Pereira SP, Deheragoda MG, et al. Autoimmune pancreatitis: clinical and radiological features and objective response to steroid therapy in a UK series. Am J Gastroenterol 2007;102:2417–25.

82. Corazziari E. Sphincter of Oddi dysfunction. Dig Liver Dis 2003;35:S26–9.

83. Geenen JE, Hogan WJ, Dodds WJ, et al. The efficacy of endoscopic sphincterotomy after cholecystectomy in patients with sphincter of Oddi dysfunction. N Engl J Med 1989;320:82–7.

84. Lehman GY, Sherman S. Sphincter of Oddi dysfunction. Int J Pancreatol 1996;20:11–25.

85. Freeman ML, Gill M, Overby C, et al. Predictors of outcomes after biliary and pancreatic sphincterotomy for sphincter of Oddi dysfunction. J Clin Gastroenterol 2007;41:94–102.

12

Malignant lesions of the biliary tract

Shishir K. Maithel
William R. Jarnagin

Introduction

Malignant lesions of the biliary tract, specifically arising from the gallbladder or biliary epithelium, are rare and only account for approximately 15% of hepatobiliary neoplasms. Gallbladder cancer is the most common site, accounting for 60% of all biliary tract cancers, while the remaining 40% are distributed throughout the extrahepatic and intrahepatic biliary tree, with the next most common site occurring at the extrahepatic biliary confluence.[1] Complete resection is associated with the best survival and is the most effective therapy, but is usually only possible in a minority of patients. Palliating the effects of biliary obstruction is thus often the primary therapeutic goal. Chemotherapy and radiation therapy have not been proved to reduce the incidence of recurrence after resection nor to improve survival. Unfortunately, due to the rarity of these tumours and their frequently advanced stage at presentation, randomised prospective trials assessing different treatment regimens have not been performed. This chapter focuses on the current management of cholangiocarcinoma, specifically hilar, intrahepatic and distal bile duct cancers, as well as gallbladder carcinoma.

Cholangiocarcinoma

General considerations

Epidemiology

Cholangiocarcinoma is an uncommon cancer with an incidence of 1–2 per 100 000 in the USA and approximately 5000–8000 new cases diagnosed each year.[2]

Overall, men are affected 1.5 times as often as women and the majority of patients are greater than 65 years of age, with the peak incidence occurring in the eighth decade of life.[2] Cholangiocarcinomas are classified according to their site of origin within the biliary tree, with those involving the biliary confluence, or hilar cholangiocarcinoma, being the most common and accounting for approximately 60% of all cases.[3-6] Twenty to thirty per cent of cholangiocarcinomas originate in the distal bile duct, while approximately 10% arise within the intrahepatic biliary tree.[7-9] Rarely, patients will present with multifocal or diffuse involvement of the biliary tree.[10] More recent studies have documented the marked increase in incidence of intrahepatic cholangiocarcinoma, which may become the more common variant (see below).[11-14]

Natural history

The vast majority of patients with unresectable bile duct cancer die within 6 months to 1 year of diagnosis, usually from liver failure or infectious complications secondary to biliary obstruction.[3,15-17] The prognosis is often worse for hilar lesions and better for lesions of the distal bile duct, which probably reflects the greater complexity and difficulty in effectively managing proximal lesions, more so than differences in tumour biology. Indeed, it has been shown that location within the biliary tree (proximal versus distal) has no impact on survival provided that complete resection is performed.[4] That being said, patients with intrahepatic cholangiocarcinoma often present with advanced lesions due to the absence of symptoms, such as jaundice or biliary tract-related sepsis.

218

Aetiology

Most cases of cholangiocarcinoma in the West are sporadic and have no obvious risk factors. However, certain pathological conditions are associated with an increased incidence, the most common of which is primary sclerosing cholangitis (PSC). The majority of patients (70–80%) with PSC have associated ulcerative colitis, while a minority of patients with ulcerative colitis develop PSC.[18] The natural history of PSC is variable, and the true incidence of cholangiocarcinoma is unknown. In a Swedish series of 305 patients followed over several years, 8% of patients eventually developed cancer. On the other hand, occult cholangiocarcinoma has been reported in up to 40% of autopsy specimens and in up to 36% of liver explants from patients with PSC.[18,19] Patients with cholangiocarcinoma associated with PSC are often not candidates for resection because of multifocal disease or severe underlying hepatic dysfunction.

Congenital biliary cystic disease (i.e. choledochal cysts) is also associated with an increased risk for the development of biliary tract cancer.[20,21] This appears to be related to the finding that these patients have an abnormal choledochopancreatic duct junction, which predisposes to reflux of pancreatic secretions into the biliary tree, chronic inflammation and bacterial contamination.[21–24] A similar mechanism may also explain the increased incidence of cholangiocarcinoma reported in patients subjected to transduodenal sphincteroplasty or endoscopic sphincterotomy. In a series of 119 patients subjected to this procedure for benign conditions, Hakamada et al. found a 7.4% incidence of cholangiocarcinoma over a period of 18 years.[25]

Hepatolithiasis is a well-known risk factor for the development of cholangiocarcinoma in Japan and parts of southeast Asia, arising in 10% of those affected. Chronic portal bacteraemia and portal phlebitis lead to intrahepatic pigment stone formation, obstruction of intrahepatic ducts, and recurrent episodes of cholangitis and stricture formation.[26,27] This recurrent inflammatory state is likely the main contributing factor to cholangiocarcinogenesis. Biliary parasites (*Clonorchis sinensis*, *Opisthorchis viverrini*) are also prevalent and endemic in parts of Asia, such as Thailand, and are similarly associated with an increased risk of cholangiocarcinoma.[19] Finally, exposure to several radionuclides and chemical carcinogens, such as thorium, radon, nitrosamines, dioxin and asbestos, may also increase the risk of cholangiocarcinoma.

Histopathology

Three macroscopic subtypes of extrahepatic cholangiocarcinoma are described: sclerosing, nodular and papillary, of which the first two are often combined into one (i.e. nodular-sclerosing) since features of both types are often seen together.[28] The histopathology is distinct between cholangiocarcinomas arising from the extrahepatic and intrahepatic biliary system. For extrahepatic cholangiocarcinoma, the overwhelming majority is adenocarcinoma, and most are firm, sclerotic tumours with a paucity of cellular components within a dense fibrotic, desmoplastic background. As a consequence, a non-diagnostic preoperative biopsy is not uncommon.[2,28,29] Papillary tumours represent a less common morphological variant, accounting for approximately 10% of tumours arising from the extrahepatic biliary tree.[28] Papillary tumours are soft and friable, may be associated with little transmural invasion, and are characterised by a mass that expands rather than contracts the duct (**Fig. 12.1**). Although papillary tumours may grow to significant size, they often arise from a well-defined stalk, with the bulk of the tumour mobile within the ductal lumen. Despite this histological variant being the minority of cases, recognition of this entity is important since they are more often resectable and have a more favourable prognosis than the other types.[19,30]

✓✓ The prognosis related to papillary bile duct tumours is related to the extent of the invasive component. Tumours with ≤10% invasive cancer have a much more favourable outcome after resection, while those with >10% behave similarly to the more common nodular-sclerosing lesions.

Hilar cholangiocarcinoma is typically highly invasive within the hepatoduodenal ligament. Direct invasion of the liver or perihepatic structures, such as the portal vein or hepatic artery, is a common feature and has important clinical implications regarding resectability.[28] The liver is also a common site of metastatic disease, as are the regional lymph node basins, but spread to distant extra-abdominal sites is uncommon at initial presentation.[3,31] These tumours also have a propensity for longitudinal spread along the duct wall and periductal tissues, which is an important pathological feature of cholangiocarcinomas as it pertains to the margin of resection.[28] There may be substantial extension of tumour beneath an intact epithelial lining, as much as 2 cm proximally and 1 cm distally, thus predisposing to a radiographic underestimation of tumour extent.[32] This predilection for submucosal extension underscores the difficulty in achieving a complete resection. Frozen section analysis of the duct margin during operation may be helpful in this regard but caution is necessary when interpreting the results. Indeed, the authors recently analysed their experience with intraoperative frozen sections and

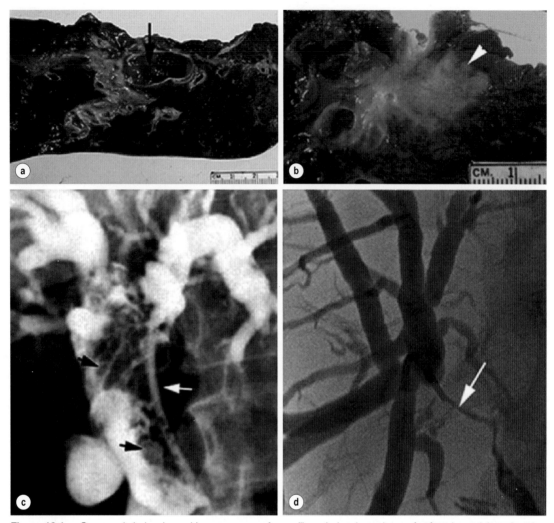

Figure 12.1 • Gross and cholangiographic appearance of a papillary cholangiocarcinoma **(a,c)** and a nodular-sclerosing tumour **(b,d)**. In **(a)** and **(c)**, note that the papillary tumour occupies the lumen and expands the duct (black arrow). A biliary stent is visualised (white arrow). In **(b)** and **(d)**, the nodular-sclerosing variant constricts the lumen, nearly obliterating it (white arrow). Reprinted with permission from Blumgart LH (ed.) Surgery of the liver, biliary tract, and pancreas, 4th edn. Elsevier Saunders, 2006.

found a substantial false-negative rate. In addition, the benefits of extending the resection with a positive frozen section result were questionable.[33]

> ✅ A frozen section evaluation of the bile duct margins may help guide the extent of resection, but caution should be used when interpreting the results.

Gross examination of intrahepatic cholangiocarcinoma reveals a grey scirrhous mass, often infiltrative into the liver parenchyma.[34] These tumours are adenocarcinomas and the diagnosis of intrahepatic or peripheral cholangiocarcinoma should be considered

in all patients presenting with a presumptive diagnosis of metastatic adenocarcinoma with an unknown primary, particularly in the setting of a large, solitary hepatic mass. A small number show different patterns with focal areas of papillary carcinoma with mucous production, signet-ring cells, squamous cell, mucoepidermoid and spindle cell variants.[35] The Liver Cancer Study group of Japan established a subclassification of these tumours based on morphology: (1) mass forming type; (2) periductal infiltrating type; (3) intraductal growth type.[36] Although some studies have suggested a correlation with outcome based on morphological subtype, this classification scheme has not gained wide acceptance. Positive immunohistochemical staining usually includes carcinoembryonic antigen (CEA), and tumour markers CA50 and CA19-9. K-ras mutations have also been detected in up to 70% of intrahepatic cholangiocarcinomas, although the frequency of this mutation is quite variable.[37,38] Metastatic disease at the time of exploration is not an infrequent finding. Tumours with both hepatocellular and cholangiocellular differentiation (combined tumours) are rare but well described. Their clinical behaviour more closely approximates that of cholangiocarcinoma than hepatocellular carcinoma, and they tend to display aggressive biology.[39]

Cholangiocarcinoma involving the proximal bile ducts (hilar cholangiocarcinoma)

Clinical presentation and diagnosis

The early symptoms of hilar cholangiocarcinoma are often non-specific, with abdominal pain, discomfort, anorexia, weight loss and/or pruritus seen in about one-third of patients.[6,19,40,41] Most patients present with jaundice or incidentally discovered abnormal liver function tests. Pruritus may precede jaundice by some weeks, and this symptom should prompt an evaluation, especially if associated with abnormal liver function tests. Patients with papillary tumours of the hilus may give a history of intermittent jaundice, perhaps due to the ball-valve effect of a pedunculated mass within the lumen or, more likely, small fragments of tumour having passed into the common bile duct. Clinical findings are often non-specific but may provide some useful information. Jaundice is usually obvious, and patients with pruritus often have multiple excoriations of the skin. The liver may be enlarged and firm as a result of biliary tract obstruction. The gallbladder is usually decompressed and non-palpable with hilar obstruction. Thus, a palpable gallbladder suggests a more distal obstruction or an alternative diagnosis. Rarely, patients with long-standing biliary obstruction and/or portal vein involvement may have findings consistent with portal hypertension.

In patients with no previous biliary intervention, cholangitis is rare at initial presentation, despite a 30% incidence of bacterial contamination.[42,43] Endoscopic or percutaneous instrumentation significantly increases the incidence of bacterial contamination and the subsequent risk of clinical infection. In fact, the incidence of bacterobilia approaches 100% after endoscopic biliary intubation, thus making cholangitis more common.[43] It should be noted that bacterial contamination of the biliary tract in partial obstruction is not always clinically apparent. The presence of overt or subclinical infection

at the time of surgery is a major source of postoperative morbidity and mortality. Thus, endoscopic and percutaneous intubations are both associated with greater morbidity and mortality following surgical resection or palliative bypass for hilar cholangiocarcinoma. In an analysis of 71 patients who underwent either resection or palliative biliary bypass for proximal cholangiocarcinoma, all patients stented endoscopically and 62% of those stented percutaneously had bacterobilia. Postoperative infectious complications were doubly increased in patients stented before operation compared to non-stented patients, while non-infectious complications were equal in both groups.[43] *Enterococcus, Klebsiella, Escherichia coli, Streptococcus viridans* and *Enterobacter aerogenes* are the most common organisms, and this spectrum of bacteria must be considered when administering perioperative antibiotics; it is imperative to take intraoperative bile specimens for culture in order to guide selection of postoperative antibiotic therapy.

While gallstones or even common bile duct stones may coexist with bile duct cancer, in the absence of certain predisposing conditions (e.g. PSC, recurrent pyogenic cholangitis (previously referred to as Oriental cholangiohepatitis)), it is uncommon for choledocholithiasis to cause obstruction at the biliary confluence. Furthermore, the degree of bilirubin elevation tends to be higher (e.g. 10–18 mg/dL) for malignant obstruction compared to benign stone disease (e.g. 2–10 mg/dL). That being said, other conditions may mimic hilar cholangiocarcinoma on imaging studies, such as benign idiopathic focal stenosis of the hepatic ducts (malignant masquerade), Mirizzi's syndrome resulting from a large stone impacted in the neck of the gallbladder, and gallbladder cancer.[44] Nevertheless, it is imperative to fully investigate and delineate the level and nature of any obstructing lesion causing jaundice to avoid missing the diagnosis of carcinoma.

However, the histopathological diagnosis of hilar cholangiocarcinoma is often not made until the specimen is removed at operation. As mentioned previously, due to the dense desmoplastic reaction associated with the sclerosing variant of cholangiocarcinoma, non-diagnostic preoperative biopsies or brushings are the usual clinical scenario. In the authors' view, histological confirmation of malignancy is not mandatory prior to exploration. With no prior suggestive history (i.e. prior biliary tract operation, PSC, hepatolithiasis), the finding of a focal stenotic lesion combined with the appropriate clinical presentation is sufficient for a presumptive diagnosis of hilar cholangiocarcinoma, which is correct in most instances.[45] Furthermore, the alternative conditions that one may encounter are often best assessed and treated at operation. It is dangerous to rely entirely on a negative result from a needle biopsy or biliary brush cytology, since they are often misleading, particularly in the face of compelling radiographic evidence of malignant disease.[46] The use of spy glass technology via endoscopic guidance has facilitated direct visualisation of the bile duct lumen and allows for targeted biopsies of the affected area.

Once a diagnosis of cholangiocarcinoma is suggested, radiological studies are crucial to determine the extent of the tumour to appropriately design a therapeutic plan.

✓✓ Preoperative biopsies or intraluminal brushings should not be relied upon to make a diagnosis of cholangiocarcinoma, as these are not always reliable, and negative results may significantly delay appropriate treatment.

Radiological investigation

High-quality radiological studies are necessary to accurately select patients for resection. Until recently, computed tomography (CT), percutaneous transhepatic cholangiography (PTC) and angiography were considered standard investigations. With improvements in the quality of non-invasive modalities, the authors' current practice relies almost exclusively on magnetic resonance cholangiopancreatography (MRCP) and duplex ultrasonography (US) for preoperative assessment, which provide similar information with less risk to the patient.

Direct cholangiography

Cholangiography demonstrates the location of the tumour and the extent of biliary disease, both of which are critical in surgical planning. Although endoscopic retrograde cholangiography (ERC) may provide helpful information, percutaneous transhepatic cholangiography (PTC) displays the intrahepatic bile ducts more reliably and has been the preferred approach. However, there is often a knee-jerk reflex to proceed with invasive cholangiography before a complete radiographic assessment has been made, which can lead to unnecessary patient morbidity and infectious complications.

Computed tomography

Cross-sectional imaging provided by CT remains an important study for evaluating patients with biliary obstruction and can provide valuable information regarding the level of obstruction, vascular involvement and liver atrophy. As portal venous inflow and bile flow are important in the maintenance of liver cell size and mass, segmental or lobar atrophy may be evident on CT that would suggest portal venous occlusion or biliary obstruction.[47]

CT angiography is particularly helpful for assessing portal venous and hepatic arterial involvement. However, CT imaging tends to underestimate the proximal extent of tumour within the bile duct and is thus not ideal as the primary determinant of resectability.[48]

Duplex ultrasonography

Ultrasonography is a non-invasive, but operator dependent, study that often precisely delineates the level of the tumour within the bile duct (**Fig. 12.2**). It can also provide information regarding tumour extension within the bile duct and in the periductal tissues.[49–51] In a series of 19 consecutive patients with malignant hilar obstruction, ultrasonography with colour spectral Doppler technique was equivalent to angiography and CT portography in diagnosing lobar atrophy, level of biliary obstruction, hepatic parenchymal involvement and venous invasion.[51] Duplex ultrasonography is particularly useful for assessing portal venous invasion. In a series of 63 consecutive patients from Memorial Sloan-Kettering Cancer Center (MSKCC), duplex ultrasonography predicted portal vein involvement in 93% of cases with a specificity of 99% and a 97% positive predictive value. In the same series, angiography with CT angio-portography had a 90% sensitivity, 99% specificity and a 95% positive predictive value.[52]

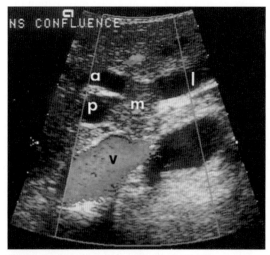

Figure 12.2 • Ultrasonographic view of a hilar cholangiocarcinoma showing a papillary tumour (m) extending into the right anterior (a) and posterior (p) sectoral ducts and the origin of the left duct (l). The adjacent portal vein (v) is not involved and has normal flow. Reprinted with permission from Blumgart LH (ed.) Surgery of the liver, biliary tract, and pancreas, 4th edn. Elsevier Saunders, 2006.

Magnetic resonance cholangiopancreatography (MRCP)

In the authors' practice, MRCP has largely replaced endoscopic and percutaneous cholangiography to assess biliary tumour extent in hilar cholangiocarcinoma. Several studies have demonstrated its utility in evaluating patients with biliary obstruction.[53–56] MRCP may not only identify the tumour and the level of biliary obstruction, but may also reveal obstructed and isolated ducts not appreciated at endoscopic or percutaneous study. By virtue of being an axial imaging modality, MRCP has further advantages over standard cholangiography by also providing information regarding the patency of hilar vascular structures, the presence of nodal or distant metastases, and the presence of lobar atrophy (**Fig. 12.3**). Furthermore, because it does not require biliary intubation, it is not associated with the same incidence of bacterobilia and infectious complications that is frequently associated with standard cholangiography.[43]

> ✔✔ Non-invasive imaging with MRCP, US and CT should be performed prior to proceeding with preoperative invasive cholangiography in order to avoid unnecessary interventions that may increase patient morbidity and infectious complications.

Preoperative evaluation and assessment of resectability

Evaluation of patients with hilar cholangiocarcinoma is principally an assessment of resectability, since resection is the only effective therapy. First and

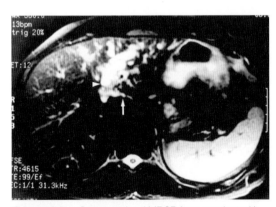

Figure 12.3 • Cross-sectional MRCP from a patient with hilar cholangiocarcinoma extending into the left hepatic duct and left lobe atrophy. The bile ducts appear white. The left lobe is small with dilated and crowded ducts (arrowhead). The principal caudate lobe duct, seen joining the left hepatic duct, is also dilated (arrow). Reprinted with permission from Blumgart LH (ed.) Surgery of the liver, biliary tract, and pancreas, 4th edn. Elsevier Saunders, 2006.

foremost, the surgeon must assess the patient's general condition, fitness for operation and liver function, since a complete resection usually includes a partial hepatectomy. The presence of significant comorbid conditions, chronic liver disease and/or portal hypertension generally precludes resection. In these patients, biliary drainage is the most appropriate intervention, and the diagnosis should be confirmed histologically if chemotherapy or radiation therapy is planned.

The preoperative evaluation must address four critical determinants of resectability: extent of tumour within the biliary tree, vascular invasion, hepatic lobar atrophy and the presence of metastatic disease.[3] The presence of lobar atrophy is often overlooked; however, its importance in determining resectability cannot be overemphasised, since it implies portal venous involvement, suggests a more locally advanced lesion, and compels the surgeon to perform a partial hepatectomy, if the tumour is indeed resectable.[47] While longstanding biliary obstruction may cause moderate atrophy, concomitant portal venous compromise results in rapid and severe atrophy of the involved segments.

Appreciation of gross atrophy on preoperative imaging is important since it often influences both operative and non-operative therapy.[47] If the tumour is not resectable, percutaneous biliary drainage through an atrophic lobe, unless necessary to control sepsis, should be avoided since it will not effect a reduction in bilirubin level. Atrophy is apparent on cross-sectional imaging as a small, often hypoperfused lobe with crowding of the dilated intrahepatic ducts (Fig. 12.3). Tumour involvement of the portal vein is usually present if there is compression/narrowing, encasement or occlusion seen on imaging studies.[3,57]

The staging systems currently used for hilar cholangiocarcinoma do not account fully for all of the tumour-related variables that influence resectability, namely biliary tumour extent, lobar atrophy and vascular involvement. The modified Bismuth–Corlette classification stratifies patients solely based on the extent of biliary duct involvement by tumour.[58] Although useful to some extent, it is not indicative of resectability or survival. Similarly, the previous AJCC T-stage system (sixth edition) was based largely on pathological criteria and had little applicability for preoperative staging. The ideal staging system should accurately predict resectability and the likelihood of associated metastatic disease, and also correlate with survival. The authors have proposed such a preoperative staging system.[3,57] This staging system places the finding of portal venous involvement and lobar atrophy into the proper context for determining resectability, especially when

Table 12.1 • Proposed T-stage criteria for hilar cholangiocarcinoma

Stage	Criteria
T1	Tumour involving biliary confluence ± unilateral extension to second-order biliary radicles
T2	Tumour involving biliary confluence ± unilateral extension to second-order biliary radicles AND *ipsilateral* portal vein involvement ± *ipsilateral* hepatic lobar atrophy
T3	Tumour involving biliary confluence + bilateral extension to second-order biliary radicles OR unilateral extension to second-order biliary radicles with *contralateral* portal vein involvement OR unilateral extension to second-order biliary radicles with *contralateral* hepatic lobar atrophy OR main or bilateral portal venous involvement

Reprinted with permission from Jarnagin WR, Fong Y, DeMatteo RP et al. Staging, resectability, and outcome in 225 patients with hilar cholangiocarcinoma. Ann Surg 2001; 234:507–19.

Box 12.1 • Criteria of unresectability

Patient factors

Medically unfit or otherwise unable to tolerate a major operation

Hepatic cirrhosis

Local tumour-related factors

Tumour extension to secondary biliary radicles bilaterally

Encasement or occlusion of the main portal vein proximal to its bifurcation

Atrophy of one hepatic lobe with contralateral portal vein branch encasement or occlusion

Atrophy of one hepatic lobe with contralateral tumour extension to secondary biliary radicles

Unilateral tumour extension to secondary biliary radicles with contralateral portal vein branch encasement or occlusion

Metastatic disease

Histologicalally proven metastases to distant lymph node basins*

Lung, liver or peritoneal metastases

*Includes peripancreatic, periduodenal, coeliac, superior mesenteric or posterior pancreaticoduodenal lymph nodes.
Reprinted with permission from Jarnagin WR, Fong Y, DeMatteo RP et al. Staging, resectability, and outcome in 225 patients with hilar cholangiocarcinoma. Ann Surg 2001; 234:507–19.

partial hepatectomy is an important component of the operative approach (Table 12.1). For example, a tumour with unilateral extension into second-order bile ducts that is associated with ipsilateral portal vein involvement and/or lobar atrophy would still be considered potentially resectable, while such involvement on the contralateral side would preclude a resection. The authors have found that this staging system correlated well with resectability, the likelihood of associated distant metastatic disease, and median survival (Table 12.2).[57] Independent confirmation of the utility of this classification scheme (the Blumgart clinical staging system) was recently reported in a series of 85 patients from China.[59] The authors' criteria for unresectability are detailed in Box 12.1. This staging scheme is now incorporated in the seventh edition of the AJCC staging system for hilar cholangiocarcinoma.

✓✓ The Bismuth–Corlette classification system is minimally helpful in guiding preoperative decision making. A modified system (the Blumgart clinical staging system) reclassifies the T stage based on the extent of bile duct and portal vein involvement, as well as the presence or absence of lobar atrophy, which is highly correlated with tumour resectability and survival. This proposed system can aid with preoperative decision making and is now incorporated in the seventh edition of the AJCC staging system.

Table 12.2 • Resectability, incidence of metastatic disease, and survival stratified by T stage

T stage	n	Explored with curative intent	Resected	Negative margins	Hepatic resection	Portal vein resection	Metastatic disease	Median survival (months)
1	87	73 (84%)	51 (59%)	38	33	2	18 (21%)	20
2	95	79 (83%)	29 (31%)	24	29	7	40 (43%)	13
3	37	8 (22%)	0	0	0	0	15 (41%)	8
Total	219	160 (71%)	80 (37%)	62	62	9	73 (33%)	16

Reprinted with permission from Jarnagin WR, Fong Y, DeMatteo RP et al. Staging, resectability, and outcome in 225 patients with hilar cholangiocarcinoma. Ann Surg 2001; 234:507–19.

Treatment options

In patients with operable disease, the principal objective is a complete resection, obtaining negative histological margins with subsequent restoration of biliary-enteric continuity. Complete resection is associated with 5-year survival rates of approximately 25–40%, which is far superior to that obtainable with non-operative therapies. Clearly, patient selection contributes largely to this finding, as patients treated non-operatively typically have more advanced disease, and no comparative trials have been performed equating stage for stage. Nevertheless, given the relatively poor response rates with chemotherapy and chemoradiation therapy, resection has emerged as the most effective treatment.

Orthotopic liver transplantation has been attempted for unresectable hilar tumours. Klempnauer et al. reported four long-term survivors out of 32 patients who underwent transplantation for hilar cholangiocarcinoma.[60] The same group also reported a 17.1% 5-year survival for their overall transplant group.[61] Comparable results were reported by Iwatsuki et al.[62] The results of transplantation have previously not been sufficiently adequate to justify its use, and most centres now do not perform liver transplantation for cholangiocarcinoma. More recently, data from the Mayo Clinic have emerged suggesting good results with transplantation in highly selected patients with low-volume unresectable disease and combined with an intensive pre-transplant treatment regimen.[63,64] Although the data are compelling, routine use of vascular resection, even when there is no obvious tumour infiltration, will likely lead to higher perioperative morbidity; this approach would therefore seem applicable to a very small proportion of patients.

Resection

Resection is the most effective therapy for patients with potentially resectable tumours, with the primary objective being complete removal of all gross disease with clear histological margins (R0 resection). The importance of an R0 resection is clear from previous studies showing that incomplete (R1 or R2) resections do not improve survival beyond that of patients with unresectable tumours (**Fig. 12.4**).[3,57] There is now overwhelming evidence to support the observation that partial hepatectomy, combined with excision of the extrahepatic biliary system, is usually required to achieve this goal (Table 12.3). A review of several series in the literature shows a close correlation between the proportion of patients who underwent concomitant partial hepatectomy and the proportion of

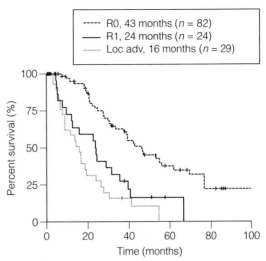

Figure 12.4 • Survival curves after resection of hilar cholangiocarcinoma. R0 indicates complete resection with histologically negative resection margins (median survival 43 months). R1 indicates histologically involved resection margins (median survival 24 months; $P < 0.001$, R0 vs. R1). Loc Adv indicates patients explored, but found to have unresectable tumours owing to local invasion (no metastatic disease) (median survival 16 months; $P < 0.19$, R1 vs. Loc Adv). Reprinted with permission from Blumgart LH (ed.) Surgery of the liver, biliary tract, and pancreas, 4th edn. Elsevier Saunders, 2006.

Table 12.3 • Summary of selected studies showing the relationship between the rate of partial hepatectomy and proportion of negative histological margins achieved

Author	Complete gross resection (n)	Partial hepatectomy (%)	Negative margin (%)
Tsao (2000)	25	16	28
Cameron (1990)	39	20	15
Gerhards (2000)	112	29	14
Hadjis (1990)	27	60	56
Jarnagin (2001)	80	78	78
Klempnauer (1997)	147	79	79
Neuhaus (2000)	95	85	61
Nimura (1990)	55	98	83

R0 resections achieved. For tumours extending into the left hepatic duct, en bloc caudate lobectomy is usually necessary to obtain a complete resection, since the principal biliary drainage of the caudate lobe is via the left hepatic duct.[65,66] A dilated caudate duct, suggesting tumour involvement, may occasionally be visualised on preoperative imaging (Fig. 12.3).

Despite improvements in preoperative imaging, a considerable number of patients are still found to have unresectable disease at the time of exploration. In a recent report from MSKCC, this number approached 50% of patients with cholangiocarcinoma explored with curative intent.[30] In an effort to minimise the number of non-curative laparotomies performed, staging laparoscopy has been utilised. Two recent studies specifically analysing patients with biliary cancer have shown that laparoscopy can identify a large proportion of patients with unresectable disease primarily in the form of radiographically occult metastases, the yield of which is greatest in locally advanced tumours.[67,68] Weber et al. evaluated 56 patients with potentially resectable hilar cholangiocarcinomas; 33 were ultimately determined to have unresectable disease, of which 14 (42%) were identified at laparoscopy and spared an unnecessary laparotomy. Additionally, a number of recent reports have suggested a potential role for fluoro-2-D-glucose positron emission tomography (FDG-PET) scanning as a means of identifying occult metastatic disease. However, most of these studies include small numbers of patients, and further evaluation is needed before PET can be recommended as a routine screening study for this disease.[69–71] In the authors' experience with FDG-PET for all biliary tract cancer, the information provided influenced management in 24% of patients.[72]

✅✅ In order to achieve an R0 resection, a concomitant partial hepatectomy is almost always necessary due to tumour extension into second-order biliary radicles or ipsilateral portal vein involvement. A caudate lobe resection in particular is often necessary, especially for left-sided tumours, in order to obtain negative margins. Staging laparoscopy should be undertaken prior to open exploration in an effort to minimise the number of non-curative laparotomies performed.

Technical aspects of intraoperative tumour assessment, exposure and resection are outside the scope of this chapter. The reader is referred to specialty texts for a detailed description of surgical techniques.[73] The authors' general approach involves the use of staging laparoscopy, followed by a full exploration of the abdomen and pelvis, including intraoperative ultrasonography. Resection of the tumour involves, at a minimum, removal of the entire extrahepatic biliary tract from just above the pancreas distally to beyond the biliary confluence with a complete porta hepatis lymphadenectomy. Also, for the reasons cited above, en bloc partial hepatectomy is required in nearly every case in order to achieve complete tumour clearance. Tumour involvement of the main portal vein proximal to its bifurcation additionally requires a vascular resection and reconstruction if technically feasible. Some authors advocate a 'no-touch' technique where a hilar en bloc resection is performed that entails resection of the portal vein bifurcation with reconstruction.[74] The authors report a 5-year survival advantage of 58% versus 29% ($P = 0.02$) associated with this approach compared to a conventional hepatectomy. This is clearly an aggressive surgical approach that is likely best applied to a select population.

The extent of lymphadenectomy that should be performed remains an area of controversy. Some surgeons advocate an extended nodal dissection as some studies have demonstrated measurable 5-year actuarial survival in the presence of metastatic disease to distant nodal basins (e.g. para-aortic).[75,76] However, an analysis of studies specifically reporting 5-year survival in patients would suggest that any nodal involvement is a powerful adverse factor and that very few patients benefit from such an aggressive approach (Table 12.4). Thus, while a complete porta hepatis lymphadenectomy should be routinely performed when attempting complete resection, the authors do not advocate an extended lymph node dissection. As is the case in other tumours, the clinical implication of a negative lymph node on histopathological analysis is likely dependent on the total number of lymph nodes sampled. A study from MSKCC reported that seven lymph nodes appears to be the target sampling number in order to accurately stage hilar cholangiocarcinoma.[77] This must be weighed against the reality that, in most series, the median number of nodes sampled from a porta hepatis lymphadenectomy is usually around three.

Results of resection

Long-term survival after resection of hilar cholangiocarcinoma can be achieved and has improved over recent years.[3,4,6,65,78,79] It is clear, however, that the results of resection depend critically on the status of the resection margins. The authors firmly believe that an increase in the use of hepatic resection is responsible for the increase in the percentage of R0 resections (negative histological margins) and the observed improvement in survival after resection. This point is emphasised by

Table 12.4 • Summary of selected series showing proportion of number of patients surviving 5 years after resection of hilar cholangiocarcinoma with metastatic disease to regional lymph nodes

Author	Resections (n)	Node positive (%)	Five-year survivors with positive nodes (n)
Sugiura (1994)	83	51	3
Klempnauer (1997)	151	29	2
Nakeeb (1996)	109	–	0
Ogura (1998)	66	52	0
Iwatsuki (1998)	72	35	0
Kosuge (1999)	65	46	4
Jarnagin (2001)	80	24	3
Kitagawa (2001)	110	53	5
Total	802	–	17 (2.1%)

a reported series of 269 patients accumulated over a 20-year period demonstrating a progressive increase in the proportion of patients subjected to partial hepatectomy, with a corresponding increase in the incidence of negative histological margins and in survival.[80] A more recent study from MSKCC reported results of resection in 106 consecutive patients and showed a median survival of 43 months in patients who underwent an R0 resection compared to 24 months in those with involved resection margins.[30] Multivariate analysis showed that an R0 resection, a concomitant hepatic resection, well-differentiated histology and papillary tumour phenotype were independent predictors of long-term survival.

Adjuvant therapy

The rarity of cholangiocarcinoma has prevented any meaningful clinical trials evaluating the use of adjuvant therapy. Several small, single-centre studies have attempted to investigate the benefit of postoperative adjuvant chemoradiation therapy in patients with hilar cholangiocarcinoma. Cameron et al. and Pitt et al. from Johns Hopkins, in two separate reports, provided data suggesting no benefit of adjuvant external beam or intraluminal radiation therapy.[81,82] In contrast, Kamada et al. suggested that radiation may improve survival in patients with histologically positive hepatic duct margins.[83] Additionally, in a small series of patients, five with hilar cholangiocarcinoma, resectability was reportedly greater in patients given neoadjuvant radiation therapy prior to exploration.[84] It must be noted, however, that none of these studies were randomised and most consisted of a small, heterogeneous group of patients. At the present time, there are no data to support the routine use of adjuvant or neoadjuvant radiation therapy, except in the context of a controlled trial.

The only phase III trial investigating adjuvant chemotherapy, which used mitomycin/5-fluorouracil (5-FU), included 508 patients with resected bile duct tumours (n = 139), gallbladder cancers (n = 140), pancreatic cancers (n = 173) and ampullary tumours (n = 56).[85] On subset analysis, there were no significant differences in overall or disease-free survival for bile duct tumours. As with radiation therapy, there are no data to support the routine use of chemotherapy in the adjuvant setting, until newer agents, such as oxaliplatin, are tested in a randomised controlled fashion.

> ✓ Adjuvant chemotherapy or radiation therapy has not been shown to prolong survival beyond that of complete surgical resection alone for hilar cholangiocarcinoma. Large prospective randomised controlled trials have not been performed. However, patients at high risk of recurrence (i.e. node positive, margin positive) may benefit from treatment, and the authors usually recommend consultation with a medical oncologist in such cases.

Palliation

All patients should be properly assessed for possible resection; however, unfortunately the majority of patients with hilar cholangiocarcinoma are not candidates for resection. In this setting, the management goals include biliary decompression and/or supportive care. Jaundice alone is not necessarily an indication for biliary decompression, given the associated morbidity and mortality. The indications for biliary decompression include intractable pruritus, recurrent cholangitis, the need for access for intraluminal radiotherapy and finally to allow recovery of hepatic parenchymal function in patients receiving chemotherapeutic agents. In fact, supportive care alone is probably the best approach for elderly patients with significant comorbid conditions, provided that pruritus is not a major feature. In patients who are found to be unresectable at operation, an operative biliary decompression can be performed and can be so constructed as to provide access to the biliary tree for postoperative irradiation.[3,86]

If the patient is deemed unresectable, the diagnosis should be confirmed with a biopsy. Biliary decompression can be obtained either by a percutaneous transhepatic route or by endoscopic stent placement, although hilar tumours are more difficult to transverse endoscopically. Moreover, the failure rates and incidence of subsequent cholangitis associated with endoscopic decompression are high.[87] Thus, most are probably better palliated via a percutaneous approach.

Percutaneous biliary drainage

Although more difficult than in those with distal bile duct tumours, percutaneous transhepatic biliary drainage and subsequent placement of a self-expandable metallic endoprosthesis (Wallstent) can be successfully performed in most patients with hilar obstruction.[88–90] Frequently, hilar tumours involve all three major hilar ducts (left hepatic, right anterior sectoral hepatic and right posterior sectoral hepatic), and thus may require two or more stents for adequate drainage.[91] Jaundice secondary to portal vein occlusion without intrahepatic biliary dilatation, however, is not correctable with biliary stents. In addition, the presence of lobar atrophy is an important factor and biliary decompression of an atrophic lobe does not usually provide much palliative benefit.

The median patency of metallic endoprostheses placed at the hilus is approximately 6 months, which is significantly lower than that reported for similar stents placed in the distal bile duct.[92] Becker et al. reported 1-year patency rates of 46% and 89% for Wallstents placed at the hilus and the distal bile duct, respectively.[88] Due to this higher occlusion rate, 25% of patients will require re-intervention. This concurs with our findings of a mean patency of 6.1 months in 35 patients palliated for malignant high biliary obstruction by placement of expandable metallic endoprostheses. The periprocedural mortality was 14% at 30 days, and seven patients (24%) had documented stent occlusion requiring repeated intervention.[92]

Intrahepatic biliary-enteric bypass

Patients found to be unresectable at operation, particularly after the bile duct has been divided, may be candidates for intrahepatic biliary-enteric bypass. The segment III duct is usually the most accessible and is our preferred approach, but the right anterior or posterior sectoral hepatic ducts can also be used.[93] Segment III bypass provides excellent biliary drainage and is less prone to occlusion since the anastomosis can be placed remote from the tumour. The 1-year bypass patency can approach 80%

without any perioperative deaths.[93] Decompression of only one-third of the functioning hepatic parenchyma is usually sufficient to relieve jaundice. Furthermore, provided that the undrained lobe has not been percutaneously drained or otherwise contaminated, communication between the right and left hepatic ducts is not necessary.[94] As discussed for stenting, bypass to an atrophic lobe or a lobe heavily involved with tumour is generally not effective.

Radiation therapy

Patients with locally unresectable tumours without evidence of widespread disease may be candidates for palliative radiation therapy. Typically, external beam radiation (EBRT) alone is used, although a combination of EBRT (5000–6000 cGy) and intraluminal iridium-192 (2000 cGy) delivered percutaneously can be administered safely and may be more effective. However, despite its feasibility, improved survival compared to biliary decompression alone has not been documented in a controlled study.[81,86,95,96] In a group of 12 patients treated with this regimen over a 3-year period at MSKCC, the median survival was 14.5 months. Episodes of cholangitis and intermittent jaundice were relatively common but the incidence of serious complications was low and there were no treatment-related deaths.[86] Given the increased morbidity and minimal benefit associated with radiation therapy, it is clearly not indicated for most patients with unresectable hilar cholangiocarcinoma.

Photodynamic therapy

Ortner, as well as others, has evaluated the efficacy of photodynamic therapy in unresectable hilar cholangiocarcinoma and reported a median survival of 439 days.[97,98] The technique involves first injecting a photosensitiser into the biliary tract, then direct illumination via cholangioscopy activates the compound, causing tumour cell death. Ortner treated nine patients in this fashion who had failed endoscopic stenting. No mortality was reported for the procedure; however, there was a 25% mortality related to the initial endoscopic stenting, which must be considered. The indication for biliary drainage or specific reasons for tumour unresectability were not mentioned, despite this information being important to assess the true extent of disease, thus making it difficult to interpret the extended survival with this palliative therapy. Since this study, two small randomised studies have reported an improvement in survival for patients with unresectable tumours treated with stenting and photodynamic therapy compared to stenting alone; however, the control groups were not comparable, since the biliary drainage procedures were suboptimal, which likely accounts for the differences in outcome.[99,100]

Chemotherapy

In cases of advanced biliary tract cancers where curative surgical resection is not an option, palliative chemotherapy has been used to potentially improve quality of life, reduce symptoms and increase survival. Only one randomised study has addressed such a role for chemotherapy, where 37 patients with advanced biliary tract cancers were randomised to receive chemotherapy (5-FU/leucovorin with or without etoposide) or best supportive care.[101] Short-term improvements in survival (6.5 vs. 2.5 months) were noted among the chemotherapy group. In addition, the treatment group also demonstrated improvement in quality of life as measured by the EORTC QLQ-C30 instrument.

Many agents (5-FU, gemcitabine, capecitabine, cisplatin, oxaliplatin, interferon) alone or in combination continue to be evaluated in phase I and II trials. Partial disease responses are consistently in the range of 10–30%. Since no consensus had been reached regarding the standard use of chemotherapy in cases of advanced biliary tract cancer, gemcitabine as a single agent had emerged as the treatment regimen of choice given its more favourable profile in both toxicity and disease response.[102] However, recently the ABC-02 Trial Investigators reported the superior survival of patients with advanced biliary cancers when treated with a doublet regimen of gemcitabine with cisplatin compared to gemcitabine alone (11.7 vs. 8.1 months; $P <0.001$).[103] The use of gemcitabine with a platinum agent, barring any contraindications, has now become the treatment regimen of choice for patients with advanced disease. This finding now raises the question of whether appropriately selected patients might benefit from this regimen in the adjuvant setting as well.

Cholangiocarcinoma involving the distal bile duct

Tumours of the lower bile duct, namely mid- and distal bile duct, are classified according to their anatomical location, although there may be considerable overlap. Mid-bile duct tumours arise between the upper border of the duodenum and the cystic duct, while distal bile duct tumours are those arising anywhere from the duodenum to the papilla of Vater.[5] Tumours of the distal bile duct may represent approximately 20–30% of all cholangiocarcinomas and 5–10% of all periampullary tumours.[6,104–106] True mid-duct tumours are distinctly uncommon, and thus Nakeeb et al. have proposed an alternative classification scheme that divides cholangiocarcinomas into intrahepatic, perihilar and distal subgroups, thereby eliminating the mid-duct group, which is often difficult to classify accurately.[6] As is

true throughout the biliary tree, adenocarcinoma is the principal histological type in the lower bile duct, and it has previously been suggested that the papillary variant is more common at this location compared to the biliary confluence.[5]

Clinical presentation and diagnosis

The clinical presentation of distal bile duct cancer is generally indistinguishable from that of hilar cholangiocarcinoma or other periampullary malignancies. Progressive jaundice is seen in 75–90% of patients, with serum bilirubin levels often exceeding 10 mg/dL.[107] Abdominal pain, weight loss, fever or pruritus occurs in one-third or fewer.[6,104] Distal bile duct tumours are frequently mistaken for adenocarcinoma of the pancreas, the most common periampullary malignancy. Endoscopic retrograde cholangiopancreatography (ERCP) can provide valuable information regarding the level of obstruction, may show that the obstruction is arising from the bile duct without involvement of the pancreatic duct, and can be both diagnostic and therapeutic in cases of choledocholithiasis. Percutaneous transhepatic cholangiography is generally less useful for tumours of the distal bile duct. A good-quality cross-sectional imaging study is also required, usually a CT with angiography to assess for vascular involvement and/or metastatic disease. It is not uncommon that CT does not reveal a mass given the frequent small tumour size at presentation. Increasingly, magnetic resonance cholangiopancreatography (MRCP) is being used to evaluate periampullary tumours. As is true for hilar lesions, MRCP can provide information of the distal bile duct previously obtainable only with the combination of ERCP and CT.[108]

In patients with a stricture of the distal bile duct and a clinical presentation consistent with cholangiocarcinoma (or any other periampullary malignancy), histological confirmation of malignancy is generally unnecessary, unless non-operative therapy is planned. Benign strictures do occur in the lower bile duct, but these are difficult to differentiate definitively from malignant strictures without resection. In addition, endoscopic brushings of the bile duct have an unacceptably low sensitivity, making a negative result virtually useless.[109] Excessive reliance on the results of percutaneous or brush biopsies serves only to delay therapy.

✓✓ The decision of whether or not to attempt resection of a presumed distal cholangiocarcinoma should not be delayed waiting for a preoperative histological diagnosis, as current methods of obtaining a preoperative tissue diagnosis are not reliable.

Staging and assessment of resectability

Carcinomas of the distal common bile duct are staged according to the AJCC system (seventh edition) for tumours of the extrahepatic bile ducts. This system is of limited clinical use, as it is based on pathological information and does not provide any information pertaining to factors that define resectability. The most important of these is the presence of tumour involvement of the portal vein, superior mesenteric artery or common hepatic artery. Tumours involving a short segment of the portal vein (<2 cm) may be resected with reconstruction of the vein. Metastatic disease to distant sites, such as the liver or peritoneum, represents an absolute contraindication to proceeding with resection; the involvement of regional nodal basins should perhaps be viewed as a relative contraindication, given the poor survival in patients with node-positive disease. Along with good-quality preoperative imaging, staging laparoscopy may help to reduce the number of non-curative laparotomies performed. Endoscopic ultrasonography (EUS) can provide additional staging information (nodal or vascular involvement) and allows an opportunity to biopsy the lesion, if necessary; however, EUS is generally not required if resection is planned based on the results of high-quality cross-sectional imaging studies.

Treatment options

Complete resection is the only effective therapy for cancers of the distal bile duct.[4–6,104–106] Reported 5-year survival rates range from 14% to 40% after complete resection, and in most studies survival beyond 1 year was uncommon in patients with tumours not amenable to resection.[5,38,104,105] Nearly all distal bile duct cancers require a pancreaticoduodenectomy for complete excision. In a series from MSKCC, 13% of patients (6 of 45) underwent bile duct excision alone, while in the Veterans Hospital study this figure was only 9% (3 of 34).[104,105] In addition to resection margin status (i.e. an R0 resection), metastatic disease to regional lymph nodes is a critical determinant of outcome. Fong et al. found that lymph node status was the only independent predictor of long-term survival after complete resection, with positive nodes conferring a 6.7 times greater likelihood of recurrence and death.[104] Ito et al. reported that 11 lymph nodes needed to be evaluated to accurately assess lymph node involvement for distal cholangiocarcinoma.[77]

Survival after resection of distal bile duct tumours is comparable to, and maybe better than, that for pancreatic cancer.[6,104,105] Furthermore, it has been erroneously assumed that survival is greater than that after resection of hilar cholangiocarcinomas as well.[5] However, if adjusted for stage and completeness of resection, the survival rates between the two are similar.[4] Adjuvant therapy after resection (chemotherapy and radiation therapy) has not been proved to improve survival, although this issue has not been evaluated in a prospective fashion.[6]

Surgical bypass (hepaticojejunostomy or choledochojejunostomy) or biliary endoprostheses can be used for palliation of symptomatic biliary obstruction. Endoprostheses for distal biliary obstruction are easier to place and have a greater long-term patency than those placed for hilar obstruction.[88] Surgical bypass provides excellent relief of jaundice, but is typically used when unresectability is found at laparotomy. The authors generally use biliary endoprostheses in patients with clear-cut unresectable disease, discovered preoperatively or at staging laparoscopy, and in those unfit for operation. Laparoscopic biliary enteric bypass is also an option, but the expertise needed to perform this procedure is not widely available.

Cholangiocarcinoma involving the intrahepatic bile ducts

Clinical presentation

Intrahepatic cholangiocarcinoma (IHC), also referred to as peripheral cholangiocarcinoma, originates from the intrahepatic biliary radicles. IHC is rare in Western countries, accounts only for approximately 10% of all cholangiocarcinomas and is less frequently associated with underlying liver parenchymal disease than hepatocellular carcinoma, although an association appears to exist. Recently, a marked increase in the incidence and age-adjusted mortality has been identified, the reasons for which are unclear but may be related to the rising incidence of obesity-related, non-alcoholic fatty liver disease or chronic hepatitis C infection.[12,13] The presenting symptoms are subtle and often only include pain either directly or indirectly related to a large lesion. Malaise, weight loss and fever are uncommon, but jaundice and pruritus may be seen in up to one-third of cases, which is generally indicative of compression or invasion of the biliary confluence. Small lesions often present as incidental findings on imaging studies undertaken for unrelated symptoms.

Diagnosis

A solitary, intrahepatic tissue mass at first raises concern for hepatocellular carcinoma, a more common disease than IHC. However, in the absence of chronic hepatic parenchymal disease, chronic hepatitis or an elevated serum α-fetoprotein level, IHC must be considered. Percutaneous needle biopsy is often performed and will demonstrate adenocarcinoma; however, a definitive diagnosis of intrahepatic cholangiocarcinoma often cannot be made based on a needle biopsy alone. Patients should be investigated for evidence of a primary tumour elsewhere (gastrointestinal tract, lung, breast), since the most common diagnosis for adenocarcinoma in the liver is metastatic disease. In the absence of an extrahepatic primary site, patients with biopsy-proven adenocarcinoma in the liver should be considered to have an intrahepatic cholangiocarcinoma. Immunohistochemical staining of the biopsy specimen may further support the diagnosis by demonstrating a lesion of pancreaticobiliary origin.

Radiological investigations

The radiological features of IHC on cross-sectional imaging are well described, and when combined with histological findings from a needle biopsy, can be virtually diagnostic. On MRI, these tumours are generally hypointense on T1-weighted images and heterogeneously hyperintense on T2-weighted images. These lesions demonstrate initial rim enhancement characterised by progressive and concentric enhancement post-administration of contrast material. Generally the lesions do not completely enhance post-contrast. In the absence of a separate primary source of disease, a lesion in the liver with this morphology on MRI evaluation can be considered virtually diagnostic of cholangiocarcinoma without a tissue diagnosis. On contrast-enhanced CT, variable rim-like enhancement is also seen, predominantly on the arterial phase images with gradual centripetal enhancement on delayed imaging (**Fig. 12.5**). Intrahepatic cholangiocarcinomas may only enhance completely on delayed imaging obtained hours after

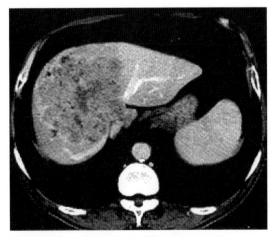

Figure 12.5 • Characteristic CT appearance of intrahepatic cholangiocarcinoma demonstrating heterogeneous enhancement.

contrast administration, a finding related to the desmoplastic nature of the tumour. Capsular retraction may also be seen.[110,111]

Staging and assessment of resectability

Currently, there is no useful clinical staging system for intrahepatic cholangiocarcinoma. The AJCC TNM classification for primary liver cancers is applied both to hepatocellular carcinoma and IHC, but is of little clinical value. Because IHCs tend to be relatively silent lesions, they are often large at presentation. Thirty per cent of patients will have peritoneal or hepatic metastases at presentation and many of these will not be detected until staging laparoscopy or exploratory laparotomy is performed. In a review of 53 peripheral cholangiocarcinomas treated at MSKCC over an 8-year period, the median tumour diameter was 7.1 cm at presentation.[112] Twenty patients were found to be unresectable at exploration for a 62% overall resectability rate. Operative findings precluding resection were intrahepatic metastases (35%), peritoneal metastases (30%), coeliac lymph node metastases (25%) and portal vein involvement (10%). Staging laparoscopy was conducted in 22 patients, of whom six were spared laparotomy secondary to findings of peritoneal and intrahepatic metastases. In a more recent review at the authors' institution, a total of 270 IHC patients were seen over a 16-year period, representing an average annual increase of 14% in patients with this diagnosis over the study period. Of the patients treated at MSKCC, 54% had unresectable disease at presentation; ultimately, 34% of the entire cohort underwent a potentially curative resection (70% of those explored with curative intent).[14]

Treatment options

Hepatic resection with negative histological margins remains the only potentially curative treatment for this disease. Unfortunately, only about one-third to one-half of patients have potentially resectable lesions at the time of presentation. Additionally, a significant proportion of these patients will have findings at operation that preclude resection.[14,112] Median survival after resection was approximately 36 months in a recent study by Endo et al., compared to 9 months for patients with advanced disease.[14] Unfortunately, even after a complete resection, recurrence was common and was predicted by tumour size >5 cm, the presence of multiple liver tumours or metastatic disease to regional lymph nodes; the liver was the single most common site of recurrence.

An international study group for IHC has recently advocated routine portal lymph node dissection at the time of resection, as approximately

30% of patients who underwent evaluation were found to have lymph node involvement.[113] Although this does not seem to provide any therapeutic benefit, it may allow for better prognostication and patient selection for adjuvant therapy. The idea of adjuvant therapy needs to be revisited, given the promising results from the ABC-02 trial that reported improved survival with gemcitabine plus cisplatin.[103] Appropriate patient selection will likely play a paramount role in the application of these data and practice to the adjuvant setting. Given the low yield of lymph nodes from a portal lymphadenectomy (median 3), the accuracy of lymph node evaluation is questionable, and thus its use as a selection criteria for adjuvant therapy is controversial. Perhaps pathological criteria from evaluation of the primary tumour, such as lymphovascular invasion and perineural invasion, should be used instead as selection criteria for adjuvant therapy, as the presence of these factors has been associated with poor survival that is similar to lymph node-positive disease.[114]

Orthotopic liver transplantation has been utilised in the management of some patients.[115,116] However, many of these lesions are suitable for resection, which would likely produce similar results. Given the critical shortage of liver grafts, transplantation for IHC is not performed in most centres, unless it is done in the context of a clinical trial. The use of chemotherapy has not been shown to improve survival, either as adjuvant therapy following resection or in patients with unresectable lesions.[117] However, as mentioned above, given the results of the ABC-02 trial for advanced disease, administration of the double regimen in the adjuvant setting needs to be evaluated. External beam radiation therapy, intraoperative radiation and intraluminal radiation therapy have all been evaluated as well, albeit in small, not well controlled, primarily retrospective studies. Similar to chemotherapy, none have shown a significant survival benefit in patients with unresectable disease. However, Ibrahim et al. reported a median survival of 31.8 months in patients with unresectable IHC treated with yttrium-90 (Y-90) who had a performance status of ECOG 0. This study included only 24 patients and a positive effect of Y-90 was not observed in patients with ECOG performance status of 1 or 2.[118] The senior author has also reported the experience using hepatic arterial infusion pump therapy (FUDR) with and without bevacizumab for advanced disease. The median survival of patients treated with intra-arterial therapy was 29.5 months, better than that usually achieved with systemic chemotherapy.[119] It also appeared that the addition of bevacizumab increased the incidence of biliary toxicity without any improvement in survival (31.1 vs. 29.5 months; P = NS).[120]

✔✔ Complete surgical resection is the best treatment for intrahepatic cholangiocarcinoma. Chemotherapy and/or radiation therapy, whether in an adjuvant or palliative setting, have not been shown to provide any significant survival benefit.

Gallbladder cancer

Gallbladder cancer is an uncommon malignancy with approximately 5000 new cases per year in the USA.[1] Historically, clinical attitudes toward gallbladder cancer have been largely based on pessimism and nihilism. This frustration spawns from the usual late presentation, lack of effective therapy and the resultant dismal prognosis. In fact, most older series reported a median survival of 2–5 months for untreated gallbladder cancers, and a less than 5% 5-year survival for treated gallbladder cancers. However, improved understanding of the disease and its treatment has led to prolonged survival and cure in selected patients. Currently, the only chance of cure is with complete surgical extirpation of the cancer.

Epidemiology/aetiology

Worldwide, the highest incidence of gallbladder cancer is found among people indigenous to the Andes Mountains of South America. In North America, the incidence is approximately 1.2 per 100 000, the highest being among native American Indians and Mexican Americans. It occurs in women almost three times more often than in men across all populations studied.[121]

As with other biliary tract tumours, chronic inflammation leading to high cellular turnover is a common denominator of associated risk factors. The most common risk factor is cholelithiasis; other factors include the presence of a cholecystoenteric fistula, typhoid bacillus infection and an anomalous pancreaticobiliary junction.[121,122] As with other gastrointestinal malignancies, the adenoma to carcinoma sequence has been demonstrated within adenomatous polyps of the gallbladder as well.[123] Gallbladder polyps are noted in 3–6% of the population undergoing ultrasonography, although the vast majority are cholesterol polyps or adenomyomatosis, both of which are benign and have no malignant potential. However, about 1% of cholecystectomy specimens contain adenomatous polyps, which do have malignant potential.[124] Conditions that increase the risk of malignancy include polyp size >1 cm, patient age >50 years and the presence of multiple lesions.[125] The conservative recommendation is to perform a prophylactic cholecystectomy for polypoid lesions greater than 0.5 cm in size, although the likelihood of malignancy in polyps even up to 1 cm appears to be extremely low. This is in contrast to gallbladder polyps arising in the setting of primary sclerosing cholangitis, which are more often neoplastic.[126] The authors' practice is to recommend cholecystectomy for polyps >1 cm, although carcinoma in such lesions appears to be much lower than previously thought. Polypoid lesions <0.5 cm have an extremely low likelihood of harbouring malignancy and are safe to follow with serial ultrasounds for evidence of growth or change in character.[123,124,127]

A gallbladder with a calcified wall, also known as a 'porcelain gallbladder', is associated with an increased risk of developing cancer (**Fig. 12.6**). The deposition of calcium most likely reflects a state of chronic inflammation. Although the risk of malignancy in a porcelain gallbladder previously was considered to be extremely high (10–50%), recent studies demonstrate a much lower incidence (<10%), with stippled calcification actually carrying a higher risk than diffuse intramural calcification.[128,129] Nevertheless, the current recommendation for patients with a porcelain gallbladder is to perform a cholecystectomy, which in most cases can be safely done laparoscopically.

> ✔✔ Although most gallbladder polyps identified at ultrasonography are benign, true adenomatous polyps do have a malignant potential. Cholecystectomy should be performed for adenomatous polyps >1 cm in size, and those <1 cm should be followed closely with serial ultrasound to detect any growth or change. A calcified gallbladder wall, likely a reflection of chronic inflammation, is also an indication for cholecystectomy.

Clinical presentation and diagnosis

Many patients present late in the course of their disease, and 75% of patients present with unresectable disease.[130] Two-thirds of patients present with abdominal pain/biliary colic. Approximately one-third will present with jaundice and 10% will have significant weight loss.[131] For early stage cancers, the diagnosis is usually made on pathological examination of a cholecystectomy specimen resected for symptoms presumed to be benign biliary colic. Preoperative diagnosis should be suspected for any mass or irregularity of the gallbladder wall noted on radiological investigation (CT or ultrasound). In any patient suspected of having a gallbladder malignancy, a duplex ultrasound should be performed to evaluate the extent of disease and possible involvement of the portal vasculature. In addition, abdominal cross-sectional imaging (CT or MRI) should be performed to evaluate for nodal disease or M1 disease. For those patients suspected of having gallbladder cancer on preoperative imaging, a tissue diagnosis is not necessary prior to exploration, and both the surgeon and patient should be prepared for an appropriate resection, knowing that the final pathology may in fact reveal benign disease.

> ✔ Imaging findings of asymmetric gallbladder wall thickening, intralumenal papillary projections, or any other finding suggesting a mass must be taken very seriously, particularly when noted on ultrasonography. Any such findings should immediately raise the concern for a possible gallbladder cancer and treated accordingly.

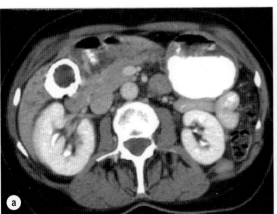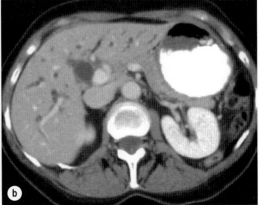

Figure 12.6 • Axial CT images of a porcelain gallbladder. Note the marked circumferential calcification of the gallbladder wall **(a)** and the intrahepatic biliary ductal dilatation **(b)**. This patient had a gallbladder cancer arising in the setting of a porcelain gallbladder, which had progressed to involve the common hepatic duct.

Histopathology and staging

The overwhelming majority of gallbladder cancers are adenocarcinomas, with a papillary subtype being associated with a relatively better prognosis compared to others.[132] Other histological subtypes, such as adenosquamous carcinoma or pure squamous cell carcinoma, are seen in the gallbladder more commonly than at any other site within the biliary tree. The AJCC staging system was updated in 2002 (sixth edition) and was based on the standard TNM classification, of which the T stage has the greatest clinical impact on the extent of surgery performed, because it is dependent on the depth of invasion into the gallbladder wall and adjacent organs. The wall of the gallbladder consists of a mucosa and lamina propria, a thin muscular layer, perimuscular connective tissue and a serosa. However, it should be noted that the gallbladder wall lacks a serosal covering along its border with the liver and the perimuscular connective tissue is continuous with the liver connective tissue. T1 tumours are divided into T1a and T1b lesions, where the former is limited to the lamina propria and the latter has invaded the muscle layer. T2 tumours have invaded through the muscle layer into the perimuscular connective tissue. T3 tumours have penetrated the serosa and directly invade either the liver or another single extrahepatic organ. T4 tumours reflect locally unresectable tumours due to invasion into the main portal vein, hepatic artery or multiple extrahepatic organs. Of note, in patients with a new diagnosis of gallbladder cancer, the presence of jaundice is an ominous finding, generally implying advanced disease that is beyond resectability. Previously, the N stage was divided into locoregional and distant lymph node involvement, but due to the powerful adverse negative impact of any positive lymph node, the sixth edition staging system simply divided tumours into being either node negative or positive, i.e. N0 or N1, respectively. Metastatic disease refers to distant metastasis. This AJCC sixth edition staging system is detailed in Table 12.5. The seventh edition of the AJCC staging system has reverted back to stratifying nodal involvement based on location, thus creating an N1 and N2 designation, and considers T4 tumours as stage IV disease (Table 12.6). It should be noted that the majority of studies referenced in this chapter utilise previous editions of the staging system, where the major difference is that T4 tumours were not deemed as unresectable.

Preoperative staging should be aimed at assessing the local extent of disease and excluding distant metastases. Cross-sectional imaging (CT or MRCP) is the mainstay of investigation, while duplex ultrasonography is helpful to assess the gallbladder lesion and can provide

Table 12.5 • AJCC staging system (sixth edition) for gallbladder cancer (TNM classification)

Primary tumour (T)

TX:	Primary tumour cannot be assessed
T0:	No evidence of primary tumour
Tis:	Carcinoma in situ
T1:	Tumour invades lamina propria or muscle layer
T1a:	Tumour invades lamina propria
T1b:	Tumour invades muscle layer
T2:	Tumour invades perimuscular connective tissue: no extension beyond serosa or into liver
T3:	Tumour perforates serosa (visceral peritoneum) or directly invades the liver and/or one other adjacent organ or structure, e.g. stomach, duodenum, colon pancreas, omentum, extrahepatic bile ducts
T4:	Tumour invades main portal vein or hepatic artery, or invades two or more extrahepatic organs or structures

Regional lymph nodes (N)

NX:	Regional lymph nodes cannot be assessed
N0:	No regional lymph node metastasis
N1:	Regional lymph node metastasis

Distant metastasis (M)

MX:	Presence of distant metastasis cannot be assessed
M0:	No distant metastasis
M1:	Distant metastasis

Stage grouping

Stage 0:	Tis, N0, M0
Stage IA:	T1, N0, M0
Stage IB:	T2, N0, M0
Stage IIA:	T3, N0, M0
Stage IIB:	T1, N1, M0
	T2, N1, M0
	T3, N1, M0
Stage III:	T4, any N, M0
Stage IV:	Any T, any N, M1

Reprinted with permission from Sobin LH, Wittekind C (eds) TNM classification of malignant tumours, 6th edn. Wiley-Liss, 2002.

some insight as to the likelihood of a malignancy; in addition, US may be helpful in assessing possible vascular involvement. FDG-PET has been shown to be helpful in identifying additional disease that changes management; Corvera et al. reported such findings in nearly one-quarter of patients.[72] In addition, staging laparoscopy is helpful for identifying distant disease, thereby avoiding non-therapeutic laparotomies.[68]

Table 12.6 • AJCC staging system for gallbladder cancer (TNM classification)

Primary tumour (T)

TX:	Primary tumour cannot be assessed
T0:	No evidence of primary tumour
Tis:	Carcinoma in situ
T1:	Tumour invades lamina propria or muscular layer
T1a:	Tumour invades lamina propria
T1b:	Tumour invades muscular layer
T2:	Tumour invades perimuscular connective tissue; no extension beyond serosa or into liver
T3:	Tumour perforates the serosa (visceral peritoneum) and/or directly invades the liver and/or one other adjacent organ or structure, such as the stomach, duodenum, colon, pancreas, omentum or extrahepatic bile ducts
T4:	Tumour invades main portal vein or hepatic artery or invades two or more extrahepatic organs or structures

Regional lymph nodes (N)

NX:	Regional lymph nodes cannot be assessed
N0:	No regional lymph node metastasis
N1:	Metastases to nodes along the cystic duct, common bile duct, hepatic artery and/or portal vein
N2:	Metastases to periaortic, pericaval, superior mesenteric artery and/or coeliac artery lymph nodes

Distant metastasis (M)

M0:	No distant metastasis
M1:	Distant metastasis

Stage grouping

Stage 0:	Tis, N0, M0
Stage I:	T1, N0, M0
Stage II:	T2, N0, M0
Stage IIIA:	T3, N0, M0
Stage IIIB:	T1, N1, M0
	T2, N1, M0
	T3, N1, M0
Stage IVA:	T4, N0, M0
	T4, N1, M0
Stage IVB:	Any T, N2, M0
	Any T, any N, M1

From Sobin LH, Wittekind C (eds) TNM Classification of Malignant Tumors, 6th edition. Wiley-Liss, 2002. This material is reproduced with permission of John Wiley & Sons, Inc.

Evidence for an aggressive surgical approach

Over the past three decades, decreasing morbidity and mortality associated with radical en bloc resections including hepatectomy, bile duct resection and regional lymphadenectomy have allowed for broader application of surgical resection in selected patients.[131,133] The current surgical approaches generally employ segmental resections (segments IVb/V) or major resections (hemihepatectomy or extended hepatectomy) when necessary. In most cases, it is the involvement of major hepatic vascular structures rather than actual depth of tumour invasion into the liver that dictates the extent of hepatic resection that must be performed.

In a series from MSKCC, Bartlett et al. reported on 149 cases in which complete surgical radical resection yielded an actuarial 5-year survival of 83% for stage II, 63% for stage III and 25% for stage IV.[131] Many contemporary studies have reported similar results, even for stage III and IV disease.[134–137] The improved survival reported in these studies relative to historical studies, in which the survival rates were dismal, demonstrates the importance of achieving negative margins at the time of resection.

Regional lymphadenectomy is currently employed as part of an aggressive surgical approach, but evidence to support an associated survival benefit is controversial. The chance of nodal involvement increases with increasing T stage. Bartlett et al. found nodal disease associated with 46% of resected T2 tumours and 54% of resected T3 tumours.[131] Node status was found to be the most powerful predictor of outcome and no patient with node-positive disease experienced long-term survival. Poor outcome for node-positive disease has been consistently reported throughout the Western literature. Again, the value of a negative lymph node is dependent on the number of lymph nodes sampled, and a study from MSKCC suggests that six lymph nodes are needed to accurately assess for lymph node involvement.[138]

Surgical therapy

Patients with gallbladder cancer will present as one of three different clinical scenarios where malignancy is (1) suspected preoperatively, (2) found at the time of exploration or (3) diagnosed after simple cholecystectomy. Contraindications to resection include distant spread (peritoneum, discontiguous liver lesions), tumour involvement of the hepatic vasculature or biliary tree that would preclude a complete resection, and presence of disease in distant lymph node groups (peripancreatic, periduodenal, periportal, coeliac and/or superior mesenteric).

The goal of resection should always be complete tumour extirpation with negative histological margins (R0). Patients with cancer identified preoperatively typically have relatively larger tumours and more extensive disease than is seen in patients diagnosed post-cholecystectomy. Gallbladder cancer identified intraoperatively is an uncommon but difficult situation, since one will have limited staging information; however, it is reasonable to proceed with definitive surgical management, since this is the only effective therapy. When the diagnosis is made after simple cholecystectomy, the need for further resection is primarily dictated by the T stage.

It is important to remember that the incidence of lymph node and distant metastases is directly related to T stage. Fong et al. reported a progressive increase in distant and nodal metastases from 16% to 79% and from 33% to 69%, respectively, on going from T2 to T4 tumours, which resulted in a progressive decline in resectability, from 58% to 13%.[139]

T1 tumours

T1a tumours, or those that are confined to the lamina propria, are most often discovered after, and adequately treated with, a simple cholecystectomy. Because the potential for nodal involvement is small, cure rates approach 85–100% if negative margins are achieved.[140,141] T1b tumours, i.e. those tumours that have extended into, but not through, the muscle layer, in theory should be cured by a simple cholecystectomy as well. However, there have been reports in the literature documenting recurrence and death following a simple cholecystectomy for T1b tumours.[142] Given the limited data regarding T1b gallbladder cancers in the literature, the decision to perform a simple cholecystectomy versus a more radical procedure should be made on a case-by-case basis.

T2 tumours

T2 lesions, or tumours that extend into the perimuscular connective tissues, should be treated with an aggressive resection, including removal of adjacent liver, lymphadenectomy of the hepatoduodenal ligament and a bile duct resection only if necessary to obtain a negative margin on the cystic duct. As discussed above, the extent of hepatic resection required depends on whether or not there is tumour involvement of the right portal pedicle (i.e. major inflow vascular structures or right hepatic duct). In the absence of such involvement, the authors prefer to perform a segmental resection of segments IVb and V, and most T2 tumours are amenable to such an approach. It should be noted that the normal plane of dissection of simple cholecystectomy, open or laparoscopic, is within the perimuscular connective tissue intimately associated with the liver. Thus, a simple cholecystectomy will not achieve tumour clearance with certainty. A lymphadenectomy is performed in the treatment of T2 tumours given that up to 50% of these lesions have associated lymph node metastases.[131] The benefit of an extended resection over simple cholecystectomy is supported by data that demonstrate improved survival. This is underscored by the fact that liver involvement can be found after radical resection in up to a quarter of patients with presumed T2 disease after cholecystectomy alone, a finding that is associated with markedly reduced recurrence-free and disease-specific survival.[138] De Aretxabala et al. reported 5-year survival rates of 70% compared with only 20% after simple cholecystectomy alone.[143]

T3 tumours

T3 tumours penetrate the serosa and may extend into the liver parenchyma or a single extrahepatic organ. These tumours require a hepatic resection and porta hepatis lymphadenectomy at a minimum. As with T2 tumours, if a limited partial hepatectomy can be performed to achieve the objectives, then this is preferred; however, one should not hesitate to perform a more extensive partial hepatectomy and/or bile duct resection if necessary. When a complete resection is achieved, 5-year survival rates of 30–50% can be obtained in this patient population.[131,136,139]

T4 tumours

T4 lesions, as defined by the sixth edition staging system, generally reflect unresectable disease.

Preoperative suspicion of malignancy

If gallbladder cancer is suspected on preoperative imaging studies, a staging laparoscopy prior to laparotomy is helpful to assess the abdomen for evidence of peritoneal spread or discontiguous liver disease. In general, however, performing a laparoscopic cholecystectomy should be avoided.[67,68,144] One needs to be prepared to proceed with resection of an invasive malignancy, unless proven otherwise. It is not unreasonable to obtain intraoperative frozen section histology to prove malignancy before proceeding with hepatic resection.

Unsuspected malignancy at exploration

It should be routine to inspect the gallbladder mucosa after simple cholecystectomy. Suspicious lesions should be sent immediately for frozen section. If a carcinoma is diagnosed, the need to perform additional surgery is dictated by the T stage on frozen section, although the information will be limited since a full histopathological evaluation is not available at the time of operation. The authors prefer to perform an oncologically correct resection, suitable for an invasive lesion, at the time it is discovered, unless there are extenuating circumstances that mandate otherwise. However, if the surgeon is not comfortable with performing a radical cholecystectomy/hepatic resection, the patient is best served by transferring them to a centre/surgeon with experience in performing the appropriate operation. A delayed radical and appropriate resection does not negatively influence the patient's outcome.[139]

Malignancy diagnosed post-cholecystectomy

When the cancer is diagnosed by postoperative histology, the need for a more radical resection will be based on T stage, as outlined above. As mentioned above, Fong et al. demonstrated a much improved 5-year survival rate in patients undergoing a second operation compared to those who did not. Five-year survival rates of 61% were achieved in patients who were re-resected compared to 19% for patients who did not undergo a radical second operation.[139] However, prior to undertaking a second operation, high-quality cross-sectional imaging (CT/MRI) should be obtained to appropriately stage the disease. Postoperative inflammatory changes may be indistinguishable from tumour and thus may necessitate bile duct resection or a more aggressive hepatic resection to ensure complete tumour eradication.

Given that inadvertent cholecystotomy during cholecystectomy is rarely documented, it is difficult to predict who is at increased risk for peritoneal dissemination and, specifically, port site recurrence. In the past, routine resection of laparoscopic port sites was recommended, in an effort to ensure clearance of microscopic disease that may have implanted during the laparoscopic procedure. However, there is little evidence to support the efficacy of routine resection of all port sites at re-operation.[145] In the authors' experience, recurrence at the port sites is a harbinger of generalised peritoneal recurrence that will not be prevented with resection of these limited areas.

> ✔ When exploring a patient for gallbladder cancer after a non-curative laparoscopic cholecystectomy has been performed, a finding of disease at the port sites is a sign of generalised peritoneal spread of disease.

Adjuvant therapy

In order to provide a rational framework upon which to develop adjuvant therapies for patients having undergone resection, Jarnagin et al. investigated the initial pattern of recurrence after resection of biliary tract cancers. Sixty-six per cent of patients with gall-bladder cancers who underwent a potentially curative resection recurred within a median follow-up of 24 months. Only 15% of patients developed a locoregional recurrence as the first site of failure, while the majority of patients (85%) had recurrence that involved a distant site.[146] Thus, local therapies targeted at locoregional disease, such as radiotherapy, are unlikely to significantly impact the course of this disease, further emphasising the importance of developing effective systemic adjuvant therapies.

Most data for the use of adjuvant therapy are derived from phase II trials in which treated patients are compared with historical controls. Most of these trials are limited by small numbers, combine chemotherapy with radiation treatment, and are confounded by inclusion of patients with less than an R0 resection.[147,148] Thus, minimal conclusions can be drawn regarding the use of external beam radiation/chemotherapy in the adjuvant setting. In cases of incomplete resection, there remains a theoretical benefit to adding an additional locoregional therapy such as external beam radiation therapy for disease control.

One phase III multi-institutional trial of adjuvant chemotherapy was performed in Japan as reported by Takada et al.[85] It should be noted that this trial included 508 patients with biliary and pancreatic cancers. However, on subset analysis, this study included 140 patients with gallbladder cancer who were randomised to undergo surgical resection alone or resection plus adjuvant mitomycin and 5-FU. In considering only the patients with gallbladder cancer, the actuarial 5-year disease-free survival favoured the adjuvant chemotherapy group in comparison to the surgery-alone group (20.3% vs. 11.6%). From these data it is reasonable to offer adjuvant chemotherapy with 5-FU and mitomycin; however, no consensus has been reached regarding routine use of adjuvant chemotherapy.[102]

Palliation

Most gallbladder cancer patients present with advanced, incurable disease. Their symptoms may include pain, jaundice or gastrointestinal obstruction. Given the dismal prognosis of approximately 2–5 months' survival, non-surgical methods of palliation including both percutaneous and endoscopic techniques to relieve intestinal or biliary obstruction should be considered first. If unresectable disease is discovered at the time of exploration, a segment III bypass can be performed to relieve jaundice, but in general patients are best served by avoiding a major operative procedure and proceeding with percutaneous biliary drainage postoperatively.[149] Intestinal bypass should be performed only in patients who have symptomatic obstruction.

Key points

Cholangiocarcinoma

Hilar

- Preoperative assessment is mainly a decision of resectability. Attention should be paid to the extent of bile duct involvement, portal vein involvement and to the presence or absence of hepatic atrophy.
- Most complete resections for hilar disease necessitate a hepatectomy.
- Chemotherapy and radiotherapy have not been shown to be beneficial beyond complete surgical resection alone.

Distal

- The clinical presentation is very similar to that of other periampullary tumours.
- Similar to hilar disease, a preoperative tissue diagnosis is not necessary to proceed with surgical resection.
- When possible, endoscopic palliation is the preferred method to relieve symptomatic jaundice in the setting of unresectable disease.

Intrahepatic

- Hepatocellular carcinoma must be excluded in patients with an intrahepatic mass.
- Metastatic adenocarcinoma to the liver from a remote primary, such as lung, breast or gastrointestinal, must be excluded.
- Similar to all other locations of cholangiocarcinoma, complete surgical resection is the optimal treatment and only chance for cure.

Gallbladder cancer

- Duplex ultrasonography should be part of the preoperative imaging to properly assess the tumour within the gallbladder wall and its relation to the bile duct and hepatic vasculature.
- A cholecystectomy should be performed for adenomatous polyps greater than 1 cm, or those that are smaller but growing and changing in character. Cholesterol polyps and adenomyomatosis are not premalignant conditions.
- Complete surgical resection is the goal, whether the diagnosis is made preoperatively, intraoperatively or after a non-curative laparoscopic cholecystectomy.

References

1. Landis SH, Murray T, Bolden S, et al. Cancer statistics, 1998. CA Cancer J Clin 1998;48(1):6–29.
2. Carriaga MT, Henson DE. Liver, gallbladder, extrahepatic bile ducts, and pancreas. Cancer 1995;75(1, Suppl.):171–90.
3. Burke EC, Jarnagin WR, Hochwald SN, et al. Hilar cholangiocarcinoma: patterns of spread, the importance of hepatic resection for curative operation, and a presurgical clinical staging system. Ann Surg 1998;228(3):385–94.
4. Nagorney DM, Donohue JH, Farnell MB, et al. Outcomes after curative resections of cholangiocarcinoma. Arch Surg 1993;128(8):871–9.
5. Tompkins RK, Thomas D, Wile A, et al. Prognostic factors in bile duct carcinoma: analysis of 96 cases. Ann Surg 1981;194:447–57.
6. Nakeeb A, Pitt HA, Sohn TA, et al. Cholangiocarcinoma. A spectrum of intrahepatic, perihilar, and distal tumors. Ann Surg 1996;224(4):463–75.
7. Berdah SV, Delpero JR, Garcia S, et al. A Western surgical experience of peripheral cholangiocarcinoma. Br J Surg 1996;83(11):1517–21.
8. Chu KM, Lai EC, Al-Hadeedi S, et al. Intrahepatic cholangiocarcinoma. World J Surg 1997;21(3):301–6.
9. Harrison LE, Fong Y, Klimstra DS, et al. Surgical treatment of 32 patients with peripheral intrahepatic cholangiocarcinoma. Br J Surg 1998;85(8):1068–70.
10. Saunders K, Longmire Jr W, Tompkins R, et al. Diffuse bile duct tumors: guidelines for management. Am Surg 1991;57(12):816–20.
11. Patel T, Steer CJ, Gores GJ. Apoptosis and the liver: a mechanism of disease, growth regulation, and carcinogenesis. Hepatology 1999;30(3):811–5.

12. Welzel TM, Graubard BI, El-Serag HB, et al. Risk factors for intrahepatic and extrahepatic cholangiocarcinoma in the United States: a population-based case–control study. Clin Gastroenterol Hepatol 2007;5(10):1221–8.

13. Welzel TM, Mellemkjaer L, Gloria G, et al. Risk factors for intrahepatic cholangiocarcinoma in a low-risk population: a nationwide case–control study. Int J Cancer 2007;120(3):638–41.

14. Endo I, Gonen M, Yopp AC, et al. Intrahepatic cholangiocarcinoma: rising frequency, improved survival, and determinants of outcome after resection. Ann Surg 2008;248(1):84–96.

15. Kuwayti K, Baggenstoss AH, Stauffer MH, et al. Carcinoma of the major intrahepatic and the extrahepatic bile ducts exclusive of the papilla of Vater. Gynecol Obstet 1957;104:357–66.

16. Sako K, Seitzinger GL, Garside E. Carcinoma of the extrahepatic bile ducts; review of the literature and report of six cases. Surgery 1957;41(3):416–37.

17. Okuda K, Kubo Y, Okazaki N, et al. Clinical aspects of intrahepatic bile duct carcinoma including hilar carcinoma: a study of 57 autopsy-proven cases. Cancer 1977;39(1):232–46.

18. Broome U, Olsson R, Loof L, et al. Natural history and prognostic factors in 305 Swedish patients with primary sclerosing cholangitis. Gut 1996;38(4):610–5.

19. Pitt HA, Dooley WC, Yeo CJ, et al. Malignancies of the biliary tree. Curr Probl Surg 1995;32(1):1–90.

20. Hewitt PM, Krige JE, Bornman PC, et al. Choledochal cysts in adults. Br J Surg 1995;82(3):382–5.

21. Vogt DP. Current management of cholangiocarcinoma. Oncology (Williston Park) 1988;2(6):37–44, 54.

22. Lipsett PA, Pitt HA, Colombani PM, et al. Choledochal cyst disease. A changing pattern of presentation. Ann Surg 1994;220(5):644–52.

23. Tanaka K, Ikoma A, Hamada N, et al. Biliary tract cancer accompanied by anomalous junction of pancreaticobiliary ductal system in adults. Am J Surg 1998;175(3):218–20.

24. Jeng KS, Ohta I, Yang FS, et al. Coexisting sharp ductal angulation with intrahepatic biliary strictures in right hepatolithiasis. Arch Surg 1994;129(10):1097–102.

25. Hakamada K, Sasaki M, Endoh M, et al. Late development of bile duct cancer after sphincteroplasty: a ten- to twenty-two-year follow-up study. Surgery 1997;121(5):488–92.

26. Chu KM, Lo CM, Liu CL, et al. Malignancy associated with hepatolithiasis. Hepatogastroenterology 1997;44(14):352–7.

27. Kubo S, Kinoshita H, Hirohashi K, et al. Hepatolithiasis associated with cholangiocarcinoma. World J Surg 1995;19(4):637–41.

28. Weinbren K, Mutum SS. Pathological aspects of cholangiocarcinoma. J Pathol 1983;139(2):217–38.

29. Rodgers CM, Adams JT, Schwartz SI. Carcinoma of the extrahepatic bile ducts. Surgery 1981;90(4):596–601.

30. Jarnagin WR, Bowne W, Klimstra DS, et al. Papillary phenotype confers improved survival after resection of hilar cholangiocarcinoma. Ann Surg 2005;241(5):703–14.

31. Tsuzuki T, Ogata Y, Iida S, et al. Carcinoma of the bifurcation of the hepatic ducts. Arch Surg 1983;118(10):1147–51.

32. Shimada H, Niimoto S, Matsuba A, et al. The infiltration of bile duct carcinoma along the bile duct wall. Int Surg 1988;73(2):87–90.

33. Endo I, House MG, Klimstra DS, et al. Clinical significance of intraoperative bile duct margin assessment for hilar cholangiocarcinoma. Ann Surg Oncol 2008;15(8):2104–12.

34. Craig JR, Peters RL, Edmondson HA. Tumor liver and intrahepatic ducts. Armed Forces Institute of Pathology; 1989.

35. The Liver Cancer Study Group of Japan. Primary liver cancer in Japan. Sixth report. Cancer 1987;60(6):1400–11.

36. Yamamoto J, Kosuge T, Shimada K, et al. Intrahepatic cholangiocarcinoma: proposal of new macroscopic classification. Nippon Geka Gakkai Zasshi 1993;94(11):1194–200.

37. Levi S, Urbano-Ispizua A, Gill R, et al. Multiple K-ras codon 12 mutations in cholangiocarcinomas demonstrated with a sensitive polymerase chain reaction technique. Cancer Res 1991;51(13):3497–502.

38. Nakeeb A, Lipsett PA, Lillemoe KD, et al. Biliary carcinoembryonic antigen levels are a marker for cholangiocarcinoma. Am J Surg 1996;171(1):147–53.

39. Jarnagin WR, Weber S, Tickoo SK, et al. Combined hepatocellular and cholangiocarcinoma: demographic, clinical, and prognostic factors. Cancer 2002;94(7):2040–6.

40. Farley DR, Weaver AL, Nagorney DM. "Natural history" of unresected cholangiocarcinoma: patient outcome after noncurative intervention. Mayo Clin Proc 1995;70(5):425–9.

41. Vatanasapt V, Uttaravichien T, Mairiang EO, et al. Cholangiocarcinoma in north-east Thailand. Lancet 1990;335(8681):116–7.

42. McPherson GA, Benjamin IS, Hodgson HJ, et al. Pre-operative percutaneous transhepatic biliary drainage: the results of a controlled trial. Br J Surg 1984;71(5):371–5.

43. Heslin MJ, Brooks AD, Hochwald SN, et al. A preoperative biliary stent is associated with increased complications after pancreatoduodenectomy. Arch Surg 1998;133(2):149–54.

44. Corvera CU, Blumgart LH, Darvishian F, et al. Clinical and pathologic features of proximal biliary strictures masquerading as hilar cholangiocarcinoma. J Am Coll Surg 2005;201(6):862–9.

45. Wetter LA, Ring EJ, Pellegrini CA, et al. Differential diagnosis of sclerosing cholangiocarcinomas of the common hepatic duct (Klatskin tumors). Am J Surg 1991;161(1):57–63.

46. Rabinovitz M, Zajko AB, Hassanein T, et al. Diagnostic value of brush cytology in the diagnosis of bile duct carcinoma: a study in 65 patients with bile duct strictures. Hepatology 1990;12(4, Pt 1):747–52.

47. Hadjis NS, Blumgart LH. Role of liver atrophy, hepatic resection and hepatocyte hyperplasia in the development of portal hypertension in biliary disease. Gut 1987;28(8):1022–8.

48. Tillich M, Mischinger HJ, Preisegger KH, et al. Multiphasic helical CT in diagnosis and staging of hilar cholangiocarcinoma. Am J Roentgenol 1998;171(3):651–8.

49. Gibson RN, Yeung E, Thompson JN, et al. Bile duct obstruction: radiologic evaluation of level, cause, and tumor resectability. Radiology 1986;160(1):43–7.

50. Okuda K, Ohto M, Tsuchiya Y. The role of ultrasound, percutaneous transhepatic cholangiography, computed tomographic scanning, and magnetic resonance imaging in the preoperative assessment of bile duct cancer. World J Surg 1988;12(1):18–26.

51. Hann LE, Greatrex KV, Bach AM, et al. Cholangiocarcinoma at the hepatic hilus: sonographic findings. Am J Roentgenol 1997;168(4):985–9.

52. Bach AM, Hann LE, Brown KT, et al. Portal vein evaluation with US: comparison to angiography combined with CT arterial portography. Radiology 1996;201(1):149–54.

53. Itoh K, Fujita N, Kubo K, et al. MR imaging of hilar cholangiocarcinoma – comparative study with CT. Nippon Igaku Hoshasen Gakkai Zasshi 1992;52(4):443–51.

54. Guthrie JA, Ward J, Robinson PJ. Hilar cholangiocarcinomas: T2-weighted spin-echo and gadolinium-enhanced FLASH MR imaging. Radiology 1996;201(2):347–51.

55. Schwartz LH, Coakley FV, Sun Y, et al. Neoplastic pancreaticobiliary duct obstruction: evaluation with breath-hold MR cholangiopancreatography. Am J Roentgenol 1998;170(6):1491–5.

56. Lee MG, Lee HJ, Kim MH, et al. Extrahepatic biliary diseases: 3D MR cholangiopancreatography compared with endoscopic retrograde cholangiopancreatography. Radiology 1997;202(3):663–9.

57. Jarnagin WR, Fong Y, DeMatteo RP, et al. Staging, resectability, and outcome in 225 patients with hilar cholangiocarcinoma. Ann Surg 2001;234(4):507–19.

58. Bismuth H, Nakache R, Diamond T. Management strategies in resection for hilar cholangiocarcinoma. Ann Surg 1992;215(1):31–8.

59. Chen RF, Li ZH, Zhou JJ, et al. Preoperative evaluation with T-staging system for hilar cholangiocarcinoma. World J Gastroenterol 2007;13(43):5754–9.

60. Klempnauer J, Ridder GJ, Werner M, et al. What constitutes long-term survival after surgery for hilar cholangiocarcinoma? Cancer 1997;79(1):26–34.

61. Pichlmayr R, Weimann A, Klempnauer J, et al. Surgical treatment in proximal bile duct cancer. A single-center experience. Ann Surg 1996;224(5):628–38.

62. Iwatsuki S, Todo S, Marsh JW, et al. Treatment of hilar cholangiocarcinoma (Klatskin tumors) with hepatic resection or transplantation. J Am Coll Surg 1998;187(4):358–64.

63. Heimbach JK, Haddock MG, Alberts SR, et al. Transplantation for hilar cholangiocarcinoma. Liver Transpl 2004;10(10, Suppl. 2):S65–8.

64. Lazaridis KN, Gores GJ. Cholangiocarcinoma. Gastroenterology 2005;128(6):1655–67.

65. Nimura Y, Hayakawa N, Kamiya J, et al. Hepatic segmentectomy with caudate lobe resection for bile duct carcinoma of the hepatic hilus. World J Surg 1990;14(4):535–44.

66. Mizumoto R, Suzuki H. Surgical anatomy of the hepatic hilum with special reference to the caudate lobe. World J Surg 1988;12(1):2–10.

67. Vollmer CM, Drebin JA, Middleton WD, et al. Utility of staging laparoscopy in subsets of peripancreatic and biliary malignancies. Ann Surg 2002;235(1):1–7.

68. Weber SM, DeMatteo RP, Fong Y, et al. Staging laparoscopy in patients with extrahepatic biliary carcinoma. Analysis of 100 patients. Ann Surg 2002;235(3):392–9.

69. Kluge R, Schmidt F, Caca K, et al. Positron emission tomography with [^{18}F]fluoro-2-deoxy-D-glucose for diagnosis and staging of bile duct cancer. Hepatology 2001;33(5):1029–35.

70. Fritscher-Ravens A, Bohuslavizki KH, Broering DC, et al. FDG PET in the diagnosis of hilar cholangiocarcinoma. Nucl Med Commun 2001;22(12):1277–85.

71. Anderson CD, Rice MH, Pinson CW, et al. Fluorodeoxyglucose PET imaging in the evaluation of gallbladder carcinoma and cholangiocarcinoma. J Gastrointest Surg 2004;8(1):90–7.

72. Corvera CU, Blumgart LH, Akhurst T, et al. ^{18}F-Fluorodeoxyglucose positron emission tomography influences management decisions in patients with biliary cancer. J Am Coll Surg 2008;206(1):57–65.

73. Jarnagin WR, Blumgart LH, Saldinger P. Cancer of the bile ducts. In: Blumgart LH, Fong Y, editors. Surgery of the liver and biliary tract. London: WB Saunders; 2000. p. 1017.

74. Neuhaus P, Thelen A, Jonas S, et al. Oncological superiority of hilar en bloc resection for the treatment of hilar cholangiocarcinoma. Ann Surg Oncol 2012;19(5):1602–8.

75. Kitagawa Y, Nagino M, Kamiya J, et al. Lymph node metastasis from hilar cholangiocarcinoma: audit of 110 patients who underwent regional and paraaortic node dissection. Ann Surg 2001;233(3):385–92.

76. Tojima Y, Nagino M, Ebata T, et al. Immunohistochemically demonstrated lymph node micrometastasis and prognosis in patients with otherwise node-negative hilar cholangiocarcinoma. Ann Surg 2003;237(2):201–7.

77. Ito K, Ito H, Allen PJ, et al. Adequate lymph node assessment for extrahepatic bile duct adenocarcinoma. Ann Surg 2010;251(4):675–81.

78. Hadjis NS, Blenkharn JI, Alexander N, et al. Outcome of radical surgery in hilar cholangiocarcinoma. Surgery 1990;107(6):597–604.

79. Baer HU, Stain SC, Dennison AR, et al. Improvements in survival by aggressive resections of hilar cholangiocarcinoma. Ann Surg 1993;217(1):20–7.

80. Saldinger PF, Blumgart LH. Resection of hilar cholangiocarcinoma – a European and United States experience. J Hepatobiliary Pancreat Surg 2000;7(2):111–4.

81. Cameron JL, Pitt HA, Zinner MJ, et al. Management of proximal cholangiocarcinomas by surgical resection and radiotherapy. Am J Surg 1990;159(1):91–8.

82. Pitt HA, Nakeeb A, Abrams RA, et al. Perihilar cholangiocarcinoma. Postoperative radiotherapy does not improve survival. Ann Surg 1995;221(6):788–98.

83. Kamada T, Saitou H, Takamura A, et al. The role of radiotherapy in the management of extrahepatic bile duct cancer: an analysis of 145 consecutive patients treated with intraluminal and/or external beam radiotherapy. Int J Radiat Oncol Biol Phys 1996;34(4):767–74.

84. McMasters KM, Tuttle TM, Leach SD, et al. Neoadjuvant chemoradiation for extrahepatic cholangiocarcinoma. Am J Surg 1997;174(6):605–9.

85. Takada T, Amano H, Yasuda H, et al. Is postoperative adjuvant chemotherapy useful for gallbladder carcinoma? A phase III multicenter prospective randomized controlled trial in patients with resected pancreaticobiliary carcinoma. Cancer 2002;95(8):1685–95.

86. Kuvshinoff BW, Armstrong JG, Fong Y, et al. Palliation of irresectable hilar cholangiocarcinoma with biliary drainage and radiotherapy. Br J Surg 1995;82(11):1522–5.

87. Liu CL, Lo CM, Lai EC, et al. Endoscopic retrograde cholangiopancreatography and endoscopic endoprosthesis insertion in patients with Klatskin tumors. Arch Surg 1998;133(3):293–6.

88. Becker CD, Glattli A, Maibach R, et al. Percutaneous palliation of malignant obstructive jaundice with the Wallstent endoprosthesis: follow-up and reintervention in patients with hilar and non-hilar obstruction. J Vasc Interv Radiol 1993;4(5):597–604.

89. Cheung KL, Lai EC. Endoscopic stenting for malignant biliary obstruction. Arch Surg 1995;130(2):204–7.

90. Miyazaki M, Ito H, Nakagawa K, et al. Aggressive surgical approaches to hilar cholangiocarcinoma: hepatic or local resection? Surgery 1998;123(2):131–6.

91. Schima E. Surgery of the biliary tract in geriatric patients (author's transl.). Zentralbl Chir 1977;102(14): 858–68.

92. Glattli A, Stain SC, Baer HU, et al. Unresectable malignant biliary obstruction: treatment by self-expandable biliary endoprostheses. HPB Surg 1993;6(3):175–84.

93. Jarnagin WR, Burke E, Powers C, et al. Intrahepatic biliary enteric bypass provides effective palliation in selected patients with malignant obstruction at the hepatic duct confluence. Am J Surg 1998;175(6):453–60.

94. Baer HU, Rhyner M, Stain SC, et al. The effect of communication between the right and left liver on the outcome of surgical drainage for jaundice due to malignant obstruction at the hilus of the liver. HPB Surg 1994;8(1):27–31.

95. Bowling TE, Galbraith SM, Hatfield AR, et al. A retrospective comparison of endoscopic stenting alone with stenting and radiotherapy in non-resectable cholangiocarcinoma. Gut 1996;39(96):852–5.

96. Vallis KA, Benjamin IS, Munro AJ, et al. External beam and intraluminal radiotherapy for locally advanced bile duct cancer: role and tolerability. Radiother Oncol 1996;41(1):61–6.

97. Ortner M. Photodynamic therapy for cholangiocarcinoma. J Hepatobiliary Pancreat Surg 2001;8(2):137–9.

98. Ortner M. Photodynamic therapy in the biliary tract. Curr Gastroenterol Rep 2001;3(2):154–9.

99. Ortner ME, Caca K, Berr F, et al. Successful photodynamic therapy for nonresectable cholangiocarcinoma: a randomized prospective study. Gastroenterology 2003;125(5):1355–63.

100. Zoepf T, Jakobs R, Arnold JC, et al. Palliation of nonresectable bile duct cancer: improved survival after photodynamic therapy. Am J Gastroenterol 2005;100(11):2426–30.

101. Glimelius B, Hoffman K, Sjoden PO, et al. Chemotherapy improves survival and quality of life in advanced pancreatic and biliary cancer. Ann Oncol 1996;7(6):593–600.

102. Daines WP, Rajagopalan V, Grossbard ML, et al. Gallbladder and biliary tract carcinoma: a comprehensive update, Part 2. Oncology (Williston Park) 2004;18(8):1049–59; discussion 1060, 1065–6, 1068.

103. Valle J, Wasan H, Palmer DH, et al. Cisplatin plus gemcitabine versus gemcitabine for biliary tract cancer. N Engl J Med 2010;362(14):1273–81.

104. Fong Y, Blumgart LH, Lin E, et al. Outcome of treatment for distal bile duct cancer. Br J Surg 1996;83(12):1712–5.

105. Wade TP, Prasad CN, Virgo KS, et al. Experience with distal bile duct cancers in U.S. Veterans Affairs hospitals: 1987–1991. J Surg Oncol 1997;64(3):242–5.

106. Yeo CJ, Cameron JL, Sohn TA, et al. Six hundred fifty consecutive pancreaticoduodenectomies in the 1990s: pathology, complications, and outcomes. Ann Surg 1997;226(3):248–60.

107. Way LW. Biliary tract. In: Current surgical diagnosis and treatment. 10th ed. East Norwark, CT: Appleton & Lange; 1994. p.537–66.

108. Georgopoulos SK, Schwartz LH, Jarnagin WR, et al. Comparison of magnetic resonance and endoscopic retrograde cholangiopancreatography in malignant pancreaticobiliary obstruction. Arch Surg 1999;134(9):1002–7.

109. Ryan ME. Cytologic brushings of ductal lesions during ERCP. Gastrointest Endosc 1991;37(2):139–42.

110. Maetani Y, Itoh K, Watanabe C, et al. MR imaging of intrahepatic cholangiocarcinoma with pathologic correlation. Am J Roentgenol 2001;176(6):1499–507.

111. Lim JH. Cholangiocarcinoma: morphologic classification according to growth pattern and imaging findings. Am J Roentgenol 2003;181(3):819–27.

112. Weber SM, Jarnagin WR, Klimstra D, et al. Intrahepatic cholangiocarcinoma: resectability, recurrence pattern, and outcomes. J Am Coll Surg 2001;193(4):384–91.

113. de Jong MC, Nathan H, Sotiropoulos GC, et al. Intrahepatic cholangiocarcinoma: an international multi-institutional analysis of prognostic factors and lymph node assessment. J Clin Oncol 2011;29(23):3140–5.

114. Patel SH, Kooby DA, Staley 3rd CA, et al. The prognostic importance of lymphovascular invasion in cholangiocarcinoma above the cystic duct: a new selection criterion for adjuvant therapy? HPB (Oxford) 2011;13(9):605–11.

115. Schlinkert RT, Nagorney DM, Van Heerden JA, et al. Intrahepatic cholangiocarcinoma: clinical aspects, pathology and treatment. HPB Surg 1992;5(2):95–102.

116. Ringe B, Canelo R, Lorf T. Liver transplantation for primary liver cancer. Transplant Proc 1996;28(3):1174–5.

117. Falkson G, MacIntyre JM, Moertel CG. Eastern Cooperative Oncology Group experience with chemotherapy for inoperable gallbladder and bile duct cancer. Cancer 1984;54(6):965–9.

118. Ibrahim SM, Mulcahy MF, Lewandowski RJ, et al. Treatment of unresectable cholangiocarcinoma using yttrium-90 microspheres: results from a pilot study. Cancer 2008;113(8):2119–28.

119. Jarnagin WR, Schwartz LH, Gultekin DH, et al. Regional chemotherapy for unresectable primary liver cancer: results of a phase II clinical trial and assessment of DCE-MRI as a biomarker of survival. Ann Oncol 2009;20(9):1589–95.

120. Kemeny NE, Schwartz L, Gonen M, et al. Treating primary liver cancer with hepatic arterial infusion of floxuridine and dexamethasone: does the addition of systemic bevacizumab improve results? Oncology 2011;80(3–4):153–9.

121. Lazcano-Ponce EC, Miquel JF, Munoz N, et al. Epidemiology and molecular pathology of gallbladder cancer. CA Cancer J Clin 2001;51(6):349–64.

122. Serra I, Serra I, Diehl AK. Number and size of stones in patients with asymptomatic and symptomatic gallstones and gallbladder carcinoma. J Gastrointest Surg 2002;6(2):272–3; author reply 273.

123. Kozuka S, Tsubone N, Yasui A, et al. Relation of adenoma to carcinoma in the gallbladder. Cancer 1982;50(10):2226–34.

124. Fong Y, Malhotra S. Gallbladder cancer: recent advances and current guidelines for surgical therapy. Adv Surg 2001;35:1–20.

125. Yeh CN, Jan YY, Chao TC, et al. Laparoscopic cholecystectomy for polypoid lesions of the gallbladder: a clinicopathologic study. Surg Laparosc Endosc Percutan Tech 2001;11(3):176–81.

126. Buckles DC, Lindor KD, Larusso NF, et al. In primary sclerosing cholangitis, gallbladder polyps are frequently malignant. Am J Gastroenterol 2002;97(5):1138–42.

127. Yang HL, Sun YG, Wang Z. Polypoid lesions of the gallbladder: diagnosis and indications for surgery. Br J Surg 1992;79(3):227–9.

128. Stephen AE, Berger DL. Carcinoma in the porcelain gallbladder: a relationship revisited. Surgery 2001;129(6):699–703.

129. Kwon AH, Inui H, Matsui Y, et al. Laparoscopic cholecystectomy in patients with porcelain gallbladder based on the preoperative ultrasound findings. Hepatogastroenterology 2004;51(58):950–3.

130. Adson M. Carcinoma of the gallbladder. In: Moody FG, editor. Advances in diagnosis and surgical treatment of biliary tract disease. Chicago: Year Book; 1983.

131. Bartlett DL, Fong Y, Fortner JG, et al. Long-term results after resection for gallbladder cancer. Implications for staging and management. Ann Surg 1996;224(5):639–46.

132. Henson DE, Albores-Saavedra J, Corle D. Carcinoma of the gallbladder. Histologic types, stage of disease, grade, and survival rates. Cancer 1992;70(6):1493–7.

133. Nakamura S, Sakaguchi S, Suzuki S, et al. Aggressive surgery for carcinoma of the gallbladder. Surgery 1989;106(3):467–73.

134. Shirai Y, Yoshida K, Tsukada K, et al. Radical surgery for gallbladder carcinoma. Long-term results. Ann Surg 1992;216(5):565–8.

135. Donohue JH, Nagorney DM, Grant CS, et al. Carcinoma of the gallbladder. Does radical resection improve outcome? Arch Surg 1990;125(2):237–41.

136. Chijiiwa K, Tanaka M. Carcinoma of the gallbladder: an appraisal of surgical resection. Surgery 1994;115(6):751–6.

137. Onoyama H, Yamamoto M, Tseng A, et al. Extended cholecystectomy for carcinoma of the gallbladder. World J Surg 1995;19(5):758–63.

138. Ito H, Ito K, D'Angelica M, et al. Accurate staging for gallbladder cancer: implications for surgical therapy and pathological assessment. Ann Surg 2011;254(2):320–5.

139. Fong Y, Jarnagin W, Blumgart LH. Gallbladder cancer: comparison of patients presenting initially for definitive operation with those presenting after prior noncurative intervention. Ann Surg 2000;232(4):557–69.

140. Shirai Y, Yoshida K, Tsukada K, et al. Inapparent carcinoma of the gallbladder. An appraisal of a radical second operation after simple cholecystectomy. Ann Surg 1992;215(4):326–31.

141. Yamaguchi K, Tsuneyoshi M. Subclinical gallbladder carcinoma. Am J Surg 1992;163(4):382–6.

142. Kimura W, Shimada H. A case of gallbladder carcinoma with infiltration into the muscular layer that resulted in relapse and death from metastasis to the liver and lymph nodes. Hepatogastroenterology 1990;37(1):86–9.

143. De Aretxabala XA, Roa IS, Burgos LA, et al. Curative resection in potentially resectable tumours of the gallbladder. Eur J Surg 1997;163(6):419–26.

144. Callery MP, Strasberg SM, Doherty GM, et al. Staging laparoscopy with laparoscopic ultrasonography: optimizing resectability in hepatobiliary and pancreatic malignancy. J Am Coll Surg 1997;185(1):33–9.

145. Shoup M, Fong Y. Surgical indications and extent of resection in gallbladder cancer. Surg Oncol Clin North Am 2002;11(4):985–94.

146. Jarnagin WR, Ruo L, Little SA, et al. Patterns of initial disease recurrence after resection of gallbladder carcinoma and hilar cholangiocarcinoma: implications for adjuvant therapeutic strategies. Cancer 2003;98(8):1689–700.

147. Kresl JJ, Schild SE, Henning GT, et al. Adjuvant external beam radiation therapy with concurrent chemotherapy in the management of gallbladder carcinoma. Int J Radiat Oncol Biol Phys 2002;52(1):167–75.

148. Mahe M, Stampfli C, Romestaing P, et al. Primary carcinoma of the gall-bladder: potential for external radiation therapy. Radiother Oncol 1994;33(3):204–8.

149. Kapoor VK, Pradeep R, Haribhakti SP, et al. Intrahepatic segment III cholangiojejunostomy in advanced carcinoma of the gallbladder. Br J Surg 1996;83(12):1709–11.

13

Acute pancreatitis

Colin J. McKay
Euan J. Dickson
C. Ross Carter

General description

Acute pancreatitis is a common cause for emergency hospital admission, with approximately 40 cases per year for each 100 000 population in Scotland,[1] Norway[2] and Sweden.[3] There has been a steady increase in the incidence and a slight reduction in case mortality, although not population mortality, over the past 45 years.[4] In approximately 80% of patients, acute pancreatitis is a rapidly-resolving condition requiring little more than analgesia and a short period of intravenous fluid resuscitation, with the remainder developing a multisystem illness characterised by a systemic inflammatory response with a variable degree of organ dysfunction.

Pathophysiology

The mechanism by which gallstones trigger an attack of acute pancreatitis has not been clearly defined. The bile reflux theory, proposed by Opie in 1901, suggested that obstruction of the common bile duct/pancreatic duct common channel by a gallstone caused reflux of bile into the pancreatic duct resulting in acute pancreatitis. While there is no doubt that passage of and at least transient obstruction by a gallstone is the initial step in biliary acute pancreatitis, there is little evidence that bile reflux is involved.

Experimental models have shed some light on the mechanism by which pancreatic duct obstruction induces acute pancreatitis. Changes in the pattern of enzyme secretion within pancreatic acinar cells, coupled with intracellular zymogen activation, are considered the important early events in the development of acute pancreatitis. Disruption of the paracellular barrier allows release of pancreatic enzymes into the paracellular space. Inflammatory cells and inflammatory mediators may further exacerbate the acinar cell injury.[4] Research has shown that many of these early events can be triggered by an increase in intracellular calcium.[5]

The mechanism of alcohol-induced acute pancreatitis is less clear, but alcohol has been shown to increase the sensitivity of acinar cells to cholecystokinin hyperstimulation, resulting in enhanced intracellular protease activation.[6] Alcohol also influences acinar cell calcium homeostasis, but several alternative theories have been proposed.

Natural history

Acute pancreatitis varies from a mild, self-limiting attack to a severe life-threatening illness and, for this reason, patients are often classified as having either mild or severe acute pancreatitis (see Box 13.1). This rather simplistic description ignores the wide variety of clinical behaviour that can be observed in these patients but helps to focus attention on the subgroup of patients who develop complications. Currently, the internationally accepted classification of acute pancreatitis and its

Box 13.1 • Definitions

Acute pancreatitis

Acute pancreatitis is an acute inflammatory process of the pancreas, with variable involvement of other regional tissues or remote organ systems.

Mild acute pancreatitis

Mild acute pancreatitis is associated with minimal organ dysfunction and an uneventful recovery. The predominant feature is interstitial oedema of the gland.

Severe acute pancreatitis

Severe acute pancreatitis is associated with organ failure and/or local complication such as necrosis (with infection), pseudocyst or abscess. Most often this is an expression of the development of pancreatic necrosis, although patients with oedematous pancreatitis may manifest clinical features of a severe attack.

Systemic inflammatory response syndrome

Response to a variety of severe clinical insults, manifested by two or more of the following conditions:

- Temperature >38 or <360 °C
- Heart rate >90 beats/min
- Respiratory rate >20/min or $PaCO_2$ <32 mmHg (<4.3 kPa)
- White blood cell count (WBC) >12 000 cells/mm³, <4000 cells/mm³ or >10% immature (band) forms

Multiple organ dysfunction syndrome

Presence of altered organ function in an acutely ill patient such that homeostasis cannot be maintained without intervention.

An **acute pseudocyst** is a collection of pancreatic juice enclosed in a wall of fibrous or granulation tissue that arises following an attack of acute pancreatitis. Formation of a pseudocyst requires 4 or more weeks from the onset of acute pancreatitis.

A **pancreatic abscess** is a circumscribed intra-abdominal collection of pus, usually in proximity to the pancreas, containing little or no pancreatic necrosis, which arises as a consequence of acute pancreatitis.

complications is set out in the paper arising from the Atlanta Conference.[7] Improved understanding of treatment concepts and the dynamic nature of the pathophysiology has rendered a number of the concepts outlined in the Atlanta Conference outdated and a revision has recently been published.[8]

Within this framework different patterns of disease have emerged. Multicentre trials in acute pancreatitis have enabled prospective study of severe acute pancreatitis and several important points have emerged. Firstly, the majority of patients who develop severe acute pancreatitis have evidence of early systemic organ dysfunction.[9] It is exceptional for a patient to have no evidence of organ failure in the first week of illness and to subsequently develop a significant late local complication. Secondly, most patients who develop organ failure have evidence of this at the time of admission or very shortly thereafter.[10] Thirdly, while the tendency is for early organ dysfunction to recover without further problems, worsening organ failure is associated with a high mortality.[9,11,12]

These observations have important implications for patient management. The presence of early organ dysfunction identifies a high-risk group of patients who merit close observation for both early and late clinical complications. In particular, deteriorating organ failure carries a high mortality and should prompt early involvement of the intensive care team and consideration of transfer to a specialist unit if possible. The fact that organ dysfunction is present at, or shortly after, admission in the majority of patients in whom it develops means that efforts should be directed at early recognition of this rather than employing prediction systems of disease severity.

The majority of patients with severe early organ dysfunction will have pancreatic necrosis on computed tomography (CT) scan. A significant proportion (30–40%) of patients with pancreatic necrosis will develop secondary pancreatic infection, usually in the second to third week after admission,[13] which may be associated with a deterioration in organ failure. Patients who have infected pancreatic necrosis complicated by multiple organ failure represent a formidable management challenge.

Diagnosis

In the majority of patients the diagnosis of acute pancreatitis is relatively easy, characterised by a clinical presentation of sudden severe epigastric pain radiating through to the back. Vomiting within the first 24 hours is very frequently severe and contributes to dehydration. Other signs and symptoms such as tachycardia, tachypnoea and circulatory collapse are dependent on the severity of the attack. A raised serum amylase (at least three times the upper limit of normal) supports the diagnosis in >95% of cases. Serum amylase estimation may be inaccurate in association with hyperlipidaemia, where a raised urinary amylase can be diagnostic. Serum lipase may be marginally more accurate but is not commonly available in routine clinical practice. CT can confirm the diagnosis where doubt exists, or in patients with delayed presentation, and it should therefore be very uncommon for the diagnosis to be made at laparotomy (**Fig. 13.1**).

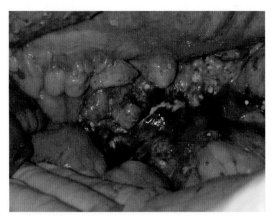

Figure 13.1 • Extensive fat necrosis in the infracolic compartment in a patient with severe acute pancreatitis.

Aetiology

Obstructive factors

Biliary disease

The mechanism by which the migration of gallstones results in acute pancreatitis is not fully understood but involves the mechanisms outlined above. Transient hold-up or impaction in the ampullary area is associated with between 35% and 65% of episodes of acute pancreatitis in most prospective studies.

Benign pancreatic duct stricture

Secondary fibrosis affecting the pancreatic duct can result in recurrent attacks of pancreatitis. Congenital or developmental anatomical abnormalities can occasionally present with pancreatitis (choledochal cyst, duodenal duplication, anomalous pancreaticobiliary junction). The role of pancreas divisum is probably overstated unless associated with ductal obstruction.

Tumours of the ampulla or pancreas

These can result in ductal obstruction and acute pancreatitis, and should be considered in an older patient where no other cause is identified, particularly if there is an antecedent history of weight loss. A dilated distal pancreatic duct may be the only sign of underlying malignancy on CT and should prompt further investigation, such as endoscopic ultrasound.

Toxic factors

Alcohol is the second most common aetiology and may predominate in certain populations. It is most commonly seen in men drinking in excess of 80 g alcohol per day, but unlike alcoholic liver disease there is no clear dose-dependent increase in risk, and it is likely that other genetic and environmental cofactors are important.

Viral infection, particularly mumps, coxsackie B and viral hepatitis, can cause acute pancreatitis. One clinical feature that may prove useful is prodromal diarrhoea, which is rare in all other types of acute pancreatitis.

Metabolic factors

Hyperparathyroidism may be associated with pancreatitis but is extremely rare (0.1%). Patients with hyperlipoproteinaemia (types I and V) may develop acute pancreatitis, but hyperlipidaemia is more commonly a secondary phenomenon seen during an acute attack.

Genetic defects

Genetic familial defects of the cationic trypsinogen gene[14] (N29I, RII7H) and the cystic fibrosis gene (CTFR) may be associated with recurrent pancreatitis, but severe acute inflammatory changes are uncommon.

Trauma

Hyperamylasaemia may occur after blunt abdominal trauma, usually from a crush injury to the body of the pancreas against the vertebral column, and is suggestive of pancreatic injury. Investigation is by contrast-enhanced CT to determine the extent of pancreatic and associated visceral injury.

Iatrogenic causes

Hyperamylasaemia may follow surgical or endoscopic procedures on the pancreas, and is usually self-limiting. The risk increases following a therapeutic endoscopic retrograde cholangiopancreatography (ERCP; 3%), especially when a sphincterotomy has been performed. Where a patient has significant symptoms or clinical signs, the possibility of iatrogenic duodenal perforation should be considered and where necessary excluded by CT.

Drug-induced acute pancreatitis may occur following ingestion of a number of drugs;[15] those most commonly implicated are valproic acid, azathioprine, L-asparaginase and corticosteroids. However, unless gallstone disease has been excluded with confidence it is unwise to ascribe acute pancreatitis to a particular drug. Repeat exposure to the same drug again causing acute pancreatitis is the strongest evidence of a direct association.

Inflammatory

Autoimmune pancreatitis is a rare condition, considered part of the IgG4-related autoimmune disease spectrum.[16] This presents as abdominal pain associated with homogeneous gland enlargement with a well-defined edge on CT, an increased IgG4/IgG ratio and a periductal lymphoplasmocytic infiltrate on biopsy. This may also be associated with abnormalities in the extrahepatic biliary tree resembling sclerosis cholangitis and a response to steroids is diagnostic. Focal autoimmune pancreatitis may prove difficult to differentiate from carcinoma. There are established associations with other autoimmune diseases (polyarteritis nodosa, systemic lupus erythematosus, vasculitis) and inflammatory bowel disease (Crohn's and ulcerative colitis), and many are now considered part of the autoimmune spectrum, although only a small proportion appear to have an association with IgG4 serum or tissue abnormalities.

Physiological

Sphincter manometric abnormalities

Type 1 pancreatic sphincter dysfunction[17] may be associated with hyperamylasaemia and abnormalities on sphincter manometry, as part of a global gut dysmotility spectrum. Managament of sphincter spasm may only partly resolve the patient's symptoms. Conventional treatment involves endoscopic sphincterotomy, but the risk of post-ERCP pancreatitis in these patients is high (30%).

Assessment of severity

The dynamic nature of organ dysfunction in patients presenting with acute pancreatitis has been well described,[9] and for over 30 years authors have explored ways of 'predicting' those patients with more severe disease. Overall mortality, whether early or late, is also associated with the development and persistence of organ failure.[18] This was indirectly shown, if not recognised, 25 years previously with the development of the predictive multifactorial scoring systems – Ranson,[19] Glasgow[20] and APACHE II[21] – which, rather than predicting the subsequent development of organ failure, more accurately identified established multisystem organ dysfunction. Their principal use is to remind the inexperienced of the multisystem nature of the disease process, or as a method of stratifying patients within a study protocol. Of the multiple factor scoring systems, APACHE II provides the best prediction of

mortality but the mainstay of assessment remains repeated, careful clinical observation.[22]

Single biochemical measures

Many studies have attempted to find a single biochemical or clinical marker that would allow adequate prediction of severity without the need for cumbersome scoring systems. In addition, the need for an objective marker of severity at the point of hospital admission is well recognised and would greatly facilitate the entry of patients with severe acute pancreatitis into clinical studies.

C-reactive protein (CRP)

The most widely studied single predictive marker is serum CRP. The major advantage of CRP is its routine availability in clinical practice. Patients with clinically severe pancreatitis usually have a CRP >200 mg/L, with a practical cut-off being 150 mg/L, but its serum peak is not reached for 36–48 h. The positive predictive value of CRP is similar to that of APACHE II[22] but its major use is in monitoring the clinical course during the acute and recovery phase.

Other single predictive markers

Peak levels of interleukin-6 (IL-6) occur within 24 h and this has aroused interest in its use as a predictor of outcome. IL-6 is a pro-inflammatory cytokine induced by stimuli such as tumour necrosis factor (TNF) and interleukin-1 (IL-1). Other single predictive markers that have been studied include trypsinogen activation peptide (TAP), leucocyte polymorph neutrophil (PMN) elastase, TNF and serum procalcitonin. Procalcitonin is the precursor of the hormone calcitonin and is raised in the presence of an inflammatory response, particularly where this is bacterial in origin. Serum procalcitonin is a promising marker of both severe acute pancreatitis and of infected pancreatic necrosis in the later phase.[22,23]

Intra-abdominal hypertension (IAH)

IAH is recognised as a contributing factor to organ dysfunction in the context of a variety of acute abdominal processes. Most of the literature to date focuses on trauma patients, but there is increasing interest in its role in patients with severe acute pancreatitis (SAP). There are data to suggest that raised intra-abdominal pressure (IAP) may be associated with disease severity,[24] organ failure and mortality in SAP.[25] There are, however, no data to suggest improved outcome following surgical decompression for raised IAP in acute pancreatitis, and indeed this may be harmful. At present the monitoring of IAP cannot be recommended outside of a clinical trial.

Repeated clinical assessment

In the absence of clinically useful predictive systems, our own practice is to monitor patients for the development of systemic organ dysfunction by repeated clinical and biochemical assessment. The presence of a systemic inflammatory response syndrome (SIRS; defined as two or more of the following: fever, tachycardia, tachypnoea or leucocytosis) identifies patients at risk of multiple organ dysfunction syndrome (MODS), particularly when three or four SIRS criteria are present or when SIRS persists for 48 h or more after admission. Patients without SIRS at admission are at very low risk. The development of systemic organ dysfunction (usually clinically manifest as hypoxaemia) mandates careful monitoring in a high-dependency or intensive care unit environment.

Imaging

Role of ultrasound (US)

> ✅ All patients with acute pancreatitis should have an ultrasonic assessment of the biliary tree within 24 h of admission.[26]

All patients with acute pancreatitis should have an ultrasonic assessment of the biliary tree within 24 h of admission.[26] In those with gallstones, the majority will have mild disease, and this will facilitate definitive treatment of cholelithiasis prior to discharge. In the emergency situation, ultrasonography can be difficult due to a number of factors, including the presence of intraluminal bowel gas or lack of patient cooperation. Therefore, in patients with a negative initial US, and no other obvious aetiological factor, the US should be repeated prior to discharge before excluding gallstones as a potential aetiological factor.

Role of CT

The main role of CT in the early phase of acute pancreatitis is to clarify the diagnosis in cases where there is diagnostic uncertainty. In patients with severe acute pancreatitis, particularly when complicated by MODS, early CT helps to exclude other pathology such as intestinal perforation, gut ischaemia or dissecting aortic aneurysm. Dynamic contrast-enhanced CT can also be used to assess disease severity (**Fig. 13.2**) and predict the potential for complications.[27] Although not widely used for this purpose clinically in the UK, it is routinely used in many other countries, and can be useful for stratification of patients in clinical trials. The CT Severity Index (CTSI)[27] combines a score for the radiological pancreatic and peripancreatic abnormalities with a weighting for the extent of necrosis. More recently there are reports of perfusion CT, which may be a useful modality for detecting early, subclinical ischaemic changes in the pancreas that then lead to pancreatic necrosis.

Role of magnetic resonance (MR)/magnetic resonance cholangiopancreatography (MRCP)

Magnetic resonance imaging (MRI) offers a realistic alternative to contrast-enhanced CT[28] in the assessment of patients with acute pancreatitis. The avoidance of cumulative radiation exposure, potentially

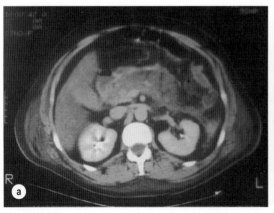 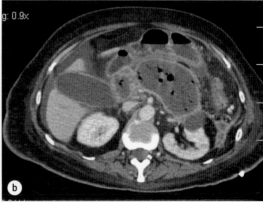

Figure 13.2 • CT scan showing acute pancreatitis with necrosis **(a)** and retroperitoneal gas **(b)**.

nephrotoxic iodinated contrast media, and the excellent contrast sensitivity and spatial resolution would make it an attractive alternative. Axial T1- and T2-weighted scans produce images analogous to those of CT. Gadolinium contrast enhancement can infer viability and improve anatomical definition. Heavily T2-weighted image acquisition, using a single breath hold and long repetition (TR) and echo (TE) times, results in little signal being produced by solid tissue, and a high signal from static fluid in the biliary and pancreatic ducts, enabling images anatomically comparable to those of ERCP to be produced.

Whilst technically feasible in most centres, the MR environment is unsuitable for patients requiring significant circulatory or respiratory support, and at present few centres have the capability to perform MR-guided intervention. Contrast-enhanced CT therefore remains the imaging modality of choice for assessment and intervention in severe acute pancreatitis. However, MR has a role in the follow-up of acute inflammatory collections, where it is superior to CT in determining the extent of solid material within a collection (**Fig. 13.3**), and in excluding choledocholithiasis in selected patients.

Endoscopic ultrasound (EUS)

EUS has rapidly emerged as an important tool in diagnostic and therapeutic algorithms for patients with acute pancreatitis. Its main areas of use are in the diagnosis of microlithiasis in patients with idiopathic pancreatitis and for linear EUS-guided drainage of peripancreatic collections, as discussed in the relevant sections below.

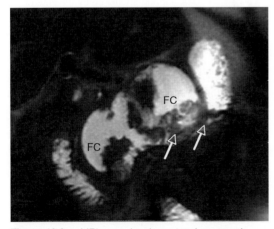

Figure 13.3 • MRI scan showing extensive necrosis (arrowed) within a post-acute fluid collection (FC).

Management

Initial management

Management of acute pancreatitis in the UK is still based on two key guideline documents, now 7[26] and 10[29] years old, respectively. The initial management of patients presenting with acute pancreatitis should be directed at the early identification and management of organ failure, most frequently renal and respiratory dysfunction.

> ✅ The initial management of patients presenting with acute pancreatitis should be directed at the early identification and management of organ failure, most frequently renal and respiratory dysfunction.

At present there are no established end-points of resuscitation to confirm that tissue perfusion and oxygen delivery have been restored adequately in patients with acute pancreatitis. Aggressive fluid resuscitation is often required, and monitoring the response to this relies upon traditional markers, in particular urine output, blood pressure and pulse oximetry. Physiological markers of resuscitation, for example acid–base balance from an arterial blood gas, may be helpful in detecting clinically occult hypoperfusion. Patients who do not respond to initial resuscitation, or who have evidence of organ dysfunction, should be transferred to a critical care environment for more invasive and intensive monitoring with central venous and arterial catheters. Respiratory failure should be treated with humidified oxygen, and this will be guided by continuous pulse oximetry and arterial blood gas analysis. Deteriorating respiratory function is a sign of disease progression. As many as half of all deaths from acute pancreatitis occur in less than 7 days, and the majority of these occur within 72 h of admission.[1] There is evidence that patients managed in specialist institutions have a reduced risk of early death and this may be an indication that management of early MODS could be improved.

Supportive management

> ✅ All patients with severe pancreatitis should be managed within a high-dependency/intensive care environment with the potential for organ support.[26]

Where possible, patients with severe acute pancreatitis should be managed by a designated multidisciplinary team who have an interest in pancreaticobiliary pathology. Facilities should be available for patients to undergo ERCP/sphincterotomy when indicated (see below). Management of these patients is complex and should be discussed with a specialist unit at an early stage. Specific measures will be determined by the clinical situation. However, therapeutic interventions are aimed at restoring tissue perfusion as rapidly as possible. This is achieved initially with volume resuscitation titrated to haemodynamic and physiological response, rather than the early use of vasopressors or inotropes in patients who are still intravascularly deplete. Acute dialysis for acidosis has not been shown to improve outcome but is required for established renal failure. Currently there is no specific therapy to reverse respiratory failure other than ventilatory support.

Specific medical management

There have been many attempts to introduce specific medical treatments for acute pancreatitis and these broadly fall into the following categories.

Prevention of infection

In patients who survive the early, systemic complications of acute pancreatitis, secondary infection of pancreatic necrosis is the most important late complication. Infection occurs in 30–40% of patients with a minimum 30% pancreatic necrosis[13] and is responsible for the majority of late deaths from acute pancreatitis. Secondary infection manifests as escalating sepsis or a deterioration in organ failure scores, usually in the second (36%) and third (71%) weeks of the illness.[30]

The role of prophylactic antibiotics to prevent secondary infection has been widely studied. The most recent Cochrane review[31] found no evidence of a significant reduction in mortality with antibiotic prophylaxis and no difference in the incidence of infected pancreatic necrosis. Even non-pancreatic infections showed no significant difference with antibiotic therapy. It was noted, however, that all of the studies were underpowered and a definitive answer to this question will require better quality clinical trials. The most recent meta-analysis of 14 trials including 841 patients also found no evidence of benefit with antibiotic prophylaxis.[32]

✅✅ Prophylactic antibiotics should not be used in the management of acute pancreatitis.[31,32]

Nutritional support

There are two main, and very separate, considerations in determining the mode of nutritional support. Severe acute pancreatitis is often a prolonged and profoundly catabolic illness, and there is no doubt that, throughout the illness, nutritional integrity should be maintained – the question in these patients is not whether nutritional support is necessary, but rather how it can be best administered.

The second consideration relates to the potential of modulating the disease process by the mode of delivery, either through maintenance of host defences or through the use of immunomodulating feeds. The first issue is a practical problem faced by clinicians on a daily basis, the second remains somewhat speculative, with interesting but inconclusive evidence so far. These will be dealt with separately.

Nutritional delivery in the patient with acute pancreatitis

The key study in this regard was the randomised study of Kalfarentzos et al. in 1996, who randomised 38 patients with severe acute pancreatitis to total parenteral nutrition (TPN) or nasojejunal feeding.[33] The most recent Cochrane review, including eight randomised trials, demonstrated a reduction in mortality, systemic complications and surgical intervention in patients given enteral nutrition.[34]

Most experience to date has been with enteral feeding distal to the duodenojejunal flexure. More recently, four randomised studies have shown nasogastric feeding to be a practical alternative to jejunal feeding.[35] All studies in this area are underpowered and it is therefore difficult to recommend this feeding route in routine clinical practice.

It is important to recognise that there are situations where parenteral nutrition must be considered, such as where complex fistulas develop, and sometimes a combination of enteral and parenteral routes is required. Combined feeding is most commonly required when enteral feed is not adequately absorbed, leading to intractable diarrhoea and fluid losses.

✅✅ Nutritional support should be by the enteral route where possible.[34]

Disease modulation through content or mode of delivery

There has been interest in the role of the intestine in the pathophysiology of multiple organ failure in critical illness, with loss of gut barrier function potentially leading to endotoxaemia and the systemic inflammatory response syndrome (SIRS). In a small study from Leeds,[36] the authors reported a reduction in the inflammatory response and organ failure in those receiving enteral support, but unfortunately there were only 13 patients with severe disease, limiting the validity of the conclusions. There have been several trials comparing so-called 'immunonutrition' with standard enteral feeding in critically ill patients, but so far no evidence of benefit has been demonstrated in acute pancreatitis.[37] Similarly, there has been interest in the role of 'probiotics', but a randomised trial from the Netherlands found an increase in fatal complications in the probiotic group, with an unexpectedly high incidence of intestinal necrosis.[38]

Other medical therapies

Inhibition of pancreatic secretion

Pharmacological attempts to suppress pancreatic function have included intravenous glucagon, somatostatin and, more recently, the somatostatin analogue octreotide. On the basis of the available literature there is no justification for the use of octreotide or any other pharmacological inhibitor of pancreatic secretion in acute pancreatitis.

Inhibition of pancreatic enzymes

Many studies have evaluated the concept of supporting the endogenous antiprotease defence mechanisms. Randomised trials of intravenous aprotinin (Trasylol), gabexatemesilate, intraperitoneal aprotinin, and both low- and high-dose fresh frozen plasma (FFP) have shown no therapeutic benefit.

Inhibition of the inflammatory response

Following initial promising results with the platelet-activating factor antagonist, lexipafant, a multicentre, randomised, placebo-controlled study of anticytokine therapy recruited 1518 patients. This study recruited only those patients with symptoms of less than 48 h duration and was restricted to those with predicted severe attacks. Not only was there no difference in mortality between groups, the incidence of local complications, length of ICU stay, hospital stay and change in organ failure scores were all similar in the three study groups.

The potential for other agents that modify the inflammatory response to influence outcome in acute pancreatitis has only been assessed in experimental models.

Role of ERCP

There have now been three published randomised trials addressing this issue, and four smaller studies. Contradicting an earlier Cochrane review,[39] the most recent meta-analysis[40] has shown early ERCP in patients with either predicted mild or severe acute biliary pancreatitis without acute cholangitis did not lead to a significant reduction in the risk of overall complications and mortality. There is no role for urgent ERCP in patients with mild disease. All patients with jaundice who exhibit signs of sepsis should undergo urgent ERCP and sphincterotomy as cholangitis may coexist with acute pancreatitis and hyperamylasaemia, but there appears to be little role for early ERCP outside this scenario.

☑☑ In the non-jaundiced patient there is no role for urgent ERCP and sphincterotomy.[40]

Definitive management issues

The definitive management issues may be considered as, firstly, those designed to prevent further attacks once a mild attack has subsided, and secondly those specifically related to the management of early and late complications.

Prevention of recurrent acute pancreatitis

Management of gallstones

The timing of cholecystectomy will obviously depend on the clinical situation. In patients recovering from mild acute biliary pancreatitis, definitive management of the gallstones to prevent a further attack should ideally be achieved during the same admission, and certainly no later than 4 weeks following discharge from hospital.[26] This will normally involve a cholecystectomy (laparoscopic or open) with intraoperative cholangiography, or alternatively duct imaging by MRCP (or EUS) followed by cholecystectomy. Elderly patients or those with significant medical comorbidity may be managed by an endoscopic sphincterotomy, although this may not be as effective as definitive surgery in preventing further attacks.

In severe acute pancreatitis, interval cholecystectomy should be performed when the inflammatory process has subsided and the procedure is potentially easier.[29]

☑ Definitive management of cholelithiasis in uncomplicated acute pancreatitis should be achieved within 4 weeks of discharge from hospital.

Investigation of non-gallstone-associated pancreatitis

Following resolution of an attack of acute pancreatitis, an assessment of potential aetiological factors is an important aspect of care, and a diagnosis of idiopathic pancreatitis should be made in less than 20% of patients.[26] Evaluation of the initial acute attack should include an adequate history (alcohol/drugs/familial), biochemical tests (liver function tests/lipids (hypertriglyceridaemia)/calcium) and biliary ultrasound. If these investigations are normal, axial imaging (CT or MR/MRCP) may be appropriate to exclude a mechanical cause. Patients in whom no cause is identified following these investigations should be considered for EUS, as a cause will be identified in the majority of cases.[41] A cholecystectomy or biliary sphincterotomy is justified in patients with recurrent idiopathic pancreatitis in whom microlithiasis or biliary sludge is identified. With the increasing use of EUS in these patients, it is increasingly recognised that many of these patients will have changes consistent with early chronic pancreatitis,[41] rather than biliary microlithiasis as suggested by earlier studies. The prevalence of microlithiasis appears to be higher in regions where gallstone disease is the predominant aetiology.

Peripancreatic fluid collections

Management of an early fluid collection

In the early stages of acute pancreatitis, up to 25% of patients with acute pancreatitis will develop a fluid collection in the peripancreatic area identifiable on CT. In themselves, these collections are of little significance and require no intervention. There are significant risks associated with aspiration and especially external drainage, in particular the development of secondary infection, fistula and recurrence, and they therefore cannot be recommended.

> ✓ Aspiration or drainage of sterile acute fluid collections should be discouraged.

Management of a pseudocyst

Management of pseudocysts is determined by an understanding of the anatomy (based on CT), the degree of necrosis (MR/EUS) and the clinical condition of the patient. As a general rule, definitive management should be delayed until all organ dysfunction has resolved and can often be performed simultaneously with management of cholelithiasis (see above).

In our experience, it is helpful to characterise pseudocysts associated with acute pancreatitis as either fluid predominant or necrosis predominant.

In each case the collection may be sterile or infected and associated with varying degrees of systemic disturbance. The size of the collection and its relationship to adjacent structures, in particular the stomach, are also important factors when considering treatment options.

Asymptomatic pseudocysts do not require treatment, and many will eventually resolve spontaneously. Acute pseudocysts are most commonly retrogastric, and may or may not link to a disrupted pancreatic duct. Three-quarters will be associated with a mild to moderate hyperamylasaemia. In symptomatic cysts, a conservative policy may be

warranted for up to 12 weeks from the onset of acute pancreatitis. This policy is not, however, without risk as pseudocyst rupture, bleeding or abscess formation may occur. The likelihood of resolution is related, at least in part, to pseudocyst size. Should conservative treatment fail, the options are percutaneous, endoscopic or surgical drainage.

Percutaneous drainage

Results of percutaneous drainage suggest wide variation in success (40–96%)[42] and the introduction of infection is a risk that must be considered. In practical terms, the risk of pancreatic fistula limits this approach and there is evidence that it can make subsequent surgical intervention more hazardous if this becomes necessary.[43] In our practice we restrict the use of percutaneous drainage to occasional patients with infected, fluid-predominant collections, particularly where there is a degree of systemic organ dysfunction. Increasingly, however, endoscopic or laparoscopic drainage is employed.

Endoscopic drainage

The technique of endoscopic cystgastrostomy as first described by Baron et al.,[44] initially by blind puncture of a cyst bulging into the stomach wall using a side-viewing endoscope, has been subsequently refined using endoscopic ultrasound guidance. EUS guidance enables drainage of cysts where no intraluminal bulge is present and also helps avoid intervening vessels. Further procedures may be required to facilitate drainage, particularly where cysts are large or where there is much necrotic debris, but we have not found it necessary to pursue active endoscopic necrosectomy in this group of patients. Where disruption of the pancreatic duct has occurred, transpapillary duct stenting can aid resolution. Baron and colleagues have recently updated their experience in 104 patients with walled-off pancreatic necrosis with successful resolution in 95 patients (91%). The mean time to intervention was 63 days and mean duration of treatment was 4.1 months. The complication rate, mainly haemorrhage and perforation, was 14%.[45]

Surgical drainage of an acute post-inflammatory collection

Surgery may be considered as a primary mode of intervention in selected patients, particularly for patients with large, necrosis-predominant collections without infection or systemic organ dysfunction. This can be readily achieved by a laparoscopic transgastric procedure, or a direct cyst-enterostomy, and allows simultaneous laparoscopic cholecystectomy where appropriate. In those patients in whom endoscopic drainage fails to achieve complete resolution, or a cyst recurs, simple surgical drainage is rarely an option as this often results from separation of the head/body and tail of the pancreas due to prior necrosis of the central pancreas – termed a 'disconnected tail'. These patients often require a challenging distal pancreatico-splenectomy.

Symptomatic or persistent pseudocysts following acute pancreatitis should be managed in a specialist unit where the full range of interventional procedures is available.

✔ Failure of percutaneous or endoscopic management is associated with the need for complex surgery and should therefore only be undertaken by or following consultation with a pancreatic specialist.[43]

Management of a pancreatic duct fistula

This complication most commonly follows prior intervention for an acute post-inflammatory collection or infected necrosis, and manifests as persistent drainage of amylase-rich opalescent fluid, in the absence of significant sepsis. Management is similar to that of a communicating pseudocyst, initially by transpapillary stenting where possible. Intraperitoneal rupture of a pseudocyst can result in pancreatic ascites or pleural effusion. More invasive management of a persistent fistula, either inaccessible or failing to respond to ductal stenting, should be delayed by percutaneous or endoscopic control, until the patient has made a full recovery, and again often requires surgical resection (distal pancreatico-splenectomy).

Management of necrosis

The management algorithm surrounding necrotising pancreatitis has altered radically in the last 15 years in response to evolving concepts, improved understanding and the development of minimally invasive techniques, including percutaneous necrosectomy and laparoscopic or EUS-guided cystgastrostomy, as an alternative to conventional open debridement. A multidisciplinary approach has evolved, and it is now common for several techniques to be utilised in an individual patient, as the indications and clinical condition of the patient alter during the course of the disease process.

The development of secondary septic complications is the usual initiator demanding invasive treatment. The choice of intervention technique is underpinned by an understanding of the dynamic evolution of post-acute, necrosis-associated collections in pancreatitis. The previously held concept that recovery would not occur until almost complete removal of necrosis had been achieved has been progressively challenged and the focus of intervention is now on

the 'adequate and maintained control of sepsis'. The success of various approaches will be dependent on the anatomical position and particularly the ratio of solid to fluid components within the collection.

The process of maturation or 'organisation', with separation and partial liquefaction of the solid components within a collection, takes in excess of 12 weeks to complete, during which four stages can be recognised:

1. True pancreatic necrosis – minimal separation of devitalised tissue with a high solid/fluid ratio.
2. Transitional pancreatic necrosis with partial but incomplete separation.
3. Organised pancreatic necrosis (OPN) – good separation of devitalised tissue within a fluid-filled cavity and formation of a fibrous wall lined with granulation tissue.
4. Pseudocyst – almost complete resolution of any solid component and a well-formed fibrous wall lined with granulation tissue.

The necrotic process associated with pancreatitis tends to involve both the pancreatic parenchyma and surrounding adipose tissue. Indeed, significant quantities of necrotic peripancreatic tissue can be present with an essentially viable gland. Complications relate to the extent of the necrotic process, and in particular the extent of parenchymal necrosis. Early aggressive debridement in the absence of infection has been advocated. However, mortality in this series was 25% overall, and the only randomised study of early versus late (> 12 days) necrosectomy was discontinued as a result of the mortality rate in the early treatment group (56% vs. 27%).[46] The general principle is now to withhold surgery in the early phase of disease, operating for complications ideally once the acute inflammatory insult has subsided.

✔✔ There is no role for early surgical intervention other than for the management of complications.

Management of sterile necrosis

The development of retroperitoneal necrosis secondary to acute pancreatitis is not in itself an indication for intervention. Pancreatic necrosis, where sterile, can usually be adequately treated by conservative means.[47] There remains debate regarding the role of debridement in patients failing to respond to conservative treatment. Early debridement does not improve outcome; however, some specialists advocate debridement in patients with continuing organ dysfunction after several weeks, but this may also be detrimental.[48] The majority of sterile post-inflammatory fluid collections progress into organised pancreatic necrosis, which can be managed with low morbidity and mortality, and our policy is to delay intervention where possible. The management of these patients is discussed in the section dealing with fluid collections associated with necrosis.

> ✔ Sterile necrosis should initially be treated conservatively where possible, allowing delayed definitive treatment.

Management of infected necrosis (early phase, 2–6 weeks)

Infected pancreatic necrosis has previously been described as the most feared surgical complication of acute pancreatitis. This led to the development of protocol-driven management in the 1990s, aimed at the early identification of secondary infection within necrosis. The presence of a persistent SIRS response made clinical differentiation between SIRS and sepsis difficult and this led to CT- or US-guided fine-needle aspiration (FNA) of the pancreatic or peripancreatic collections as a diagnostic test. FNA was considered the cornerstone of management as it was thought infected necrosis mandated radical surgical intervention.[49,50]

Our own approach has progressed from one based on the presence or absence of infection to one based on organ dysfunction. Infected collections, even those containing gas, may be observed when the patient is clinically well and recovering with conservative treatment. Patients with profound organ dysfunction in whom we suspect secondary infection, with a drainable peripancreatic collection, will undergo percutaneous drainage aimed at sepsis control, with later staged percutaneous or open management of the necrosis as clinically appropriate, and we no longer perform diagnostic FNA. Decision-making in these patients is extremely difficult and is best carried out within an experienced multidisciplinary team.

Methods of necrosectomy

The traditional approach to infected necrosis was open laparotomy/debridement. These approaches are falling from favour with increasing evidence that minimally invasive intervention may reduce morbidity/mortality;[51–53] however, they remain the method of choice in some countries.

Open laparotomy/debridement

The technique of pancreatic debridement involves a wide exposure of the abdomen, usually through a bilateral subcostal/rooftop incision. Both colonic flexures are mobilised to expose the retroperitoneum and the lesser sac entered via the gastrocolic omentum, or occasionally the transverse mesocolon. Pus is aspirated from the abscess cavity, leaving the solid component behind, which is then removed by 'blunt finger' dissection (**Fig. 13.4**). Tissue that

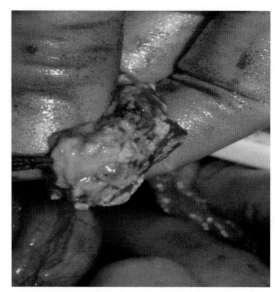

Figure 13.4 • Solid necrotic material removed at open necrosectomy by blunt finger dissection.

will not come away by finger teasing should be left in situ to demarcate and subsequent removal at a later procedure. The procedure may also include a cholecystectomy, operative cholangiogram and feeding jejunostomy.

Methods for postoperative management of the debridement cavity after laparotomy are as follows:

- **With drainage/'closed packing'.** Simple drainage, often with multiple retroperitoneal tube drains, was the conventional approach to the postoperative management of the debrided pancreatic and peripancreatic bed. Whilst mortality was less than with resective procedures, multiple second-look laparotomies were often required for residual sepsis. The initial results of Warshaw and colleagues reported respectable mortality figures of 24% using this technique. Their technique has been modified using multiple soft Penrose drains containing cotton gauze to pack the cavity following completion of the necrosectomy.[54] These are subsequently removed at intervals, allowing the cavity to collapse around the drains. Their reported mortality rate using this technique is the lowest in the literature (6.2%), although the series included patients with sterile necrosis (11%) and pancreatic abscess (39%), and only 14% had both sepsis syndrome and a positive culture requiring early intervention, which is indicative of the difficulties in interpretation of the available literature.

- **With open packing.** Bradley and colleagues from Atlanta have been the principal proponents of the open laparostomy technique.[55] In this, at the conclusion of the debridement, the lesser sac is packed with lubricated cotton gauze and the abdomen left open, allowing planned re-explorations every few days until granulation tissue forms. Enteric fistula and secondary haemorrhage are not uncommon, and the technique is rarely performed as a first option. Surgical packing and planned re-operation is, however, sometimes required to control blood loss from the retroperitoneum following the development of an intraoperative coagulopathy, a lavage system being created, following correction of the coagulopathy, at the time of subsequent pack removal.

- **With closed lavage.** Postoperative closed lavage as described by Beger et al.[56] is the most popular method for postoperative sepsis control following open debridement, the aim of the lavage being the continuous removal of devitalised necrotic material and bacteria. Several (four to six) large-diameter tube drains are inserted in the lesser sac and throughout the abdomen, and the abdomen closed. Continuous lavage is then commenced, our own preference being for CAPD dialysis fluid (Dianil 7, Baxter Healthcare, potassium free, Iso-osmolar) warmed through a blood warmer and delivered at 500 mL/h. The lavage is continued, for around 3–4 weeks on average, until the return fluid is clear and the patient has no residual signs of systemic sepsis. This technique has been adopted with minor variations by centres on both sides of the Atlantic.

Minimally invasive approaches to infected necrosis

Minimally invasive surgery has been shown consistently to be associated with a lesser activation of the inflammatory response than equivalent open surgery, and there is experimental evidence suggesting that local sepsis and the inflammatory response may be lessened by a minimally invasive rather than an open technique. The widespread belief that formal necrosectomy is required has recently been challenged and there is evidence that patients can resolve following simple percutaneous drainage or following limited necrosectomy. The PANTER trial and several prospective cohort series[51–53] have suggested that by minimising the massive inflammatory

'hit' of open pancreatic necrosectomy, a minimally invasive approach to the management of infected pancreatic necrosis may lessen the risk of post-procedural organ failure, respiratory and wound morbidity in these patients. However, there is as yet no evidence that one minimal approach is superior to another.

- **Percutaneous drainage.** Freeny et al.,[57] combining aggressive CT-guided percutaneous drainage with continuous post-drainage lavage, showed that nearly half the pancreatic abscesses may resolve. However, more than half of these patients required subsequent surgical intervention for residual sepsis. Drain occlusion is common due to necrotic debris and repeated drains may be necessary. Simple drainage, even with small-diameter drains, may be associated with complete resolution and within the PANTER trial 'step-up' arm, 35% of patients were successfully managed by small-bore (4-mm) percutaneous drainage alone.

- **Minimally invasive surgery.** Simple percutaneous or endoscopic drainage alone may result in complete resolution; however, they also have a useful role providing initial sepsis control, associated with an improvement in organ dysfunction. Careful drain management is required to recognise drain blockage early and to prevent recurrent sepsis. As a result of the difficulties in maintaining drain patency, we have developed a technique[58] to allow minimally invasive drainage, and in addition removal of the necrotic component. This involves the intraoperative dilatation of a previously placed CT-guided percutaneous drain tract and subsequent necrosectomy using a urological rigid-rod lens system (**Fig. 13.5**). Complete resolution of sepsis and necrosis can occur without recourse to further surgery, with a reduced need for postoperative organ support compared to the open procedures. In other centres as well as within our own patient cohort, this technique has significantly reduced mortality.[52] The Dutch Pancreatitis study group have popularised a video-assisted retroperitoneal debridement technique (VARD variation of the Fagniez technique) through a small 5-cm incision in the left flank. Their management approach has evolved from being initially performed on all patients with infected

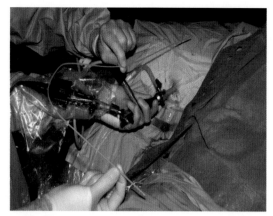

Figure 13.5 • Percutaneous necrosectomy showing the rod lens scope and a guiding catheter to ensure accurate drain placement.

necrosis, to now being used as a 'step-up' approach should initial percutaneous drainage fail to control sepsis. The Dutch group have completed a randomised trial[51] comparing this minimally invasive two-stage 'step-up' approach with open necrosectomy and have shown a reduction in early organ failure (respiratory) and late morbidity, but the study was underpowered to address mortality.

• **Endoscopic necrosectomy.** The principle of tract dilatation and minimally invasive necrosectomy has also been used with the endoscopic approach. Seifert et al.[59] have reported the dilatation of an endocyst-gastrotomy tract, allowing insertion of the endoscope into the retroperitoneum and subsequent piecemeal debridement. More recently the use of multiple transgastric cyst gastrostomy puncture sites has been reported, allowing nasocystic lavage and stent-assisted drainage through alternative drainage sites with good sepsis control.[60]

There is currently no evidence that one minimally invasive technique has any advantage over another and choice is often determined by local expertise and resources.

Management of pancreatic abscess

A pancreatic abscess by definition is an infected, fluid-predominant acute collection (pseudocyst) with little or no necrosis, and is therefore suitable for minimally invasive drainage. The endoscopic technique of Baron described above has been used in this situation with reasonably good effect, but there is a significant risk of haemorrhage from blind puncture

of the abscess wall. The EUS-guided endoscopic technique appears to be associated with a lower morbidity and has a reported resolution of sepsis of nearly 90%.[61] Laparoscopic cyst gastrostomy may be an effective alternative.

Specific late complications

Haemorrhage

Life-threatening haemorrhage may rarely occur acutely in pancreatic necrosis within the first week following presentation and requires mesenteric embolisation or surgical exploration. Haemorrhage is, however, a relatively common problem following prior necrosectomy as a postoperative reactionary haemorrhage due to a combination of having a large raw surface, partly controlled sepsis and exposed major vessels, leading to reactionary haemorrhage (**Fig. 13.6**). Bleeding may be arterial or venous. Urgent surgical intervention and ligation of proximal visceral vessels may be suggested; however, the combination of haemorrhage and subsequent laparotomy frequently precipitates escalating organ failure and death. Angiography and embolisation, with endovascular metal coils, is therefore the treatment of choice.

Segmental portal hypertension and gastrointestinal haemorrhage

Splenic vein thrombosis is associated with up to 15% of patients dying with acute pancreatitis. In those patients with thrombosis that survive the acute attack, the splenic venous drainage diverted through the short gastric vessels may result in patients developing large venous collaterals. Short

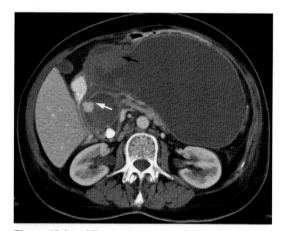

Figure 13.6 • CT scan showing large acute fluid collection with a pseudoaneurysm (indicated by white arrow) and haematoma (black arrow) within the collection.

gastric and lienocolic varices may make surgery on late complications of an acute pancreatitic episode hazardous. When necessary, splenectomy is curative. Despite the frequency of venous collaterals on follow-up CT, late gastrointestinal haemorrhage due to gastric varices is rare in practice.

Pancreatic duct stricture

Pancreatic duct stricture can occur following resolution of an attack of acute pancreatitis as a result of local tissue damage and fibrotic repair. More commonly, complete occlusion occurs, resulting in a disconnected duct syndrome should a remnant of viable tail remain, the treatment of which is described above. A pancreatic duct stricture may be present on its own, or in association with a duct disruption causing a pseudocyst or pancreatic fistula. Isolated pancreatic duct stricture can result in recurrent attacks of abdominal pain, sometimes with hyperamylasaemia and with dilatation of the distal duct system. Management of the stricture may be by simple dilatation and temporary stenting, by surgical resection of the stricture along with the pancreatic tail, or by surgical drainage of the pancreatic duct system into a Roux loop.

Gastric outlet obstruction

Gastric outlet obstruction resulting in persistent vomiting or high-volume gastric aspirates from nasogastric suction may complicate up to 10% of patients with severe acute pancreatitis. The recent trend towards nasojejunal intubation has rendered this complication less troublesome and the majority of patients can be treated by nasoenteric feeding until the local oedema/ileus settles. Occasionally, a gastroenterostomy is required for long-standing gastric stasis.

Key points

- Initial assessment and resuscitation should take account of the multisystem nature of the disease, and patients with organ dysfunction should be managed within a high-dependency environment.
- All patients with acute pancreatitis should have ultrasonic assessment of the biliary tree within 24 h of admission.
- Prophylactic antibiotics are not recommended as part of standard management in patients with acute pancreatitis, and when used should be for a defined period. No drug therapy has been shown to be beneficial.
- Nutritional support should be by the enteral route where possible.
- In the non-jaundiced patient there is no role for urgent ERCP and sphincterotomy.
- Definitive management of cholelithiasis should be within 4 weeks of discharge, in uncomplicated cases.
- Failure of percutaneous or endoscopic management is associated with the need for complex surgery and should therefore only be undertaken by, or following consultation with, a pancreatic specialist.
- There is no role for early surgical intervention other than for the management of complications.
- Sterile necrosis should be treated conservatively.
- Surgery for infected necrosis should aim to achieve the adequate and maintained control of sepsis.

References

1. McKay CJ, Evans S, Sinclair M, et al. High early mortality rate from acute pancreatitis in Scotland, 1984–1995. Br J Surg 1999;86(10):1302–5.

2. Appelros S, Borgstrom A. Incidence, aetiology and mortality rate of acute pancreatitis over 10 years in a defined urban population in Sweden. Br J Surg 1999;86(4):465–70.

3. Halvorsen FA, Ritland S. Acute pancreatitis in Buskerud County, Norway. Incidence and etiology. Scand J Gastroenterol 1996;31(4):411–4.

4. Yadav D, Lowenfels AB. Trends in the epidemiology of the first attack of acute pancreatitis: a systematic review. Pancreas 2006;33(4):323–30.

5. Criddle DN, McLaughlin E, Murphy JA, et al. The pancreas misled: signals to pancreatitis. Pancreatology 2007;7(5–6):436–46.

6. Katz M, Carangelo R, Miller LJ, et al. Effect of ethanol on cholecystokinin-stimulated zymogen conversion in pancreatic acinar cells. Am J Physiol 1996;270(1, Pt 1):G171–5.

7. Bradley 3rd EL. A clinically based classification system for acute pancreatitis. Summary of the International Symposium on Acute Pancreatitis, Atlanta, GA, September 11 through 13, 1992. Arch Surg 1993;128(5):586–90.

8. Banks PA, Bollen TL, Dervenis C, et al. Acute Pancreatitis Classification Working Group. Classification of acute pancreatitis–2012: revision of the Atlanta classification and definitions by international consensus. Gut 2013;62(1):102–11.

9. Buter A, Imrie CW, Carter CR, et al. Dynamic nature of early organ dysfunction determines outcome in acute pancreatitis. Br J Surg 2002;89(3):298–302.

10. McKay CJ, Curran F, Sharples C, et al. Prospective placebo-controlled randomized trial of lexipafant in predicted severe acute pancreatitis. Br J Surg 1997;84(9):1239–43.

11. Isenmann R, Rau B, Beger HG. Early severe acute pancreatitis: characteristics of a new subgroup. Pancreas 2001;22(3):274–8.

12. Johnson CD, Abu-Hilal M. Persistent organ failure during the first week as a marker of fatal outcome in acute pancreatitis. Gut 2004;53(9):1340–4.

13. Beger HG, Bittner R, Block S, et al. Bacterial contamination of pancreatic necrosis. A prospective clinical study. Gastroenterology 1986;91(2):433–8.

14. Whitcomb DC, Ulrich 2nd CD. Hereditary pancreatitis: new insights, new directions. Bailliere's Best Pract Res Clin Gastroenterol 1999;13(2):253–63.

15. Underwood TW, Frye CB. Drug-induced pancreatitis. Clin Pharm 1993;12(6):440–8.

16. Chari ST. Current concepts in the treatment of autoimmune pancreatitis. JOP 2007;8(1):1–3.

17. Hogan WJ, Geenen JE, Dodds WJ. Dysmotility disturbances of the biliary tract: classification, diagnosis, and treatment. Semin Liver Dis 1987;7(4):302–10.

18. McKay CJ, Buter A. Natural history of organ failure in acute pancreatitis. Pancreatology 2003;3(2):111–4.

19. Ranson JH, Rifkind KM, Roses DF, et al. Prognostic signs and the role of operative management in acute pancreatitis. Surg Gynecol Obstet 1974;139(1):69–81.

20. Blamey SL, Imrie CW, O'Neill J, et al. Prognostic factors in acute pancreatitis. Gut 1984;25(12):1340–6.

21. Wilson C, Heath DI, Imrie CW. Prediction of outcome in acute pancreatitis: a comparative study of APACHE II, clinical assessment and multiple factor scoring systems. Br J Surg 1990;77(11):1260–4.

22. Gravante G, Garcea G, Ong SL, et al. Prediction of mortality in acute pancreatitis: a systematic review of the published evidence. Pancreatology 2009;9(5):601–14.

23. Mofidi R, Suttie SA, Patil PV, et al. The value of procalcitonin at predicting the severity of acute pancreatitis and development of infected pancreatic necrosis: systematic review. Surgery 2009;146(1):72–81.

24. Al-Bahrani AZ, Abid GH, Holt A, et al. Clinical relevance of intra-abdominal hypertension in patients with severe acute pancreatitis. Pancreas 2008;36(1):39–43.

25. Zhang WF, Ni YL, Cai L, et al. Intra-abdominal pressure monitoring in predicting outcome of patients with severe acute pancreatitis. Hepatobiliary Pancreat Dis Int 2007;6(4):420–3.

26. UK guidelines for the management of acute pancreatitis. Gut 2005;54(Suppl. 3):iii1–9.

27. Balthazar EJ, Robinson DL, Megibow AJ, et al. Acute pancreatitis: value of CT in establishing prognosis. Radiology 1990;174(2):331–6.

28. Viremouneix L, Monneuse O, Gautier G, et al. Prospective evaluation of nonenhanced MR imaging in acute pancreatitis. J Magn Reson Imaging 2007;26(2):331–8.

29. Uhl W, Warshaw A, Imrie C, et al. IAP guidelines for the surgical management of acute pancreatitis. Pancreatology 2002;2(6):565–73.

30. Beger HG, Rau B, Mayer J, et al. Natural course of acute pancreatitis. World J Surg 1997;21(2):130–5.

31. Villatoro E, Mulla M, Larvin M. Antibiotic therapy for prophylaxis against infection of pancreatic necrosis in acute pancreatitis. Cochrane Database Syst Rev 2010;(5);CD002941.

32. Wittau M, Mayer B, Scheele J, et al. Systematic review and meta-analysis of antibiotic prophylaxis in severe acute pancreatitis. Scand J Gastroenterol 2011;46(3):261–70.
   Most recent review of the role of antibiotics in acute pancreatitis.

33. Kalfarentzos F, Kehagias J, Mead N, et al. Enteral nutrition is superior to parenteral nutrition in severe acute pancreatitis: results of a randomized prospective trial. Br J Surg 1997;84(12):1665–9.
   This initial randomised trial has since been supported by seven others.

34. Al-Omran M, Albalawi ZH, Tashkandi MF, et al. Enteral versus parenteral nutrition for acute pancreatitis. Cochrane Database Syst Rev 2010;(1);CD002837.

35. Petrov MS, Correia MI, Windsor JA. Nasogastric tube feeding in predicted severe acute pancreatitis. A systematic review of the literature to determine safety and tolerance. JOP 2008;9(4):440–8.

36. Windsor AC, Kanwar S, Li AG, et al. Compared with parenteral nutrition, enteral feeding attenuates the acute phase response and improves disease severity in acute pancreatitis. Gut 1998;42(3):431–5.

37. Petrov MS, Loveday BP, Pylypchuk RD, et al. Systematic review and meta-analysis of enteral nutrition formulations in acute pancreatitis. Br J Surg 2009;96(11):1243–52.

38. Besselink MG, van Santvoort HC, Buskens E, et al. Probiotic prophylaxis in predicted severe acute pancreatitis: a randomised, double-blind, placebo-controlled trial. Lancet 2008;371(9613):651–9.

39. Ayub K, Imada R, Slavin J. Endoscopic retrograde cholangiopancreatography in gallstone-associated acute pancreatitis. Cochrane Database Syst Rev 2004;(4);CD003630.

40. Petrov MS, van Santvoort HC, Besselink MG, et al. Early endoscopic retrograde cholangiopancreatography versus conservative management in acute biliary pancreatitis without cholangitis: a meta-analysis of randomized trials. Ann Surg 2008;247(2):250–7.
    The most recent review of the role of ERCP in acute pancreatitis.

41. Yusoff IF, Raymond G, Sahai AV. A prospective comparison of the yield of EUS in primary vs. recurrent idiopathic acute pancreatitis. Gastrointest Endosc 2004;60(5):673–8.

42. Bhattacharya D, Ammori BJ. Minimally invasive approaches to the management of pancreatic pseudocysts: review of the literature. Surg Laparosc Endosc Percutan Tech 2003;13(3):141–8.

43. Nealon WH, Walser E. Surgical management of complications associated with percutaneous and/or endoscopic management of pseudocyst of the pancreas. Ann Surg 2005;241(6):948–60.

44. Baron TH, Thaggard WG, Morgan DE, et al. Endoscopic therapy for organized pancreatic necrosis. Gastroenterology 1996;111(3):755–64.

45. Gardner TB, Coelho-Prabhu N, Gordon SR, et al. Direct endoscopic necrosectomy for the treatment of walled-off pancreatic necrosis: results from a multicenter U.S. series. Gastrointest Endosc 2011;73(4):718–26.

46. Mier J, Leon EL, Castillo A, et al. Early versus late necrosectomy in severe necrotizing pancreatitis. Am J Surg 1997;173(2):71–5.
    The only randomised trial of early surgery in acute pancreatitis.

47. Buchler MW, Gloor B, Muller CA, et al. Acute necrotizing pancreatitis: treatment strategy according to the status of infection. Ann Surg 2000;232(5):619–26.

48. Uomo G, Visconti M, Manes G, et al. Nonsurgical treatment of acute necrotizing pancreatitis. Pancreas 1996;12(2):142–8.

49. Rau B, Pralle U, Mayer JM, et al. Role of ultrasonographically guided fine-needle aspiration cytology in the diagnosis of infected pancreatic necrosis. Br J Surg 1998;85(2):179–84.

50. Gerzof SG, Banks PA, Robbins AH, et al. Early diagnosis of pancreatic infection by computed tomography-guided aspiration. Gastroenterology 1987;93(6):1315–20.

51. van Santvoort HC, Besselink MG, Bakker OJ, et al. A step-up approach or open necrosectomy for necrotizing pancreatitis. N Engl J Med 2010;362(16):1491–502.

52. Raraty MG, Halloran CM, Dodd S, et al. Minimal access retroperitoneal pancreatic necrosectomy: improvement in morbidity and mortality with a less invasive approach. Ann Surg 2010;251(5):787–93.

53. van Santvoort HC, Bakker OJ, Bollen TL, et al. A conservative and minimally invasive approach to necrotizing pancreatitis improves outcome. Gastroenterology 2011;141(4):1254–63.

54. Fernandez-del Castillo C, Rattner DW, Makary MA, et al. Debridement and closed packing for the treatment of necrotizing pancreatitis. Ann Surg 1998;228(5):676–84.

55. Bradley 3rd EL. Management of infected pancreatic necrosis by open drainage. Ann Surg 1987;206(4):542–50.

56. Beger HG, Buchler M, Bittner R, et al. Necrosectomy and postoperative local lavage in necrotizing pancreatitis. Br J Surg 1988;75(3):207–12.

57. Freeny PC, Hauptmann E, Althaus SJ, et al. Percutaneous CT-guided catheter drainage of infected acute necrotizing pancreatitis: techniques and results. Am J Roentgenol 1998;170(4):969–75.

58. Carter CR, McKay CJ, Imrie CW. Percutaneous necrosectomy and sinus tract endoscopy in the management of infected pancreatic necrosis: an initial experience. Ann Surg 2000;232(2):175–80.

59. Seifert H, Faust D, Schmitt T, et al. Transmural drainage of cystic peripancreatic lesions with a new large-channel echo endoscope. Endoscopy 2001;33(12):1022–6.

60. Varadarajulu S, Phadnis MA, Christein JD, et al. Multiple transluminal gateway technique for EUS-guided drainage of symptomatic walled-off pancreatic necrosis. Gastrointest Endosc 2011;74(1):74–80.

61. Giovannini M, Pesenti C, Rolland AL, et al. Endoscopic ultrasound-guided drainage of pancreatic pseudocysts or pancreatic abscesses using a therapeutic echo endoscope. Endoscopy 2001;33(6):473–7.

14

Chronic pancreatitis

Alexandra M. Koenig
Kai Bachmann
Jakob R. Izbicki

Summary

Chronic pancreatitis (CP) is a widespread disorder with enormous personal and socioeconomic impact. This inflammatory disease is characterised by the progressive conversion of pancreatic parenchyma to fibrous tissue, predominantly in the head of the gland, with consecutive endocrine and exocrine insufficiency. Consumption of alcohol and nicotine abuse are the leading causes in the progress of the disease. The aim of therapy is primarily pain relief, improvement in the quality of life and treatment of complications. Surgical intervention encompasses drainage procedures, surgical resections or the combination of both.

Duodenum-preserving resection of the pancreatic head combines the highest safety of all surgical procedures with the maximum efficacy.

Definition

✔✔ Chronic pancreatitis is a benign inflammatory disease, characterised by an irreversible loss of pancreatic parenchyma, leading to exocrine insufficiency with maldigestion and in advanced stages finally endocrine insufficiency.

Although the lost function can be replaced with pancreatic enzymes and management of diabetes mellitus, the most challenging symptom is pain.

Ammann et al. suggested that acute pancreatitis and chronic alcoholic pancreatitis are different stages of the same disease.[1,2] Chronic pancreatitis represents the persistent damage after episodes of severe acute pancreatitis.[3,4]

The classification of CP as an separate disease was described in 1946 by Comfort et al.[5] Since then, different classifications of CP have been presented. According to the Marseille Classification, CP is characterised by histological changes, persisting after the aetiologic agent has been removed.[6] The Cambridge Classification (1983) defined CP as an ongoing inflammatory disease characterised by irreversible structural changes associated with abdominal pain and permanent loss of function.

In the Marseille–Rome classification of 1988 obstructive chronic pancreatitis, chronic inflammatory pancreatitis (with loss of exocrine parenchyma and replacement by fibrosis) and the chronic calcifying pancreatitis were described.

Recently, a new classification of CP has been suggested. Probable CP is characterised by a typical history and one or more of the following criteria: recurrent or persistent pseudocysts, ductal alterations, endocrine insufficiency (abnormal glucose tolerance test) or pathological secretin test. Definite CP is characterised by a typical history and at least one of the following criteria: typical histology from an adequate surgical specimen, moderate or marked ductal alterations, pancreatic calcification, marked exocrine insufficiency defined as steatorrhea, normalised or markedly reduced by enzyme substitution.[7]

Incidence

✔✔ Chronic pancreatitis is a disease with high personal and socioeconomic impact. The prevalence of CP is 10–30 per 100 000 population and it affects about 8 new patients per 100 000 population per year in the USA.[8,9] Autopsy series suggest a higher prevalence of 0.04–5%.

Aetiology

Chronic pancreatitis is a highly complex process that begins with episodes of acute pancreatitis and progresses to end-stage fibrosis at different rates in different people due to different mechanisms. The most frequent causes are excess alcohol consumption (70–90%),[9] cholelithiasis, autoimmune or individual genetic predisposition and anatomical variants such as pancreas divisum (Box 14.1).

In up to 20% of patients the reasons or predisposing factors are not identifiable. The peak presentation of the disease occurs in patients between 35 and 55 years of age. Long-term consumption of alcohol is associated with an increased risk of developing CP. The precise level of daily alcohol intake at which patients are at risk for developing CP has not been clearly recognised, but it is estimated at 60–80 g per day, although individual sensitivity to the toxic effects of alcohol varies. Women are at greater risk, as are non-Caucasians when compared to their Caucasian counterparts. High caloric intake of protein and fat, smoking and lack of vitamins and trace elements have been described as additional predisposing risk factors.

Clinical course

Recurrent episodes of abdominal pain is the main symptom of CP, leading to inability to work, early retirement and addiction to analgesics. Severe pain attacks are the leading causes for hospitalisation. In most patients, pain is characterised as deep, penetrating, radiating to the back, and mostly worse after meals. Pain is frequently nocturnal, usually felt centrally in the epigastric region or subcostally with radiation to the back or shoulder tip, and is often eased by leaning forward or lying down to one side with knees pulled up, the so-called 'jack-knife' position. Ammann et al. described two different types of pain. The first, type A, is characterised by recurrent bouts of short-term, relapsing pain episodes. Type B pain is characterised as prolonged and persistent, and it is associated with secondary complications of CP such as pseudocysts or biliary obstruction. The natural course of CP is characterised by a consecutive loss of pancreatic parenchyma by fibrosis leading to exocrine insufficiency with diarrhoea, steatorrhoea, malnutrition and weight loss. In advanced stages, patients may present with endocrine insufficiency (diabetes mellitus). The clinical course and histomorphological changes that characterise the disease are extremely variable. Overall, life expectancy is shortened by 10–20 years. The mortality is increased 3.6-fold compared with a population without CP. The annual treatment costs are approximately $17 000 per patient.

The inflammation leads to progressive and irreversible loss of functional parenchyma and replacement with fibrotic tissue. The ductal system displays strictures of the bile duct, and duodenal stenosis[10] or the formation of pancreatic pseudocysts. Furthermore, CP can result in intraductal or parenchymal calcifications of the pancreas.

✔ Besides pain, and exocrine/endocrine malfunction, mechanical complications occur in CP. The process of continuing organ destruction cannot be interrupted by abstinence from alcohol consumption. Despite thousands of reports that have been published in the last few decades dealing with this disease, the pathogenesis and pathophysiology of CP are poorly understood and the clinical course is unpredictable.[11]

The natural course is that most patients with longstanding CP will become pain free due to a progressive 'burning out' of the organ.[12,13] Episodes of pain may occur less frequently, whereas endocrine and exocrine insufficiency commonly worsens. The pancreatic parenchyma is irreversibly converted to fibrous tissue with associated diabetes and steatorrhoea.[14]

At the time of onset of CP, 8% of patients have at least a moderate degree of endocrine insufficiency, whereas in long-term follow-up approximately 80% have endocrine insufficiency.[15,16] Studies have shown that it takes 10–20 years of a progressive inflammatory process to cause exocrine insufficiency by destroying the pancreatic parenchyma.[17,18]

Box 14.1 • Aetiology of chronic pancreatitis

Alcohol 70–90%
Idiopathic 20–30%
Cholelithiasis
Autoimmune
Genetic
Anatomical variants
Others

✔✔ Ten years after onset of CP, 50–93% of patients with CP still suffer from abdominal pain.[19]

At least 50–68% of patients with CP need surgery for management of complications or for intractable pain.[20] Although spontaneous relief occurs, the effects of chronic pain can have lasting repercussions including depression, opiate addiction, unemployment and social alienation exacerbated by the stigma of alcoholism.

Reduction of alcohol intake does not influence the course of pain in chronic alcoholic pancreatitis, but continued alcohol abuse is associated with significantly lower survival rates. Patients that stop drinking may get some improvement in exocrine function.[21] Endocrine insufficiency does not alter the course of pain. For the individual patient, the course of the disease is unpredictable.[21–23]

Pathophysiological findings and pain mechanisms in chronic pancreatitis

Despite the advances in our understanding of pathophysiology there is still no therapy directed toward the inflammatory process that leads to the regression of the disease. Therefore, symptom control is the primary aim of treatment. Several theories about the course of pain have been proposed but it is extremely multifactorial and variable between patients.

✔✔ Alcohol consumption is the leading cause of CP in western countries (70–90%).[7]

The acinar cells are directly damaged by alcohol. A change in microcirculatory perfusion and alterations in epithelial permeability lead to an imbalance in the pancreatic juice, and decreased fluid or bicarbonate secretion. Parenchymal necrosis of the pancreas may induce perilobular fibrosis that leads to intralobular fibrosis, ductal obstruction and periductal inflammation. Altered amounts of lithostatin in the pancreatic juice can lead to formation of protein plugs and stones in ducts and ductules.[24]

Pathomorphological findings in CP such as inflammatory infiltration of the pancreatic tissue, fibrosis, atrophy of the acinar cells, calcifications, pancreatic duct strictures and pseudocysts can affect focal segments of the gland, or be a diffuse finding throughout the whole organ.

Histomorphologically different forms of CP can be distinguished.

Calcifying CP

The most common form (calcifying CP) is characterised by recurrent bouts of acute pancreatitis with abdominal pain and development of intraductal calculi, protein plugs and parenchyma calcifications. These alterations of various degrees in different stages of the disease lead to pancreatic duct stenosis and consecutively to prestenotic duct dilatation. Additionally, epithelial alterations, inflammatory periductal infiltrations, parenchymal atrophy, necrosis and fibrosis can be found.[25]

Obstructive CP is often painless and caused by blockage of the main pancreatic duct due to tumour or an inflammatory process (post-acute pancreatitis) that leads to atrophy of the pancreatic tissue and prestenotic duct dilatation. No alteration of the ductal epithelium is found.[26] Pancreatic duct stones are uncommon. Periductal fibrosis and inflammatory infiltration are mainly found around the larger ducts and in the pancreatic head. Diffuse fibrotic changes occur throughout the organ without lobular topography. Pancreatic main-duct stenosis may be caused by papillary stenosis (tumour) or inflammation, duodenal diverticula, pancreatic tumours, congenital or acquired duct abnormalities (pancreas divisum), or rarely by traumatic pancreatic duct injuries. Small-duct pancreatitis is an extremely rare form of CP that is defined as main duct diameter ≤3 mm, with fibrous and inflammatory tissue.[27]

Autoimmune pancreatitis

Autoimmune pancreatitis is characterised by the absence of typical risk factors for developing CP or hereditary factors. In the past this subtype was named primary inflammatory sclerosis of the pancreas, non-alcoholic duct destructive pancreatitis or lymphoplasmacytic sclerosing pancreatitis.[28–30] The term autoimmune pancreatitis was introduced by Yoshida et al. in 1995.[31] Autoimmune pancreatitis can present with a focal event or with multiple lesions. Pseudocysts and caliculi are rarely found. Four histological features are characteristic of autoimmune pancreatitis. Lymphoplasmacytic infiltration, consisting of lymphocytes and plasma cells (often with high levels of IgG4), macrophages, neutrophils and eosinophils result in an intestinal fibrosis.[32] Additionally, periductal inflammation and periphlebitis can lead to luminal strictures or obliterative venulitis, respectively. Obstructive jaundice is caused by an effect on the common bile duct that may extend to the gallbladder and biliary tree. An increased level of IgG4 is a sensitive marker.[33] Autoimmune pancreatitis is associated with other autoimmune disorders such as ulcerative colitis,

Crohn's disease, primary sclerosing cholangitis, Sjörgren's syndrome, lymphocytic thyroiditis and primary biliary cirrhosis.[34]

Hereditary CP

Hereditary chronic pancreatitis (HCP) is a rare form with an incidence of approximately 3.5–10 per 100 000 inhabitants.[35] The morphological findings in HCP are irregular sclerosis with focal, segmental or diffuse destruction of the parenchyma. Different mutations have been detected to be associated with HCP, most commonly *R122H*, an N291 mutation of the *PRSS1* gene, and mutations of the *CFTR* and *SPINK1* genes.[36] The risk of developing pancreatic cancer is increased in HCP with *PRSS1* mutation as compared with the normal population and chronic alcoholic pancreatitis.

Rare reasons for CP besides pancreatic duct obstruction due to tumours, strictures, diverticula and anatomical variations like pancreas divisum or annular pancreas are trauma and genetic mutation.

✅✅ In up to 20% of patients the reason for CP remains unclear.

Pathogenesis of pain in chronic pancreatitis

Pain is the cardinal symptom in patients with CP. Together with often ongoing consumption of alcohol, it is most difficult to treat. The permanent pain impairs quality of life, leads to addiction to analgesics and results frequently in unemployment or early retirement.

In the initial stage of the disease the pain is intermittent and recurrent; later it persists. Painless pancreatitis is found rarely in alcohol-induced pancreatitis (<10%), while pain-free periods are seen in late-onset idiopathic pancreatitis.[37]

The formation of duct dilatation and hypertension due to downstream obstruction of the pancreatic duct is the most widely accepted hypothesis for the cause of pain in CP.

Ebbehoj et al. found a significantly higher pancreatic tissue pressure in patients who had painful CP compared with pain-free controls. These findings are interesting but have not been reproduced by other investigators. The reason for increased pressure can be due to postinflammatory scarring of the pancreatic (main and side) ducts, pancreatic duct stones or stricture or haemosuccus pancreaticus that leads to obstruction. Other reasons are pancreatic abscess, ascites, bile duct stenosis or duodenal stenosis. Patients with a reduced intraductal pressure had better pain relief compared to patients with higher intraductal pressure.[38] The assessment of pain is very difficult. Most trials in CP use classifications for description of pre- and postoperative pain or outcome such as excellent (no pain), good (better), fair (nil) and poor (worse); therefore, no comparison between different trials is possible. Pain relief is more common in patients that quit drinking. The underlying mechanism for pain in CP is poorly understood. Different concepts have been hypothesised, but none of them can completely explain the pain in this disease.

✅✅ The impact of various factors for the pathogenesis of pain remains unclear and can vary between patients.

Additionally, it has been reported that phenotypic modification of primary sensory neurons may play a role in causing persistent pain. Focal release and uptake of mediators in the peptidergic nerves have been shown to be changed by initial pancreatic inflammation. Previous trials revealed that the number and diameter of the pancreatic nerves, as well as activity, are significantly increased in patients with CP. A correlation between pain and expression of growth-associated protein 43 and level of methionine-enkephalin was detected. It is hypothesised that increased pressure facilitates the influx of pain mediators into the nerves and causes a neuritis resulting in pain.

Another hypothesis is that pancreatic ischaemia is responsible for the pain. Ischaemia activates xanthine oxygenase, leading to toxic oxygen metabolites. An increased level of cytochrome P450 in patients with CP was found in several trials but treatment with an inhibitor of xanthine oxygenase did not reduce the pain.

It is also likely that an individual's genetics plays a role in the overall pain experience. Genetic polymorphisms have been associated with disparate postoperative pain sensation and response to narcotics. Unfortunately, examination of candidate gene polymorphisms in visceral pain syndromes has been less convincing and clear evidence is lacking (Box 14.2).

Box 14.2 • Pathogenesis of pain in chronic pancreatitis

- Inflammation
- Duct obstruction
- Intra- and extrapancreatic causes (pseudocysts, common bile ducts, duodenal stenosis)
- High pancreatic tissue pressure
- Ischaemia of the pancreatic tissue
- Genetic factors
- Fibrotic encasement of sensory nerves
- Neuropathy

Preoperative assessment and investigations

A thorough history and physical examination is pivotal for the diagnosis and adequate therapy of patients with CP. The evaluation of aetiological factors is essential to select patients for the different therapeutic options.

Laboratory evaluation

Beside routine variables, laboratory data should include cholestasis parameters and tumour markers for pancreatic carcinoma. Endocrine and exocrine function has to be evaluated. Typically, serum lipase and amylase levels are markedly elevated in the acute setting, but may be normal in CP as a result of severe acinar atrophy. The presence of leucopenia and thrombocytopenia suggests that splenic vein thrombosis may have resulted in hypersplenism. Some studies have shown an elevated serum cholecystokinin (CCK) level in CP patients. It is proposed that CCK may increase pancreatic enzyme secretion. Trypsin levels are particularly high in patients with alcoholic pancreatitis, even when amylase levels are normal. In patients with auto-immune pancreatitis, the IgG and in particular its subtype IgG4 will be raised, the latter having a sensitivity and specificity as high as 95–97%, respectively.

Imaging studies

For tailored therapy and especially for planning surgical therapy, imaging studies play a central role in the diagnostic work-up of CP patients.

Abdominal ultrasound is an effective method that may help to establish the diagnosis. The use of endoscopic ultrasound is more sensitive and specific. Many patients undergo multiple endoscopic retrograde cholangiopancreatography (ERCP) procedures for diagnosis and therapeutic interventions. The gold standard in diagnosis of CP and for the planning of surgical therapy is contrast-enhanced computed tomography (CT) and magnetic resonance imaging (MRI). MRI offers the additional possibility to evaluate the ductal system by magnetic resonance cholangiopancreatography (MRCP). The advantage of CT is the better visualisation of parenchymal calcifications. Positron emission tomography (PET) may be helpful to differentiate between CP and pancreatic cancer (Box 14.3).

Treatment

The treatment of CP and its complications remains a major challenge. The most distressing symptom is intractable pain with continual abuse of analgesics.

Box 14.3 • Preoperative assessment and investigations

Medical history
Evaluation of aetiological factors
Symptoms
Previous treatment
Laboratory data
Routine
IgG4
CEA, CA 19-9
Imaging studies
Ultrasound
Endoscopic ultrasound
Fine-needle aspiration
ERCP
CT
MRI
(PET)

✅ The primary therapy for CP should be a conservative, symptom-related treatment.

Conservative therapy

The basis of adequate management of CP includes reduction of risk factors, replacement therapy for exocrine and endocrine insufficiency and nutritional supplementation, as well as pain therapy. Medical therapies such as dietary alterations, analgesics (non-steroidal anti-inflammatory drugs, paracetamol, prednisolone, dextropropoxiphene, tricylic antidepressives and in the late stages opioids), oral enzyme supplements and somatostatin analogues may improve symptoms. An important aspect in the treatment of CP patients is a multidisciplinary approach. Alternative therapies such as psychiatric or psychological input, transcutaneous electronic nerve stimulation, acupuncture, intrathecal pumps for opioids and spinal cord stimulation may be beneficial as adjunctive treatment (Box 14.4).

Endoscopic and interventional treatment

✅✅ Endoscopic treatment in patients with CP may provide effective pain relief or allow treatment of local complications, especially drainage of pancreatic pseudocysts.

Box 14.4 • Conservative treatment in chronic pancreatitis

Causal therapy
Reduction of risk factors
Autoimmune pancreatitis
Corticosteroid treatment and re-evaluation
Adjunct treatment
Antioxidant therapy
Pain therapy
Diet and treatment of exocrine insufficiency
Substitution with pancreatic enzymes
Analgesia according to the WHO scheme
Therapy of endocrine insufficiency
Diet
Oral antidiabetic medication
Insulin therapy
Alternative therapies
Psychiatric, psychological treatment
Nerve stimulation
Acupuncture

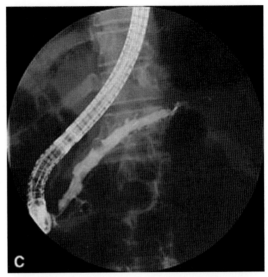

Figure 14.1 • Endoscopic retrograde pancreatogram and stenting in a patient with chronic pancreatitis.

Pancreatic ductal obstruction is the most frequent indication for endoscopic therapy to decompress and drain the pancreatic ductal system. Additionally, percutaneous catheter drainage is available as a temporising measure in high-risk surgical patients with complicated or infected pancreatic pseudocysts. For pain control, endosonography-guided or percutaneous coeliac nerve block with alcohol or steroids and thoracoscopic splanchnicectomy have been described. Pain relief and response rates range from 20% to 87%, but published data are rare and there are no prospective randomised trials. These procedures are associated with severe complications and recurrent symptoms with re-hospitalisation are common.

Up to 60% of patients with CP have pancreatic duct stones, which cause obstruction and an increase of intraductal pressure. Extracorporal shockwave lithotripsy (ESWL) can be used in painful, chronic, calcified pancreatitis with low morbidity and mortality rate.

Endoscopy

Different endoscopic procedures have been used in the treatment of CP, including sphincterotomy, endoscopic stone extraction (in some trials combined with extracorporal shockwave lithotripsy) and stenting of the pancreatic duct (**Fig. 14.1**).

Endoscopic pancreatic sphincterotomy in CP is technically challenging. Indications are sphincter of Oddi dysfunction or papillary stenosis/stricture. Another indication is to gain better access to the pancreatic duct for dilatation, transpapillary drainage and stenting (**Fig. 14.2**). Endoscopic stenting with regular changes resulted in complete pain relief in 45–95% of patients. Early complications (pancreatitis, cholangitis) occurred in 10–15% and late complications (strictures, ductal changes) in 10–30% of patients,[39,40] but initial pain relief was 89%. In a further trial, pain control was achieved following stenting in 70% of patients after 12 months' follow-up and in 62% of patients after 27 months' follow-up, with an overall morbidity rate of 25%.

✓ Endoscopic stenting plays a role in patients who are unfit for surgery, but it is not recommended as definitive therapy, mainly with regard to the necessity for repeated endoscopic interventions due to infection, stent displacement or stent occlusion (Box 14.5).

Surgical therapy, timing and indications

The major indication for surgical treatment in patients with CP is to relieve pain followed by treatment of local complications. The purpose is to preserve as much pancreatic parenchyma as possible.

Two randomised controlled trials have demonstrated the superiority of surgical versus endoscopic therapy in primary success rate, pain relief[42,43] and quality of life. The results show that, in patients with advanced calcifying CP and symptomatic pancreatic duct obstruction, surgery is more effective than endoscopy. Surgery was not only more effective but

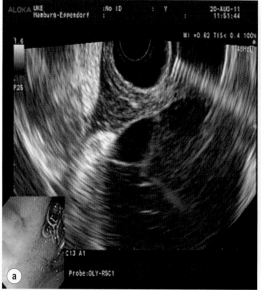

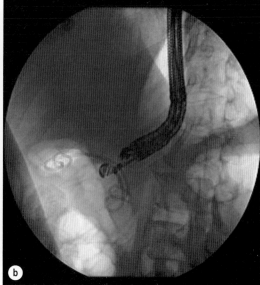

Figure 14.2 • Endoscopic drainage of pancreatic pseudocyst.

it also required fewer interventions. For most of the surgically treated patients a single operation resulted in immediate and permanent pain relief. Therefore the timing of the intervention should take these facts into consideration.[41–45]

✔✔ Endoscopically treated patients usually undergo multiple procedures and almost half subsequently require surgery.

Nealon and Thompson concluded in their study that early operative drainage should be performed before the gland is functionally and morphologically irreversibly damaged.[46] They suggested that patients with obstructive CP-related dilation or obstruction of the pancreatic duct and with biliary pancreatitis should undergo early surgical treatment before nutritional or metabolic disorders occur.

✔ Because CP is an inflammatory process resulting in irreversible damage of the pancreas, it is recommended that early intervention should be considered.

Box 14.5 • Interventional and endoscopic therapy

Interventional external drainage

Temporary treatment of abscess

Infected pseudocyst

If internal drainage is not possible

Often followed by surgery

Internal drainage

Therapy of pseudocysts

Less invasive than surgery

High recurrence rate

Endoscopic ductal drainage

Pancreas divisum

Proximal pancreas duct stenosis

Pancreaticolithiasis

Bile duct stenosis

Surgical techniques

Selection of the surgical intervention

The surgical technique should be adjusted to the pathomorphological changes in the pancreas. Several surgical strategies have been suggested for treatment of CP. The vast majority of patients present with a ductal obstruction located in the pancreatic head. In these patients, pancreatic head resection is the procedure of choice. In cases with predominant involvement of the tail of the pancreas, left-sided resection is favoured.

In general, surgical intervention should be safe and associated with low mortality and morbidity. Additionally, it should be effective in treatment of the underlying disease. An optimal surgical intervention should manage the intractable pain, resolve complications affecting adjacent organs and drain the main pancreatic duct.

✔✔ An optimal procedure should guarantee a low relapse rate, preserve maximal endocrine and exocrine function and, most importantly, restore quality of life.

Concern about underlying malignancy should be ruled out by frozen section analysis, as differentiating an inflammatory mass from a malignant tumour preoperatively may be challenging. It must be emphasised that in approximately 10% of patients, the initial diagnosis of a pancreatic carcinoma is based on the histological specimen at time of operation.[47,48]

The rationale for performing pancreatico-duodenectomy, essentially an 'oncological' procedure for treatment of a benign condition, is that

the majority of patients with CP present with an inflammatory pseudotumour of the pancreatic head as the dominant morphological pathology. This may be accompanied by duodenal and distal common bile duct obstruction. Such cephalic masses are widely assumed to trigger pain development, thereby representing the pacemaker of the disease. In patients with an inflammatory pseudotumour of the pancreatic head, ductal dilatation to the left of the mesenterico-portal axis is regarded as a secondary event not requiring surgical therapy, once the head has been sufficiently decompressed.

Simple drainage procedures that represent the other end of the scale aim to drain a dilated pancreatic duct. The indication is ductal ectasia and suspicion of intraductal hypertension without enlargement of the pancreatic head. Whether such simple drainage procedures are combined with a limited or subtotal resection of the pancreatic head depends on the presence or absence of inflammatory enlargement.[49]

Coffey and Link were the first to describe ductal drainage procedures by opening the main pancreatic duct. Subsequently, DuVal and Zollinger independently performed decompression of the main pancreatic duct by resection of the pancreatic tail and retrograde drainage of the pancreatic duct via a terminoterminal or terminolateral pancreatico-jejunostomy. A further operation is decompression of the main pancreatic duct with resection of the pancreatic tail, splenectomy and longitudinal laterolateral pancreatico-jejunostomy, as described by Puestow and Gillesby. Partington and Rochelle reported a spleen-preserving longitudinal pancreatico-jejunostomy without pancreatic tail resection.[50]

For many years the longitudinal pancreatico-jejunostomy introduced by Partington and Rochelle was the favoured surgical option for treatment of CP. Duodenum-preserving pancreatic head resections combine resectional aspects addressing the pancreatic head without sacrificing the gastroduodenal and bilioduodenal passage with drainage aspects comparable to the Partington–Rochelle procedure. The rationale for duodenum-preserving resection is to prevent loss of uninvolved organs and achieve optimal control of symptoms, especially pain. Due to minimising the loss of normal pancreatic tissue this procedure therefore has the potential to reduce loss of pancreatic function. The indication is patients with CP suffering from pain with multiple strictures of the main pancreatic duct, intraductal caliculi and an enlarged fibrotic pancreatic head and uncinate process. In addition, main duct dilatation with associated pseudocysts or obstruction of the duodenum or common bile duct is a further indication for this procedure.

Pancreatico-duodenectomy

The extent of resection in the Kausch–Whipple procedure includes pancreatic head resection with the duodenum and distal third of the stomach, or it can be modified as a pylorus-preserving pancreatico-duodenectomy (Longmire/Traverso). It offers improvement of the quality of life and pain relief in short- and long-term follow-up in about 90% of patients. The major disadvantage of pancreatico-duodenectomy is the sacrifice of surrounding non-diseased organs with loss of natural bowel continuity. Furthermore, pancreatic exocrine and endocrine function is significantly reduced. Comparing the classic Whipple procedure with the pylorus-preserving pancreatico-duodenectomy, a significantly higher rate of pain and nausea and lower quality of life have been reported.[51] Nowadays the procedures can be performed with low mortality (0–5%) in experienced centres, but morbidity rates of 20–40% remain high.[52,53]

Distal and total pancreatectomy

Near total pancreatico-duodenectomy and total pancreatectomy have been proposed in the treatment of CP. Due to high morbidity and mortality and deleterious effects on pancreatic function, these procedures have essentially been abandoned. In patients with complications after pancreatic surgery (pancreatic fistula or anastomotic leakage) or intractable pain after sufficient resection and/or drainage procedure, total pancreatectomy may be indicated as a last resort procedure. Resections of the distal part of the pancreas are often associated with endocrine insufficiency and they offer only short-term pain relief. The only suitable indications are localised severe complications of the pancreatic tail such as a pseudoaneurysm.

Partington–Rochelle procedure

The operation according to Partington and Rochelle is a spleen-preserving longitudinal pancreatico-jejunostomy without pancreatic tail resection. It is the most important simple drainage procedure and can be performed with low mortality and morbidity (approximately 3% and 20%, respectively). A maximum volume of pancreatic tissue is preserved. In most patients the main pancreatic duct can be effectively drained. In short-term follow-up, pain relief is found in approximately 75% of patients, but frequently it fails to provide long-lasting pain relief. The reason for persisting or recurrent pain has been attributed to an incomplete decompression of the main pancreatic duct, especially in the head of the pancreas.

Nowadays, the only suitable indication for a simple drainage procedure (Partington–Rochelle) with longitudinal pancreatico-jejunostomy is an isolated dilatation of the pancreatic ductal (>7 mm) or 'chain of lakes', without an inflammatory mass in the pancreatic head.

Longitudinal pancreatico-jejunostomy and cyst drainage

Nealon and co-workers analysed patients with CP and pseudocysts. They compared longitudinal pancreatico-jejunostomy alone and in combination with cystojejunostomy.

The operating time in longitudinal pancreatico-jejunostomy alone was shorter and the complication rates were comparable (11% vs. 16%). In long-term follow-up, the percentage of pain-free patients was good in both groups (87% and 89%, respectively).

Beger procedure

Beger and colleagues introduced the first duodenum-preserving resection of the pancreatic head as an organ-sparing procedure. This method consists of a subtotal resection of the pancreatic head after transection of the pancreas above the portal vein (**Fig. 14.3**). The pancreas is drained by an end-to-end or end-to-side pancreatico-jejunostomy using a Roux-en-Y loop.

An advantage of this procedure is that physiological gastroduodenal passage and common bile duct continuity are preserved.[54,55] The mortality rate in experienced centres is low (0–3%), with morbidity rates of 15–32% and the procedure provides long-term pain relief in 75–95% of patients.[56]

Frey procedure

In 1985, Frey and colleagues developed a modification of the duodenum-preserving pancreatic head resection (DPPHR). This combined a longitudinal pancreatico-jejunostomy of the body and tail of the pancreas (Partington–Rochelle procedure) with a limited duodenum-preserving excision of the pancreatic head. In contrast to the Beger procedure, the pancreas is not divided over the superior mesenteric portal vein (**Fig. 14.4**) and reconstruction can be performed with one single anastomosis. The head

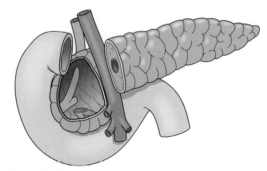

Figure 14.3 • Beger procedure.

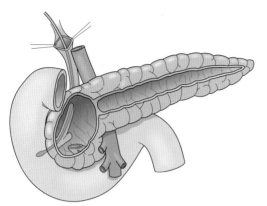

Figure 14.4 • Frey procedure.

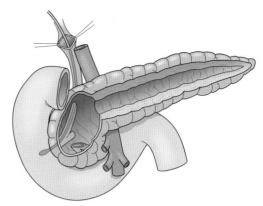

Figure 14.5 • Hamburg procedure.

of the pancreas is cored out, leaving a small cuff along the duodenal wall. Drainage of the cavity of the pancreatic head and the opened main duct of the body and tail is performed with a longitudinal pancreatico-jejunostomy using a Roux-en-Y loop. The Frey procedure can be performed with low mortality (< 1%) and acceptable morbidity (9–39%). In a prospective trial, 56% of patients were pain free and 32% had substantial pain relief. Exocrine and endocrine pancreatic functions are preserved and the procedure can be combined with procedures to treat complications of adjacent organs such as common bile duct stenosis, duodenal stenosis and internal pancreatic fistulas.[57]

Berne procedure

The Berne variation derives from a similar idea and combines the advantages of the Frey and Beger procedures.[58] This operation avoids the delicate division of the pancreatic neck anterior to the portal vein as in Beger's procedure, but compared to a Frey procedure, the extent of pancreatic resection is much greater and the common bile duct is decompressed. No longitudinal drainage of the pancreatic duct, as described by Frey and Izbicki, is performed. In patients with common bile duct obstruction, a longitudinal opening in the cavity of the pancreatic head is performed for bile drainage. The Berne procedure has been shown to be feasible, effective and safe with a mortality of 0–1% and a morbidity rate of 20–23%.[59]

Hamburg procedure

The Hamburg procedure is a further established modification of a DPPHR that combines aspects of the Beger and Frey procedures (**Fig. 14.5**). Subtotal excision of the pancreatic head including the uncinate process is performed. The extent of the cephalic decompression is comparable to the Beger procedure but avoids transection of the gland over the superior mesenteric portal vein as in a Frey procedure.

Drainage of the body and tail of the organ is achieved by excision of the ventral aspect of the pancreas into the pancreatic duct followed by longitudinal pancreatico-jejunostomy of the body and tail of the pancreas, which is comparable to the Partington–Rochelle procedure. The major advantage of this technique is that the extent of the resection can be customised to the individual morphology of the pancreas. It has been established as an effective and safe procedure, especially in patients with the sclerosing form of pancreatitis or extensive parenchymatous calcifications.[60] The V-shaped excision creates a trough-like new duct system; the underlying principle is the drainage of second- and third-order pancreatic duct side branches.

V-shaped excision

The sclerosing entity of CP, e.g. small-duct disease, is characterised by a non-dilated Wirsung duct with narrowing or even 'pseudo-vanishing'. For this disease, the authors suggest a longitudinal V-shaped excision of the ventral aspect of the pancreas combined with a longitudinal pancreatico-jejunostomy (**Fig. 14.6**). If this condition is accompanied by an enlarged pancreatic head, pancreatic head resection should be performed.

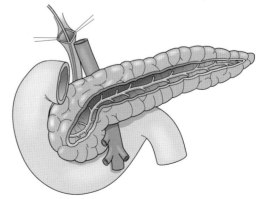

Figure 14.6 • V-shaped excision.

Excellent results have been reported after V-shaped excision, with pain relief in 89% of patients. Additionally, the mortality and morbidity of this procedure were low (0% and 19.6%, respectively).

Selection of the procedure

To date, four prospective randomised trials comparing duodenum-preserving resection and pancreatico-duodenectomy have been published. Results of long-term follow-up (>5 years) are available in two trials. No prospective randomised trials comparing simple drainage procedures or comparing drainage to resection exist.

In summary, duodenum-preserving resection of the pancreatic head is a less invasive technique compared to pancreatico-duodenectomy, with benefits especially concerning pain relief and improvement of quality of life during the first 2 years postoperatively. The comparable results of the different technique of duodenum preserving pancreatic head resections (Beger, Frey, Hamburg and Berne) are not surprising considering that all procedures involve the removal of a portion of the pancreatic head and effectively decompress the main pancreatic duct.[61] The major difference is the transection of the pancreatic neck in the Beger procedure and the additional longitudinal drainage of the pancreatic duct in the body and tail of the organ in the Frey and Hamburg procedures.

> ✔ Surgery offers good results in patients with CP, with pain relief in up to 90%. In short-term follow-up, the duodenum-preserving resections are superior to pancreatico-duodenectomy, but in long-term follow-up the outcome is comparable.

Salvage procedures

Due to improvement of surgical techniques and patient selection, pancreatic surgery for CP can be associated with excellent results. Recurrence may develop, most frequently in the remnant of the pancreatic head, indicating either insufficient surgical resection of the head of the pancreas or aggressive disease. In these patients 'redo' pancreas head resections are indicated. The procedures that should be considered are partial pancreatico-duodenectomy (Whipple procedure, pylorus-preserving pancreato-duodenectomy) and in selected patients (i.e. re-recurrence) even total spleno-pancreatico-duodenectomy. This procedure is indicated in patients that have undergone partial pancreatico-duodenectomy, and additional interventional nerve blocks or surgical denervation failed to achieve definitive pain relief.

Table 14.1 • Surgical therapy

Indications	Pain
	Complications
	Unsuccessful other treatment
	Suspicion of malignancy
Surgical techniques	
Pure drainage	
Cystojejunostomy	Isolated pseudocyst
Pancreatico-jejunostomy	
Partington–Rochelle procedure	Ductal dilation (>7 mm) Without inflammatory mass
Resection procedures	
Pancreatic head resection	Inflammatory mass in the head of pancreas
PD and ppPD	Suspicion of malignancy
	Irreversible duodenal stenosis
DPPHR	
Beger	Inflammatory mass in head
Bern	Less difficult than Beger
Frey	Ductal obstruction in head and tail
Hamburg	Combines aspects of Beger and Frey
	Sclerosing pancreatitis
	Extensive parenchymatous calcification
V-shaped excision	Small-duct disease (<3 mm)
Left resection	Isolated CP in tail (rare)
	Pseudoaneurysms
Segmental resection	Isolated ductal stenosis in body
Total pancreatectomy	Changes in entire pancreas (rare)

In patients that have previously undergone DPPHR or partial pancreatico-duodenectomy with recurrence of the CP in the body or tail, a V-shaped drainage procedure is indicated (Table 14.1).

Complications of chronic pancreatitis

In the course of CP, several potentially life-threatening complications may occur. In 12% of patients that underwent surgery for CP, duodenal obstruction was detected, often associated with common bile duct stenosis. Duodenal obstruction can also occur secondarily to development of a pancreatic pseudocyst. Patients typically suffer from nausea, vomiting, upper abdominal pain and weight loss. If duodenal obstruction does not resolve within 1–2 weeks of conservative therapy, interventional/surgical treatment is indicated.

Common bile duct (CBD) stenosis is due to the close anatomical relationship of the distal common bile duct with the head of the pancreas. In patients with CP, bile duct strictures are found in 5–9% of patients and in up to 35% after surgical procedures for CP. Patients with a CBD stricture can present with elevated liver enzymes, jaundice or with sepsis due to cholangitis. Patients with CBD strictures secondary to CP will invariably require surgical intervention. Excluding a local malignancy is of greatest importance in patients with duodenal or CBD obstruction.

Pancreatic ascites (**Fig. 14.7**) is found in approximately 4% of patients with CP and in 6–14% of those with a pancreatic pseudocyst (**Fig. 14.8**). It is defined as massive accumulation of pancreatic fluid in the peritoneal cavity. The amylase level in the ascitic fluid is typically above 1000 IU/L. ERCP should be performed to localise the site of leakage and to perform endoscopic pancreatic duct stenting. Additional treatment with somatostatin

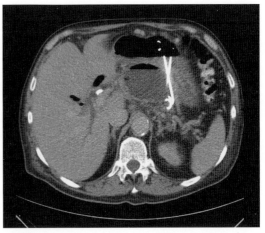

Figure 14.8 • Pancreatic pseudocyst and external drainage.

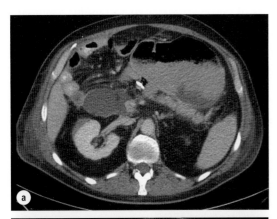

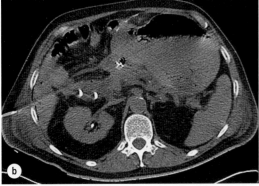

Figure 14.7 • Pancreatic ascites and drainage.

or octreotide together with diuretics and repeated paracentesis may be beneficial for some patients. In patients with persistent or recurrent accumulation of ascites and/or sudden deterioration of clinical status, surgery may be indicated.

The treatment of pancreatic pseudocysts should consider several aspects. Within 6 weeks a spontaneous resolution may occur in 40% of patients, whereas the pseudocyst-related complication rate, especially haemorrhage and infection (**Fig. 14.9**), is 20%. After 6 weeks, the rate of spontaneous remission is 4% and the complication rate increases to 56%. Therefore, intervention should be delayed for 6 weeks after diagnosis in patients with an uncomplicated pseudocyst. However, in patients with haemorrhage, abscess or infection, immediate intervention is mandatory. Surgery is only indicated if internal (transgastric) or CT-guided drainage fails.

In patients with complications of adjacent organs, such as duodenal stenosis or thrombosis of the portal vein with cavernous transformation, surgery should be performed as soon as they are diagnosed.

Pancreatico-pleural fistulas result from a disruption of the pancreatic duct or leakage from a pseudocyst. They are rare, but associated with significant morbidity and mortality. Three main types of thoracic manifestations are mediastinal pseudocyst formation, pancreatico-pleural fistula and pancreatico-bronchial fistula. Once a pancreatico-pleural fistula is suspected, the concentration of amylase in the pleural effusion should be measured. Conservative treatment has an efficacy of 30–60%, a recurrence rate of 15% and a mortality rate of 12%.[62] If conservative therapy fails, endoscopic sphincterotomy or stenting and surgery

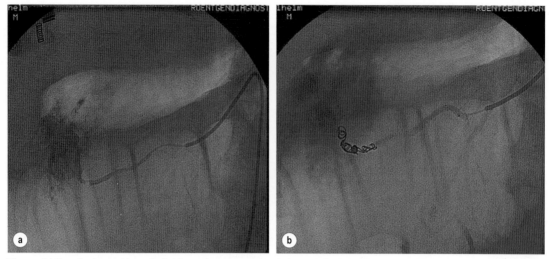

Figure 14.9 • Angiographic embolisation using a coaxial technique and microcoils.

should be considered, aiming to reduce the intra-ductal hypertension as this inhibits the spontaneous closure of fistula.

Extrahepatic portal hypertension is a less common complication of CP. It may be confined to either the superior mesenteric or splenic venous branch or may involve the whole spleno-mesenterico-portal axis.[63] It is defined as extrahepatic hypertension of the portal venous system in the absence of liver cirrhosis. The pathogenesis of extrahepatic portal hypertension in CP may include several factors. The inflammatory process is capable of causing initial damage to vascular walls and generating venous spasm, venous stasis and thrombosis.

Fibrosis of the pancreas can lead to progressive constriction of the spleno-mesenterico-portal axis. Other reasons are considerable pancreatic head enlargement or compression by pancreatic pseudocysts or inflammatory swelling of the gland. At present, extrahepatic portal hypertension per se is not an indication for surgical intervention in CP, because there is no evidence of an increased risk of haemorrhage, even though a potential risk of oesophageal or gastric varices exists. Additionally, these patients have a considerably increased surgical risk. If varices start to bleed, therapeutic options include interventional measures such as sclerotherapy, variceal ligation, and interventional (transjugular intrahepatic portosystemic shunts, TIPSS) or surgical portosystemic shunting procedures. In patients with thrombosis of the portal vein with cavernous transformation, a transection of the pancreatic parenchyma above the portal vein as required for the Beger procedure and pancreatico-duodenectomy should be avoided as this is associated with unpredictable risks.

Key points

- Consumption of alcohol and nicotine abuse are the leading causes of CP.
- Surgery is superior to endoscopic management regarding pain relief and quality of life.
- Pancreatic surgery should be undertaken by specialists in high-volume units.
- Duodenum-preserving resection of the pancreas is safe and effective and offers the best short-term outcome.

References

1. Ammann RW, Akovbiantz A, Largiader F, et al. Course and outcome of chronic pancreatitis. Longitudinal study of a mixed medical-surgical series of 245 patients. Gastroenterology 1984;86(5, Pt 1):820–8.

2. Strate T, Yekebas E, Knoefel WT, et al. Pathogenesis and the natural course of chronic pancreatitis. Eur J Gastroenterol Hepatol 2002;14(9):929–34.

3. Kloppel G, Maillet B. Pathology of acute and chronic pancreatitis. Pancreas 1993;8(6):659–70.

4. Kloppel G, Maillet B. The morphological basis for the evolution of acute pancreatitis into chronic

pancreatitis. Virchows Arch A Pathol Anat Histopathol 1992;420(1):1–4.

5. Kloppel G. Chronic pancreatitis, pseudotumors and other tumor-like lesions. Mod Pathol 2007;20(Suppl. 1):S113–31.

6. Banks PA. Classification and diagnosis of chronic pancreatitis. J Gastroenterol 2007;42(Suppl. 17): 148–51.

7. Ammann RW. Diagnosis and management of chronic pancreatitis: current knowledge. Swiss Med Wkly 2006;136(11–12):166–74.
This paper reviews the literature on CP. Based on experience, some of the discussed features such as aetiology and staging may help to predict in a given patient what is the risk for having a good or bad outcome without or with a surgical (or endoscopic) intervention.

8. Lohr JM. Medical treatment of pancreatic cancer. Expert Rev Anticancer Ther 2007;7(4):533–44.

9. Mayerle J, Lerch MM. Is it necessary to distinguish between alcoholic and nonalcoholic chronic pancreatitis? J Gastroenterol 2007;42(Suppl. 17):127–30.

10. Pessaux P, Varma D, Arnaud JP. Pancreaticoduodenectomy: superior mesenteric artery first approach. J Gastrointest Surg 2006;10(4):607–11.

11. Knoefel WT, Eisenberger CF, Strate T, et al. Optimizing surgical therapy for chronic pancreatitis. Pancreatology 2002;2(4):379–84.

12. Ammann RW. Alcoholic pancreatitis with special reference to clinical course, diagnosis and differential diagnosis. Schweiz Rundsch Med Prax 1984;73(18): 573–7.

13. Ammann RW, Akovbiantz A, Largiader F. Pain relief in chronic pancreatitis with and without surgery. Gastroenterology 1984;87(3):746–7.

14. Chari ST. Chronic pancreatitis: classification, relationship to acute pancreatitis, and early diagnosis. J Gastroenterol 2007;42(Suppl. 17):58–9.

15. Malka D, Hammel P, Sauvanet A, et al. Risk factors for diabetes mellitus in chronic pancreatitis. Gastroenterology 2000;119(5):1324–32.

16. Malka D, Vasseur S, Bodeker H, et al. Tumor necrosis factor alpha triggers antiapoptotic mechanisms in rat pancreatic cells through pancreatitis-associated protein I activation. Gastroenterology 2000;119(3): 816–28.

17. Lankisch PG, Lohr-Happe A, Otto J, et al. Natural course in chronic pancreatitis. Pain, exocrine and endocrine pancreatic insufficiency and prognosis of the disease. Digestion 1993;54(3):148–55.

18. Lankisch PG. Enzyme treatment of exocrine pancreatic insufficiency in chronic pancreatitis. Digestion 1993;54(Suppl. 2):21–9.

19. Layer P, Yamamoto H, Kalthoff L, et al. The different courses of early- and late-onset idiopathic and alcoholic chronic pancreatitis. Gastroenterology 1994;107(5):1481–7.

20. Parc R, Frileux P, Tiret E, et al. Acute necroticohemorrhagic pancreatitis. Why, when and how to drain? Apropos of 106 cases. Chirurgie 1989;115(9):651–5.

21. Lankisch MR, Imoto M, Layer P, et al. The effect of small amounts of alcohol on the clinical course of chronic pancreatitis. Mayo Clin Proc 2001;76(3): 242–51.

22. Lankisch PG. Natural course of chronic pancreatitis. Pancreatology 2001;1(1):3–14.

23. Lankisch PG, Assmus C, Lehnick D, et al. Acute pancreatitis: does gender matter? Dig Dis Sci 2001;46(11):2470–4.

24. Sarles H. Epidemiology and physiopathology of chronic pancreatitis and the role of the pancreatic stone protein. Clin Gastroenterol 1984;13(3):895–912.

25. Kloppel G. Pathology of chronic pancreatitis and pancreatic pain. Acta Chir Scand 1990;156(4): 261–5.

26. Lehnert P. Etiology and pathogenesis of chronic pancreatitis. Internist (Berl) 1979;20(7):321–30.

27. Yekebas EF, Bogoevski D, Honarpisheh H, et al. Long-term follow-up in small duct chronic pancreatitis: a plea for extended drainage by "V-shaped excision" of the anterior aspect of the pancreas. Ann Surg 2006;244(6):940–6.

28. Ectors N, Maillet B, Aerts R, et al. Non-alcoholic duct destructive chronic pancreatitis. Gut 1997;41(2): 263–8.

29. Strate T, Taherpour Z, Bloechle C, et al. Long-term follow-up of a randomized trial comparing the Beger and Frey procedures for patients suffering from chronic pancreatitis. Ann Surg 2005;241(4): 591–8.

30. Strate T, Mann O, Kleinhans H, et al. Microcirculatory function and tissue damage is improved after therapeutic injection of bovine hemoglobin in severe acute rodent pancreatitis. Pancreas 2005; 30(3):254–9.

31. Yoshida K, Toki F, Takeuchi T, et al. Chronic pancreatitis caused by an autoimmune abnormality. Proposal of the concept of autoimmune pancreatitis. Dig Dis Sci 1995;40(7):1561–8.

32. Toomey DP, Swan N, Torreggiani W, et al. Autoimmune pancreatitis: medical and surgical management. JOP 2007;8(3):335–43.

33. Choi EK, Kim MH, Lee TY, et al. The sensitivity and specificity of serum immunoglobulin G and immunoglobulin G4 levels in the diagnosis of autoimmune chronic pancreatitis: Korean experience. Pancreas 2007;35(2):156–61.

34. Agrawal S, Daruwala C, Khurana J. Distinguishing autoimmune pancreatitis from pancreaticobiliary cancers: current strategy. Ann Surg 2012;255(2): 248–58.

35. Barkin JS, Fayne SD. Chronic pancreatitis: update 1986. Mt Sinai J Med 1986;53(5):404–8.

36. Whitcomb DC, Gorry MC, Preston RA, et al. Hereditary pancreatitis is caused by a mutation in the cationic trypsinogen gene. Nat Genet 1996;14(2): 141–5.

37. Fasanella KE, Davis B, Lyons J, et al. Pain in chronic pancreatitis and pancreatic cancer. Gastroenterol Clin North Am 2007;36(2):335–64.ix.

38. Ebbehoj N, Borly L, Bulow J, et al. Pancreatic tissue fluid pressure in chronic pancreatitis. Relation to pain, morphology, and function. Scand J Gastroenterol 1990;25(10):1046–51.

39. Buscaglia JM, Kalloo AN. Pancreatic sphincterotomy: technique, indications, and complications. World J Gastroenterol 2007;13(30):4064–71.

40. Buscaglia JM, Kalloo AN, Jagannath SB. Endoscopic versus surgical treatment for chronic pancreatitis. N Engl J Med 2007;356(20):2102–4.

41. Liao Q, Wu WW, Li BL, et al. Surgical treatment of chronic pancreatitis. Hepatobiliary Pancreat Dis Int 2002;1(3):462–4.

42. Dite P, Ruzicka M, Zboril V, Novotny I. A prospective, randomized trial comparing endoscopic and surgical therapy for chronic pancreatitis. Endosc 2003 July;35(7):553–8.

43. Cahen DL, Gouma DJ, Nio Y, Rauws EA, Boermeester MA, Busch OR, et al. Endoscopic versus surgical drainage of the pancreatic duct in chronic pancreatitis. N Engl J Med 2007 February 15;356(7):676–84.

44. Cahen DL, Gouma DJ, Laramee P, et al. Long-term outcomes of endoscopic vs surgical drainage of the pancreatic duct in patients with chronic pancreatitis. Gastroenterology 2011;141(5):1690–5.

45. Strobel O, Buchler MW, Werner J. Surgical therapy of chronic pancreatitis: indications, techniques and results. Int J Surg 2009;7(4):305–12.

46. Nealon WH, Thompson JC. Progressive loss of pancreatic function in chronic pancreatitis is delayed by main pancreatic duct decompression. A longitudinal prospective analysis of the modified Puestow procedure. Ann Surg 1993;217(5):458–66.

47. Ihse I, Borch K, Larsson J. Chronic pancreatitis: results of operations for relief of pain. World J Surg 1990;14(1):53–8.

48. Ihse I, Gasslander T. Surgical treatment of pain in chronic pancreatitis: the role of pancreaticojejunostomy. Acta Chir Scand 1990;156(4):299–301.

49. Buchler M, Uhl W, Beger HG. Surgical strategies in acute pancreatitis. Hepatogastroenterology 1993;40(6):563–8.

50. Partington PF, Rochelle RE. Modified Puestow procedure for retrograde drainage of the pancreatic duct. Ann Surg 1960;152:1037–43.

51. Mobius C, Max D, Uhlmann D, et al. Five-year follow-up of a prospective non-randomised study comparing duodenum-preserving pancreatic head resection with classic Whipple procedure in the treatment of chronic pancreatitis. Langenbecks Arch Surg 2007;392(3):359–64.

52. Warshaw AL. Pain in chronic pancreatitis. Patients, patience, and the impatient surgeon. Gastroenterology 1984;86(5, Pt 1):987–9.

53. Strate T, Bachmann K, Busch P, et al. Resection vs drainage in treatment of chronic pancreatitis: long-term results of a randomized trial. Gastroenterology 2008;134(5):1406–11.

54. Izbicki JR, Bloechle C, Knoefel WT, et al. Complications of adjacent organs in chronic pancreatitis managed by duodenum-preserving resection of the head of the pancreas. Br J Surg 1994;81(9): 1351–5.

55. Frey CF, Amikura K. Local resection of the head of the pancreas combined with longitudinal pancreaticojejunostomy in the management of patients with chronic pancreatitis. Ann Surg 1994;220(4):492–504.

56. Buchler MW, Friess H, Muller MW, et al. Duodenum preserving resection of the head of the pancreas: a new standard operation in chronic pancreatitis. Langenbecks Arch Chir Suppl Kongressbd 1997;114:1081–3.

57. Beger HG, Buchler M, Bittner RR, et al. Duodenum-preserving resection of the head of the pancreas in severe chronic pancreatitis. Early and late results. Ann Surg 1989;209(3):273–8.

58. Gloor B, Friess H, Uhl W, et al. A modified technique of the Beger and Frey procedure in patients with chronic pancreatitis. Dig Surg 2001;18(1):21–5.

59. Koninger J, Seiler CM, Sauerland S, et al. Duodenum-preserving pancreatic head resection – a randomized controlled trial comparing the original Beger procedure with the Berne modification (ISRCTN No. 50638764). Surgery 2008;143(4):490–8.

60. Bachmann K, Mann O, Izbicki JR, et al. Chronic pancreatitis – a surgeon's view. Med Sci Monit 2008;14(11):RA198–205.

61. Diener MK, Rahbari NN, Fischer L, et al. Duodenum-preserving pancreatic head resection versus pancreatoduodenectomy for surgical treatment of chronic pancreatitis: a systematic review and meta-analysis. Ann Surg 2008;247(6):950–61.

62. Kaman L, Behera A, Singh R, et al. Internal pancreatic fistulas with pancreatic ascites and pancreatic pleural effusions: recognition and management. Aust N Z J Surg 2001;71(4):221–5.

63. Izbicki JR, Yekebas EF, Strate T, et al. Extrahepatic portal hypertension in chronic pancreatitis: an old problem revisited. Ann Surg 2002;236(1):82–9.

15

Pancreatic adenocarcinoma

Michael E. Kelly
Kevin C. Conlon

Introduction

Adenocarcinoma of the pancreas accounts for 3% of new cancer cases per annum,[1] yet it is the fourth leading cause of cancer-related death in Western countries. The insidious nature of the disease and its vagueness of presentation contribute to late diagnosis. Eighty per cent of patients have unresectable tumours at initial diagnosis. The overall survival at 5 years still remains at 6%, unchanged over the last four decades.[1] However, in recent years improvements in preoperative imaging and staging modalities, coupled with advancements in adjuvant therapies with the use of immunomodulators and monoclonal antibodies, have resulted in some degrees of optimism. Progress has been made as the molecular basis of the disease is better understood. With such poor survival rates and recent high-profile media attention, a renewed interest in tackling this elusive cancer has arisen.

Around 95% of pancreatic tumours are adenocarcinoma, originating from the exocrine part of the pancreas. Nearly all of these are ductal adenocarcinomas, which is the focus of this chapter.

Epidemiology

An estimated 44 000 new cases of adenocarcinoma of the pancreas occurred in the USA in 2011, and almost 38 000 died in the same year.[2] In the UK, 8085 people were diagnosed with pancreatic cancer and 8020 people died during 2009.[3] The incidence of pancreatic cancer varies with age, sex and ethnicity.

In 2008, the standardised incidence rate of pancreatic cancer was 3.9 per 100 000 population, while the standardised mortality rate was slightly lower at 3.7 per 100 000 population. Pancreatic cancer is the eleventh commonest cancer in males and eighth commonest cancer in females.[4] The peak incidence for the disease occurs between the seventh and eighth decades of life, and is rare under the age of 30. In the American population, African and Hawaiian ethnicities confer a higher incidence than Caucasian, whereas Asian and Hispanic ethnic groups have a lower risk of developing the disease. The incidence of pancreatic cancer is rising, particularly in Europe, although this observation is subject to reporting bias related to improved diagnostics. However, pancreatic neoplasm must be detected at an early stage to enable the potential for curative treatment.

Risk factors (see Box 15.1)

Smoking

Tobacco smoking is by far the leading preventable cause of pancreatic cancer, with an estimated 2.5-fold increase in risk when compared to non-smokers.[5] In 1986, the International Agency for Research on Cancer (IARC) classified smoking as a proven carcinogen with respect to cancer of the pancreas. Observational studies suggest that a dose-dependent relationship exists, necessitating long-term exposure.[5] However, smokers who have quit for more than 10 years no longer experience an increased risk.[5] While the chemical cause is unclear,

Box 15.1 • Risk factors for pancreatic cancer

Age (above 60 years)
Smoking
Obesity
High-fat diets
Alcohol abuse
Pancreatitis
• Chronic pancreatitis
• Hereditary pancreatitis
Diabetes
Family history of pancreatic cancer
Genetic predisposition
• Peutz–Jeghers syndrome
• Li–Fraumeni syndrome
• Fanconi syndrome
• Familial adenomatous polyposis
• Lynch syndrome
• Gardner syndrome
• Multiple endocrine neoplasia
• BRCA1
• Von Hippel–Lindau syndrome

it is hypothesised that N-nitroso compounds in tobacco are carried to the pancreas in the blood. The time in which cigarette smoking exerts its negative influence is also subject to debate; however, observational studies seem to point towards the latter stages of carcinogenesis, particularly in the 15 years preceding development.

Diet and alcohol

Excessive body weight appears to increase the risk of pancreatic cancer. It has been shown that obesity has a positive association, with a relative risk of 1.72.[6] Diets high in saturated fat have a suggested contributing role in carcinogenesis,[6] although data are limited. Caffeine and meat preservatives have been suggested to have a negative association, but in recent years this has become more debated due to the studies having methodological flaws, and more recent studies demonstrating the opposite. Vitamin C, vitamin D and high-fibre diets have suggested protective associations with pancreatic neoplasm.[7–9]

The role of heavy alcohol consumption in the development of pancreatic cancer still remains controversial.

Occupation

Workers exposed to ionising radiation, insecticides, aluminium, nickel, acrylamide and halogenated hydrocarbons are reported to have an increased risk of developing pancreatic adenocarcinoma. There is evidence of increased risk in people exposed to chlorinated hydrocarbon solvents (metal degreasing workers and dry cleaners), and those working in the paint and varnish industry and the textiles industry.[10]

Past medical history

Chronic pancreatitis is a progressive inflammatory process with associated irreversible histological changes. It is highly linked to excessive alcohol consumption, with up to an 18-fold increase in risk of pancreatic cancer compared to the general population. Quantifying the risk is still difficult due to confounding factors such as smoking, alcohol and diet.[11]

Diabetes has a positive association for pancreatic cancer. Meta-analysis has shown that type 2 diabetes increases the risk of pancreatic cancer by 82%.[11] The high prevalence of diabetes in society excludes hyperglycaemia as a screening tool for pancreatic cancer.

Other conditions linked with pancreatic cancer include Gardner's syndrome, cystic fibrosis and multiple endocrine neoplasia type 1 (neuroendocrine cancers).

Hereditary pancreatic cancer

The accurate incidence of familial pancreatic cancer remains elusive, despite various reports of pancreatic cancer families.

✔✔ The ongoing National Familial Pancreas Tumour Registry estimates the risk of developing pancreatic neoplasm in an individual with two affected family member to be approximately 6.4-fold, increasing to 32-fold if three family members are affected.[12]

Pancreatic carcinogenesis has an established genetic predisposition. Familial conditions such as Peutz–Jeghers syndrome, germ-line mutation in the *STK11/LKB11* gene,[13] *BRCA2* expression[14] and familial atypical multiple mole melanoma (*p16/CDKN2A* germ-line mutation) may predispose to pancreatic cancer.[14] Links with hereditary non-polyposis colorectal cancer (Lynch syndrome), *BRCA1* and von Hippel–Lindau have been suggested but not confirmed, as conferring increased risk.[15] With the speed of developing technology, matched with reduced genetic diagnostic expense, one can foresee the potential for the discovery of further genes relating to familial pancreatic cancer.

Precursor lesions

Histologically distinct precursor lesions have been attributed to pancreatic carcinogenesis. Preneoplastic lesions are usually asymptomatic and can be incidentally discovered at the time of resection. They appear to follow a multi-step progression to invasive carcinoma.[15] These precursor lesions include pancreatic intraepithelial neoplasia (PanIN), intraductal papillary mucinous neoplasm (IPMN) and mucinous cystic neoplasm (MCN).[16] Because of their small size (usually <5 mm), they are difficult to detect, making them elusive to computerised tomography (CT) or magnetic resonance imaging (MRI).[15]

Pan-INs are the most frequent preneoplastic lesions, observed in approximately 82% of pancreas with neoplasm.[17] They are subclassified into PanIN-1, PanIN-2 and PanIN-3 depending upon the degree of cytological and architectural atypia.[17] Each of these precursor lesions harbours a unique repertoire of clinicopathological and genetic characteristics that has an impact on the natural history and prognosis of these lesions.

Workers in Johns Hopkins University proposed pancreatic intraepithelial neoplasms (PanIN; 1A→1B→2→3) as the precursor lesions to invasive carcinoma.[18] The model is analogous to that of ductal carcinoma in situ (DCIS) of the breast or adenomatous polyps in colorectal cancer. The lesions display atypical mucinous epithelium replacing the physiological cuboidal epithelium. The evidence for PanIN being a true premalignant state is largely circumstantial. These lesions were first described adjacent to resected adenocarcinoma. The more atypical PanIN-2 and -3 were seen exclusively in neoplastic pancreas. These lesions also display similar genetic aberrations to the frankly invasive samples. In particular, the percentage of p16 and K-ras mutations increases with the more atypical PanIN. These data have heralded development of a tumour genesis model involving sequential progression from PanIN-1a to invasive adenocarcinoma.[19]

Classically, evolution from precursor lesions to pancreatic neoplasm (ductal adenocarcinoma) involves diverse molecular changes (**Fig. 15.1**). Recent studies indentified at least 119 independent loci that may potentially play a role in tumour progression, including K-ras, TP53, p16/CDKN2A, MYC and AKT2.[20] The K-ras gene product mediates signal transduction in a number of growth factor receptors. K-ras single point mutation is observed in 90–95% of pancreatic ductal adenocarcinoma, representing the most common mutation in this disease.[21] K-ras is currently the focus of multiple ongoing studies to see if it can be utilised as a diagnostic tool.[13] Altered epidermal growth factor receptor expression (EGFR) causing overexpression is thought to be an early event in pancreatic carcinogenesis.[22]

Inactivation of numerous tumour suppressor genes, including p16/CDKN2A and TP53, plays a pivotal role in the development of pancreatic cancer. Loss of tumour suppression is noted in 70–95% of pancreatic neoplasm.[17] Other targets including transforming growth factor-β (TGF-β) receptor genes, BRCA2, HER-2/NEU, DPC4, MKK4 and EBER-1 are currently under investigation. The discussion about these genes is outside the scope of this chapter. However, the best chance for cure in the treatment of pancreatic cancer lies with detecting these non-invasive lesions before progression to invasive carcinoma.

Presentation

The majority of patients present with vague and non-specific symptoms (Box 15.2). As a result, the disease is commonly widespread at diagnosis, and approximately 80% of patients present with unresectable disease.

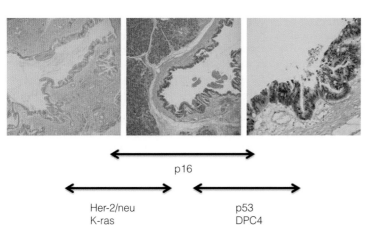

Figure 15.1 • Diagrammatic representation of the multi-step progression to invasive carcinoma from low-grade neoplasm on the left to high-grade on the right. Images courtesy of Dr Paul Crotty.

- Early satiety
- Obstructive jaundice (with or without pain)
- Unexplained weight loss
- Endoscopy negative epigastric/back pain
- Late-onset diabetes
- Signs of malabsorption without defined cause
- None

Tumours in the body and tail of the pancreas usually present late. Pain is the most consistent symptom. Painless jaundice is seen in 13% of patients while 34% present with only pain and 46% present with both pain and jaundice. Weight loss and anorexia are observed in 7% of patients. Rarely, tumour invasion into stomach or duodenum can present as haematemesis and malaena. Patients may also present with late-onset diabetes mellitus and acute pancreatitis.[23] Limited series have examined the screening of asymptomatic cohorts, with little evidence to support the introduction of population screening for pancreatic cancer.[14] However, there may be a place for targeted screening of high-risk groups in the near future.

The classical Courvoisier sign (palpable gallbladder in the presence of painless jaundice) occurs in less than 25% of patients. Jaundice may represent either primary disease causing biliary obstruction or external compression of the biliary system by metastatic nodal disease. Pain is a more common symptom than physicians usually appreciate, occurring due to the involvement of the visceral afferent nerves or relating to an induced local pancreatitis. Pain on initial presentation is synonymous with a higher incidence of unresectability. Weight loss is common, often associated with early satiety, nausea or vomiting. The latter symptom may be due to gastric outlet obstruction.

Virchow's node (left supraclavicular node associated with upper gastrointestinal (GI) malignancy), thrombophlebitis migrans (non-specific paraneoplastic sign named after Trousseau) and Sister Mary Joseph nodule (umbilical metastatic lesion via the falciform ligament) are well-described features of advanced disease. Hepatomegaly is seen in 65% of patients and may indicate liver metastases. Blumer's shelf (rectally palpable rectovesical or rectovaginal mass) rarely occurs and is not usually sought as part of routine examination.

The most useful aid in disease diagnosis is a high index of suspicion. Vague epigastric symptoms and weight loss in the presence of normal endoscopy and preliminary radiology should initiate further detailed investigation.

Investigation

Serology

Haematological and hepatic biochemical measurements are largely unhelpful in diagnosis. A mild normochromic anaemia may be present secondary to occult blood loss; thrombocytosis is also sometimes observed. Elevated serum bilirubin and alkaline phosphatase confirm obstructive jaundice; amylase and lipase may be elevated in patients presenting with pancreatitis (5%). A raised prothrombin time suggests hepatic dysfunction secondary to metastases. Hyperglycaemia is non-specific and occurs in approximately 20% of patients. This could be related to the fact that type 2 diabetes confers an increased risk for pancreatic cancer. Patients with malnutrition have hypoalbuminaemia and low cholesterol level.

Markers

There still remains no ideal tumour marker for pancreatic carcinoma. Carbohydrate antigen 19-9 (CA 19-9; 0–37 U/mL) exists in tissue as an epitope of sialylated Lewis a-type blood group antigen, and is the most widely utilised tumour marker. It was based on a monoclonal antibody to colorectal cancer cell lines. CA 19-9 is elevated in only approximately 50% of cases.[24] Among symptomatic patients, CA 19-9 has a sensitivity of 81–85% and specificity of 81–90%.[24] However, the positive predictive value remains low among the asymptomatic population, making it a very poor screening test. Falsely elevated CA 19-9 is documented in other neoplasms including gastric, colorectal, cholangiocarcinoma and urothelial malignancies, as well as benign conditions such as pancreatitis, hepatitis, thyroiditis and biliary obstruction. In addition patients expressing Lewis blood group antigens (a and b) may have elevated levels.[25] CA 19-9 may be used to assess recurrence of disease, with a level higher than 500 U/mL signifying advanced disease.[25] A level exceeding 243 U/mL for patients undergoing primary chemoradiotherapy for locoregionally advanced disease also indicates poorer median survival (7.1 vs. 12.3 months).[26]

Several other tumour markers are currently being investigated including carcinoembryonic antigen (CEA), K-ras, p53, CA242, CA50, SPAN-1, DU-PAN2, CAM-17.1 and a number of mucins (MUC1, MUC3, MUC4 and MUC5AC). They are proposed as having application in pancreatic neoplasms, although none of these markers are sensitive enough to be recommended for clinical use. CA242 shows promise as an independent prognostic factor.[27]

Diagnosis

Imaging studies

Transabdominal (TA) ultrasound (US) is the initial investigation in the jaundiced patient. It is noted for its superior sensitivity for determining cholelithiasis over CT. Common bile duct dilatation (>7 mm; >10 mm in post-cholecystectomy patients) is an indirect sign, together with pancreatic duct dilatation (>2 mm). The primary pancreatic lesion is often visible together with liver metastases and ascites if present. For lesions >3 cm TAUS has approximately 95% sensitivity; however, this is considerably lower for smaller lesions.[28] The main criticism of TAUS is machine quality difference and operator experience; thus it is user dependent.[29] The role of colour Doppler US has been suggested to examine portal vein or superior mesenteric involvement. Ultrasound remains a useful imaging modality for the initial screening of the jaundiced patient, but further radiological modalities are necessary to examine the pancreas and assess resectability.

CT remains the most common staging modality. Conventional CT has been replaced by more sensitive dynamic CT with thinner slice/cuts (1–3 mm) with multidetector and 3D reconstruction. The sensitivity is approximately 90% for lesions greater than 2 cm, decreasing to approximately 60% for smaller lesions.[30,31] CT allows for assessment of the primary lesion, its relationship to the remainder of the pancreas and peripancreatic vasculature, and determination of resectability (**Figs 15.2** and **15.3**). Direct evidence of a tumour is often seen as a hypodense mass, with other subtle signs such as pancreatic atrophy, deformity of the glandular contour or dilatation

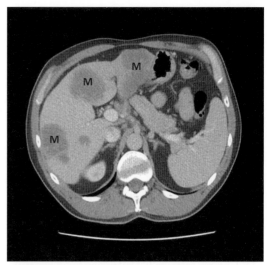

Figure 15.3 • CT scan showing multiple hepatic metastases (M) from pancreatic neoplasm.

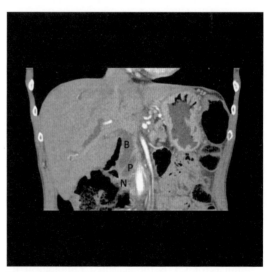

Figure 15.4 • CT scan of coronal view demonstrating biliary duct (B), pancreatic duct (P), obstruction by pancreatic neoplasm (N) denoting the double duct sign.

of the common bile and pancreatic ducts (**Fig. 15.4**). Metastatic lesions can be detected, and portal vein or superior mesenteric artery involvement can be determined.

✓✓ However, despite advances, CT imaging is limited at detecting small liver or peritoneal neoplastic deposits of occult disease.[31,32]

MRI is mainly used as an adjuvant to other imaging modalities for planning treatment options. The combination of T1/T2-weighted imaging with magnetic

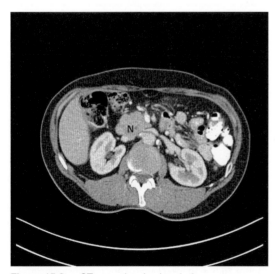

Figure 15.2 • CT scan showing head of pancreas neoplasm (N).

resonance cholangiopancreatography (MRCP) is useful to visualise the primary tumour and its relationship to the biliary and pancreatic ducts, as well as peripancreatic vasculature. MRI/MRCP is considered to be equivalent to CT for assessing primary disease.[33,34]

Positron emission tomography (PET) shows accumulation of [^{18}F]2-fluoro-2-deoxy-D-glucose (FDG) by tumour cells, and has the advantage of combining metabolic activity and imaging characteristics. PET-CT scanners are able to detect small pancreatic neoplasms up to 7 mm in diameter, and to diagnose metastatic disease in about 40%.[35] PET is becoming a more common method of measuring tumour response to treatment and may help predict prognosis. However, FDG-PET is not accurate in pancreatic disease due to its reliance on normal glucose haemostasis. The combination of PET-CT has a sensitivity of 92%, and is superior to either modality alone.[36,37]

Endoscopic retrograde cholangiopancreatography (ERCP) is reserved mainly to assess obstructive intraductal lesions and to relieve biliary obstruction in selected cases. MRCP has replaced ERCP as a diagnostic modality of choice.

Endoscopic ultrasound (EUS) is becoming more commonly used in staging pancreatic cancer. It provides high-quality images and is noted to be more sensitive than CT for detecting small pancreatic lesions. EUS is also accurate in determining cancer involvement of the portal or splenic vein.[38] It has similar efficacy to ERCP in defining small periampullary lesions. EUS may also help clarifying benign conditions mimicking cancer such as sclerosing pancreatitis or atypical choledocholithiasis. Fine-needle aspiration (FNA) of a lesion can be achieved with similar sensitivity and specificity to CT-guided FNA. However, the main drawbacks of EUS include cost, invasiveness and operator dependency.

Cytology/histology

Multidetector CT is the accepted radiological investigation of choice in the staging and diagnosis of pancreatic cancer. In selected cases, histological confirmation of neoplasm may not be established prior to resection. However, in patients selected for neoadjuvant treatment, histological confirmation is essential via FNA by EUS/ERCP or percutaneously by CT guidance.

Advanced staging techniques

Laparoscopy

Despite advances in non-invasive imaging, laparoscopic staging and ultrasound have a role in selected cases.[38,39] Laparoscopy can be performed immediately before conversion to laparotomy[40,41] or as an interval staging measure.[42]

The role of staging laparoscopy is dependent on institution protocol, and there still exists some considerable controversy regarding its use. Its aim is to identify radiographically occult metastatic disease via a minimally invasive approach to prevent non-therapeutic laparotomies. Laparoscopic examination allows for direct visualisation of intra-abdominal organs. It has been shown to be very sensitive in detecting small metastatic deposits <3 mm on peritoneal and hepatic structures[43] (**Figs 15.5** and **15.6**). The added value of laparoscopy over state-of-the-art dynamic multislice CT remains up to 20%.[42]

Those who oppose minimal access staging suggest that a significant proportion of patients require surgical bypass and therefore laparoscopic staging should only be used if this would not be contemplated at laparotomy.[43] Single-centre studies suggest that the need for subsequent operative palliation is less than 5%.[44]

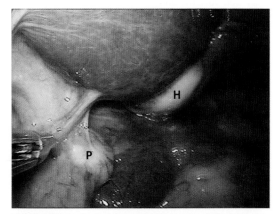

Figure 15.5 • Staging laparoscopy demonstrating hepatic metastatic deposit (H) and peritoneal metastatic deposit (P).

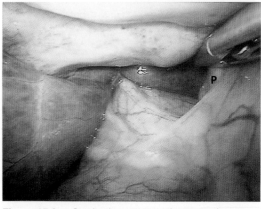

Figure 15.6 • Staging laparoscopy demonstrating a peritoneal deposit (P).

✓✓ However, two randomised prospective studies have reported that approximately 20% of patients who had been randomised not to have prophylactic gastroenterostomy at the time of their initial surgery required subsequent operative intervention for duodenal obstruction.[45,46]

General laparoscopy is performed with an angled (usually 30°) lens looking for small-volume peritoneal and liver metastases. The liver is examined systematically and usually all but segment 7 can be viewed. Biopsy of hepatic or peritoneal deposits for frozen section histology is taken, and the procedure is terminated if positive. If metastases are not seen, the hepaticoduodenal ligament is inspected for nodal disease. The lesser sac is opened by incising the gastrocolic omentum to inspect for tumour, and biopsies of the primary may be performed. This is achievable in approximately 80%. In certain centres, mobilisation of the duodenum is performed, but in the majority of cases this is unnecessary. With more efficacious neoadjuvant therapies, it is important to use laparoscopic strategies to define patients who may be suitable for downstaging similar to advanced rectal lesions.

✓✓ Laparoscopic ultrasound (LUS) has been utilised as an additional aid to detect intrahepatic metastases, lymph node or vascular involvement to determine resectability[40,47] (**Fig. 15.7**). However, the added value is less than 10% and therefore LUS should only be used in selective cases in which there is considerable concern of vascular invasion.

Peritoneal cytology taken at the time of laparoscopic staging may also improve the accuracy of laparoscopic staging. In a prospective study of 150 consecutive patients with pancreatic carcinoma, unexpected metastases were found in 5–10%.[48] Positive cytology is associated with advanced disease; it predicts unresectability of pancreatic adenocarcinoma and a decreased survival. As both radiological and endoscopic imaging will continue to advance, staging laparoscopy and LUS will have a selective role, especially in cases of equivocal findings.

Pathology

Ductal adenocarcinomas account for >85% of all pancreatic neoplasms.

Other types of malignant tumours include the following:

- adenosquamous carcinoma;
- mucinous non-cystic (colloid) carcinoma;
- mucinous cystic neoplasms;
- intraductal papillary mucinous neoplasm with an associated invasive carcinoma;
- solid pseudopapillary neoplasm;
- acinar cell carcinoma;
- pancreatoblastoma;
- serous cystadenocarcinoma;
- undifferentiated (anaplastic) carcinoma;
- signet-ring cell carcinoma;
- giant cell carcinoma.

Treatment

Treatment options should be discussed at a multidisciplinary level, with emphasis on established guidelines. The American Joint Committee on Cancer TMN staging is outlined in Table 15.1. **Figure 15.8** outlines our current treatment algorithm for patients with pancreatic cancer.

Resection

Surgical treatment remains the only potential cure for pancreatic cancer, yet patient selection remains key.

If jaundice is present, then the controversy is whether preoperative biliary decompression should be undertaken. Evidence suggests an increased risk of perioperative sepsis, pancreatic fistula and wound infection.[49,50] However, a recent meta-analysis questioned these previous findings.[51] The authors' practice is not to decompress the bile duct preoperatively, unless symptoms and signs of cholangitis or secondary signs of hyperbilirubinaemia are present. If a neoadjuvant approach is being considered, biliary stenting is required prior to commencing chemo/radiotherapy. Coagulopathy, if present, is treated with vitamin K prior to resection.

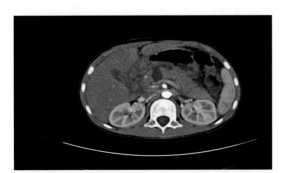

Figure 15.7 • Laparoscopic ultrasound showing head of pancreas cystic mass with multiple septations and solid nodule.

Table 15.1 • American Joint Committee on Cancer TNM staging, 2010

Tumour (T)	Node (N)	Metastasis (M)
Tx: Primary tumour cannot be assessed	Nx: Regional lymph nodes cannot be assesed	
T0: No evidence of primary tumour	N0: no regional nodes	M0: no metastases
Tis: Carcinoma in situ		
T1: <2 cm within pancreas	N1: Regional lymph node metastasis	M1: spread to distant organs or non-regional nodes (e.g. aortocaval)
T2: >2 cm within pancreas		
T3: Tumour extends beyond the pancreas but without involvement of the coeliac axis or the SMA		
T4: Tumour involves the coeliac axis or the SMA (unresectable primary tumour)		
Stage 0: Tis, N0, M0		
Stage IA: T1, N0, M0		
Stage IB: T2, N0, M0		
Stage IIA: T3, N0, M0		
Stage IIB: T1, N1, M0/T2, N1, M0/T3, N1, M0		
Stage III: T4, Any N, M0		
Stage IV: Any T, Any N, M1		

Used with the permission of the American Joint Committee on Cancer (AJCC), Chicago, Illinois. The original source for this material is the AJCC Cancer Staging Manual, Seventh Edition (2010) published by Springer Science and Business Media LLC, www.springer.com

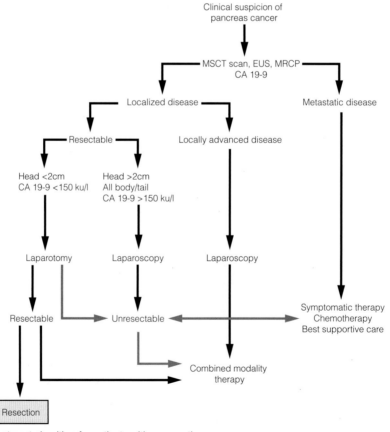

Figure 15.8 • Treatment algorithm for patients with pancreatic cancer.

Patient selection is paramount, including cardio-vascular and respiratory evaluation. Surgery with curative intent is associated with a median survival of 11–23 months, with approximately 10–18% alive at 5 years.[52] Previously, pancreatic resections were associated with significant mortality; however, with advances in perioperative supportive care, mortality rates have now been reduced to less than 5% in high-volume centres.[53]

Pancreatico-duodenectomy

Kausch first described pancreatico-duodenectomy in 1912, later popularised by Whipple in 1935. The classical Whipple procedure (two-stage) was an en-bloc resection of the pancreatic head, duodenum, common bile duct, with the distal stomach and surrounding lymph nodes. Later being preformed as a one-stage operation, it still remains the mainstay of surgical therapy for tumours of the pancreatic head and neck.

The right colon is mobilised, exposing the third and fourth parts of the duodenum, and an extended Kocherisation is performed. This allows a tumour in the head of the pancreas to be palpated and views of the left renal vein. The aortocaval and portal vein (PV) nodal packages are dissected and the respective vessels are skeletonised. Resectability is finally assessed as extensive involvement of the confluence of the PV/superior mesenteric vein (SMV) may herald termination of the procedure. It is important to remember that short segments of the PV can be resected if necessary, and therefore an involved PV does not necessarily denote unresectability.

The remaining porta hepatis is dissected, and nodes are cleared. Cholecystectomy facilitates higher ligation of the bile duct, which is transected just proximal to the insertion of the cystic duct. It is our practice to send a biliary aspirate for routine culture and sensitivity as postoperative infective complications tend to involve enteric organisms.[54]

The common bile duct is mobilised distally and the hepaticoduodenal ligament is dissected along its length, taking care to identify and preserve the common hepatic artery and PV. The gastroduodenal artery is ligated while care is taken not to damage an aberrant right hepatic artery.

In a conventional Whipple, the distal stomach is resected. This is the authors' favoured approach as resection includes the nodes along the greater and lesser curves, reduces stomach-emptying dysfunction postoperatively, diminishes the density of parietal cells and theoretically reduces the risk of gastritis. The stomach is transected at the antrum along with the attached omentum. The proximal jejunum along with its mesentery is transected and the mobilised duodenum and jejunum is delivered back under the ligament of Treitz.

The pancreas is transected between four stay sutures (to facilitate haemostasis in the marginal arteries) after the uncinate process is dissected from the superior mesenteric vessels. Retroperitoneal dissection allows the tumour and nodal package to be delivered en bloc. If any doubt exists regarding the adequacy of tumour clearance, the pancreatic resection margin should be sent for frozen section histology.

 Verbeke and Menon have shown that a discrepancy between margin status and clinical outcome is due to frequent under-reporting of microscopic margin involvement. The lack of a standardised pathological examination, with confusing nomenclature and controversy regarding the definition of microscopic margin involvement, results in a wide variation of reported R1 rates (between 0% and 83%).[55]

Reconstruction is undertaken with the biliary anastomosis followed by the pancreatic and finally the gastric. The most significant cause of morbidity is the development of pancreatic fistula, observed in up to 10–20% of cases.[56]

Pancreatico-jejunostomy and pancreatico-gastrostomy are the most commonly employed techniques for pancreatico-enteric reconstruction. These suggest a marginal decrease in fistula rates with the former, although differences are not clinically significant and have not induced a change in operative strategy, with jejunal reconstruction still favoured.[57]

The nature of the pancreatic reconstruction is subject to individual variation. The authors favour a two-layered pancreatico-jejunal anastomosis with mucosa-to-mucosa reconstruction. Choledocho-jejunostomy is performed in a similar manner (end to side), leaving the gastro-jejunostomy until the end.

 Abdominal drains are not placed routinely.[58]

Morbidity following resection varies, with the majority of complications being minor; however, pancreatic fistula can occur in 10–20% of cases. Most complications can be dealt with either conservatively or using drains placed by interventional radiology. Less than 5% of cases require re-operation.

Pylorus-preserving pancreatico-duodenectomy (PPPDR)

Many centres recommend a PPPDR approach, first described by Watson in 1942. It is believed to retain a functioning pylorus with an intact neurovascular supply, thus ensuring good gastrointestinal function and diminishing nutritive, dumping and bile reflux sequelae.[59] Both pancreatico-duodenectomy and PPPDR have similar perioperative adverse events; however, in overall analysis PPPDR has decreased operating times, fewer blood transfusions, lower mortality and improved long-term patient survival.[59] Detractors of PPPDR point to delayed gastric emptying as a potential cause for concern with this procedure.[60]

The procedure dictates conventional mobilisation up to where the stomach requires transection. In PPPDR the right gastric artery is preserved and the duodenum is transected at least 2 cm distal to the pylorus. Reconstruction is usually accomplished by duodeno-jejunostomy or gastro-jejunostomy.

Extended lymph node and vascular dissection

It is the authors' practice to perform extended dissection including aortocaval nodal clearance in the majority of cases. At presentation, most tumours have involvement of lymph nodes beyond the gland. Ishikawa et al. demonstrated increased median (but not long-term) survival following extended lymph node dissection.[61] However, outside of Japan, findings of increased survival have not been validated. Studies have failed to demonstrate increased morbidity that one would expect with a radical operation, although in our experience there is invariably increased ascites in those who undergo extended lymphadenectomy. We believe that clearance of the left gastric and aortocaval nodes increases the specificity of staging and therefore predicted prognosis, and increases the likelihood of a negative surgical margin, although this remains controversial.

The role of extensive vascular resection has been proposed in certain cases. Pancreatico-duodenectomy with major vascular resection had been reported in recent years with acceptable outcomes, despite the increased challenging nature. Survival benefits are slight, and require further investigation.[62]

Distal pancreatectomy

Distal pancreatectomy is the procedure of choice for tumours of the body and tail of the pancreas. The pancreatic neck is dissected from the portal vein and the splenic flexure of the colon is taken down. In the majority of ductal cancers, the spleen is also resected in order to achieve an en-bloc clearance. Splenic preservation is generally limited to patients with benign or borderline neoplasms. Patients undergoing distal pancreatectomy and splenic resection are vaccinated prophylactically preoperatively against encapsulated organisms such as *Haemophilus influenzae* B, meningococcus C and pneumococcus.

Laparoscopic pancreatectomy

Laparoscopic pancreatectomy remains one of the most challenging laparoscopic abdominal operations, and hence case series have low numbers. Two centres have shown total laparoscopic pancreatico-duodenectomy to be safe and feasible, with comparable results to the open approach.[63,64] However, laparoscopic distal pancreatic resection is currently the most frequently performed laparoscopic pancreatic operation. It is associated with a higher likelihood of splenic preservation, increased operative time, decreased blood loss and decreased length of stay.[63] With the further development of robot-assisted surgery, minimally invasive pancreatico-duodenectomy is likely to become more common.

Total pancreatectomy

Some suggest that pancreatic cancer is a multicentric disease and therefore advocate total pancreatectomy. Total pancreatectomy for neoplasm was initially proposed to avoid the risk of pancreatico-enteric leaks and to remove potential undetectable synchronous disease in other parts of the gland. Although total pancreatectomy can be carried out safely, the survival benefit is so dismal it questions the indication for the operation.

Central pancreatectomy

The role of central pancreatectomy (CP) is rare and limited due to a low spectrum of indications. The surgery is historically reserved for chronic pancreatitis and traumatic injuries. More recently, it has been advocated for use in lesions of the pancreatic neck. Critics of its role cite higher rates of pancreatic anastomotic leakage. However, CP offers preserved functional elements (endocrine and exocrine) of the pancreas.[65]

Surgical palliation

Obstructive jaundice

In the majority of patients, biliary obstruction can be adequately relieved by endoscopic measures. However, in selected cases surgical palliation may be required. Cholecysto-jejunostomy may be performed in cases where the cystic duct is patent and the tumour is not within 1 cm of the cystic duct. Alternatively, choledocho-jejunostomy may be used, which has been shown to be equivalent.

Upper GI tract outflow obstruction

Gastric and duodenal outlet obstruction is said to occur in up to 20% of patients. Once jaundice has been addressed, persistent nausea and vomiting should alert the attending physician that upper

GI obstruction is present. If biliary obstruction is being dealt with at open operation, prophylactic duodenal bypass should be considered. Minimal access laparoscopic gastro-jejunostomy is becoming the management of choice when warranted. Luminal endoscopic stent placement is associated with more favourable short-term results, whereas gastro-jejunostomy may be a better treatment option in patients with a predicted more prolonged survival.

Adjuvant therapies

✓✓ Despite surgery with curative intent, the 5-year survival rates remain low. There is evidence to support the use of adjuvant chemotherapy after resection. Randomised controlled trials including ESPAC-3 and CONKO-001 show an overall trend towards increased survival.[66,67]

Gemcitabine is becoming more favoured than 5-fluorouracil (5-FU) because its safety profile is better with similar efficacy.[68]

The role of adjuvant chemoradiation is less well defined, with conflicting outcomes from the trials. The Gastrointestinal Study Group (GITSG) showed a survival with 5-FU and radiotherapy, but the study size (n=43) was criticised.[69] The European Organization of Research and Treatment of Cancer (EORTC) trial showed no statistical survival benefit for those treated with adjuvant chemoradiation compared with an observation group.[70] More recently, the Johns Hopkins–Mayo Clinic Collaborative study demonstrated that chemoradiation post pancreatico-duodenectomy was associated with improved survival.[71]

Despite the role of adjuvant therapy, survival remains poor, with the need to discover more efficacious treatment and further studies to elucidate the optimum therapy protocol, with consideration of timing and the need for more individualised treatment regimens.

Neoadjuvant therapy

In recent years, many centres support the role of neoadjuvant therapy in the treatment of pancreatic cancer. Theoretical advantages include the delivery of chemotherapy or radiotherapy to well-oxygenated tissue, and hence early treatment of micrometastatic disease. Neoadjuvant therapy may help to identify patients who have more aggressive disease, and therefore would not be ideal surgical candidates. There is speculation that neoadjuvant chemoradiation decreases the risk of pancreatic leaks and makes pancreatic reconstruction easier.[72] Detractors of neoadjuvant therapy claim that the delay in surgery may allow local disease to progress; however, this is difficult to prove. It has been suggested recently that neoadjuvant treatment should be targeted at patients with borderline pancreatic cancer with the aim to downstage the disease, allowing for resection at later date, with evidence of improved survival rates.[72,73]

Future areas of interest

The last decade has seen considerable improvements in diagnosis, as well as advances in minimally invasive and endoscopic management of pancreatic cancer. Biological agents like erlotinib (epidermal growth factor receptor inhibitor), cetuximab, bevacizumab and axitinib are currently being investigated for their role in the treatment of pancreatic cancer. Unfortunately, so far none have shown a significant survival benefit.

Despite recent radiological developments, there remains a limited ability to detect pancreatic cancer at an early stage. Therefore, an emphasis on better understanding of cancer genetics, predisposing factors and the role of tumour markers in aiding the diagnosis is crucial. Further trials will help utilise neoadjuvant or adjuvant therapy in appropriate cases. Surgical techniques, especially oncological dissection methods, will need to be standardised to ensure stricter quality control and better data comparison.

Key points

- Prognosis remains poor since the majority of patients present with advanced unresectable disease.
- Multidetector row CT is the radiological staging modality of choice.
- Laparoscopic staging has a role in selected patients.
- Resectional surgery is associated with <5% mortality and 30–50% morbidity rates.
- The majority of patients re-occur with distal disease, hence the need for novel neoadjuvant treatments.

References

1. Jemal A, Siegel R, Xu J, et al. Cancer statistics 2010. CA Cancer J Clin 2010;60:277–300.

2. American Cancer Society. Cancer facts and figures 2011. Available online: http://www.cancer.org/research/cancerfactsfigures/cancerfactsfigures/cancer-facts-figures-2011.

3. Cancer Research UK. Cancer statistics. London: CRUK; 2008.

4. Holly EA, Chaliha I, Bracci PM, et al. Signs and symptoms of pancreatic cancer: a population based control study in the San Francisco Bay area. Clin Gastroenterol Hepatol 2004;2:510–7.

5. Iodice S, Gandini S, Maisonneuve P, et al. Tobacco and the risk of pancreatic cancer: a review and meta-analysis. Langenbecks Arch Surg 2008;393(4):535–45.

6. Michaud DS, Giovannucci E, Willett WC, et al. Physical activity, obesity, height, and the risk of pancreatic cancer. JAMA 2001;286:921–9.

7. Dong J, Zou J, Yu XF. Coffee drinking and pancreatic cancer risk: a meta-analysis of cohort studies. World J Gastroenterol 2011;17(9):1204–10.

8. Bulathsinghala P, Syrigos KN, Saif MW. Role of vitamin D in the prevention of pancreatic cancer. J Nutr Metab 2010;721365.

9. Olsen GW, Mandel JS, Gibson RW, et al. A case control study of pancreatic cancer and cigarettes, alcohol, coffee and diet. Am J Public Health 1989;79:1016–9.

10. Ojajarvi IA, Partanen TJ, Ahlbom A, et al. Occupational exposures and pancreatic cancer: a meta-analysis. Occup Environ Med 2000;57:316–24.

11. Hurley R, Ansary-Moghaddam A, Berrington de Gonazalez A, et al. Type II diabetes and pancreatic cancer: a meta-analysis of 36 studies. Br J Cancer 2005;92:2076–83.

12. Hruban RH, Canto M, Goggins M, et al. Update on familial pancreatic cancer. Adv Surg 2010;44:293–311.

13. Hemminski A, Markie D, Tomlinson I, et al. A serine/threonine kinase gene defective in Peutz–Jegers syndrome. Nature 1998;391:184–7.

14. Ozcelik H, Schmocker B, Di Nicola N, et al. Germline BRCA2 6174delT mutations in Ashkenazi Jewish pancreatic cancer patients. Nat Genet 1997;16:17–8.

15. Koorstra JB, Hustinx SR, Offerhaus GJ, et al. Pancreatic carcinogenesis. Pancreatology 2008;8:110–25.

16. Maitra A, Fukushima N, Takarori K, et al. Precursors to invasive pancreatic cancer. Adv Anat Pathol 2005;12:81–91.

17. Hruban RH, Maitra A, Goggins M. Update on pancreatic intra-epithelial neoplasia. Int J Clin Exp Pathol 2008;1:306–16.

18. Singh M, Maitra A. Precursor lesions of pancreatic cancer: molecular pathology and clinical implications. Pancreatology 2007;7:9–19.

19. Cubilla AL, Fitzgerald PJ. Morphological lesions associated with human primary invasive non-endocrine pancreas cancer. Cancer Res 1976;36:2690–8.

20. Aguirre AJ, Brennan C, Bailey G, et al. High resolution characterization of pancreatic adenocarcinoma genome. Proc Natl Acad Sci U S A 2004;101:9067–72.

21. Delpu Y, Hanoun N, Lulka H, et al. Genetic and epigenetic alterations in pancreatic carcinogenesis. Curr Genomics 2011;12(1):15–24.

22. Ozaki N, Ohmuraya M, Hirota M, et al. Serine protease inhibitor Kazal type 1 promotes proliferation of pancreatic cancer cells through epidermal growth factor receptor. Mol Cancer Res 2009;7:1572–81.

23. Gullo L, Tomassetti P, Migliori M, et al. Do early symptoms of pancreatic cancer exist that can allow an earlier diagnosis? Pancreas 2001;22:210–3.

24. Goonetilleke KS, Siriwardena AK. Systematic review of carbohydrate antigen (CA19-9) as a biochemical marker in the diagnosis of pancreatic cancer. Eur J Surg Oncol 2007;33:266–70.

25. Safi F, Schlosser W, Kolb G, et al. Diagnostic value of CA 19-9 in patients with pancreatic cancer and nonspecific gastrointestinal symptoms. J Gastrointest Surg 1997;1:106–12.

26. Micke O, Bruns F, Kurowski R, et al. Predictive value of carbohydrate antigen 19-9 in pancreatic cancer treated with radiochemotherapy. Int J Radiat Oncol Biol Phys 2003;57:90–7.

27. Moossa AR, Gamagami RA. Diagnosis and staging of pancreatic neoplasms. Surg Clin North Am 1995;75:871–90.

28. Gandolfi L, Torresan F, Solmi L, et al. The role of ultrasound in biliary and pancreatic disease. Eur J Ultrasound 2003;16:141–59.

29. Karlson BM, Ekbom A, Lindgren PG, et al. Abdominal US for diagnosis of pancreatic tumor: prospective cohort analysis. Radiology 1999;213:107–11.

30. Barreiro CJ, Lillemoe KD, Koniaris LG. Diagnostic laparoscopy for peri-ampullary and pancreatic cancer. What is the true benefit? J Gastrointest Surg 2002;6:75–81.

31. Valls C, Andia E, Sanchez A. Dual phase helical CT of pancreatic adenocarcinoma assessment of resectability before surgery. AJR Am J Roentgenol 2002;178:821–6.

32. Katz MH, Savides TJ, Moossa AR, et al. An evidence-based approach to the diagnosis and staging of pancreatic cancer. Pancreatology 2005;5(6):576–90.

33. Schima W, Függer R, Schober E, et al. Diagnosis and staging of pancreatic cancer: comparison of mangafodipir trisodium-enhanced MR imaging and contrast-enhanced helical hydro-CT. AJR Am J Roentgenol 2002;179:717–24.

34. Park HS, Lee JM, Choi HK, et al. Pre-operative evaluation of pancreatic cancer; comparison of gadolinium enhanced dynamic MRI with MRCP versus MDCT. J Magn Reson Imaging 2009;30:586–95.

35. Maemura K, Takao S, Shinchi H, et al. Role of positron emission tomography in decisions on treatment strategies for pancreatic cancer. J Hepatobiliary Pancreat Surg 2006;13:435–41.

36. Wakabayashi H, Nishiyama Y, Otani T, et al. Role of ^{18}F-fluorodeoxyglucose positron emission tomography imaging in surgery for pancreatic cancer. World J Gastroenterol 2008;14:64–9.

37. DeWitt J, Devereaux B, Chriswell M, et al. Comparison of endoscopic ultrasonography and multidetector computed tomography for detecting and staging pancreatic cancer. Ann Intern Med 2004;141:753–63.

38. van Dijkum EJ, de Wit LT, van Delden OM, et al. Staging laparoscopy and laparoscopic ultrasonography in more than 400 patients with upper gastrointestinal carcinoma. J Am Coll Surg 1999;189:459–65.

39. Pisters PW, Lee JE, Vauthey JN, et al. Laparoscopy in the staging of pancreatic cancer. Br Surg 2001;88:325–37.

40. White R, Winston C, Gonen M, et al. Current utility of staging laparoscopy for pancreatic and peripancreatic neoplasm. J Am Coll Surg 2008;206:445–50.

41. Holzman MD, Reintgen KL, Tyler DS, et al. The role of laparoscopy in the management of suspected pancreatic and periampullary malignancies. J Gastrointest Surg 1997;1:236–44.

42. Jimenez RE, Warshaw AL, Rattner DW, et al. Impact of laparoscopic staging in the treatment of pancreatic cancer. Arch Surg 2000;135:409–15.

43. Conlon KC, Dougherty E, Klimstra DS, et al. The value of minimal access surgery in the staging of patients with potentially resectable peripancreatic malignancy. Ann Surg 1996;223(2):134–40.

44. Espat NJ, Brennan MF, Conlon KC. Patients with laparoscopically staged unresectable pancreatic adenocarcinoma do not require subsequent surgical biliary or gastric bypass. J Am Coll Surg 1999;188:649–57.

45. Jeurnink SM, Eijck C, Steyerberg EW, et al. Stent versus gastrojejunostomy for the palliation of gastric outlet obstruction: a systematic review. BMC Gastroenterol 2007;7:18.

46. Lillemoe KD, Cameron JL, Hardacre JM, et al. Is prophylactic gastrojejunostomy indicated for unresectable periampullary cancer? A prospective randomized trial. Ann Surg 1999;230:322–30.
Two key papers arguing the role for and against prophylactic gastroenterostomy in palliation of pancreatic cancer.

47. Barabino M, Santambrogio R, Ceretti AP, et al. Is there still a role for laparoscopy combined with ultrasonography in the staging of pancreatic cancer. Surg Endosc 2011;25:160–5.

48. Schmidt J, Fraunhofer S, Fleisch M, et al. Is peritoneal cytology a predictor of unresectability in pancreatic carcinoma? Hepatogastroenterology 2004;51(60):1827–31.

49. Pisters PW, Hudec WA, Hess KR, et al. Effect of preoperative biliary decompression on pancreaticoduodenectomy-associated morbidity in 300 consecutive patients. Ann Surg 2001;234:47–55.

50. van der Gaag NA, Kloek JJ, de Castro SM, et al. Preoperative biliary drainage in patients with obstructive jaundice: history and current status. J Gastrointest Surg 2009;13:814–20.

51. Wang Q, Gurusamy KS, Lin H, et al. Preoperative biliary drainage for obstructive jaundice. Cochrane Database Syst Rev 2008;CD005444.

52. Katz MH, Wang H, Fleming JB, et al. Long-term survival after multidisciplinary management of resected pancreatic adenocarcinoma. Ann Surg Oncol 2009;16:836–47.

53. McPhee JT, Hill JS, Whalen GF, et al. Perioperative mortality for pancreatectomy: a national perspective. Ann Surg 2007;246:246–53.

54. Povoski SP, Karpeh MS, Conlon KC, et al. Pre-operative biliary drainage: impact on intraoperative bile cultures and infectious morbidity after pancreaticoduodenectomy. J Gastrointest Surg 1999;3(5):496–505.

55. Verbeke CS, Menon KV. Redefining resection margin status in pancreatic cancer. HPB (Oxford) 2009;11(4):282–9.

56. Stojadinovic A, Brooks A, Hoos A, et al. An evidence-based approach to the surgical management of resectable pancreatic adenocarcinoma. Am Coll Surg 2003;196(6):954–64.

57. Yeo CJ, Cameron JL, Maher MM, et al. A prospective randomized trial of pancreatico-gastrostomy versus pancreatico-jejunostomy after pancreaticoduodenectomy. Ann Surg 1995;222:580–92.

58. Conlon KC, Labow D, Leung D, et al. Prospective randomized clinical trial of the value of intraperitoneal drainage after pancreatic resection. Ann Surg 2001;234:487–94.

59. Wenger FA, Jacobi CA, Haubold K, et al. Gastrointestinal quality of life after duodenopancreatectomy in pancreatic carcinoma. Preliminary results of a prospective randomized study: pancreatoduodenectomy or pylorus-preserving pancreatoduodenectomy. Chirurg 1999;7:1454–9.

60. Cooperman AM, Kini S, Snady H, et al. Current surgical therapy for carcinoma of the pancreas. J Clin Gastroenterol 2000;31:107–13.

61. Ishikawa O, Ohigashi H, Sasaki Y, et al. Adjuvant therapies in extended pancreatectomy for ductal adenocarcinoma of the pancreas. Hepatogastroenterology 1998;45:644–50.

62. Al-Haddad M, Martin JK, Nguyen J, et al. Vascular resection and reconstruction for pancreatic malignancy: a single center survival study. J Gastrointest Surg 2007;11:1168–74.

63. Kendrick ML, Cusati D. Total laparoscopic pancreaticoduodenectomy: feasibility and outcome in an early experience. Arch Surg 2010;145:19–23.

64. Palanivelu C, Jani K, Senthilnathan P, et al. Laparoscopic pancreaticoduodenectomy: technique and outcomes. J Am Coll Surg 2007;205:222–30.

65. Christein JD, Smoot RL, Farnell MB. Central pancreatectomy: a technique for the resection of pancreatic neck lesions. Arch Surg 2006;141:293–9.

66. Oettle H. Adjuvant chemotherapy with gemcitabine vs observation in patients undergoing curative-intent resection of pancreatic cancer. JAMA 2007;297:267–77.

67. Neoptolemos J, Büchler M, Stocken DD, et al. ESPAC-3(v2): a multicenter, international, open-label, randomized, controlled phase III trial of adjuvant 5-fluorouracil/folinic acid (5-FU/FA) versus gemcitabine (GEM) in patients with resected pancreatic ductal adenocarcinoma. J Clin Oncol 2009;27(Suppl. 18)Abstract.

68. Regine WF, Winter KA, Abrams RA, et al. Fluorouracil vs gemcitabine chemotherapy before and after fluorouracil-based chemoradiation following resection of pancreatic adenocarcinoma: a randomized controlled trial. JAMA 2008;299:1019–26.

69. Neoptolemos JP, Stocken DD, Friess H, et al. A randomized trial of chemoradiotherapy and chemotherapy after resection of pancreatic cancer. N Engl J Med 2004;350(12):1200–10.

70. Klinkenbijl JH, et al. Adjuvant radiotherapy and 5-fluorouracil after curative resection of cancer of the pancreas and periampullary region: phase III trial of the EORTC gastrointestinal tract cancer cooperative group. Ann Surg 1999;230(6):776–82.

71. Hsu CC, Herman JM, Corsini MM, et al. Adjuvant chemoradiation and chemotherapy for pancreatic adenocarcinoma: the Johns Hopkins–Mayo Clinic collaborative study. Ann Surg Oncol 2010;17(4):981–90.

72. Katz MH, Fleming JB, Lee JE, et al. Current status of adjuvant therapy for pancreatic cancer. Oncologist 2010;15:1205–13.

73. Callery MP, Chang KJ, Fishman EK, et al. Pretreatment assessment of resectable and borderline resectable pancreatic cancer: expert consensus statement. Ann Surg Oncol 2009;16:1727–33.

16

Cystic and neuroendocrine tumours of the pancreas

Saxon Connor

Introduction

Although pancreatic ductal adenocarcinoma accounts for the majority of patients with neoplastic disease of the pancreas, over the last two decades there has been an increasing recognition of cystic and neuroendocrine pancreatic neoplasms.[1] The aim of this chapter is to examine these tumours in more detail, with particular emphasis on intraductal papillary mucinous neoplasms (IPMNs) and pancreatic neuroendocrine tumours (NETs). Where possible, evidence-based recommendations for the investigation and management of these tumours will be provided.

Intraductal papillary mucinous neoplasms

IPMNs have only been recognised as separate entities to ductal adenocarcinoma of the pancreas since 1982,[2] subsequent to which the World Health Organisation clarified their definition.[3] They are defined as a grossly visible, mucin-producing epithelial neoplasm of the pancreas, which arises from within the main pancreatic duct (main-duct IPMN) or one of its branches (branch-duct IPMN), and most often but not always has a papillary architecture. They are distinguished from mucinous cystic neoplasms (MCNs) by the absence of ovarian-type stroma.[4]

The incidence (95% confidence interval) is estimated at 2.04 (1.28–2.80) per 100 000 population; however, this increases significantly after the sixth decade.[5] The precise aetiology remains unknown,

although an association with extrapancreatic primaries (10%), most commonly colorectal, breast and prostate, has been reported, but this is not significantly different to that seen with primary pancreatic adenocarcinoma.[6] IPMN has also been shown to be a predictor of pancreatic cancer as compared to other intra-abdominal pathologies, with an odds ratio of 7.18.[7]

Clinical presentation

IPMNs most commonly present with symptoms related to pancreatic duct obstruction. The Johns Hopkins group reported their experience comparing the presentation and demographics to those patients presenting with pancreatic adenocarcinoma.[8,9] Although the mean age of presentation was similar to that of pancreatic adenocarcinoma (seventh decade), the clinical presentation was significantly different. Of the 60 patients with IPMNs, 59% presented with abdominal pain but only 16% presented with obstructive jaundice, compared to 38% and 74% of patients with pancreatic adenocarcinoma, respectively.[8] This is in spite of the fact that only five of the 60 patients with IPMNs had tumours within the body or tail.[8] In addition, those with IPMNs were more likely to have been smokers and 14% had suffered previous attacks of acute pancreatitis (compared to 3% of those with pancreatic ductal adenocarcinoma).[8] Weight loss was a prominent factor reported in 29% of patients with IPMNs.[9] Symptoms associated with invasive malignancy included the presence of jaundice, weight loss, vomiting[9] and diabetes.[10] Patients with invasive IPMNs were a mean of 5 years older (68 vs. 63 years) compared to those with non-invasive IPMNs.[9] This led the authors to conclude that IPMN was a slow-growing tumour with a significant latency to develop invasive disease.[9] Increasingly, an important presentation is the incidental finding due to cross-sectional imaging for other medical indications. IPMN was the final diagnosis in 36% of pancreatic 'incidentalomas' that underwent pancreatico-duodenectomy.[11]

Investigation

Computed tomography (CT) and magnetic resonance imaging (MRI) form the mainstay of non-invasive radiological imaging of suspected IPMN. The classical features of main-duct IPMN are of a grossly dilated main pancreatic duct (**Fig. 16.1**), while branch-type IPMN can present with small cystic lesions that may appear in a 'grape-like' configuration.[12] Although MRI and CT have been shown to identify accurately tumour location and communication with the pancreatic duct, the detection of invasive malignancy remains problematic.[13–15] Radiological features associated with malignancy include the presence of a solid mass, biliary dilatation >15 mm and increasing size of either the tumour for branch-type IPMN (growth rate >2 mm/year)[16] or main pancreatic duct diameter for main-duct IPMN.[15] ^{18}F-labelled fluorodeoxyglucose CT/positron emission tomography (PET) has recently been shown in small case series to differentiate benign from malignant IPMNs. In a series of 29 patients, a standardised uptake value of >2.5 was shown to have a 96% accuracy in determining the presence of malignancy.[17] Differentiating IPMN from other cystic neoplasms (particularly branch-type IPMN from MCN) can be difficult and the importance of considering the clinical picture cannot be underestimated, particularly the patient's age, gender and history of pancreatitis or genetic syndromes.[18] Radiologically, localisation within the uncinate process, detection of non-gravity-dependent luminal filling defects (papillary projections) or grouped gravity-dependent luminal filling defects (mucin), and upstream dilatation of ducts (MCN ducts are normal) all favour the diagnosis of branch-type IPMN.[19] Differentiating diffuse main-duct IPMN from chronic obstructive pancreatitis can be challenging radiologically[19] (clinically, patients with IPMN tend to be 20 years

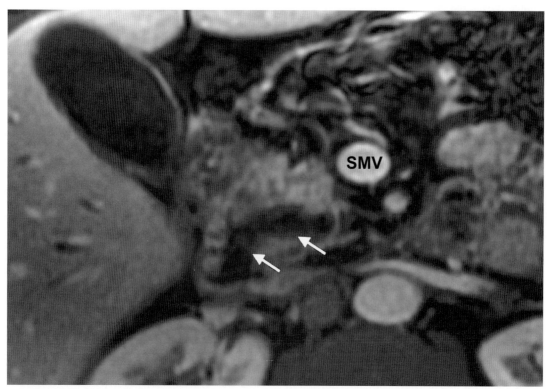

Figure 16.1 • MRI (post-gadolinium, T1-weighted, fat-saturated) image of the pancreas. The white arrows indicate a dilated pancreatic duct with a widely open ampulla consistent with a main-duct intraductal papillary neoplasm. SMV, superior mesenteric vein. Histology is shown in Fig. 16.2.

older and lack a history of heavy alcohol use), but high-quality cross-sectional imaging looking for endoluminal filling defects (either mucin or papillary proliferations), cystic dilatation of collateral branches (particularly within the uncinate process), communication of dilated ducts with normal ducts without evidence of an obstructing lesion or a widely open papilla (Fig. 16.1) all favour IPMN.[19]

Endoscopic ultrasound (EUS) has the advantage of being able to sample cystic fluid and biopsy solid lesions at the time of assessment, although its utility over cross-sectional imaging has recently been questioned.[20] Features seen at EUS suggestive of malignancy include main duct >10 mm (for main-duct IPMN), while suspicious features for branch-type IPMN include tumour diameter greater than 40 mm associated with thick irregular septa and mural nodules >10 mm.[21] In a series of 74 patients with IPMNs of which 21 (28%) had invasive carcinoma, the sensitivity, specificity and accuracy of EUS fine-needle aspiration in predicting invasive carcinoma were 75%, 91% and 86%, respectively.[22] In this particular study, the elevated levels of carcinoembryonic antigen (CEA) and carbohydrate antigen (CA) 19-9 within cyst fluid did not predict the presence of malignancy.[22] Importantly, the absence of mucin does not exclude IPMN.[23] While the presence of necrosis is the only feature that is strongly suggestive of invasive carcinoma, abundant background inflammation and parachromatin clearing are suspicious for carcinoma in situ.[23]

Endoscopic retrograde cholangiopancreatography (ERCP) can be used in the diagnosis of IPMN, although MRI (including the use of gadolinium) is increasingly replacing it (Fig. 16.1). The observation at ERCP of mucin protruding from a widely open papilla is diagnostic.[24] Biopsies and aspiration of ductal contents can be obtained; however, the yield is less than 50%.[24]

Although there are no tumour markers specific to IPMN, serum CA19-9 but not CEA has been shown to be an independent predictor of malignancy.[10]

Given the increasing frequency of diagnosis and relatively low rate of malignancy within branch-duct IPMN, clinicoradiological scoring systems have been proposed.[10,25] Fujino et al. have proposed a clinicoradiological scoring system for predicting the presence of invasive malignancy in patients with both branch- and main-duct IPMNs (based on an analysis of 64 patients who underwent resection).[10] It consists of seven factors (Table 16.1), each with an assigned score. A cut-off of 3 or more predicts malignancy with a sensitivity, specificity, positive predictive value, negative predictive value and overall accuracy of 95%, 82%, 91%, 90% and 91%, respectively. No patient with a score of >4 had benign lesions, while no patient with a score of <2 had malignancy.

Table 16.1 • Proposed scoring system[10] to predict malignancy in patients with suspected intraductal papillary mucinous neoplasms of the pancreas

Variable	Score
Patulous papilla	1
Jaundice	1
Diabetes mellitus	1
Tumour size ≥42 mm	1
Main-duct type	2
Main duct ≥6.5 mm	3
CA 19-9 ≥35 units/mL	3

A cut-off of 3 or more predicts malignancy with a sensitivity, specificity, positive predictive value, negative predictive value and overall accuracy of 95%, 82%, 91%, 90% and 91%, respectively.

Clearly, if this system is validated and further refined with larger numbers of patients, this may prove a very simple and useful predictor of underlying malignancy. In a large study by Hwang et al.,[25] 237 patients with branch-duct IPMN who underwent resection were studied. Using multivariate analysis to identify independent predictors of either malignancy or invasiveness, formulae were created. However, the presence of a mural nodule, elevated serum CEA or cyst size greater than 28 mm was sufficient to conclude that there was underlying malignant change or invasion and an indication for surgery.[25] An important point when considering the use of these scoring systems is that the radiological measurement varies by scan modality and may not correlate well with the final pathological measurement.[26]

Pathology

IPMNs involve the head of the gland in 70% of cases, while 5–10% are spread diffusely throughout the gland, and the rest are located within the body and tail.[27] On sectioning, the involvement can be diffuse or segmented, with projections of papillary epithelium (**Fig. 16.2**) and tenacious thick mucin within the involved dilated ducts. The projections and mucin can extend along the ducts and into the surrounding structures, including the ampulla, duodenum and bile duct. Communication of the main pancreatic duct with the cystic lesion can usually be established. IPMNs are subclassified into main duct, branch type or mixed, depending on site of origin. This is important as branch-type neoplasms are less likely to be associated with malignancy.[24] Surrounding pancreatic parenchyma may appear firm and hard due to scarring and atrophy from obstructive chronic pancreatitis secondary to the

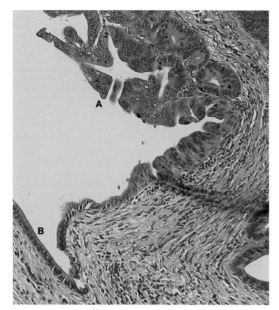

Figure 16.2 • Haematoxylin-and-eosin-stained section from the pancreatico-duodenectomy specimen of the patient in Fig. 16.1. Label A is in the lumen of the proximal pancreatic duct with adjacent proliferation of severely dysplastic glandular epithelium with intraluminal papillary growth, but no stromal invasion in this area. Elsewhere in the specimen focal stromal invasion was identified. Label B indicates remnant low columnar non-neoplastic epithelium of the duct.

tumour. The presence of gelatinous or solid nodules should raise the suspicion of an invasive component. Microscopically, the most typical appearance is of mucin-secreting columnar epithelium with variable atypia (low-, moderate-, high-grade dysplasia or invasive carcinoma).[27] The growth pattern varies from flat ducts (ectasia) through to prominent papillae. The tumour tends to follow the pancreatic ducts and can be multifocal in 20–30% of patients.[27] IPMNs can contain intestinal, gastric or, less commonly, pancreatico-biliary type differentiation. The gastric type are more often associated with branch-type IPMN and would seem to be associated with a different (lower) malignant potential, growth pattern and type of mucin production compared to the intestinal type.[28,29] Invasive carcinoma occurs focally and is thought to result from a stepwise progression through increasingly dysplastic lesions.[27] The invasive growth pattern can be muconodular (colloid) or a conventional ductal pattern and would appear to be related to the underlying cellular differentiation (intestinal vs. pancreatico-biliary, respectively).[27,29]

Pathologically, differentiating IPMN from other cystic neoplasms of the pancreas is important. The absence of ovarian stroma helps to separate IPMN from MCN.[4] For lesions between 0.5 and 1 cm, differentiating pancreatic intraepithelial neoplasia (PanIN) from IPMN is difficult. IPMNs tend to have taller and more complex papillae and are associated with abundant luminal mucin.[27] The presence of coarse and stippled chromatin with a smooth nuclear membrane will differentiate cystic pancreatic endocrine neoplasms from IPMNs.[27]

Management

In determining the most appropriate management of patients with IPMNs, the following should be considered. Given the preponderance for these to present in older patients and the fact that the majority will be located within the head of the pancreas, it is important to assess for comorbidities and general fitness for major pancreatic surgery. If the patient is deemed not fit enough for surgery, then simple medical management of symptoms is appropriate. Equally, in the event of an incidental diagnosis, intensive follow-up regimens are not indicated if tumour progression would not lead to surgical intervention. Presuming the patient is a suitable candidate for surgery (if required), then appropriate staging to determine surgical resectability (criteria equivalent to those for pancreatic adenocarcinoma) should be performed.

> ✅ For main-duct IPMNs, a consensus document (International Association of Pancreatology (IAP) guidelines)[4] recommended that all such patients should undergo resection. This was based on reviewing available evidence, which concluded the following: the incidence of malignancy (in situ or invasive disease) in main-duct tumours is between 60% and 92%; it is thought that most main-duct IPMNs will undergo transformation into malignant disease if left untreated; a significant survival advantage is seen for those who are resected with in situ or benign disease compared to those with invasive disease; the ability to exclude malignancy on clinicoradiological criteria is limited.

The same IAP guidelines[4] recommended that all patients with symptomatic branch-duct IPMNs underwent resection on the basis that it would alleviate symptoms and because the literature would suggest that there is a higher rate of malignancy in patients who are symptomatic (risk of invasive malignancy 30%).[4] For asymptomatic patients[4] it was recommended that patients with tumours ≥30 mm or with mural nodules underwent resection due to the increased risk of malignancy. Although risk factors for malignancy have been identified by more than one study using multivariate analysis,[10,30] these have been based on small numbers of patients. Nagai et al. have challenged this approach, advocating aggressive surgical resection for branch-type IPMNs, arguing that the identified risk factors do not have a high enough negative predictive value, that survival is significantly compromised in those with invasive disease, and that pancreatic surgery can be performed with a low morbidity and mortality in experienced centres.[31]

Since publication of the IAP guidelines,[4] a large dual-centre study[32] consisting of 145 patients with branch-duct IPMNs who underwent resection has been reported. Of these 145 patients, 22% had malignant disease (in situ or invasive) and 40% were asymptomatic. Although symptoms per se were not found to be a predictor of malignancy on univariate analysis, jaundice and abdominal pain were more likely to be associated with malignancy. Radiologically malignant tumours were larger, and on pathological analysis the presence of a thick wall, nodularity and size ≥30 mm were all significantly associated with malignancy. It is important to note, however, that other than size these factors were not assessed radiologically. In addition, there was a significant discrepancy between radiologically and pathologically measured size (radiological measurement was consistently 15% greater). The authors concluded that their results supported the IAP guidelines, particularly with regard to non-surgical management of those that were asymptomatic with no concerning features of malignancy.

Given that even branch-duct IPMN would appear to be a premalignant lesion, albeit a slow-growing one, one has to know the outcome from long-term follow-up if conservative management is to be successful. In two large prospective contemporary studies[33,34] of branch-duct IPMNs, in which indications for resection were based on IAP guidelines, patients were allocated to a surgical or intensive follow-up arm. In both studies 18% of patients met the criteria for surgery at initial presentation. Of these patients, the final histology was malignant (in situ or invasive disease) in 3 of 20[33] and 8 of 34[34] patients. In those patients submitted to follow-up, intensive regimens (3–6 monthly for the first 2 years) were used in both studies, including combinations of CT, EUS and MRI. Between 5% and 12% of patients subsequently progressed to surgery during follow-up (median 12–18 months). Of these patients, 0 of 5[33] and 2 of 18[34] had malignant disease. All remaining patients (*n* = 84[33] and *n* = 132[34]) that were followed remained alive during median follow-up periods of 30 months, with no deaths attributable to their disease.

The methodology of the follow-up regimen of both these studies raises further questions. Both used state-of-the-art imaging at a frequency that many health systems may struggle to provide. Both studies showed that although the current recommendations for branch-duct IPMN are very sensitive in detecting malignancy, the specificity remains low and hence many patients are followed intensively and subjected to surgery without clear benefit. Further work will be required to try and identify subgroups of patients at high risk of change so that the specificity of intervention can be improved.

✔ For branch-duct IPMNs a selective approach to resection should be undertaken based on symptoms, CA19-9 >25 U/mL, tumour size >3.5 cm, presence of mural nodules or thick walls.[4,32,33]

For those patients in whom surgery is indicated, the decision regarding the extent of pancreatic resection and nodal dissection needs to be decided. Fujino et al. reviewed the outcome in 57 patients who underwent surgical resection for IPMN.[35] Their approach was to perform a localised resection where pre-resection imaging revealed localised disease, using intraoperative ultrasound (IOUS) to determine the point of pancreatic transection, while in patients with diffuse disease a total pancreatectomy was performed. Frozen section was performed and for patients with invasive carcinoma a radical resection was performed. Where non-invasive disease was detected, a tumour-free margin was sufficient. Of the 33 patients with main-duct IPMNs, 14 met the pre-resection criteria for total pancreatectomy. All 24 patients with branch-duct tumours underwent partial resections, although two subsequently required completion pancreatectomy for complications. Correlating the final pathological assessment with the IOUS indicated an accuracy of ductal spread of 74% for main-duct tumours and 96% for branch-duct tumours. Frozen section was performed in 30 of the patients who underwent partial resection and in 29 patients it correlated with the final result. Only one patient had invasive malignancy at the transected surface, while a further two patients who did not have frozen section assessment had invasive malignancy at the resection margin.

In reviewing the final histology of the 16 patients undergoing total pancreatectomy, resection was found to be appropriate (frankly or potentially malignant tissue throughout all segments of the pancreas) in 12 patients. Importantly, six of these 16 patients had severe long-term problems with hypoglycaemia, two of whom died as a result of this complication. For those 41 patients undergoing partial pancreatectomy, five patients had an involved margin (three with invasive carcinoma, two with dysplasia). The three patients with invasive carcinoma all died from metastatic disease. Of the patients with clear margins, 7 of 34 died from metastatic disease, while two developed metachronous pancreatic disease at 2 and 12 years. The results of this study led the authors to conclude that, if possible, partial pancreatectomy should be performed and that the risk of recurrent malignancy in the remnant is outweighed by the severe long-term complications from total pancreatectomy.

Although Fujino et al.[35] report frozen section to be very accurate, it can be a challenging undertaking for the pathologist. However, not all positive margins require resection. Current recommendations from the IAP guidelines[4] are that, in the presence of adenoma or borderline atypia, no further resection is required, but if in situ or invasive carcinoma is present, then further resection should be performed. However, what has not yet been addressed in the literature is the effect of potentially spilling invasive carcinoma cells (i.e. cutting through invasive tumour) during surgery and the effect this has on long-term outcomes. This is particularly important as increasingly limited resections are being reported for low-grade lesions within the pancreas with good long-term outcomes. However, for main-duct IPMNs, the authors have advised caution for exactly this reason, given the risk of a positive resection margin and subsequent recurrence.[36]

> ✅ For those undergoing resection, partial pancreatectomy is preferred to total pancreatectomy and intraoperative frozen section should be performed to ensure clear margins.[35]

Outcome

The main determinant of survival following resection is the presence of invasive disease (Table 16.2). The 5-year survival for those with non-invasive disease is 77–100%[9,31,33,35,37,38] vs. 13–68%[1,9,31,33,35,37–41] for those with invasive disease. Other factors that have been reported to be associated with poor survival in those with invasive disease include the presence of jaundice,[42] tumour type (tubular worse than colloid),[9,29,41,42] vascular invasion,[39,40,42] perineural invasion,[39] poorly differentiated tumours,[39] percentage of tumour that was invasive[39,42] and positive lymph node involvement,[9,37,39,42] which has been reported in up to 41%[37] of patients with invasive disease. Invasive branch-type tumours have been shown to have similar survival to those with invasive main-duct disease[42] and margin status has not been associated with worse long-term outcome.[9,39,40,42] In studies that have performed a multivariate analysis with adequate numbers of patients per variable, lymph node involvement,[39,41] invasive component >2 cm,[39] absence of weight loss,[39] morphological subtype[29] and tubular carcinoma[41] have been found to be independent predictors of poorer outcome. Invasive IPMN would

Table 16.2 • Survival following resection for intraductal papillary mucinous neoplasms by presence of invasion

Author	Number of patients	Five-year survival (%) Non-invasive	Invasive
Sohn et al.[9]	84	77	–
	52	–	43
Hardacre et al.[38]	24	90	–
	13	–	22
Wada et al.[37]	75	100	–
	25	–	46
Salvia et al.[33]	80	100	–
	58	–	60
D'Angelica et al.[42]	32	95	–
	30	–	60
Fujino et al.[35]	19	91	–
	38	–	13
Winter et al.[1]	90	–	48
Nagai et al.[31]	42	100	–
	30	–	58
Yopp et al.[41]	59		68
Kargozaran et al.[40]	641		26
Turrini et al.[39]	98		30

still appear to have a better prognosis than pancreatic ductal adenocarcinoma,[31,37,41] although the tubular subtype may not.[41] The role of adjuvant therapy for those with invasive disease has not been addressed in formal trials. Outcomes from retrospective series have been analysed,[39,41] yet the role of either radiotherapy or chemotherapy remains unclear and currently cannot be recommended as the standard of care.

Recurrence following resection can be classified as disseminated (including peritoneal disease) or local (within the pancreatic remnant). White et al. have reported on 78 patients who underwent resection for non-invasive IPMNs over a 13-year period.[43] The median follow-up was 40 months. Only six patients (7.7%) developed local recurrence, three of whom underwent further resection and remained under active follow-up. Importantly, time to recurrence was extremely variable, with a range of 8–62 months, indicating that long-term surveillance of the pancreatic remnant is required. There was a significant association of recurrence with positive margins,[43] although this has not been shown elsewhere.[9] Given the significant morbidity and late mortality associated with total pancreatectomy,[35] the authors favoured follow-up of the remnant as opposed to total pancreatectomy.[43]

In a large series of 145 patients who underwent resection for branch-type IPMNs, 6.9% of patients developed recurrence.[32] Four of 139 patients with non-invasive disease developed local recurrence at a mean follow-up of 34 months, while 6 of 16 patients with invasive carcinoma developed distant disease (three also had local recurrence) at a mean follow-up of 24 months (all died within 2 years of recurrence). These findings have been further supported by Park et al., who identified invasive disease, elevated CA19-9 and tumour location within the head as independent risk factors for recurrence.[44]

✅ There is a lack of reliable evidence regarding recommended follow-up regimens. The IAP guidelines[4] acknowledge this, but feel it is reasonable to perform yearly CT or MRI and space it out once the patient has shown no signs of change after several years. The routine use of tumour markers is currently not supported.

Given that recurrence would seem to occur most commonly within the pancreatic remnant, Tomimaru et al.[45] have proposed performing a pancreatico-gastrostomy to allow easy endoscopic follow-up of the duct. Additionally, the association of IPMNs with other gastrointestinal malignancies[4] should alert physicians to investigate new gastrointestinal symptoms promptly.

Pancreatic neuroendocrine tumours

Pancreatic neuroendocrine tumours (PNETs) are rare tumours with a reported incidence of 0.2–0.4 per 100 000, although post-mortem studies have reported PNETs in up to 10% of the population.[46] Eighty-five per cent of PNETs are non-syndromic (non-functional), with the rest comprised of syndromic tumours[47] of which carcinoid, insulinoma and gastrinoma are the most common.[48] The aetiology is poorly understood and although the majority of tumours are sporadic, there are associations with several hereditary syndromes, including Von Hippel–Lindau, multiple endocrine neoplasia-1 (MEN-1), neurofibromatosis type 1 and tubular sclerosis.[49]

Clinical presentation

The mode of presentation is dependent on the functional state of the tumour. Non-functioning tumours may present incidentally, whereas symptoms are usually related to mass effect or the presence of metastatic disease. For those tumours associated with a syndrome, this will be related to the specific hormone production (Table 16.3).

Investigations

The order of investigations will be dependent on presentation. The general principle for functional tumours is to confirm the diagnosis (biochemically) prior to localisation (radiologically).

Biochemical

Specific fasting gut hormones can be measured for functional tumours.[48] For suspected insulinoma and carcinoid, this would include fasting glucose, insulin, C-peptide and 24-hour urinary 5-hydroxyindoleacetic acid (5-HIAA).[48] In addition, in the majority of PNETs, including non-functional tumours,[48] serum chromogranin A (protein produced from cells arising from the neural crest) will be elevated. Although chromogranin A is sensitive, it is not highly specific and those interpreting the test must be aware of causes of false-positive results.[50] The degree of elevation of chromogranin A has been shown to correlate with burden of disease (although not with gastrinomas), response to treatment and recurrence.[50]

Other investigations such as calcium, parathyroid hormone, calcitonin and thyroid function tests should also be considered, particularly if there is a history that suggests MEN-1.[48] For those in whom a hereditary component is suspected, referral to an appropriate genetic service for further investigation should be initiated.

Radiology

For non-functioning tumours, where localisation is often not an issue, a high-quality arterial and portal venous phase CT will be sufficient to direct therapy, particularly in determining if surgery is indicated. Features suggestive of a PNET on CT include the presence of a hypervascular or hyperdense lesion within the pancreas; however, they can also appear cystic or contain calcifications.[51] The presence of a large incidental mass within the pancreas, particularly without vascular encasement or desmoplastic reaction, should also alert the clinician to the possibility of a PNET.[51]

Although somatostatinomas, VIPomas and glucagonomas tend to be large and easily identified and staged by contrast-enhanced CT, this is often not the case for insulinomas and gastrinomas, unless there is widespread metastatic disease. Most insulinomas are under 2 cm and solitary. On CT they tend to be hypervascular (**Fig. 16.3**) with either uniform or target enhancement; however, given that they are often non-contour conforming, detection of the vascular

Table 16.3 • Presentation, diagnosis and initial medical management of functional pancreatic neuroendocrine tumours

Tumour type	Syndrome	Symptoms	Diagnosis	Medical options for initial symptom control
Insulinoma	Whipple's triad	Neuroglycaemic or neurogenic symptoms relieved with eating	1. Insulin:glucose ratio >0.3 in presence of hypoglycaemia 2. C-peptide suppression test	Overnight feeding Diazoxide titrated to symptom resolution Somatostatin analogue
Gastrinoma	Zollinger–Ellison	Complicated peptic ulceration or gastro-oesophageal reflux, diarrhoea, abdominal pain	1. Serum fasting gastrin >1000 pg/mL (if gastric pH <2.5) 2. Secretin stimulation test	High-dose proton pump inhibition (may require up to 60 mg b.d.)
Glucagonoma	Glucagonoma syndrome	Necrolytic migratory erthyma, weight loss, diabetes mellitus, stomatitis, diarrhoea, thromboembolism	Plasma glucagon >1000 pg/mL	Somatostatin analogue Hyperalimentation Thrombosis prophylaxis
VIPoma	Verner–Morrison syndrome	Profuse watery diarrhoea, hypokalaemia	Plasma VIP >1000 pg/mL	Somatostatin analogue
Somatostatinoma		Gallstones, steatorrhoea, hypochlorhydria, glucose intolerance	Raised plasma somatostatin	
Carcinoid	Carcinoid syndrome	Abdominal pain, if metastases then flushing, palpitations, rhinorrhoea, diarrhoea, bronchospasm, pellagra	24-hour urinary 5-HIAA	Somatostatin analogue

blush is essential to localise them (the chance of detection can be maximised by timing the images 25 seconds after contrast injection).[51] MRI features include low signal intensity on T1-weighted images and they are particularly well seen on fat-suppressed (T1- and T2-weighted) images.[51] In contrast to insulinoma, gastrinoma can be multiple and extra-pancreatic (located within the gastrinoma triangle; the junction between neck and body of the pancreas medially, the junction of the second and third parts of the duodenum inferiorly and the junction of the common bile duct and cystic duct superiorly).[52] On radiological examination, they tend to be less vascular than insulinoma.[51] There is a high rate (70–80%) of lymph node and hepatic metastases.[51] The sensitivity of CT in the detection of gastrinoma is related to size and can be as low as 30–50%.[52] Although slightly better figures have been reported for insulinomas, this can be increased to 94% with the use of thin formats and, with the addition of endoscopic ultrasound, sensitivities of 100% have been reported.[52]

Endoscopic ultrasound is particularly useful for imaging the duodenal wall, regional lymph nodes and the pancreatic head, and has reported sensitivities of 79–100%, but is operator dependent.[52] Equally, the use of intraoperative ultrasound has also been shown to be useful, particularly in gastrinomas, by identifying occult multiple primaries or metastatic disease. The sensitivity for detecting small lesions in the pancreatic head is reported to be as high as 97%.[52]

PNET hepatic metastases often appear as low-attenuation lesions on pre-contrast CT and hypervascular lesions on post-contrast imaging.[52] It is, however, important to perform a hepatic arterial phase as they can be isointense with normal parenchyma on portal venous imaging. MRI appearances of hepatic metastases are usually of low signal intensity lesions on T1 and high signal intensity on T2-weighted images. Importantly, 15% of hepatic metastases were only seen on immediate post-gadolinium imaging.

In addition to standard radiological imaging, somatostatin receptor scintigraphy (SRS) is also very useful in the staging and treatment of PNETs (with the exception of insulinomas).[53] This works on the principle that PNETs express somatostatin

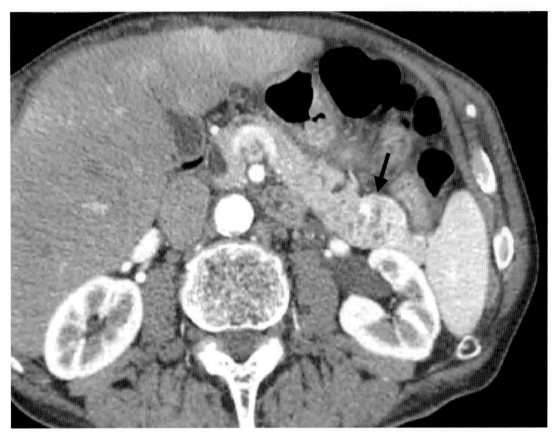

Figure 16.3 • A 78-year-old man presented with neuroglycaemic symptoms. Biochemical testing confirmed an insulinoma. Arterial phase computed tomography revealed a hypervascular lesion in the tail of the pancreas (black arrow). Laparoscopic spleen-preserving distal pancreatectomy was performed. Histology confirmed malignant, node-positive neuroendocrine tumour consistent with an insulinoma. After 4 years with no symptoms the patient re-presented with symptoms of hypoglycaemia. Further investigation revealed an isolated nodal recurrence adjacent to the superior mesenteric artery. The patient has recently undergone a completion radical antegrade modular distal pancreatico-splenectomy with resolution of hypoglycaemic symptoms.

receptors. The use of a somatostatin analogue labelled with a radioactive isotope (of which there are several) allows a functional image to be obtained but it requires somatostatin analogues to be stopped prior to the scan. As a single investigation, it is probably the most sensitive for the detection of PNETs; however, equivalence can be achieved with a combined approach of standard radiology (particularly MRI and EUS), which has the advantage of providing a detailed anatomical analysis.[54] SRS does, however, offer the advantage of reflecting functionality, which is important if treatment doses of radiolabelled somatostatin analogues or meta-iodobenzylguanidine (MIBG) are to be used. ^{18}F-labelled deoxyglucose PET has not been shown to be useful for the majority of PNETs; however, the development of newer alternatives to ^{18}F-labelled deoxyglucose would appear to be promising.[54] Invasive investigations such as selective arterial

calcium (insulinoma) and secretin (gastrinoma) stimulation with hepatic/portal venous sampling are not used routinely and are only undertaken if there is a high suspicion, but non-invasive imaging has failed to localise the tumour.[53,55]

Treatment

Once the diagnosis of a functioning tumour is established, control of the hormonal excess is the first priority in minimising symptoms and complications. Medications used for each individual tumour are shown in Table 16.3. Somatostatin analogue infusions are recommended pre- and intraoperatively for carcinoid tumours to prevent carcinoid crisis.[48] Surgery offers the only chance of cure for those with localised disease for PNETs. The approach is dependent on tumour type and the presence or absence of an inherited syndrome. The specific management of hereditary PNETs is beyond the remit of this chapter and readers are referred to more detailed reviews for an in-depth discussion.[49,53,55]

Over 80% of localised sporadic insulinomas are solitary, benign and under 2 cm in size, making them ideal for consideration of enucleation and laparoscopic resection.[53] Enucleation is considered possible if the lesion can be clearly localised pre- or intraoperatively and if the relationship to the pancreatic duct has been clearly identified.[48] Intraoperative ultrasound has been shown to be particularly valuable in helping to assess these factors.[53] Postoperatively, histological conformation of the benign nature must be confirmed.[48] Resection is required for tumours where malignancy is suspected (hard, infiltrating tumour, duct obstruction or lymph node involvement), if there is major vascular involvement or the tumour is large.[53] Patients should be assessed for resection as for any pancreatic tumour. However, if a distal pancreatectomy is being performed attempts to preserve the spleen should be made.[53] Blind pancreatic resection should be avoided.[53] Not surprisingly given the rare nature of the tumour, data in support of laparoscopic resection remain limited to small case series; however, early results indicate that although it can be performed safely, significant conversion, re-exploration and morbidity rates remain.[56]

✔✔ For localised sporadic gastrinoma, surgery has been shown to increase survival.[57]

Duodenotomy and intraoperative ultrasound combined with palpation (sensitivity 91–95%) are the key to successful intraoperative localisation.[55] For duodenal gastrinomas, small tumours (<5 mm) can be enucleated from the submucosa while larger tumours require full-thickness excision.[55] For pancreatic gastrinomas, intraoperative assessment regarding the suitability for enucleation (similar to that described above for insulinomas) should be performed. However, if the tumour is not suitable, a formal pancreatic resection (pancreatico-duodenectomy) should be performed. If enucleation is performed, consideration of peripancreatic nodal sampling should be undertaken, given the high rate of metastatic disease.[58]

Most localised non-functioning tumours will be detected at such a size that enucleation is not feasible. Given the discrepancy between the clinical and autopsy incidence of PNETs and the increasing use of cross-sectional imaging, this is likely to become a more frequent possibility. The size at which patients with asymptomatic suspected benign, non-functioning PNETs should undergo resection is not clear.[59] Although the risk of malignancy is related to size, tumours between 1 and 3 cm can harbour malignant potential[59] (**Fig. 16.4**). Currently, patients

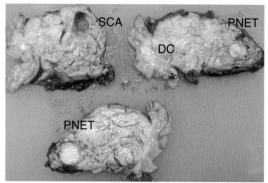

Figure 16.4 • A 30-year-old female with Von Hippel–Lindau disease underwent pancreatic screening. Radiological imaging revealed five neuroendocrine tumours within the pancreatic head. Pancreatico-duodenectomy was performed. Pathological sectioning of the pancreatic head revealed multiple neuroendocrine tumours (PNETs), including at least one well-differentiated pancreatic endocrine carcinoma (node positive) and a well-differentiated duodenal endocrine carcinoma (DC). All tumours were between 12 and 18 mm diameter. An incidental serous cyst adenoma (SCA) was also identified.

should be assessed regarding fitness for surgery and an informed decision made with the patient regarding resection or observation. Central pancreatectomy has also been shown to be feasible for selected tumours and has the advantage of reducing the risk of postoperative diabetes.[36] A formal resection with lymphadenectomy should be performed for suspected malignant tumours as lymph node metastases are common (27–83%).[59]

Resection is the treatment of choice for symptomatic patients with localised disease.[59] The median survival for those who underwent resection was significantly longer than for those with metastatic disease or locally advanced unresectable disease (7.2 years vs. 2.1 and 5.2 years, respectively).[59] Importantly, however, 48% of patients who underwent resection for localised disease developed recurrence at a median follow-up of 2.7 years.[59] Because of the long natural history of these tumours and given that many are symptomatic and difficult to palliate without resection (e.g. tumour bleeding), the criteria for what determines unresectable disease may not be the same as those for adenocarcinoma of the pancreas. The MD Anderson experience would suggest that, in high-volume centres, major venous reconstruction can be performed safely, but only rarely should arterial reconstruction (isolated hepatic artery involvement) or upper abdominal exenteration be performed, due to the associated high long-term morbidity.[59] In addition, a recent report has also indicated that an incomplete resection (R2) is associated with a high perioperative mortality and may in fact be detrimental to the patient's survival.[60]

Metastatic disease

Only 10% of patients with hepatic metastases will be suitable for potentially curative resection.[48] However, it would appear that although recurrence rates are high, a survival advantage can be achieved, although randomised data are lacking.[61] Synchronous cholecystectomy should be performed to reduce complications from adjuvant therapy such as somatostatin analogues and hepatic artery embolisation.[61] For patients with non-functioning unresectable metastatic disease, there is no evidence to support palliative or 'debulking' resections, with possibly the only exceptions being those who have significant local symptoms from the primary and low-volume hepatic metastases.[59] For those with obstruction of the gastrointestinal or biliary tract, surgical bypass should be the first-line treatment in those with well-differeniated disease, given the indolent nature of the disease.[61]

> ✅ A cytoreductive approach (surgery or ablative therapies) has been advocated in patients with hormonal excess and hepatic metastases if 90% of tumour bulk can be removed, although randomised trials are lacking.[48,53,55] Other options assessed by the UK guidelines on the management of PNETs included somatostatin analogues (short and long acting), interferon-α, hepatic artery embolisation, radiolabelled analogues (MIBG and somatostatin), liver transplantation and radiofrequency ablation.[48]

Until recently the role of chemotherapy for PNETs has been based around streptozocin and 5-fluorouracil after a randomised trial in 1979 showed a survival advantage for patients with metastatic carcinoid tumours receiving combination chemotherapy.[62] However, given the side-effects and variable behaviour of PNETs, it has not been widely accepted into clinical practice.

> ✅✅ Two recent placebo-controlled randomised trials using the novel agents sunitinib[63] and everolimus[64] have shown an increase in overall and progression-free survival, respectively. Thus, although further studies are warranted, the results of these two trials would suggest these treatments should represent the standard of care.

Pathology and outcome

PNETs are classified into four groups based on a combination of clinical, histological and molecular features.[48] Tumours confined to the pancreas are classified as well-differentiated endocrine tumours that can be subdivided into those of benign behaviour (<2 cm size), <2 mitoses per 10 high-power fields (HPFs), Ki67 index <2% (and no vascular invasion) or uncertain behaviour (if the above criteria are not met). Tumours not confined to the pancreas (gross local invasion or metastases) or that exhibit evidence of small-cell carcinoma are considered endocrine carcinoma, which are further subdivided into well-differentiated (well to moderately differentiated, mitotic rate 2–10 per 10 HPFs, Ki67 index >5%) or poorly differentiated (small-cell carcinoma, necrosis, >10 mitoses per 10 HPFs, Ki67 index >15%, prominent vascular and perineural invasion). Importantly, the diagnosis of functional tumours is not made histologically but clinically, as immunohistochemical staining of specific hormones does not correlate with the clinical picture.[48] In 2010, the seventh edition of the American Joint Committee on Cancer (AJCC) published its first TNM staging classification for PNETs.[65] Using this, Strosberg et al. retrospectively applied the staging system to a dataset of 425 patients with PNETs.[66] Five-year overall survival for stages I–IV was 92%, 84%, 81% and 57%, respectively, thus indicating the proposed system is a useful adjunct for classifying PNETs.

Other tumours

The other two main types of cystic neoplasms are serous (SCA) and mucinous (MCN) cystic neoplasms. Because of the difference in malignant potential, the management of these two tumours differs, yet clinically and radiologically there is considerable overlap. It is therefore useful to contrast and compare them. The exact incidence of serous and mucinous cystic tumours is unknown; however, in a retrospective review of 24 039 patients undergoing radiological imaging, 0.7% had pancreatic cystic neoplasms. Of the 49 (0.2%) who underwent surgery, 10 and 16 patients had a final diagnosis of SCA and MCN, respectively.[67] SCAs are more common in men (2:1), with a peak incidence in the seventh decade, and evenly distributed throughout the pancreas, with up to a third being asymptomatic.[68] In contrast, MCNs are predominantly found in women, with a peak incidence in the fifth decade, and are more likely to be located within the tail.[69] SCAs are also commonly associated with Von Hippel–Lindau syndrome[49] (Fig. 16.4), and young patients presenting with multiple cystic lesions involving the pancreas and kidneys should be genetically assessed.[68]

On cross-sectional imaging, the typical appearances of an SCA are of a microcystic (>6 cysts, each cyst <2 cm individual diameter) lesion with or without central calcification (so-called sunburst calcification).[18,70] When the classic features are present, differentiation from other tumours is not difficult; however, a rare solid type exists that radiologically can be mistaken for neuroendocrine tumour.[12] MRI may be useful in this setting.[18] The presence of a uni- or oligolocular macrocystic (>2 cm) lesion is more difficult to diagnose and a wide differential exists. Both SCAs (oligocystic type) and MCNs can fall into this group, although MCNs are less likely to be multilocular and, if calcification occurs, it does so peripherally and may be a marker of underlying malignancy.[18] The presence of solid components within a cystic lesion indicates the presence of, or high risk of, malignancy and therefore surgical resection should be considered.[18] Included within this differential would be PNET, solid pseudo-papillary neoplasm (young women) or mucinous cyst adenocarcinoma.[18] It is unusual for either SCAs or MCNs to communicate with the pancreatic duct, but it has been reported.[18]

The ability of non-interventional imaging to obtain an accurate diagnosis is limited. In a recent report of 100 SCAs from Bassi et al.,[71] the correct diagnosis was achieved in 53%, 54% and 76% by ultrasound (US), CT and MRI, respectively. An incorrect diagnosis was made in 31%, 34% and 26%, and the investigation was non-diagnostic in 16%, 12% and 0% with US, CT and MRI, respectively.

In a study[7] of solitary cystic (IPMNs were excluded) neoplasms, 71 patients underwent EUS and fluid aspiration (for mucin, viscosity, amylase, lipase, CEA, CA19-9, cytology) followed by surgery to assess its accuracy.[72] The authors concluded that an accurate algorithm using measurement of viscosity, lipase and CEA can be used to determine the diagnosis of cystic lesions. A viscosity of ≥1.6 indicates an MCN and the patient should be offered resection. If it is <1.6 and the lipase is <6000 U/mL, this indicates an SCA. If the viscosity is <1.6 and lipase is >6000 U/mL, then a CEA measurement should be performed, and if this value is less than 480 U/mL the diagnosis is a pseudocyst. If it is > 480 U/mL, a repeat EUS and fine-needle aspiration should be performed in 3–6 months. Using this algorithm, only 2 of 71 patients that underwent resection for suspected MCN had a final histology revealing a pseudocyst.

✓ The management of SCAs and MCNs differs depending on their malignant potential. It is currently recommended that all suspected MCNs undergo resection because of their malignant potential,[4] but for SCA malignant transformation is very rare and for asymptomatic lesions no intervention is required.[71] Symptomatic lesions should be resected.

Pathologically, SCAs demonstrate monomorphous cuboidal-shaped epithelium. The cells are glycogen rich with cellular cytoplasm and small regular nuclei. There is a lack of mitotic activity. The cysts appear 'empty' on microscopy. In contrast, the cyst content of MCNs is turbid and tenacious.[68] Microscopically (unlike SCAs) the cyst lining can be highly variable. The cells are mucin producing, which can be a single cell layer of flattened cuboidal epithelium or contain papillary tufting.[68] The tumours are classified as benign, borderline or malignant depending on the nuclear features of the cells.[68] It is important to examine the whole tumour as malignant invasion can occur without the presence of a mass.[68] The unique feature of MCNs, however, is the presence of ovarian stroma (highly cellular, densely packed, plump spindle cells). Current recommendations require the presence of this for a tumour to be classified as MCN.[4] This is particularly important when the differential includes IPMN, in which this type of stroma is not seen.[4]

Key points

- As the use of cross-sectional imaging has become more frequent, there has been an increase in the diagnosis of cystic neoplasms within the pancreas.
- Main-duct intraductal papillary mucinous neoplasms should be resected due to the high incidence of underlying malignancy; however, a selective approach to intervention for side-branch intraductal papillary mucinous neoplasms should be taken (dependent on the presence of symptoms, tumour markers and tumour characteristics).
- Investigation and follow-up of cystic lesions of the pancreas requires a multimodal approach, of which endoscopic ultrasound with biopsy is becoming an increasingly important component.
- While asymptomatic serous cyst adenomas do not require intervention, mucinous cystic neoplasms should be resected due to their underlying malignant potential.
- The management of pancreatic neuroendocrine tumours will be dependent on the presence or absence of an underlying genetic syndrome, whether the tumour is hormonally active, and stage of disease.
- New adjuvant therapies have been shown to increase progression-free survival in patients with advanced neuroendocrine tumours.

References

1. Winter JM, Cameron JL, Campbell KA, et al. 1423 pancreaticoduodenectomies for pancreatic cancer: a single-institution experience. J Gastrointest Surg 2006;10:1199–210.

2. Ohashi K, Murakami Y, Maruyama M, et al. Four cases of mucin producing cancer of the pancreas on specific findings of the papilla of Vater [in Japanese]. Prog Dig Endosc 1982;20:348–51.

3. Longnecker DS, Adler G, Hruban RH, et al. Intraductal papillary mucinous neoplasm of the pancreas. In: Hamilton SR, Aaltonen LA, editors. World Health Organisation classification of tumours, pathology and genetics of tumours of the digestive system. Lyon: IARC Press; 2000. p. 237–41.

4. Tanaka M, Cahri S, Adsay V, et al. International consensus guidelines for management of intraductal papillary mucinous neoplasms and mucinous cystic neoplasms of the pancreas. Pancreatology 2006;6:17–32.

5. Reid-Lombardo KM, St Sauver J, Li Z, et al. Incidence, prevalence, and management of intraductal papillary mucinous neoplasm in Olmsted County, Minnesota, 1984–2005: a population study. Pancreas 2008;37:139–44.

6. Riall TS, Stager VM, Nealon WH. Incidence of additional primary cancers in patients with invasive intraductal papillary mucinous neoplasms and sporadic pancreatic adenocarcinomas. J Am Coll Surg 2007;204:803–13.

7. Macari M, Eubig J, Robinson E, et al. Frequency of intraductal papillary mucinous neoplasm in patients with and without pancreas cancer. Pancreatology 2010;10:734–41.

8. Sohn TA, Yeo CA, Cameron JL, et al. Intraductal papillary mucinous neoplasms of the pancreas: an increasingly recognized clinicopathologic entity. Ann Surg 2001;234:313–21.

9. Sohn TA, Yeo CA, Cameron JL, et al. Intraductal papillary mucinous neoplasms of the pancreas: an updated experience. Ann Surg 2004;239:788–97.

10. Fujino Y, Matsumoto I, Ueda T, et al. Proposed new score predicting malignancy of IPMN of the pancreas. Am J Surg 2007;194:304–7.

11. Winter JM, Cameron JL, Lillemoe KD, et al. Periampullary and pancreatic incidentaloma: a single institution's experience with an increasingly common diagnosis. Ann Surg 2006;243:673–80.

12. Irie H, Yoshimutu K, Tajima T, et al. Imaging spectrum of cystic pancreatic lesions: learn from atypical cases. Curr Probl Diagn Radiol 2007;36:213–26.

13. Yamada Y, Mori H, Matsumoto S. Intraductal papillary mucinous neoplasms of the pancreas: correlation of helical CT and dynamic MR imaging features with pathologic findings. Abdom Imaging 2008;33(4):474–81.

14. Pilleul F, Rochette A, Partensky C, et al. Preoperative evaluation of intraductal papillary mucinous tumors performed by pancreatic magnetic resonance imaging and correlated with surgical and histopathologic findings. J Magn Reson Imaging 2005;21:237–44.

15. Kawamoto S, Lawler LP, Horton KM, et al. MDCT of intraductal papillary mucinous neoplasm of the pancreas: evaluation of features predictive of invasive carcinoma. Am J Roentgenol 2006;186:687–95.

16. Kang MJ, Jang JY, Kim SJ, et al. Cyst growth rate predicts malignancy in patients with branch duct intraductal papillary mucinous neoplasms. Clin Gastroenterol Hepatol 2011;9:87–93.

17. Tomimaru Y, Takeda Y, Tatsumi M, et al. Utility of 2-[^{18}F] fluoro-2-deoxy-D-glucose positron emission tomography in differential diagnosis of benign and malignant intraductal papillary-mucinous neoplasm of the pancreas. Oncol Rep 2010;24:613–20.

18. García Figuerias R, Villalba Martín C, García Figuerias A, et al. The spectrum of cystic masses of the pancreas. Imaging features and diagnostic difficulties. Curr Probl Diagn Radiol 2007; 36:199–212.

19. Procacci C, Carbognin G, Biasiutti C, et al. Intraductal papillary mucinous tumours of the pancreas: spectrum of CT and MR findings with pathologic correlation. Eur Radiol 2001;11:1939–51.

20. Cone MM, Rea JD, Diggs BS, et al. Endoscopic ultrasound may be unnecessary in the preoperative evaluation of intraductal papillary mucinous neoplasm. HPB (Oxford) 2011;13:112–6.

21. Kubo H, Chijiiwa Y, Akahoshi K, et al. Intraductal papillary-mucinous tumors of the pancreas: differential diagnosis between benign and malignant tumors by endoscopic ultrasonography. Am J Gastroenterol 2001;96:1429–34.

22. Pais SA, Attasaranya S, Leblanc JK, et al. Role of endoscopic ultrasound in the diagnosis of intraductal papillary mucinous neoplasms: correlation with surgical histopathology. Clin Gastroenterol Hepatol 2007;5:489–95.

23. Michaels PJ, Brachtel EF, Bounds BC, et al. Intraductal papillary mucinous neoplasm of the pancreas: cytologic features predict histologic grade. Cancer 2006;108:163–73.

24. Tanaka M, Kobayashi K, Mizumoto K, et al. Clinical aspects of intraductal papillary mucinous neoplasm of the pancreas. J Gastroenterol 2005;40:669–75.

25. Hwang DW, Jang JY, Lim CS, et al. Determination of invasive predictors in branch duct type IPMN of the pancreas: a suggested scoring formula. J Korean Med Sci 2011;26:740–8.

26. Maimone S, Agrawal D, Pollack MJ, et al. Variability in measurements of pancreatic cyst size among EUS, CT and MRI modalities. Gastrointest Endosc 2010;71:945–50.

27. Hruban RH, Pitman MB, Klimstra DS, editors. AFIP atlas of tumor pathology. Tumors of the pancreas. Washington, DC: ARP Press; 2007.

28. Ban S, Naitoh Y, Mino-Kenudson M, et al. IPMN of the pancreas: its histopathological difference in 2 types. Am J Surg Pathol 2006;30:1561–9.

29. Furukawa T, Hatori T, Fujita I, et al. Prognostic relevance of morphological types of IPMN of the pancreas. Gut 2011;60:509–16.

30. Sugiyama M, Izumisato Y, Abe N, et al. Predicitive factors for malignancy in IPMN of the pancreas. Br J Surg 2003;90:1244–9.

31. Nagai K, Doi R, Kida A, et al. Intraductal papillary mucinous neoplasms of the pancreas: clinicopathological characteristics and long term follow up after resection. World J Surg 2008;32:271–8.

32. Rodriguez JR, Salvia R, Crippa S, et al. Branch-duct intraductal papillary mucinous neoplasms: observations in 145 patients who underwent resection. Gastroenterology 2007;133:72–9.

33. Salvia R, Crippa S, Falconi M, et al. Branch-duct intraductal papillary mucinous neoplasms of the pancreas: to operate or not to operate? Gut 2007; 56:1086–90.

34. Bae SY, Lee KT, Lee JH, et al. Proper management and follow-up stratergy of branch duct intraductal papillary mucinous neoplasms of the pancreas. Dig Liver Dis 2012;44(3):257–60.

35. Fujino Y, Suzuki Y, Yoshikawa T, et al. Outcomes of surgery for IPMN of the pancreas. World J Surg 2006;30:1909–14.

36. Crippa S, Bassi C, Warshaw AL, et al. Middle pancreatectomy: indications, short- and long-term operative outcomes. Ann Surg 2007;246:69–76.

37. Wada K, Kozarek RA, Traverso LW. Outcomes following resection of invasive and non invasive IPMN of the pancreas. Am J Surg 2005;189:632–5.

38. Hardacre JM, McGee MF, Stellato TA, et al. An aggressive surgical approach is warranted in the management of cystic pancreatic neoplasms. Am J Surg 2007;193:374–9.

39. Turrini O, Waters JA, Schnelldorfer T, et al. Invasive IPMN: predictors of survival and role of adjuvant therapy. HPB (Oxford) 2010;12:447–55.

40. Kargozaran H, Vu V, Ray P, et al. Invasive IPMN and MCN: same organ, different outcome. Ann Surg Oncol 2011;18:345–51.

41. Yopp AC, Katabi N, Janakos M, et al. Invasive carcinoma arising in IPMN of the pancreas. A matched control study with conventional pancreatic adenocarcinoma. Ann Surg 2011;253:968–74.

42. D'Angelica M. Brennan MF, Suriawinata AA, et al. Intraductal papillary mucinous neoplasms of the pancreas. An analysis of clinicopathological features and outcome. Ann Surg 2004;239:400–8.

43. White R, D'Angelica M, Katabi N, et al. Fate of the remnant pancreas after resection of non-invasive IPMN. J Am Coll Surg 2007;204:987–95.

44. Park J, Lee KT, Jang TH. Risk factors associated with post operative recurrence of IPMN of the pancreas. Pancreas 2011;40(1):46–51.

45. Tomimaru Y, Ishikawa O, Ohigashi H, et al. Advantage of pancreaticogastrostomy in detecting recurrent intraductal papillary mucinous carcinoma in the remnant pancreas: a case of successful re-resection after pancreaticoduodenectomy. J Surg Oncol 2006;93:511–5.

46. Kimura W, Kurda A, Morioka Y. Clinical pathology of endocrine tumours of the pancreas: analysis of autopsy cases. Dig Dis Sci 2004;36:933–42.

47. Bilimoria KY, Tomlinson JS, Merkow RP, et al. Clinicopathologic features and treatment trends of pancreatic neuroendocrine tumors: analysis of 9,821 patients. J Gastrointest Surg 2007;11:1460–7.

48. Ramage JK, Davies AHG, Ardill J, et al. Guidelines for the management of gastroenteropancreatic neuroendocrine tumours. Gut 2005;54:1–16.

49. Alexakis N, Connor S, Ghaneh P, et al. Hereditary pancreatic endocrine tumours. Pancreatology 2004; 4:417–33.

50. Lawrence B, Gustafsson BL, Kidd M, et al. The clinical relevance of chromogranin A as a biomarker for gastroenteropancreatic neuroendocrine tumors. Endocrinol Metab Clin North Am 2011; 40(1):111–34.

51. Rha SE, Jung SE, Lee KH, et al. CT and MR imaging of endocrine tumour of the pancreas according to WHO classification. Eur J Radiol 2007;62:371–7.

52. Rockall AG, Reznek RH. Imaging of neuroendocrine tumours. Best Pract Clin Endocr Metab 2007;21:43–68.

53. Tucker ON, Crotty PL, Conlon KC. The management of insulinoma. Br J Surg 2006;93:264–75.

54. Sundin A, Garske U, Orlefors H. Nuclear imaging of neuroendocrine tumours. Best Pract Clin Endocr Metab 2007;21:69–85.

55. Fendrich V, Langer P, Waldmann J, et al. Management of sporadic and multiple endocrine neoplasia type 1 gastrinomas. Br J Surg 2007;94:1331–41.

56. Mabrut JY, Fernandez-Cruz L, Azagra JS, et al. Laparoscopic pancreatic resection; results of a multicentre European study of 127 patients. Surgery 2005;137:597–605.

57. Norton JA, Fraker DL, Alexander HR, et al. Surgery increases survival in patients with gastrinoma. Ann Surg 2006;244:410–9.

In a study of 160 patients with gastrinomas, 35 patients (with similar staged localised disease) who did not undergo resection were compared to those who underwent resection. After 12 years' follow-up, 29% of those who did not undergo surgery had developed hepatic metastases compared to 5% in the resected group ($P < 0.001$).

58. Akerstrom G, Hellman P. Surgery on neuroendocrine tumours. Best Pract Clin Endocr Metab 2007;21:87–109.

59. Kouvaraki MA, Solorzano CC, Shapiro SE, et al. Surgical treatment of non functioning pancreatic islet cell tumours. J Surg Oncol 2005;89:170–85.

60. Bloomston M, Muscarella P, Shah MH, et al. Cytoreduction results in high perioperative mortality and decreased survival in patients undergoing pancreatectomy for neuroendocrine tumors of the pancreas. J Gastrointest Surg 2006;10:1361–70.

61. Minter RM, Simeone DM. Contemporary management of nonfunctioning pancreatic neuroendocrine tumors. J Gastrointest Surg 2012;16(2):435–46.

62. Moertel CG, Hanley JA. Combination chemotherapy trials in metastatic carcinoid tumor and the malignant carcinoid syndrome. Cancer Clin Trials 1979;2:327–34.

63. Raymond E, Dahan L, Raoul JL, et al. Sunitinib malate for the treatment of pancreatic neuroendocrine tumors. N Engl J Med 2011;364:501–13.
    One hundred and seventy-one patients with advanced and progressive PNETs were randomised in double-blind fashion to placebo or sunitinib. The trial was stopped early due to increased complications and death in the placebo group. An improved progression-free survival (11.5 vs. 5.5 months, $P < 0.001$) and reduced risk of death (105 vs. 255, $P = 0.02$) were seen in the treatment group.

64. Yao JC, Shah MH, Ito T, et al. Everolimus for advanced pancreatic neuroendocrine tumours. N Engl J Med 2011;364:514–23.
    In a placebo-controlled randomised crossover design trial, 410 patients with advanced and progressive PNETs were enrolled to placebo or everolimus. In those patients who received everolimus there was a 65% reduction in risk of progression (median progression-free survival was 11 months vs. 4.6 months) as compared to placebo. In addition, tolerance was high.

65. Edge SB, Byrd DR, Compton CC, et al., editors. AJCC cancer staging manual. 7th ed. Chicago, IL: Springer; 2010.

66. Strosberg JR, Cheema A, Weber J, et al. Prognostic validity of a novel American Joint Committee on Cancer Staging Classification for pancreatic neuroendocrine tumors. PNETs. J Clin Oncol 2011;29:3044–9.

67. Spinelli KS, Fromwiller TE, Daniel RA, et al. Cystic pancreatic neoplasms: observe or operate. Ann Surg 2004;239:651–9.

68. Compton CC. Histology of cystic tumours of the pancreas. Gastroint Endosc Clin North Am 2002;12:673–96.

69. Sarr MG, Kendrick ML, Nagorney DM, et al. Cystic neoplasms of the pancreas. Surg Clin North Am 2001;81:497–509.

70. Megibow AJ, Lavelle MT, Rofsky NM. Cystic tumors of the pancreas. The radiologist. Surg Clin North Am 2001;81:489–95.

71. Bassi C, Salvia R, Molinari E, et al. Management of 100 consecutive cases of pancreatic serous cystadenoma: wait for symptoms and see at imaging or vice versa? World J Surg 2003;27:319–23.

72. Linder JD, Geenen JE, Catalano MF. Cyst fluid analysis obtained by EUS-guided FNA in the evaluation of discrete cystic neoplasms of the pancreas: a single centre experience. Gastrointest Endosc 2006;64:697–702.

17

Hepatobiliary and pancreatic trauma

Rowan W. Parks

Introduction

Despite its relatively protected location, the liver is the most frequently injured intra-abdominal organ, although splenic injuries are more common following blunt abdominal trauma. Associated injuries to other organs, uncontrolled haemorrhage from the liver and subsequent development of septic complications contribute significantly to morbidity and death.

This chapter will address the presentation, initial assessment and management of patients with liver, non-iatrogenic biliary and pancreatic injuries. The selection criteria for conservative management will be discussed together with the indications for operative intervention. The factors guiding operative decision-making and the available therapeutic options at operation will be examined. The spectrum of complications and likely outcomes following trauma will also be reviewed. It is not always possible in clinical practice to separate these injuries into clearly distinct categories; however, practical guidance based on the evidence available will be presented.

Liver trauma

Mechanisms of liver injury

Blunt and penetrating trauma are the two principal mechanisms of liver injury. Road traffic accidents account for the majority of blunt injuries, whereas knife and gunshot wounds constitute the major cause of penetrating injuries. In the UK, blunt trauma predominates by a ratio of approximately 2:1 as documented in a large Scottish epidemiological study.[1] Whilst this is typical for other European centres,[2] it differs from the experience in South Africa, where penetrating injuries account for 66% of liver trauma,[3] and in North America, where up to 86% of liver injuries are penetrating wounds.[4,5]

Two types of blunt liver trauma have been described – deceleration (shearing) trauma and crush injury. Deceleration injuries occur in road traffic accidents and in falls from a height where there is movement of the liver relative to its diaphragmatic attachments.[6] Crush injuries are caused by direct trauma to the liver area. The two types of injury may coexist but tend to produce somewhat different types of liver injury. Deceleration or shearing injuries create lacerations in the hepatic parenchyma, typically between the right posterior section (segments 6 and 7) and the right anterior section (segments 5 and 8), which can extend to involve major vessels. In contrast, a direct blow to the abdomen may lead to a crush injury, with damage to the central portion of the liver (segments 4, 5 and 8). Compression between the right lower ribs and the spine may also cause bleeding from the caudate lobe (segment 1). Blunt trauma can rupture Glisson's capsule and can also lead to subcapsular or intraparenchymal haematoma formation. Penetrating injuries are usually associated with gunshot or stab wounds, with the former usually resulting in more tissue damage due to the cavitation effect as the bullet traverses the liver substance.

Injury to the hepatic veins and juxtahepatic vena cava can occur as a result of shearing stress in blunt trauma. It is worth noting that there may not be initial exsanguinating haemorrhage as the weight of the liver may provide some compression.

Classification of liver injury

The severity of liver trauma ranges from a minor capsular tear, with or without parenchymal injury, to extensive disruption involving both lobes of the liver with associated hepatic vein or vena caval injury. The American Association for the Surgery of Trauma has adopted for general use the classification of liver injury described initially in 1989 by Moore and colleagues, and revised subsequently in 1994[7] (Table 17.1). The hepatic injury grade is calculated from assessment of the liver injury using information derived from radiological study, operative findings or autopsy report. Where there are multiple injuries to the liver, the grade is advanced by one stage. Grade I or II injuries are considered minor; they represent 80–90% of all cases and usually require minimal or no operative treatment. Grade III–V injuries are generally considered severe and may require surgical intervention, while grade VI lesions are regarded as incompatible with survival. Schweizer et al. have described a protocol-based liver trauma management system employing this classification system that permits lesser injuries to be treated non-operatively and allows more appropriate selection of patients for operative treatment.[8]

The initial assessment and management of an injured patient should proceed according to the Advanced Trauma Life Support (ATLS) guidelines of the American College of Surgeons Committee on Trauma. The initial focus of attention is on the patient's airway, breathing and circulation. The airway is secured, intravenous access established and fluid resuscitation commenced.

The role of 'aggressive' high-volume fluid replacement in trauma victims has been questioned, with evidence suggesting that excessive fluid replacement is associated with adverse outcome.[9] As this evidence came from an American series that included a large proportion of relatively young, previously fit adults suffering from penetrating trauma to the torso, with ready access to trauma centres, the results may not necessarily be applicable to practice in other countries.

Diagnosis of liver injury

In penetrating abdominal trauma, hepatic injury should be considered in any patient with a wound to the abdomen. Hepatic injury should also be considered in patients with penetrating low thoracic wounds and also in posterior penetrating wounds below a coronal plane at the tips of the scapulae.

Patients with major hepatic injury may present with profound clinical shock and abdominal distension. Hypotension resistant to fluid resuscitation combined with gross abdominal distension is an indication for immediate laparotomy. The operative management options for patients in this situation will be discussed in detail subsequently. Emergency room thoracotomy with cross-clamping of the descending thoracic aorta is a dramatic intervention, but even in centres where this technique is advocated the outcome is poor.

Table 17.1 • Hepatic injury scale used by the American Association for the Surgery of Trauma

Grade		Description
I	Haematoma	Subcapsular, <10% surface area
	Laceration	Capsular tear, <1 cm parenchymal depth
II	Haematoma	Subcapsular, 10–50% of surface area
	Laceration	Intraparenchymal <10 cm in diameter, 1–3 cm parenchymal depth, <10 cm in length
III	Haematoma	Subcapsular, >50% surface area or expanding; ruptured subcapsular or parenchymal haematoma; intraparenchymal haematoma >10 cm or expanding
	Laceration	>3 cm parenchymal depth
IV	Laceration	Parenchymal disruption involving 25–75% of hepatic lobe or 1–3 Couinaud segments within a single lobe
V	Laceration	Parenchymal disruption involving >75% of hepatic lobe or >3 Couinaud segments within a single lobe
	Vascular	Juxtahepatic venous injuries – retrohepatic cava, major hepatic veins
VI	Vascular	Hepatic avulsion

Note: advance one grade for multiple injuries up to grade II.

In Feliciano et al.'s series of 1000 patients with liver trauma treated during a 5-year period, 45 patients underwent emergency room thoracotomy for control of haemorrhage related to their liver injury and all died.[4] Similarly, in an 11-year review of 783 patients who sustained liver trauma in Scotland, 11 patients underwent an unsuccessful laparotomy or thoraco-laparotomy in the emergency room.[1]

✔ Emergency room surgery remains a potentially life-saving manoeuvre in patients with significant intrathoracic injury who may have a coexistent liver injury. However, there is little place for this intervention in patients with a predominant abdominal injury. These patients are better served by rapid assessment and transport to the operating theatre.

In less dramatic situations, with a patient who is haemodynamically stable or responds to fluid resuscitation, appropriate investigations can be employed to obtain more information regarding the liver injury and to ascertain whether there is coexisting intra-abdominal visceral injury. During the initial survey a detailed clinical history is taken. Particular attention is paid to the mechanism of a road traffic accident, with supplemental information from ambulance crew, witnesses or police being used to piece together a picture of the accident. Speed of vehicle, position of occupant in vehicle, use of seatbelts, employment of airbag restraint systems and a history of ejection of the patient from the vehicle are important items of information. Conscious patients may complain of abdominal pain. Shoulder tip pain may arise from blood in the subdiaphragmatic space causing phrenic nerve irritation.

As resuscitation proceeds, a detailed physical examination is carried out. On inspection, attention is paid to the presence of anterior abdominal wall bruising, which may indicate compression from a seatbelt, and flank bruising, which may indicate retroperitoneal extravasation of blood. Signs of localised or generalised peritonitis are recorded in the conscious patient. In this context it should be noted that although there is evidence that the use of opiate analgesia will not significantly obscure physical signs in patients with acute abdominal pain, these findings have not been confirmed in abdominal trauma patients where the situation may be complicated by head injury, alcohol intoxication or the requirement for assisted ventilation.

Baseline investigations consist of a full blood count (for haemoglobin and haematocrit), serum urea and electrolytes, serum amylase, a coagulation screen, and blood for crossmatching. An erect chest radiograph and a plain abdominal film can be taken if the patient is sufficiently stable. In the context of diagnosing liver injury, features that may be of relevance include fractures of the lower ribs, elevation of the right hemidiaphragm and loss of the psoas shadow suggesting retroperitoneal bleeding. Retroperitoneal perforation of the duodenum may give rise to soft tissue shadowing in the right upper quadrant, loss of the psoas shadow and occasionally extraluminal gas may be noted.

Following initial assessment, patients who are conscious but have haemodynamic instability resistant to fluid resuscitation and with clinical signs of peritonitis should undergo laparotomy. In patients who are haemodynamically stable and have suspected liver injury, further diagnostic tests may be undertaken at this stage to define the nature of the injuries. An ideal test will establish the presence and extent of any liver injury together with providing information on concomitant visceral injury.

Formerly, diagnostic peritoneal lavage (DPL) was the procedure of choice for the quick diagnosis of haemoperitoneum, particularly in patients with an impaired level of consciousness and equivocal physical signs. However, DPL is invasive and a positive result for blood provides no information regarding either the site or the nature of the injury, and in the context of liver injury may lead to patients undergoing surgery where they may be better treated non-operatively.

An alternative investigation that has been advocated in initial trauma evaluation is focused assessment with sonography for trauma (FAST).[10] This involves ultrasonographic assessment of the pericardium, right upper quadrant including Morrison's pouch, left upper quadrant and pelvis. This evaluation is not designed to identify the degree of organ injury, but rather the presence of blood. A large meta-analysis of the use of emergency ultrasonography for blunt abdominal trauma reported sensitivity rates ranging from 28% to 97% and specificity rates close to 100%.[11]

Rozycki et al. demonstrated a significant correlation between haemoperitoneum in the right upper quadrant and injury to the liver, and suggested that adherence to a pre-agreed protocol increased the reliability of ultrasound assessment of abdominal trauma.[12] Other centres have also reported that ultrasound is a reliable 'first' test for the assessment of a patient with suspected liver trauma.[13] However, an important cautionary note comes from the study carried out by Richards et al.[14] In a series of 1686 abdominal ultrasound scans for trauma, 71 patients had bowel or mesenteric injury and 30 patients had a negative ultrasound scan (43% false-negative rate). Limitations of FAST include operator dependence, poor assessment of the retroperitoneum, unreliable detection of pneumoperitoneum and difficulty in scanning obese patients or those with overlying wounds.

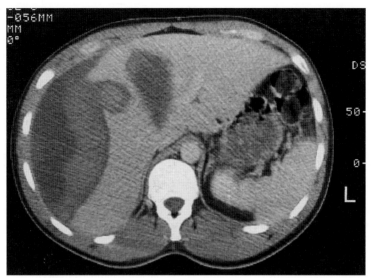

Figure 17.1 • CT image of a 25-year-old male who sustained a blunt injury to the right chest wall but was admitted to hospital haemodynamically stable. The scan shows a substantial subcapsular haematoma associated with an intraparenchymal laceration. This patient was managed successfully without operation.

Computed tomography (CT) is the 'gold standard' investigation for the evaluation of a patient with suspected liver trauma (**Fig. 17.1**). The use of intravenous contrast may help in the detection of non-viable parenchyma. CT has high sensitivity and specificity for detecting liver injuries; these attributes increase as the time between injury and scanning increases, as haematomas and lacerations become better defined. Specific CT features of liver trauma have been reported by a number of authors. Fang et al. described intraparenchymal 'pooling' of intravenous contrast that correlated strongly to the presence of ongoing haemorrhage.[15] Yokota and Sugimoto documented 'periportal tracking' to consist of a circumferential area of low attenuation around the portal triad.[16] Periportal tracking is thought to represent blood or fluid within the condensation of the Glissonian sheath around the portal structures and indicates the presence of injury to structures in the portal triad. If the sign is present in the periphery of the liver it may alert the clinician to the presence of a peripheral bile duct injury that in turn may present as a bile leak. Addition of oral contrast does not appear to add to the diagnostic yield of CT in the assessment of liver injury.[17]

In order to maintain a balanced perspective, it is worthwhile considering some of the limitations of CT in the assessment of liver trauma. The CT-defined grade of injury may differ from the grade of liver injury found at operation, with the predominant tendency being to overdiagnose the grade of injury on CT as compared with subsequent operative findings. Croce et al. concluded that CT should not be used in isolation to estimate blood loss and that CT may not provide an accurate assessment of the extent of a liver laceration in some areas of the liver – specifically in the vicinity of the falciform ligament.[18]

Bearing the above limitations in mind, CT will help define the extent of the liver injury and will be of value in the detection of injury to other intra-abdominal viscera, in particular pancreatic injury. CT will allow the liver injury to be graded and thus will provide objective information that is mandatory if non-operative treatment is to be contemplated. Further refinements now permit accurate three-dimensional image reconstruction, and technical modifications such as helical CT combined with intravenous contrast allow demonstration of the biliary tree (CT cholangiography) or vascular anatomy (CT angiography).

Some authors recommend performing a whole-body CT as the standard diagnostic tool during the early phase for patients with polytrauma, advocating that this will alter treatment in up to 34% of patients with blunt trauma.[19] A 30% reduction in mortality using this approach has also been reported.[20] Other arguments in favour of an imaging survey are the reduction in time from admission to intervention and consistency in managing haemodynamically unstable patients.[21] However, at present the logistics of such an approach are not universally applicable as it requires a CT scanner in, or very close to, the emergency department.

Other diagnostic/therapeutic modalities for the assessment and treatment of liver injury

Non-invasive imaging techniques such as magnetic resonance imaging (MRI) have the advantage of being free of ionising radiation, but increased cost aside, the time taken to produce a scan means that this technique is not yet widely used in the trauma setting.

Angiography plays a vital role in the conservative management of liver injuries. Extravasation of contrast seen on CT requires emergency angiography and therapeutic angiographic embolisation for ongoing blood loss or haemobilia.[22] Angioembolisation is also reported following damage control surgery prior to removal of packs if rebleeding is suspected.[23,24]

Other diagnostic modalities may be used in specific situations. Endoscopic retrograde cholangiopancreatography (ERCP) may help in delineation of the biliary tree in patients with liver trauma, and endoscopic transpapillary stents may be used as a therapeutic modality to treat biliary leaks.[25]

Diagnostic laparoscopy has been used successfully in patients with abdominal trauma, and therapeutic laparoscopic techniques for managing liver injuries using fibrin glue have also been described. However, in the specific context of liver trauma, concerns have been raised about the use of laparoscopy because general anaesthesia, muscle relaxation and the creation of a pneumoperitoneum may decompress a stable perihepatic haematoma. Furthermore, laparoscopic assessment of the injured liver may not provide sufficient detail concerning parenchymal injury. For these reasons, the role of laparoscopy has yet to be established in the assessment of liver injuries.

> ✅ FAST is reliable for the initial assessment of a patient with suspected liver trauma, but CT remains the gold standard to define the extent of injury in a stable patient.

Management of liver injury: selection of patients for non-operative management

The feasibility of non-operative management of patients with intra-abdominal solid-organ injury was first established in paediatric surgery but was subsequently extended to adult practice. Richie and Fonkalsrud described successful conservative management of four patients with liver injury in an era before the availability of CT.[26] Further indirect evidence for the feasibility of a non-operative approach came from a report published by White and Cleveland[27] in the same year. They reported a consecutive series of 126 patients with liver trauma, all of whom underwent laparotomy. Interestingly, 67 patients in this series (53%) had placement of a drain to the subhepatic space as their only liver-related surgical intervention at laparotomy. Subsequent studies have recognised that 50–80% of liver injuries stop bleeding spontaneously and this has led to a non-operative approach for blunt liver trauma in selected patients.

Non-operative management of liver trauma is now a well-established treatment option. Trunkey's group in Portland, Oregon, first defined in 1985 the following criteria for the selection of patients for non-operative management:

- haemodynamic stability;
- absence of peritoneal signs;
- availability of good-quality CT;
- an experienced radiologist;
- ability to monitor patients in an intensive care setting;
- facility for immediate surgery (and by implication, availability of an experienced liver surgeon);
- simple liver injury with <125 mL of free intraperitoneal blood;
- absence of other significant intra-abdominal injuries.[28]

Farnell et al. extended the threshold of haemoperitoneum to 250 mL and described specific liver injuries suitable for non-operative management.[29] Feliciano suggested subsequently that any blunt hepatic injury, regardless of its magnitude, should be managed without operation if the patient was haemodynamically stable and had a haemoperitoneum of less than 500 mL.[30] The degree of liver injury amenable to successful non-operative management has gradually extended over recent years, and most authors now believe that the ultimate decisive factor in favour of non-operative management is haemodynamic stability of the patient at presentation or after initial resuscitation, irrespective of the grade of liver injury on CT or the amount of haemoperitoneum.[31,32]

A 22-month prospective study from Memphis of the initial non-operative treatment of haemodynamically stable blunt hepatic trauma patients compared outcome to a matched cohort of blunt hepatic trauma patients treated operatively.[33] The study reported that of 136 patients with blunt trauma, 24 (18%) underwent emergency surgery. Of the remaining 112 patients, 12 (11%) failed conservative management (for causes not related to the liver injury in seven) and the remaining 100 patients were treated successfully without operation. Of these, 30% had minor injuries (grades I and II) but 70% had major injuries (grades III–V). This study concluded that non-operative management was safe for haemodynamically stable patients and that this was independent of the CT-delineated grade of the liver injury. The blood transfusion requirement and the incidence of abdominal complications were lower in the non-operatively treated group.

Reporting a single institutional experience, Boone et al. stated that 46 (36%) of 128 consecutive patients with blunt liver trauma were successfully treated non-operatively, including 23 patients with grade III and IV injuries.[31] A review of 495 patients from the published literature noted a success rate for non-operative treatment of 94%.[34] This was accomplished with a mean transfusion rate of 1.9 units, a complication rate of 6% and a mean hospital stay of 13 days. There were no liver-related deaths, nor were there any missed enteric injuries.

The current consensus view is that successful selection of patients for conservative treatment after blunt abdominal trauma cannot be carried out by CT alone, but that an overall assessment of suitability for such an approach must take into account the findings of careful repeated clinical examination and the results of close monitoring of haemodynamic and haematological parameters. If non-operative management is selected, haemodynamic instability is the predominant indication for intervention early in the clinical course whilst intervention (often radiological or endoscopic) may be required later for management of bile leak or intrahepatic collections.

If a non-operative strategy is selected it should be borne in mind that the risk of hollow-organ injury increases in proportion to the number of solid organs injured[35] and that there is a small but significant risk of delayed haemorrhage. However, it appears that the natural course of liver injuries is more analogous to that of lung or kidney injuries, rather than splenic injuries, in that any deterioration is usually gradual, with a fall in haemoglobin level or an increase in fluid requirement, rather than acute haemodynamic decompensation. Therefore, with close supervision, patients who fail with an initial non-operative approach can be detected early and treated appropriately.

Although non-operative management of haemodynamically stable patients with liver trauma has become the standard of care over the past decade, the role of in-hospital follow-up CT to monitor the injury remains controversial. Demetriades et al. reported that follow-up CT at a mean of 10 days after surgical intervention showed a 49% incidence of liver-related complications, most of which required subsequent intervention.[36] However, other authors suggest there is little evidence that follow-up CT provides additional information and rarely changes management.[37] In the author's practice, in-hospital follow-up scan is not employed routinely unless the patient develops relevant symptoms or signs, but a follow-up scan 4–6 weeks later is undertaken to ensure resolution of the injury.

The management policy for abdominal gunshot injuries in most centres continues to be a mandatory laparotomy, regardless of the clinical presentation;[38] however, several studies have reported successful non-operative management of selected liver gunshot injuries.[39,40] In the study by Omoshoro-Jones et al., 26.6% of patients who presented with liver gunshot injuries were managed non-operatively, with an overall success rate of 94% and a morbidity rate of 36%, of which 3% were liver related.[39] This approach is associated with the risk of failure to detect concomitant intra-abdominal visceral injury and therefore should only be considered in specialist centres with experience in management of liver trauma and appropriate facilities to deal with any complications that arise.

✅ Non-operative management is safe for haemodynamically stable patients with CT evidence of liver injury.

Operative management of liver injury

General strategy

Primary operative intervention is indicated for liver injury if the patient is haemodynamically unstable despite adequate initial resuscitation. Important prerequisites for a successful outcome are: adequate blood, platelets, fresh frozen plasma and cryoprecipitate; an intensive care unit; the necessary diagnostic facilities to monitor and detect potential complications; and an experienced liver surgeon. Although this is the ideal, patients with liver trauma often present initially to surgeons without specialist hepatobiliary experience and without the facilities available in liver surgery units. The surgeon operating on a patient in this situation should therefore attempt to control bleeding without causing further complications.

Choice of incision

A long midline incision is widely employed for an emergency laparotomy. It has the advantages that it can be made rapidly, and extended proximally (to enter the chest after median sternotomy) or distally as required. Access to the liver can be improved by converting the incision into a 'T' by adding a right transverse component or to a 'Y' by adding a right lateral thoracotomy, although extension of the incision into the chest is exceptional. In situations where an operation is being carried out after initial conservative management, for example to treat bile leakage or perform delayed resectional debridement, a subcostal incision with fixed costal margin retraction affords excellent access to the liver.

Intraoperative assessment

Once the abdomen has been entered, blood and clots should be removed and packs inserted into each quadrant of the abdomen. A thorough laparotomy is performed in a systematic manner to identify all intra-abdominal injuries. Any perforations in the bowel should be sutured immediately to minimise contamination. Significant liver haemorrhage can usually be controlled initially by direct pressure using packs, although additional techniques that may be employed include: temporary digital compression of the free edge of the lesser omentum (Pringle manoeuvre; **Fig. 17.2**); bimanual compression of the liver; or manual compression of the aorta above

the coeliac trunk. At this point, further evaluation of the extent of liver injury should be delayed until the anaesthetist has replenished adequately the intravascular volume and stabilised the blood pressure. Attempts to evaluate the liver injury before adequate resuscitation may result in further blood loss, with worsening hypotension and acidosis.

The packs can subsequently be gently removed to allow a detailed evaluation of the type and extent of the liver injury. It should be borne in mind that a subcapsular haematoma may cover an area of ischaemic tissue and that parenchymal lacerations may be associated with damage to segmental bile ducts. Many liver injuries will have stopped bleeding spontaneously by the time of surgery. However, if there is active bleeding, a Pringle manoeuvre can be used diagnostically and compression can be maintained with an atraumatic vascular clamp if haemorrhage decreases (**Fig. 17.3**). The clamp should be occluded only to the degree necessary to compress the blood vessels and not to injure the common bile duct. A normal liver can tolerate inflow occlusion for up to 1 hour; however, the ability of a damaged liver to tolerate ischaemia may be impaired. If haemorrhage

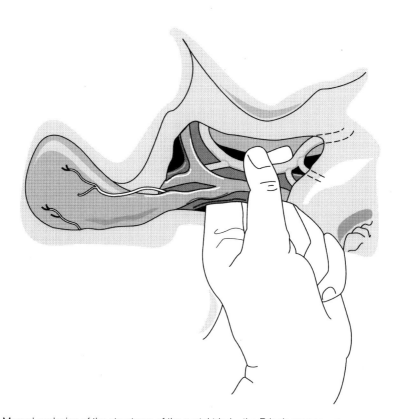

Figure 17.2 • Manual occlusion of the structures of the portal triad – the Pringle manoeuvre.

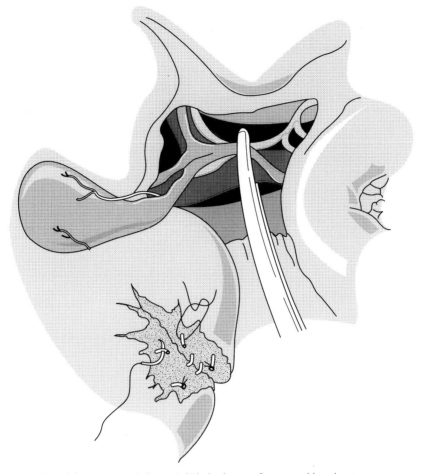

Figure 17.3 • Occlusion of the structures in the portal triad using a soft non-crushing clamp.

is unaffected by portal triad occlusion, major vena cava injury or atypical vascular anatomy should be suspected. Hepatic outflow control may also be required. Access to the suprahepatic cava can be gained by an experienced liver surgeon, and slings may be placed around the hepatic veins following mobilisation of the liver from its peritoneal attachments. Total vascular occlusion of the liver requires control of the inferior vena cava below the liver in addition to the suprahepatic cava but is likely to be poorly tolerated by an injured liver.

Perihepatic packing

In situations where it is thought that definitive control of haemorrhage cannot be obtained, or patients are deemed critically unstable, coagulopathic or acidotic and therefore would not tolerate a prolonged operative procedure, perihepatic packing can be employed. This has led to the concept of damage

control surgery – rapid perihepatic packing, closure of the abdominal incision with or without a Bogota bag and transferring the patient to ICU as soon as possible for continued resuscitation and rewarming. When the metabolic derangements have been corrected or improved, the patient can be taken back to theatre or transferred to a specialist centre for re-exploration and definitive treatment.[41]

As packing is thus a widely applicable procedure, some attention should be devoted to technical considerations. The packs should not be inserted into the liver substance itself, as this will tend to distract the edges of the parenchymal tear and encourage continued bleeding. Rather, the technique of packing involves manual closure or approximation of the parenchyma, followed by sequential placing of dry abdominal packs or a single rolled gauze around the liver and directly over the injury in an attempt to provide tamponade to a bleeding wound (**Fig. 17.4**).

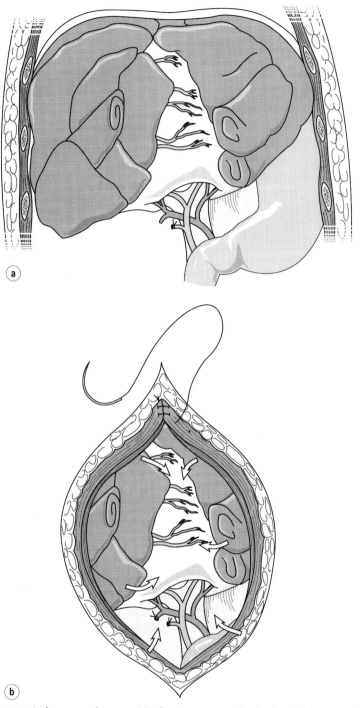

Figure 17.4 • (a) Placement of gauze packs around the liver to compress the fracture. **(b)** Closure of the incision provides additional compression. Reproduced from Berne TV, Donovan AJ. Section 10. Injury and haemorrhage. In: Blumgart LH, Fong Y (eds) Surgery of the liver and biliary tract, 3rd edn, Vol. 2. Edinburgh: Churchill Livingstone, 1994. With permission from Elsevier.

Most surgeons employ skin closure only, leaving the fascia for primary closure at the subsequent procedure for pack removal. The presence of packs, combined with massive oedema of the bowel, may lead to difficulties in wound closure. If this is encountered, a mesh can be inserted to prevent further compromise of ventilation and bowel viability, and to avoid pressure necrosis of the liver.[42]

The principal complications and limitations of perihepatic packing can be considered as 'early' or 'late'. Early complications include failure to control haemorrhage. However, this is relatively uncommon as even in patients with caval or hepatic venous injuries, packing may control haemorrhage. Concerns may also be raised about the potential for compromise of caval blood flow by packing, although this may be avoided by monitoring caval pressure if this technique is available. The principal late complications of packing are infection and multiple organ dysfunction. The risk of septic complications has led to the recommendation that liver packs should be removed as soon as possible. However, Nicol et al. reported in a series of 93 patients requiring liver packing that an early re-look laparotomy at 24 hours rather than at 48 hours or later was associated with a higher incidence of re-bleeding necessitating re-packing, without any difference in the incidence of liver-related complications or intra-abdominal collections.[43] Perihepatic packing is an indication for intravenous antibiotic administration.

> ✅ The first re-look laparotomy following packing for a liver injury should only be performed after 48 hours, when hypotension, hypothermia, coagulopathy and acidosis have been corrected.

Techniques for surgical haemostasis

Exposed bleeding vessels can be suture-ligated, clipped or repaired to achieve haemostasis. The ultrasonic dissector is useful in removing damaged and non-viable hepatic parenchyma whilst exposing blood vessels. Diathermy coagulation can also be used and in this context the argon beam coagulator, which 'sprays' the diathermy current on an argon beam, is invaluable as it produces surface eschar without the diathermy probe becoming adherent to the liver surface. The argon beam coagulator also has the advantage of producing less hepatic tissue necrosis than conventional diathermy, which is an advantage in a potentially contaminated operative field. Fibrin glue has been used as an adjunctive measure in some centres; however, there are concerns regarding the use of fibrin glue in humans. Fatal hypotension following application of fibrin glue

into a deep hepatic laceration has been reported.[44] Recently, recombinant factor VIIa has been reported as a potential adjunct in the management of liver injuries;[45] however, further controlled studies are warranted to evaluate the safety and efficiency of this drug.

Liver sutures are absorbable sutures on a large curved blunt-tipped needle often used in conjunction with a bolster of haemostatic material. These can be used to approximate a fissured parenchymal injury and thus control haemorrhage as an alternative to exploration of the depths of the injury. The disadvantages of this technique are that vessels may continue to bleed, resulting in a cavitating haematoma, bile duct injuries may not be detected, and the suture itself may cause further bleeding, ischaemia or intrahepatic bile duct injury (**Fig. 17.5**).

Stone and Lamb reported that the greater omentum could be employed as a pedicled flap to fill a defect in the liver parenchyma and may help stop oozing from the low-pressure venous system of the liver parenchyma.[46] The use of an absorbable polyglactin perihepatic mesh, particularly for major parenchymal disruptions, has also been reported.[47] This technique is not indicated where juxtacaval or hepatic vein injury is suspected. Advocates of mesh wrapping claim that it can provide the benefits of packing without the disadvantages. In particular, a second laparotomy is not required routinely and, as mesh wrapping does not increase intra-abdominal volume or pressure, abdominal closure is much easier and respiratory or renal function is less compromised. However, there is some concern about the amount of time needed to apply the mesh wrap in a haemodynamically unstable patient who might be best treated with rapid insertion of perihepatic packs, and as yet there is insufficient general experience with this technique.

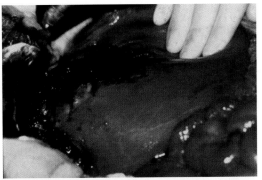

Figure 17.5 • Operative photograph demonstrating a liver injury with necrosis at the site of previously inserted liver sutures that had been applied in an attempt to arrest haemorrhage.

Resectional debridement

This technique involves removal of devitalised liver tissue down to normal parenchyma using the lines of the injury, rather than anatomical planes, as the boundaries of the resection.[48] The optimum timing may be to combine debridement with pack removal, as necrotic tissue will be well demarcated at 48 h post-injury. Resectional debridement is by definition 'non-anatomical' and may expose segmental bile ducts (**Fig. 17.6**). Disrupted bile ducts exposed in the periphery of the liver should be sutured or ligated in order to prevent postoperative bile leaks, as this troublesome complication will not necessarily be treatable by endoscopic transampullary biliary stenting. It is better to anticipate and avoid this complication.

Anatomical liver resection

The practical difficulties of undertaking formal anatomical liver resection in a patient with a significant liver injury, who will frequently have associated shock, coagulopathy and concomitant injury, are such that this type of treatment is not used widely. It is generally accepted that anatomical resections should be reserved for situations in which no other procedure adequately achieves haemostasis, such as with deep liver lacerations involving major vessels and/or bile ducts, where there is extensive devascularisation or if there is major hepatic venous bleeding.

Strong et al. reported a single-centre series of 37 patients that underwent anatomical resection for liver trauma from an institutional experience of 287 patients with liver injury treated over a 13-year period.[49] Twenty-seven of these patients underwent right hemihepatectomy and overall there were three postoperative deaths (8% mortality rate). However, these excellent results achieved by a technically skilled liver surgeon and his unit may not be reproduced if the technique were more widely used.

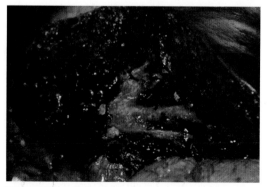

Figure 17.6 • Debridement of a liver injury managed 3 days before by packing has left the branches of the right portal pedicle exposed.

Selective ligation of the hepatic artery

Selective ligation of the hepatic artery is no longer a commonly used technique and is not mentioned frequently in contemporary reports. It may be used when intrahepatic manoeuvres have failed and when persistent re-bleeding occurs on unclamping the hepatic pedicle. In a series of 60 patients,[50] Mays reported ligation of the right hepatic artery in 36 patients, the left hepatic artery in 15 patients and the main hepatic artery in the remaining nine patients. No cases of liver failure or necrosis were observed but it seems likely that modern liver surgical approaches have rendered ligation an uncommon manoeuvre in liver injury. Hepatic arterial ligation to control haemorrhage should only be performed when other manoeuvres have failed, when selective ligation has failed and when pedicle clamping has been demonstrated to arrest haemorrhage. Acute gangrenous cholecystitis is a well-recognised complication of hepatic artery ligation, and cholecystectomy should be performed if the main hepatic artery or right hepatic artery is ligated.

Management of hepatic venous and retrohepatic caval injury

Suspicion that one of these serious injuries is present should be raised if the Pringle manoeuvre fails to arrest haemorrhage. In this situation it is vital that a systematic approach be adopted. Injudicious mobilisation of the liver can cause exsanguination or embolisation of air or detached fragments of liver parenchyma. Therefore it is important to exclude anatomical vascular variants as a source of persistent bleeding. For example, there may be bleeding from the left liver due to the presence of a left hepatic artery arising from the left gastric artery or there may be bleeding from the right liver due to an aberrant right hepatic artery. The commonest anatomical variation in the origin of the right hepatic artery (occurring in approximately 15% of cases) is the persistence of the right primordial hepatic artery where the right hepatic artery arises from the superior mesenteric artery and runs just to the right and slightly posterior to the structures in the porta hepatis. These anatomical variants should be considered and excluded. During this process, active bleeding can be reduced or arrested by perihepatic packing. Persistent bleeding despite exclusion of anatomical variants may then indicate the presence of hepatic venous or retrohepatic caval injury. These injuries account for about 10% of liver trauma cases, and there is no clear consensus on an optimal management strategy. Total vascular exclusion (clamping of the inferior vena cava and suprahepatic cava in addition to the Pringle manoeuvre) may be used. However, clamping the vena cava will seriously compromise venous return in a situation of major trauma and seems unwise. Veno-venous bypass (shunt from common femoral vein to left internal jugular or axillary vein) has the advantage of preserving venous return. Atriocaval shunting has also been described and, combined with a Pringle manoeuvre, allows total vascular isolation of the liver. Chen et al. reported on a series of 19 patients with blunt juxtahepatic venous injury from a group of 92 patients with blunt liver trauma over a 2-year period.[51] Five patients with isolated left hepatic vein injuries were treated with the use of veno-venous bypass with no mortality. Ten of the 20 patients with isolated right hepatic vein injury were treated using an atriocaval shunt but the mortality in these 20 patients was 18 (80%), with one survivor in both the shunted and non-shunted groups. Of four patients with combined right and left hepatic vein injury, one was treated by liver transplantation but all four patients in this group died. The overall mortality rate in patients with juxtahepatic vein injury was 63%. The opportunity to optimise the outcome in patients with these serious injuries probably lies in packing followed by transfer to a specialist liver surgery unit.

Ex vivo surgery and liver transplantation

Ringe and Pichlmayr[52] reported a consecutive series of eight patients with severe liver trauma treated by total hepatectomy followed by liver transplantation. These patients had all undergone prior surgery for trauma, which had been followed by severe complications – uncontrollable bleeding in four and massive necrosis in four. Where a donor liver was not immediately available a temporary portacaval shunt was used as a bridging procedure. There was a high mortality in this group, with six out of eight patients dying from multiple organ failure or sepsis. The authors conclude that total hepatectomy can be a potentially life-saving procedure in exceptional emergencies in patients with major liver injuries. Heparinised coated tubes such as the Gott shunt can be used to bridge caval defects if total hepatectomy and excision of a caval segment is required in order to obtain haemostasis.[53] The shunt acts as a temporary bridge during the anhepatic phase and has been reported to remain patent over an 18-h period. Whilst experience of this sort of surgery is extremely infrequent, awareness of the therapeutic potential is useful and small series continue to report encouraging results.[54]

Complications of liver trauma

Complications of non-operative management

Complications of non-operative management of liver trauma can be considered in three main categories. First, it should be borne in mind that complications can arise as a result of inappropriate selection of a patient for conservative management. If a patient has continued bleeding this may present as episodes of hypotension requiring fluid and blood replacement, impaired renal function, impaired respiratory function (due to diaphragmatic splinting by intra-abdominal haematoma) and there may be evidence of coagulopathy. These features represent not so much a 'complication' as the natural progression of a patient with continued active intra-abdominal bleeding, and in such a case the policy of non-operative intervention will require reappraisal.

The second group of complications are those relating to coexisting injuries that have not been recognised at the time of initial presentation or become apparent after initial delay. Bile leaks may manifest as biliary peritonitis or as a localised bile collection. ERCP is useful in diagnosing the source of a bile leak in patients with liver trauma treated non-operatively and also in postoperative patients. Perforations of the intestine are also at risk of being missed as the signs of abdominal tenderness may be attributed to intra-abdominal blood from the liver injury. The risk of missing this type of injury can be minimised by regular careful clinical observation. Intestinal perforation may become apparent on serial ultrasound or CT by the presence of free intra-peritoneal fluid or gas. In Sherman et al.'s series of patients with liver trauma treated non-operatively, 4 of 30 (13%) patients initially treated without operation required subsequent laparotomy.[32] These were due to splenic injury in three patients and renal injury in one patient. Although the grade of injury to these organs is not specified, in all cases the injuries became apparent after a period of clinical observation. However, the authors concluded that this risk of missed solid-organ injury does not obviate the benefits of initial non-operative management.

The third category of complication relates to the late complications of liver injury. Liver injury may give rise to a transient increase in liver transaminase enzymes. Their persistent elevation suggests significant liver injury. Septic complications such as intra-abdominal abscess and bile leak are recognised late complications and may require radiological, endoscopic or surgical intervention.

Postoperative complications after surgery for liver trauma

The complications after liver surgery for trauma are similar to those encountered after any form of hepatic surgery. Haemorrhage in the immediate postoperative period may be due to coagulopathy related to large-volume transfusion and may require correction with fresh frozen plasma and platelet concentrates. If there is no evidence of a significant coagulopathy and bleeding continues, CT angiography may provide diagnostic information. Selective mesenteric angiography may permit therapeutic embolisation, but if this is unsuccessful, re-laparotomy will be indicated to assess and control the source of bleeding and to remove retained blood and clot. Bleeding in the later postoperative period may be due to haemobilia or bleeding from the biliary tree into the gut. It has been reported to occur in 1.2% of patients with liver trauma.[55]

Postoperative sepsis may be due to infected collections of bile or blood, or related to devitalised segments of liver parenchyma. Ultrasound and CT are of value in diagnosis and these modalities may be used to guide placement of drains. Bile leakage from a drain site is not uncommon and usually ceases spontaneously; however, if it persists, ERCP may be all that is required to define the site of the leak and allow temporary stent placement. Arteriovenous fistula is not an uncommon complication after liver injury and can manifest as an arterioportal fistula resulting in portal hypertension.

Outcome after liver injury

The outcome after liver trauma is related not only to the severity of the injury but also to the severity of any associated injury. Most series report mortality rates of approximately 10–15%; however, the large variation in case mix between different centres makes comparison difficult. In a large series of 1000 cases of liver trauma from Houston, an overall mortality of 10.5% was reported.[4] White and Cleveland documented a similar mortality rate, with eight deaths occurring in a consecutive series of 126 patients (6.3%).[27] The results in the series reported by Schweizer et al. recorded an overall mortality rate of 12% (21 deaths in 175 patients), with a progressively higher mortality rate associated with an increasing grade of liver injury.[8] In a series of 337 patients, Kozar et al. reported 37 hepatic-related complications in 25 patients; 63% (5 of 8) of patients with grade V injuries developed complications, 21% (19 of 92) of patients had grade IV injuries, but only 1% (1 of 130) of patients had grade III injuries.[56] The mechanism of injury has an important bearing on the mortality rate, with blunt trauma carrying a higher mortality rate (10–30%) than penetrating liver trauma (0–10%). While most early deaths seem to be due to uncontrolled haemorrhage and associated injuries, most late deaths result from head injuries and sepsis with multiple organ failure.

Extrahepatic biliary tract trauma

Non-iatrogenic injury to the extrahepatic biliary tract is uncommon and encountered only rarely by surgeons outside specialist hepatobiliary centres. Most injuries are due to penetrating rather than blunt abdominal trauma. Biliary tract injury is diagnosed infrequently before operation and is often only recognised incidentally at laparotomy. Extrahepatic bile duct injury due to blunt trauma is only rarely associated with injury to the portal vein or hepatic artery. This may be explained by the increased length, tortuosity and elasticity of the vascular structures. Furthermore, a vascular injury, especially portal vein rupture, is likely to be associated with a high immediate mortality.

Incidence of biliary injury

The reported incidence of injury to the extrahepatic biliary system varies between 1% and 5% of patients who sustain abdominal trauma.[57] In a review of 5070 patients who sustained blunt and penetrating abdominal trauma, Penn reported a 1.9% incidence of gallbladder injury.[58] Soderstrom et al. identified 31 patients (2.1%) with gallbladder injury in a group of 1449 patients who sustained blunt abdominal trauma and underwent exploratory laparotomy.[59] In a further review of 949 patients undergoing laparotomy for acute trauma, there were 32 injuries to the gallbladder (3.4%) and five to the common bile duct (0.5%).[60] Burgess and Fulton reported that, over a 5-year period, 24 of 184 patients with abdominal trauma had extrahepatic bile duct or gallbladder injury as well as liver injury.[61] They reported that this injury was often seen with severe hepatic trauma and in association with multiple organ injury. Dawson et al. reviewed the results of treatment of all patients with porta hepatis injuries presenting to a level I trauma centre in Seattle over an 11-year period.[62] A total of 21 patients (0.21% of 10 500 admissions) had injuries to the portal triad, of whom 11 (52%) died. Isolated extrahepatic bile duct injury occurred in four of these patients. Injuries to the portal vein or hepatic artery, either in isolation or in association with extrahepatic bile duct injury, were associated with the worst prognosis. Of note is the fact that in none of the 21 cases was the diagnosis of the injury made preoperatively. The male to female ratio is usually reported as approximately 5:1.[63] However, Bade et al. reported a male to female ratio of 25:1, which may reflect the higher number of injuries from stab wounds seen in a South African population.[64] Most series report a median age of approximately 30 years and there are many reports in children.

Classification of biliary injury

The gallbladder is the most frequently injured part of the extrahepatic biliary tract. The largest reported series of extrahepatic biliary tract injuries consists of 53 patients, of whom 45 (85%) sustained injury to the gallbladder and eight (15%) had an injury to the bile duct.[64] Kitahama et al. reported the gallbladder to be involved in 32 (80%) of 40 patients, while ductal injury occurred in 12 (30%), some patients having multiple injuries.[63]

Injury to the gallbladder resulting from blunt trauma can be classified as contusion, avulsion or perforation. In addition to these three main types of injury, Penn added traumatic cholecystitis as a pathological entity.[58] The most common type of gallbladder injury is perforation. Avulsion of the gallbladder may refer to the organ being partially or completely torn from the liver bed while still attached to the bile duct, or it may signify complete separation from all attachments with the organ lying free in the abdomen. Contusion is probably under-reported, as it will be recognised only if laparotomy is performed. The natural course of an untreated gallbladder contusion is not known, although it is likely that the majority resolve without further complication. It has been speculated that an intramural haematoma might result in necrosis of the gallbladder wall and result in a subsequent perforation. There have been a number of reports of delayed rupture of the gallbladder, and it is plausible that unrecognised contusion of the gallbladder might lead to such a delayed presentation.

Bile duct injury is classified according to the site of injury and according to whether the transection is partial or complete. Partial duct injuries are often referred to as 'tangential' wounds. Penetrating injuries can affect any part of the extrahepatic biliary system; however, the commonest sites of injury due to blunt trauma are at the point where the common bile duct enters the pancreas and where the biliary confluence exits from the liver. These sites are at points of maximum fixation, which accounts for their propensity to injury.

Isolated injury to the extrahepatic biliary tract is very uncommon. The liver is the organ most commonly injured in association with biliary tract trauma (approximately 80% of cases), with the duodenum, stomach, colon and pancreas being the next most frequently reported. Associated vascular injuries are relatively rare; however, inferior vena cava and portal vein injuries are more commonly reported than those to the hepatic artery, renal vessels or aorta.

Presentation and diagnosis of biliary injury

Clinical presentation of the vast majority of bile duct injuries can be divided into two broad categories. The first contains patients in whom clinical signs or associated injury lead to laparotomy with early diagnosis and surgical management (early presentation); these patients generally present with hypovolaemic shock or signs of an acute abdomen. The second category of patient has a delay (greater than 24h) in diagnosis and definitive therapy (delayed presentation). These patients comprised over half the cases (53.2%) in a review of combined series.[65] In addition, a third category of patient, representing a very small proportion of those who sustain a bile duct injury, may present with obstructive jaundice months or even years after the initial trauma (late presentation). In these patients, the bile duct injury is always isolated. Compromise of the blood supply to the duct may occur either at the time of the primary injury or at operation during the Pringle manoeuvre, and this may contribute to the development of a late biliary stricture. Bourque et al. reported that the delay between clinical presentation and surgical intervention for isolated bile duct injury averaged 18 days, with a range from several hours to 60 days.[66] Michelassi and Ranson reported that biliary injury was not recognised at initial operation in 11 (12%) of 91 patients with extrahepatic biliary tract trauma,[65] whereas Dawson and Jurkovich reported that 41% of bile duct injuries were missed at initial laparotomy.[67]

If a non-operative course of management for abdominal trauma is adopted, suspicion of an extrahepatic bile duct injury may be raised by CT evidence of a central liver injury involving the porta hepatis or the head of the pancreas, the presence of fluid collections in the subhepatic space, or evidence of periportal tracking of haematoma.[16] The diagnostic procedure of choice is ERCP, and if a duct injury is identified this may be treated by endoscopic stenting.[68]

Intraoperative recognition of biliary tract injury requires a high index of suspicion. The presence of free bile in the peritoneal cavity, or the presence of bile staining in the hepatoduodenal ligament or retroperitoneum, is a sign of injury to the extrahepatic bilary tract. Biliary tract injury must also be suspected if there is profuse bleeding from the hepatic artery or portal vein, particularly following blunt trauma, as the bile duct is also likely to be injured. Penetrating wounds near the porta hepatis require careful examination. If routine dissection does not reveal the location of the injury, fine-needle intraoperative cholangiography via the gallbladder or common bile duct may identify the site. Cystic duct cholangiography should be considered after cholecystectomy for traumatic gallbladder injury to avoid missing an associated bile duct injury.

It is possible for a patient who has sustained blunt abdominal trauma to be discharged from hospital only to return days or weeks later with a combination of symptoms and signs, including jaundice, abdominal distension, nausea, vomiting, anorexia, abdominal pain, low-grade fever or weight loss – a clinical picture similar to that seen in patients with intraperitoneal bile leakage following cholecystectomy. When jaundice develops after abdominal trauma, missed extrahepatic biliary injury must be considered.

Operative management of biliary injury

Many patients with extrahepatic biliary tract injury present in shock due to associated haemorrhage, and the priority at laparotomy is to identify and control haemorrhage. The report of Dawson et al. demonstrates that these patients are at risk of exsanguinating on the operating table.[62] Injuries to the gallbladder are best treated by cholecystectomy.[69] Primary repair of a clean and simple partial or complete transection of the common duct using absorbable sutures such as 4/0 polydioxanone over a T-tube inserted through a separate choledochotomy has been described. However, this type of repair is not appropriate if there is any evidence of duct contusion, loss of ductal tissue or possible injury to the hepatic artery as this may increase the risk of late development of an ischaemic stricture. In general, it is therefore safer to recommend that most injuries should be managed by fashioning a Roux-en-Y hepatico-jejunostomy as in the management of iatrogenic bile duct injuries.

Outcome after biliary injury

Injuries of this nature are associated with a mortality rate of 10% from concomitant injuries.[63] Septic complications and bile leakage account for most of the early morbidity and may require operative intervention. Late morbidity after repair of a traumatic biliary tract injury is unusual; however, jaundice or episodes of ascending cholangitis suggest a stricture of the ductal system.

Pancreatic trauma

Injuries to the pancreas are uncommon, accounting for 1–4% of severe abdominal injuries, and usually occur in young men. In a report of 51 425 patients from the Trauma Register of the German Society of Trauma Surgery, 9268 (18%) had documented abdominal injuries and 284 (3.1%) had a pancreatic injury.[70]

Mechanisms of pancreatic injury

Deceleration injury and direct blunt trauma are major mechanisms of pancreatic trauma, with the neck of the gland being at risk of transection across the vertebral column. The deep location of the pancreas means that considerable force is needed to cause an injury and this level of force may often be sufficient to damage other organs.

Diagnosis of pancreatic injury

Pancreatic injury should be suspected in any patient with penetrating trauma to the trunk, particularly if the entry site is between the nipples and the iliac crest, and in any patient with blunt compression trauma of the upper abdomen.

In an early study, Moretz et al. found that there was no reliable correlation between serum amylase and pancreatic injury.[71] In a later report, Takashima et al. retrospectively studied admission serum amylase values in a series of 73 patients with blunt pancreatic trauma treated in a single institution over a 16-year period.[72] Sixty-one (84%) of these patients had a raised serum amylase level. Of interest, the serum amylase level was found to be abnormal in all patients admitted more than 3 hours after trauma.

Bearing in mind the practicality that patients with pancreatic injury will simultaneously be undergoing evaluation to exclude concomitant intra-abdominal visceral injury, contrast-enhanced CT has been the investigation of choice (Fig. 17.7). Reported CT features of pancreatic injury include free intraperitoneal fluid, localised fluid in the lesser sac, retroperitoneal fluid, pancreatic oedema or swelling and changes in

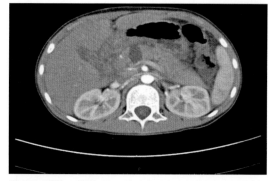

Figure 17.7 • CT image showing a complete transection of the neck of the pancreas in an 8-year-old boy who had fallen out of a tree.

the peripancreatic fat. The presence of fluid in the lesser sac between the pancreas and the splenic vein is reported by Lane et al. to be a reliable sign in blunt pancreatic injury.[73] However, Sivit and Eichelberger reported that this radiological sign was rarely the only abnormal CT finding in pancreatic injury.[74] It should be borne in mind that many of these CT features are also seen in acute pancreatitis (and furthermore that acute pancreatitis may occur as a result of blunt abdominal trauma). There is also evidence that CT tends to underdiagnose pancreatic injury. Akhrass et al. evaluated the clinical course of 72 patients with pancreatic injury admitted over a 10-year period.[75] Seventeen of these patients underwent CT as part of their initial assessment and this was reported as normal in nine. Eight of these patients underwent laparotomy (principally for suspected associated splenic injury) and three were found to have pancreatic injury requiring distal pancreatectomy. Newer, non-invasive imaging modalities such as magnetic resonance pancreatography have been reported in the assessment of patients with suspected pancreatic trauma.[76] Increased sophistication with the use of this technique may allow for accurate assessment of pancreatic ductal integrity.

Classification of pancreatic injury

Of the various proposed classification schemes, Lucas suggested in an early report that appropriate treatment be formulated according to the type of injury.[77] This classification system divides pancreatic injuries into three groups:

- grade I – superficial contusion with minimal damage;
- grade II – deep laceration or transection of the left portion of the pancreas;
- grade III – injury of the pancreatic head (**Fig. 17.8**).

A more complex system of classification taking into account the frequent coexistence of duodenal and pancreatic injuries was proposed by Frey and Wardell[78] (Table 17.2). The most common site of injury is the neck of the pancreas. The relative frequency of pancreatic injuries reported in collected reviews is represented in **Fig. 17.9**.

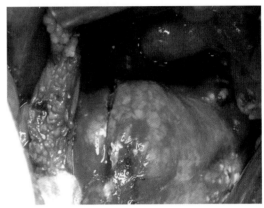

Figure 17.8 • Operative photograph of a transection injury along the neck of the pancreas resulting from a direct blow to the abdomen. This injury was managed by distal pancreatectomy and splenectomy.

Table 17.2 • Classification of pancreatic injury proposed by Frey and Wardell

Pancreatic injury	
Class I	Capsular damage, minor gland damage (P_1)
Class II	Body or tail pancreatic duct transection, partial or complete (P_2)
Class III	Major duct injury involving the head of the pancreas or the intrapancreatic common bile duct (P_3)
Duodenal injury	
Class I	Contusion, haematoma or partial-thickness injury (D_1)
Class II	Full-thickness duodenal injury (D_2)
Class III	Full-thickness injury with >75% circumference injury or full-thickness duodenal injury with injury to the extrahepatic common bile duct (D_3)
Combined pancreatico-duodenal injuries	
Type I	P_1D_1, P_2D_1 or D_2P_1
Type II	D_2P_2
Type III	D_3P_{1-2} or P_3D_{1-2}
Type IV	D_3P_3

Reproduced from Frey CF, Wardell JW. Injuries to the pancreas. In: Trede M, Carter DC (eds) Surgery of the pancreas. Edinburgh: Churchill Livingstone, 1993. With permission from Elsevier.

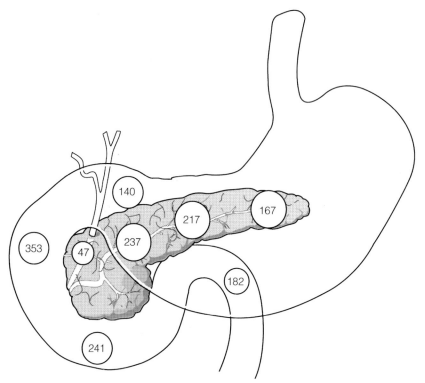

Figure 17.9 • Distribution of pancreatic injuries in the world literature. Note the preponderance of injuries in the junctional area of the neck of the gland. Reproduced from Frey CF, Wardell JW. Section 9. Injuries to the pancreas. In: Trede M, Carter DC (eds) Surgery of the pancreas. Edinburgh: Churchill Livingstone, 1993. With permission from Elsevier.

Initial management of pancreatic injury

In a major retrospective clinical casenote review of pancreatic trauma from six hospitals, Bradley et al. demonstrated a significant association between pancreas-related morbidity and injury to the main pancreatic duct.[79] Delayed intervention (due to delay in recognition of main pancreatic duct injury) was associated with high morbidity. CT was unreliable for the assessment of main pancreatic ductal integrity and an accurate assessment required ERCP.

> ✔ Assessment of the integrity of the main pancreatic duct is critical to the treatment of pancreatic injury. In patients with a suspected pancreatic injury (who are haemodynamically stable), ERCP is indicated to assess major duct integrity. Demonstration of an intact main pancreatic duct at ERCP in a patient with suspected isolated pancreatic injury may allow for a trial of non-operative management.

Operative management of pancreatic injury

The mainstay of treatment remains operative as pancreatic injuries are usually diagnosed at laparotomy. The important principles at operation are to gain good access to allow thorough inspection of the gland. Access to the lesser sac is best done by creating a window in the gastrocolic omentum outside the gastroepiploic arcade to allow examination of the body of the pancreas. A Kocher manoeuvre is necessary to permit palpation of the head of the pancreas between the thumb and fingers. A thorough inspection of the base of the transverse mesocolon is also undertaken. Injury to the pancreas is suspected if retroperitoneal haemorrhage can be seen through the base of the mesocolon or the lesser omentum. Absence of any sign of haemorrhage over the pancreas and duodenum makes injury unlikely.

Experience of patients with pancreatic injury from Durban led to the recommendation for operative treatment of patients with penetrating or gunshot injury and signs of peritoneal irritation.[80] In this large series of 152 patients with pancreatic trauma presenting during a 5-year period, 63 patients had been shot, 66 stabbed and 23 had blunt trauma. The mainstay of treatment was exploratory laparotomy followed by drainage of the pancreatic injury site. Large-bore soft silastic drains were used to minimise the risk of drain erosion into a major vessel. The mortality rates in these groups were 8% after gunshot injury, 2% after stab wounds and 10% after blunt trauma. The majority of these deaths were attributed to damage of other organs. The proportions of patients that developed pancreatic fistulas in the three groups were 14%, 9% and 13%, respectively. The authors concluded that 'conservative' surgical drainage (avoiding pancreatic resection) was justified after pancreatic injury. This large series lends weight to the treatment plan proposed by Lucas for grade I injuries, which consists of passive closed drainage using a wide-bore drain.

Simplified management guidelines based on the treatment protocols developed during the treatment of 124 pancreatic injuries at the University of Tennessee[81] also advocate simple drainage alone for proximal pancreatic injuries. There were 37 (30%) patients with proximal injuries. The 'pancreas-related' morbidity was 11% – principally the sequelae of pancreatic fistulas. Of 87 distal pancreatic injuries, the integrity of the main pancreatic duct was not established in 54 (62%). Patients thought to have a high probability of duct transection were treated by distal pancreatectomy. A concern with simple drainage for injuries in the head of the pancreas is persistent pancreatic fistula, and thus a surgical alternative is to drain the head of the pancreas into a Roux-en-Y limb of jejunum.

Moncure and Goins described their experience over a 6-year period with a consecutive series of 44 patients with pancreatic injury,[82] of which penetrating abdominal trauma accounted for the majority of cases. Class I pancreatic injuries occurred in 55% of patients and the majority were managed by simple drainage. Grade II injuries occurred in 18% and grade III injuries in 21%. Coexistent duodenal injuries were treated by primary closure in 21% and more complex duodenal exclusion techniques were used in 20%. The most frequent complications were intra-abdominal abscesses (31%) and pancreatic fistulas (16%).

Krige et al. reported on a series of 110 patients with pancreatic injuries after blunt trauma.[83] One hundred and one patients underwent a total of 123 operations, including drainage of the pancreatic injury (n=73), distal pancreatectomy (n=39) and Whipple resection (n=5). The overall complication rate was 74.5% and the mortality rate was 16.4%. Only two of the 18 deaths were attributable to the pancreatic injury. Mortality increased exponentially as the number of associated injuries increased.

Severe Lucas grade III injuries involving the head of the pancreas, duodenum and distal bile duct represent a major challenge, but fortunately are relatively rare, occurring in approximately 5% of all duodenal injuries.[84] The principles of treatment are to ensure that haemorrhage from concomitant injuries is dealt with first, as this is likely to be the major source of mortality. Similarly a prolonged operative procedure should be avoided in a potentially unstable patient and the involvement of an experienced pancreatic surgeon is desirable. Duodenal injuries can be closed primarily or drained into a Roux loop. Bile duct injuries may be repaired primarily over a T-tube or drained into a Roux limb of jejunum. The large variety of operative procedures described for these complex injuries suggests that treatment has to be tailored to the individual injury complex and that no single procedure is likely to be uniformly applicable or successful. Very rarely, pancreatico-duodenectomy may be required for complex, severe pancreatic injuries with concomitant duodenal and distal bile duct injuries. Clearly, this sort of resection should not be undertaken lightly in an individual suffering from shock and its sequelae, but rather like liver transplantation for trauma it is useful to have an index of awareness of the available therapeutic options.

Complications of pancreatic injury

The most common post-traumatic complications include necrotising pancreatitis, pseudocyst formation, pancreatic abscesses and pancreatic fistula. Cerwenka et al. reported the incidence of these complications to be 15%, 9%, 6% and 4%, respectively.[85] The principles regarding management are similar to those for treating these complications when they arise as a result of pancreatitis or pancreatic surgery. Inflammation of the pancreas after trauma behaves in much the same way as acute biliary or acute alcohol-induced pancreatitis, with the possible exception that there is a higher incidence of development of local complications such as pseudocyst – possibly relating to the nature of duct disruption in trauma. The Cape Town group reported that, of a series of 64 patients with pancreatic trauma, pseudocysts developed in 15 patients (23%), of whom eight had a duct injury demonstrated by endoscopic retrograde pancreatography.[86] Patients with pseudocysts related to distal duct injury were treated successfully by percutaneous aspiration. Three patients with duct injuries in the neck/body region underwent distal pancreatectomy. Pseudocysts related to ductal injury in the head of the pancreas were drained internally by Roux-en-Y cyst-jejunostomy. The authors concluded that traumatic pancreatic pseudocysts associated with a peripheral duct injury may resolve spontaneously, whereas those associated with injuries to the proximal duct would more likely require surgical intervention. Alternative treatment strategies include endoscopic transpapillary or transmural drainage of the pseudocyst.

The incidence of pancreatic fistula after surgery for trauma is dependent on the type of procedure, with some evidence that the fistula rate is higher after drainage procedures than after resection. Successful insertion of pancreatic duct stents has been reported for management of major pancreatic duct disruption; however, the incidence of long-term ductal stricture is high and therefore the role of pancreatic duct stenting needs to be further defined.[87]

✅ Management of post-traumatic pseudocysts and fistulas will depend on the time from injury, presence of ongoing ductal leak, site of leak and presence of debris within a pseudocyst cavity. The optimal treatment strategy should involve a multidisciplinary approach in a specialist unit employing similar principles to those of managing these complications following an attack of acute pancreatitis.

Conclusion

The contemporary management of patients with suspected liver, biliary or pancreatic injury involves detailed clinical assessment and resuscitation followed, in haemodynamically stable patients, by imaging investigations. If surgical intervention is required, the mainstay of treatment is to control haemorrhage. In European healthcare systems, the optimum care of the patient may consist of packing followed by transfer to a regional hepato-pancreatico-biliary unit. A paper by Hoyt et al. examining preventable causes of death in 72 151 admissions with abdominal trauma to North American level I trauma centres identified abdominal injury as the cause of death in 287, with liver injury being responsible for 92.[88] Delays in packing were highlighted as a preventable cause of death, as was a need for better understanding of the end-points to be achieved by packing. The conclusion of this large survey was that the management of liver injury remains a major technical challenge.

Key points

- Management of patients with suspected liver, biliary or pancreatic injury involves detailed clinical assessment and resuscitation.
- Haemodynamic instability resistant to fluid resuscitation associated with clinical signs of peritonism is an indication for immediate laparotomy.
- Patients who are haemodynamically stable or who respond to initial fluid resuscitation should undergo further imaging investigations.
- Laparotomy is generally required for patients with an abdominal gunshot wound.

Liver trauma
- Non-operative management of liver trauma is now a well-established treatment option.
- Significant liver haemorrhage can initially be controlled at operation by manual compression of the liver parenchyma, a Pringle manoeuvre or by compression of the aorta above the coeliac trunk. Perihepatic packing is a highly effective technique to control bleeding from the liver or juxtahepatic veins.
- Resectional debridement of non-viable hepatic parenchyma may be undertaken, but anatomical resection is rarely indicated.
- Other techniques to control haemorrhage include suture ligation of vessels, mesh wrapping of a liver lobe and selective hepatic arterial ligation.
- Postoperative complications include bile leakage or sepsis, and may require radiological, endoscopic or surgical intervention.

Extrahepatic biliary tract trauma
- This uncommon injury is more likely to be due to penetrating rather than blunt abdominal trauma.
- It is rarely diagnosed before operation and is usually recognised incidentally at laparotomy.
- Concomitant vascular injury of the portal vein or hepatic artery is rare.
- ERCP may demonstrate bile leakage and allow therapeutic insertion of a biliary stent.
- Definitive operative intervention for gallbladder trauma is cholecystectomy.
- Roux-en-Y hepatico-jejunostomy is the operation of choice for most injuries to the bile duct.

Pancreatic trauma

- This is most commonly diagnosed by CT; however, ERCP may be undertaken to assess pancreatic duct integrity and may allow therapeutic stenting if leakage of contrast is identified.
- Exploratory laparotomy and drainage of the pancreatic region remains the mainstay of surgical treatment.
- Selected injuries may be managed by distal pancreatectomy, pancreatico-duodenectomy or pancreatico-jejunostomy Roux-en-Y.

References

1. Scollay JM, Beard D, Smith R, et al. Eleven years of liver trauma: the Scottish experience. World J Surg 2005;29:744–9.

2. Talving P, Beckman M, Haggmark T, et al. Epidemiology of liver injuries. Scand J Surg 2003;92:192–4.

3. Krige JE, Bornman PC, Terblanche J. Liver trauma in 446 patients. S Afr J Surg 1997;35:10–5.

4. Feliciano DV, Mattox KL, Jordan GL, et al. Management of 1000 consecutive cases of hepatic trauma (1979–84). Ann Surg 1986;204:438–54.

5. Fabian TC, Croce MA, Stanford GG, et al. Factors affecting morbidity following hepatic trauma. A prospective analysis of 482 injuries. Ann Surg 1991;213:540–7.

6. Parks RW, Chrysos E, Diamond T. Management of liver trauma. Br J Surg 1999;86:1121–35.

7. Moore EE, Cogbill TH, Jurkovich GJ, et al. Organ injury scaling: spleen and liver (1994 revision). J Trauma 1995;38:323–4.

8. Schweizer W, Tanner S, Baer HU, et al. Management of traumatic liver injuries. Br J Surg 1993;80:86–8.

9. Bickell WH, Wall Jr MJ, Pepe PE, et al. Immediate versus delayed fluid resuscitation for hypotensive patients with penetrating torso injuries. N Engl J Med 1994;331:1105–9.

10. Scalea TM, Rodriguez A, Chiu WC, et al. Focused assessment with sonography for trauma (FAST): results from an international consensus conference. J Trauma 1999;46:466–72.

11. Stengel D, Bauwens K, Sehouli J, et al. Systematic review and meta-analysis of emergency ultrasonography for blunt abdominal trauma. Br J Surg 2001;88:901–12.

12. Rozycki GS, Ochsner MG, Feliciano DV, et al. Early detection of hemoperitoneum by ultrasound examination of the right upper quadrant: a multi-center study. J Trauma 1998;45:878–83.

13. McKenney MG, Martin L, Lentz K, et al. 1000 consecutive ultrasounds for blunt abdominal trauma. J Trauma 1996;40:607–12.

14. Richards JR, McGahan JP, Simpson JL, et al. Bowel and mesenteric injury: evaluation with abdominal US. Radiology 1999;211:399–403.

15. Fang JF, Chen RJ, Wong YC, et al. Pooling of contrast material on computed tomography mandates aggressive management of blunt hepatic injury. Am J Surg 1998;176:315–9.

16. Yokota J, Sugimoto T. Clinical significance of periportal tracking on computed tomographic scan in patients with blunt liver trauma. Am J Surg 1994;168:247–50.

17. Shankar KR, Lloyd DA, Kitteringham L, et al. Oral contrast with computed tomography in the evaluation of blunt abdominal trauma in children. Br J Surg 1999;86:1073–7.

18. Croce MA, Fabian TC, Kudsk KA, et al. AAST organ injury scale: correlation of CT graded liver injuries and operative findings. J Trauma 1991;31:806–12.

19. Deunk J, Dekker HM, Brink M, et al. The value of indicated computed tomography scan of the chest and abdomen in addition to the conventional radiological work-up for blunt trauma patients. J Trauma 2007;63:757–63.

20. Huber-Wagner S, Lefering R, Qvick LM, et al. The value of indicated computed tomography. Effect of whole-body CT during trauma resuscitation on survival: a retrospective, multicentre study. Lancet 2009;373:1455–61.

21. Chan O. Primary computed tomography survey for major trauma. Br J Surg 2009;96:1377–8.

22. Forlee MV, Krige JE, Welman CJ, et al. Haemobilia after penetrating and blunt liver injury: treatment with selective hepatic artery embolisation. Injury 2004;35:23–8.

23. Johnston JW, Gracias VH, Reilly PM. Hepatic angiography in the damage control population. J Trauma 2001;50:176.

24. Letoublon C, Morra I, Chen Y, et al. Hepatic arterial embolization in the management of blunt hepatic trauma: indications and complications. J Trauma 2011;70:1032–6.

25. Carrillo EH, Spain DA, Wohltmann CD, et al. Interventional techniques are useful adjuncts in the non-operative management of hepatic injuries. J Trauma 1999;46:619–22.

26. Richie JP, Fonkalsrud EW. Subcapsular haematoma of the liver: non-operative management. Arch Surg 1972;104:780–4.

27. White P, Cleveland RJ. The surgical management of liver trauma. Arch Surg 1972;104:785–6.

28. Meyer AA, Crass RA, Lim RC, et al. Selective non-operative management of blunt liver injury using computed tomography. Arch Surg 1985;120:781–4.

29. Farnell MB, Spencer MP, Thompson E, et al. Nonoperative management of blunt hepatic trauma in adults. Surgery 1988;104:748–56.

30. Feliciano DV. Continuing evolution in the approach to severe liver trauma. Ann Surg 1992;216:521–3.

31. Boone DC, Federle M, Billiar TR, et al. Evolution of management of major hepatic trauma: identification of patterns of injury. J Trauma 1995;39:344–50.

32. Sherman HF, Savage BA, Jones LM, et al. Non-operative management of blunt hepatic injuries: safe at any grade? J Trauma 1994;37:616–21.

33. Croce MA, Fabian TC, Menke PG, et al. Nonoperative management of blunt hepatic trauma is the treatment of choice for hemodynamically stable patients. Results of a prospective trial. Ann Surg 1995;221:744–53.

34. Pachter HL, Hofstetter SR. The current status of nonoperative management of adult blunt hepatic injuries. Am J Surg 1995;169:442–54.

35. Nance ML, Peden GW, Shapiro MB, et al. Solid viscus injury predicts major hollow viscus injury in blunt abdominal trauma. J Trauma 1999;43:618–22.

36. Demetriades D, Karaiskakis M, Alo K, et al. Role of postoperative computed tomography in patients with severe liver injury. Br J Surg 2003;90:1398–400.

37. Cox JC, Fanian TC, Maish GO, et al. Routine follow-up imaging is unnecessary in the management of blunt hepatic injury. J Trauma 2005;59:1175–80.

38. Cogbill TH, Moore EE, Jurkovich GJ, et al. Severe hepatic trauma: a multicenter experience with 1335 liver injuries. J Trauma 1988;28:1433–8.

39. Omoshoro-Jones JA, Nicol AJ, Navsaria PH, et al. Selective non-operative management of liver gunshot injuries. Br J Surg 2005;92:890–5.

40. Demetriades D, Hadjizacharia P, Constantinou C, et al. Selective nonoperative management of penetrating abdominal solid organ injuries. Ann Surg 2006;244:620–8.

41. Calne RY, McMaster P, Pentlon BD. The treatment of major liver trauma by primary packing with transfer of the patient for definitive treatment. Br J Surg 1978;66:338–9.

42. Cue JI, Cryer HG, Miller FB, et al. Packing and planned reexploration for hepatic and retroperitoneal hemorrhage: critical refinements of a useful technique. J Trauma 1990;30:1007–13.

43. Nicol AJ, Hommes M, Primrose R, et al. Packing for control of haemorrhage in major liver trauma. World J Surg 2007;31:569–74.

44. Berguer R, Staerkel RL, Moore EE, et al. Warning: fatal reaction to the use of fibrin glue in deep hepatic wounds. Case reports. J Trauma 1991;31:408–11.

45. Vick LR, Islam S. Recombinant factor VIIa as an adjunct in nonoperative management of solid organ injuries in children. J Pediatr Surg 2008;43:195–9.

46. Stone HH, Lamb JM. Use of pedicled omentum as an autogenous pack for control of haemorrhage in major injuries of the liver. Surg Gynecol Obstet 1975;141:92–4.

47. Brunet C, Sielezneff I, Thomas P, et al. Treatment of hepatic trauma with perihepatic mesh: 35 cases. J Trauma 1994;37:200–4.

48. Cox EF, Flancbaum L, Dauterieve AH, et al. Blunt trauma to the liver. Analysis of management and mortality in 323 consecutive patients. Ann Surg 1988;207:126–34.

49. Strong RW, Lynch SV, Wall DR, et al. Anatomic resection for severe liver trauma. Surgery 1998;123:251–7.

50. Mays ET. Hepatic trauma. Curr Probl Surg 1976;13:6–73.

51. Chen RJ, Fang JF, Lin BC, et al. Surgical management of juxtahepatic venous injuries in blunt hepatic trauma. J Trauma 1995;38:886–90.

52. Ringe B, Pichlmayr R. Total hepatectomy and liver transplantation: a life-saving procedure in patients with severe hepatic trauma. Br J Surg 1995;82:837–9.

53. Lin PJ, Jeng LB, Chen RJ, et al. Femoro-arterial bypass using Gott shunt in liver transplantation following severe hepatic trauma. Int Surg 1993;78:295–7.

54. Ginzburg E, Shatz D, Lynn M, et al. The role of liver transplantation in the subacute trauma patient. Am Surg 1998;64:363–4.

55. Maurel J, Aouad K, Martel B, et al. Post-traumatic hemobilia. How to treat? Ann Chir 1994;48:572–5.

56. Kozar RA, Moore FA, Cothren CC, et al. Risk factors for hepatic morbidity following nonoperative management: multicentre study. Arch Surg 2006;141:451–9.

57. Parks RW, Diamond T. Non-surgical trauma to the extrahepatic biliary tract. Br J Surg 1995;82:1303–10.

58. Penn I. Injuries of the gallbladder. Br J Surg 1962;49:636–41.

59. Soderstrom CA, Maekawa K, DuPriest Jr RW, et al. Gallbladder injuries resulting from blunt abdominal trauma: an experience and review. Ann Surg 1981;193:60–6.

60. Posner MC, Moore EE. Extrahepatic biliary tract injury: operative management plan. J Trauma 1985;25:833–7.

61. Burgess P, Fulton RL. Gall bladder and extrahepatic biliary duct injury following abdominal trauma. Injury 1992;23:413–4.

62. Dawson DL, Johansen KH, Jurkovich GJ. Injuries to the portal triad. Am J Surg 1991;161:545–51.

63. Kitahama A, Elliott LF, Overby JL, et al. The extrahepatic biliary tract injury: perspective in diagnosis and treatment. Ann Surg 1982;196:536–40.

64. Bade PG, Thomson SR, Hirshberg A, et al. Surgical options in traumatic injury to the extrahepatic biliary tract. Br J Surg 1989;76:256–8.

65. Michelassi F, Ranson JH. Bile duct disruption by blunt trauma. J Trauma 1985;25:454–7.

66. Bourque MD, Spigland N, Bensoussan AL, et al. Isolated complete transection of the common bile duct due to blunt trauma in a child, and review of the literature. J Pediatr Surg 1989;24:1068–70.

67. Dawson DL, Jurkovich GJ. Hepatic duct disruption from blunt abdominal trauma: case report and literature review. J Trauma 1991;31:1698–702.

68. Jenkins MA, Ponsky JL. Endoscopic retrograde cholangiopancreatography and endobiliary stenting in the treatment of biliary injury resulting from liver trauma. Surg Laparosc Endosc 1995;5:118–20.

69. Ball CG, Dixon E, Kirkpatrick AW, et al. A decade of experience with injuries to the gallbladder. J Trauma Manag Outcomes 2010;4:3.

70. Heuer M, Hussmann B, Lefering R, et al. Pancreatic injury in 284 patients with severe abdominal trauma: Outcome, course and treatment algorithm. Arch Surg 2011;396:1067–76.

71. Moretz III JA, Campbell DP, Parker DE, et al. Significance of serum amylase in evaluating pancreatic trauma. Am J Surg 1975;130:739–41.

72. Takashima T, Sugimoto K, Hirata M, et al. Serum amylase level on admission in the diagnosis of blunt injury to the pancreas: its significance and limitations. Ann Surg 1997;226:70–6.

73. Lane MJ, Mindelzun RE, Sandhu JS. CT diagnosis of blunt pancreatic trauma: importance of detecting fluid between the pancreas and the splenic vein. AJR Am J Roentgenol 1994;163:833–5.

74. Sivit CJ, Eichelberger MR. CT diagnosis of pancreatic injury in children: significance of fluid separating the splenic vein and the pancreas. AJR Am J Roentgenol 1995;165:921–4.

75. Akhrass R, Kim K, Brandt C. Computed tomography: an unreliable indicator of pancreatic trauma. Am Surg 1996;62:647–51.

76. Nirula R, Velmahos GC, Demetriades D. Magnetic resonance cholangiopancreatography in pancreatic trauma: a new diagnostic modality? J Trauma 1999;47:585–7.

77. Lucas CE. Diagnosis and treatment of pancreatic and duodenal injury. Surg Clin North Am 1977;57:49–65.

78. Frey CF, Wardell JW. Injuries to the pancreas. In: Trede M, Carter DC, editors. Surgery of the pancreas. Edinburgh: Churchill Livingstone; 1993. p. 565–89.

79. Bradley E, Young Jr PR, Chang MC, et al. Diagnosis and initial management of pancreatic trauma: guidelines from a multi-institutional review. Ann Surg 1998;227:861–9.

80. Madiba TE, Mokoena TR. Favourable prognosis after surgical drainage of gunshot, stab or blunt trauma of the pancreas. Br J Surg 1995;82:1236–9.

81. Patton Jr JH, Lyden SP, Croce MA, et al. Pancreatic trauma: a simplified management guideline. J Trauma 1997;43:234–9.

82. Moncure M, Goins WA. Challenges in the management of pancreatic and duodenal injuries. JAMA 1993;85:767–72.

83. Krige JE, Kotze UK, Hameed M, et al. Pancreatic injuries after blunt abdominal trauma: an analysis of 110 patients treated at a level 1 trauma centre. S Afr J Surg 2011;49:58–67.

84. Feliciano DV, Martin TD, Cruse PA, et al. Management of combined pancreatoduodenal injuries. Ann Surg 1987;205:673–80.

85. Cerwenka H, Bacher H, El-Shabrawi A, et al. Management of pancreatic trauma and its consequences – guidelines or individual therapy? Hepatogastroenterology 2007;54:581–4.

86. Lewis G, Krige JE, Bornman PC, et al. Traumatic pancreatic pseudocysts. Br J Surg 1993;80:89–93.

87. Lin BC, Liu NJ, Fang JF, et al. Long-term results of endoscopic stent in the management of blunt major pancreatic duct injury. Surg Endosc 2006;20:1551–5.

88. Hoyt DB, Bulger EM, Knudson MM, et al. Death in the operating room: an analysis of a multicenter experience. J Trauma 1994;37:426–38.

Index

NB: Page numbers followed by *f* indicate figures, *t* indicate tables and *b* indicate boxes.

C

H